Cardiology
1992

Cardiology

1992

WILLIAM C. ROBERTS, M.D., Editor

Chief, Pathology Branch
National Heart, Lung, and Blood Institute
National Institutes of Health, Bethesda, Maryland, and
Clinical Professor of Pathology and Medicine (Cardiology),
Georgetown University, Washington, D.C., and
Editor-in-Chief, The American Journal of Cardiology

JAMES T. WILLERSON, M.D.

Randall Professor of Medicine and
Chairman
Department of Internal Medicine
University of Texas Medical School at Houston
and
Director of Cardiology Research
At The Texas Heart Institute, Houston,
Texas

DEAN T. MASON, M.D.

Physician-in-Chief, Western Heart Institute
Chairman, Department of
Cardiovascular Medicine
St. Mary's Hospital and Medical Center
San Francisco, California
Editor-in-Chief, American Heart Journal

CHARLES E. RACKLEY, M.D.

Professor of Medicine
Division of Cardiology
Department of Medicine
Georgetown University Medical Center
Washington, D.C.

THOMAS P. GRAHAM, JR., M.D.

Professor of Pediatrics
Chief, Division of Pediatrics
Vanderbilt University
Nashville, Tennessee

Butterworth–Heinemann

Boston   London   Oxford   Singapore   Sydney   Toronto   Wellington

LC 92-071347

ISBN 0-7506-9318-5

ISSN 0275-0066

Butterworth–Heinemann
80 Montvale Avenue
Stoneham, MA 02180

10 9 8 7 6 5 4 3 2 1

Printed in the United States of America

Contents

7. Myocardial Heart Disease 359

Preface

Cardiology 1992 is the twelfth book to be published in this series. It contains summaries of 740 articles, all published in 1991. A total of 30 medical journals (Table I) were examined and at least one and usually many articles were summarized from each journal. The number of articles summarized by each of the five authors is listed in Table II. All of Rackley's submissions were from *Circulation;* Mason's from *The American Heart Journal;* and Willerson's from *The Journal of American College of Cardiology.* The contributions of Graham and Roberts were from a variety of medical journals. The summaries from each contributor were submitted

TABLE I. *Journals containing articles summarized in* Cardiology 1992.

1. American Heart Journal
2. American Journal of Cardiology
3. American Journal of Hypertension
4. American Journal of Medicine
5. Annals of Internal Medicine
6. Annals of Surgery
7. Annals of Thoracic Surgery
8. Archives of Internal Medicine
9. Archives of Pathology and Laboratory Medicine
10. Arteriosclerosis and Thrombosis
11. British Heart Journal
12. British Medical Journal
13. Catheterization and Cardiovascular Diagnosis
14. Chest
15. Circulation
16. Cleveland Clinic Journal of Medicine
17. Clinical Cardiology
18. Current Problems in Cardiology
19. European Heart Journal
20. Human Pathology
21. Journal of American College of Cardiology
22. Journal of the American Medical Association
23. Journal of Thoracic and Cardiovascular Surgery
24. Lancet
25. Mayo Clinic Proceedings
26. Medicine
27. Modern Pathology
28. Morbidity and Mortality Weekly Report
29. New England Journal of Medicine
30. Progress in Cardiovascular Disease

TABLE II. *Contributions of the Five Authors to* Cardiology 1992.

AUTHOR	CHAPTERS										Totals
	1	2	3	4	5	6	7	8	9	10	
1) WCR	86	97	65	37	48	31	17	5	10	26	422 (57.03%)
2) JTW	0	38	24	15	0	8	5	0	5	7	102 (13.78%)
3) DTM	2	32	17	8	2	10	5	5	6	2	89 (12.03%)
4) CER	7	23	13	10	1	8	1	0	4	8	75 (10.13%)
5) TPG, Jr.	0	0	0	3	0	0	3	45	0	1	52 (7.03%)
TOTALS	95	190	119	73	51	57	31	55	25	44	740 (100%)
Figures	16	32	23	9	4	9	4	0	8	11	116
Tables	11	7	3	3	2	2	0	1	0	3	32

to me, organized into the various sections in each of the 10 chapters, and each summary was copyedited by me.

A book of this type is made possible because of unselfish contributions from several individuals, none of whom is rewarded by authorship. I am enormously grateful to Marjorie Hadsell for typing perfectly the 422 summaries contributed by me; to Angie Esquivel, Leslie Flatt, Azora L. Irby, and Joy Phillips also for typing many summaries; to Kathleen Higgins for all her work obtaining permissions, and to Barbara Murphy for efficiently coordinating the publishing of the book in Boston.

William C. Roberts, M.D.
Editor

Conversion of Units

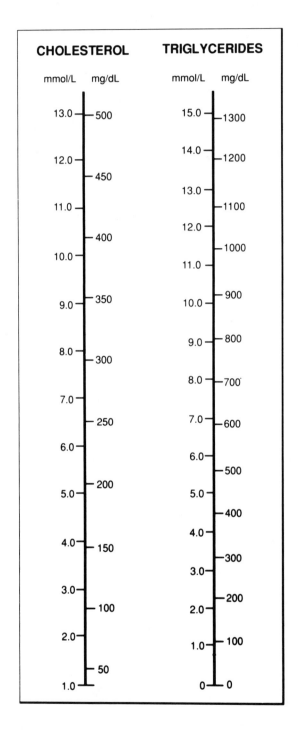

Cholesterol mg/dL = mmol/L x 38.6
Triglyceride mg/dL = mmol/L x 88.5

1

Factors Causing, Accelerating, or Preventing Coronary Artery Atherosclerosis

---

Changes in physician views of atherosclerotic risk factors

To determine recent changes in physicians' practices for cardiovascular disease risk reduction, Bostick and associates[1] from Minneapolis, Minnesota, interviewed by telephone in 1987 and again in 1989 a randomly selected sample of practicing primary care physicians in the upper Midwest. The reported mean cut-off levels for labeling a total serum cholesterol level as abnormal dropped from 5.84 to 5.43 mmol/L (226 to 210) and for initiating medication, from 7.34 to 6.54 mmol/L (284 to 253) (Figure 1-1). The proportion of physicians using diuretics as preferred step 1 antihypertensive agents dropped from 60% to 32% (Figure 1-2). Preferences became evenly divided among diuretics, angiotensin-converting enzyme inhibitors, and B-blockers. Advice about physical exercise changed little, but consensus among practicing physicians was high. Substantial improvements were found in smoking cessation activities. Practicing physicians are proving to be responsive to new scientific evidence and education in the prevention of cardiovascular disease.

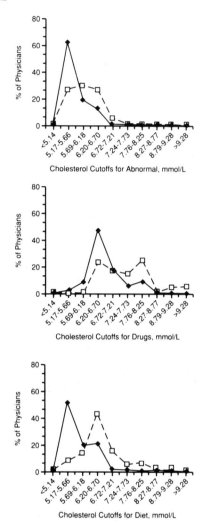

Fig. 1-1. Percentages of a cohort of physicians in 1987 (broken lines) and 1989 (solid lines) using various cutoff levels or labeling total serum cholesterol level as abnormal, requiring drug treatment and initiating dietary treatment. Levels in conventional metric units corresponding to those given in Systeme International units on the graph are as follows: less than 200, 200 to 219, 220 to 239, 240 to 259, 260 to 279, 280 to 299, 300 to 319, 320 to 339, 340 to 359, and greater than 359 mg/dl. Data for the top two graphs (abnormal and drugs) are from self-report on serial surveys 2 years apart, but data for the bottom graph (diet) are from questions asked only on the 1989 survey. Reproduced with permission from Bostick, et al.[1]

Prevalence in premature coronary artery disease

Genest and associates[2] from Boston, Massachusetts, determined the prevalence of modifiable cardiovascular risk factors (systemic hypertension, diabetes mellitus, cigarette smoking, LDL cholesterol ≥160 mg/dl and HDL cholesterol <35 mg/dl) in 321 men <60 years of age (mean 50 ± 7) with premature CAD documented at coronary angiography. The prevalence of these risk factors was markedly different than in the Framingham Offspring Study population, used here as a comparison group. In the patients with CAD, only 3% had no risk factor (other than male

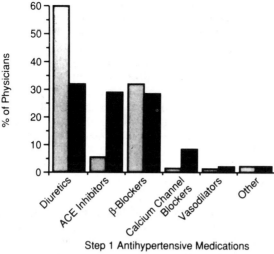

Step 1 Antihypertensive Medications

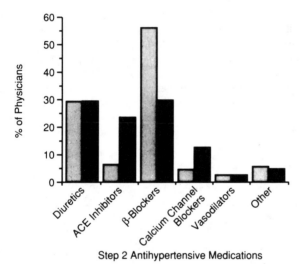

Step 2 Antihypertensive Medications

Fig. 1-2. Percentages of a cohort of physicians preferring various anti-hypertensive medications as first- and second-step agents in both 1987 (shaded bars) and 1989 (black bars). ACE indicates angiotensinconverting enzyme. Reproduced with permission from Bostick, et al.[1]

sex), compared with 31% in the Framingham Offspring Study subjects. Most patients with CAD (97%) had ≥1 additional risk factor. When the patients with CAD were divided by age groups (40 to 49 years [n = 109], 50 to 59 [n = 191]), no significant differences were observed in the prevalence of risk factors between the young and older patients. The prevalence of systemic hypertension (41 vs 19%), diabetes mellitus (12 vs 1.1%), cigarette smoking (67 vs 28%) and HDL cholesterol <35 mg/dl (63 vs 19%) was markedly higher in the patients with CAD than in Framingham Offspring Study subjects, whereas the prevalence of LDL cholesterol ≥160 mg/dl was not significantly different between patients with CAD and Framingham Offspring Study subjects (26 vs 26%). The use of B-adrenergic blockers was associated with a decreased prevalence of elevated LDL cholesterol and an increased prevalence of low HDL cholesterol, compared with patients not receiving this class of medication. When applying the guidelines of the National Cholesterol Education Program to patients with established CAD, only 52% had total cholesterol levels ≥200 mg/dl and thus nearly half (48%) would not undergo further screening for lipoprotein abnormalities. In the group of patients with a total cholesterol <200 mg/dl, 75% had a low HDL cholesterol (<35 mg/dl). It is recommended that in men with established CAD, and in those with 1 additional risk factor, fasting triglyceride and HDL cholesterol levels be determined in addition to total cholesterol.

In carotid-artery disease

Homer and associates[3] from Rochester, Minnesota, studied the effect of serum lipids and lipoproteins on extracranial carotid artery atherosclerosis in patients who underwent carotid arteriography. Serum lipid and lipoprotein values along with data on other potential predictors of extra-cranial carotid artery atherosclerosis were determined in 240 patients who had at least 1 extracranial carotid artery visualized (Table 1-1). In a multiple logistic regression analysis, the independently significant predictors of the presence of extracranial CAS were, in decreasing order of significance, duration of smoking of cigarettes, hypertension, age, and LDL cholesterol (Table 1-2). Serum cholesterol, triglycerides, HDL cholesterol, and apolipoprotein A-I did not show an independent effect. Although LDL cholesterol was an independent predictor of the presence of extracranial carotid artery atherosclerosis, its effect as a predictor was far outweighed by the effects of the duration of smoking of cigarettes and a history of hypertension.

TABLE 1-1. *Mean values of lipid and lipoprotein variables, stratified by severity of CAS.* Reproduced with permission from Homer, et al.[3]

	Arteriographic classification of CAS			
Variable	Normal (N = 104; 57 M, 47 F)	Mild (N = 36; 20 M, 16 F)	Moderate (N = 31; 19 M, 12 F)	Severe (N = 69; 52 M, 17 F)
Total cholesterol† (mg/dl)				
Male	199.9 ± 5.2	202.0 ± 7.7	223.2 ± 8.1	215.8 ± 5.4
Female	196.9 ± 5.4	199.1 ± 8.0	220.2 ± 8.6	212.8 ± 6.8
Triglycerides (mg/dl)				
Male	183.9 ± 15.5	293.9 ± 25.7	158.7 ± 33.0	215.0 ± 15.9
Female	174.0 ± 17.0	170.2 ± 28.5	199.3 ± 26.4	242.4 ± 27.7
HDL cholesterol‡ (mg/dl)				
Male	38.8 ± 1.4	35.6 ± 2.1	40.5 ± 2.2	37.0 ± 1.5
Female	48.6 ± 1.5	45.4 ± 2.2	50.3 ± 2.3	46.8 ± 1.9
LDL cholesterol†§ (mg/dl)				
Male	137.0 ± 5.4	116.7 ± 8.9	146.2 ± 9.1	141.4 ± 5.5
Female	114.5 ± 5.9	130.0 ± 9.9	151.6 ± 11.4	136.1 ± 9.6
Apolipoprotein A-I‡ (mg/dl)				
Male	143.2 ± 4.1	135.2 ± 6.7	143.1 ± 6.9	132.3 ± 4.2
Female	145.5 ± 4.5	143.5 ± 7.5	139.0 ± 8.7	156.4 ± 7.3
HDL:total cholesterol ratio†‡				
Male	0.20 ± 0.01	0.19 ± 0.01	0.18 ± 0.01	0.18 ± 0.01
Female	0.25 ± 0.01	0.23 ± 0.01	0.23 ± 0.01	0.22 ± 0.01

*Data are shown as age-adjusted means ± SE (adjusted to age = 60 years). CAS = carotid artery atherosclerosis; HDL = high-density lipoprotein; LDL = low-density lipoprotein.
†Related significantly to the presence of extracranial CAS in the individual risk factor analysis.
‡Negative association with the presence of extracranial CAS.
§The only lipid variable related independently and significantly to the presence of severe CAS in the multivariate analysis.

TABLE 1-2. *Discrete variables included in multiple logistic regression analysis and relationship to severity of CAS.* Reproduced with permission from Homer, et al.*[3]

| | Total | Arteriographic classification of CAS | | | | | | | |
| | | Normal | | Mild | | Moderate | | Severe | |
Variable	no.	No.	%	No.	%	No.	%	No.	%
Sex									
Male	148	57	39	20	14	19	13	52	35
Female	92	47	51	16	17	12	13	17	18
Cigarette use									
Never	67	45	67	8	12	8	12	6	9
Former	84	24	29	12	14	16	19	32	38
Current	89	35	39	16	18	7	8	31	35
Cigarettes/day									
0	67	45	67	8	12	8	12	6	9
1-10	8	2	25	4	50	1	12	1	12
11-20	64	22	34	8	12	9	14	25	39
21-30	47	19	40	9	19	5	11	14	30
31-40	43	14	33	7	16	4	9	18	42
>40	11	2	18	0	0	4	36	5	45
Hypertension									
Absent	125	72	58	19	15	8	6	26	21
Present	115	32	28	17	15	23	20	43	37
Diabetes									
No	207	98	47	28	14	27	13	54	26
Yes	33	6	18	8	24	4	12	15	45

*CAS = carotid artery atherosclerosis.

BLOOD LIPIDS

Changes in cholesterol awareness

The National Heart, Lung, and Blood Institute in Bethesda, Maryland[4] sponsored national telephone surveys of practicing physicians and the adult public in 1983, 1986, and 1990 to assess attitudes and practices regarding high serum cholesterol levels. Each time, approximately 1,600 physicians and 4,000 adults were interviewed. Trends show continuing change in medical practice and public health behavior relating to serum cholesterol (Figure 1-3). In 1990, physicians reported treating serum cholesterol at considerably lower levels than in 1986 and 1983 (Table 1-3). The median range of serum cholesterol at which diet therapy was initiated was 5.17 to 5.66 mmol/L (200 to 219) in 1990, down from 6.21 to 6.70 mmol/L (240 to 259) in 1986 and 6.72 to 7.21 mmol/L (260 to 279) in 1983. The median ranges for initiating drug therapy were 6.21 to 6.70 mmol/L (240 to 259) in 1990, 7.76 to 8.25 mmol/L (300 to 319) in 1986, and 8.79 to 9.28 mmol/L (340 to 359) in 1983. The number of adults who reported having had their cholesterol level checked rose from 35% to 46% to 65% in 1983, 1986, and 1990, respectively. Between 1983 and 1990, the number of adults reporting a physician diagnosis of high serum cholesterol increased from 7% to 16%; the number reporting a prescribed cholesterol-lowering diet increased from 3% to 9%. Reports of self-initiated diet efforts reached a high of 19% in 1986 and decreased to 15% in 1990. Two percent of adults reported drug prescriptions in 1990 compared with 1% in earlier years. In 1990, over 90% of physicians reported

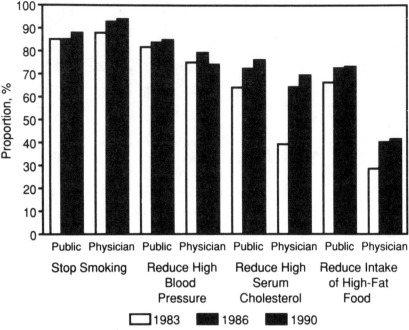

Fig. 1-3. Preventive actions with large effect on coronary heart disease. (Public: N = 4007, 1983; N = 4004, 1986; and N = 3700, 1990. Physicians: N = 1610, 1983; N = 1277, 1986; and N = 1604, 1990). Proportion responding action has "large effect" only is shown. Each action was thought to have a large or moderate effect by more than 94% of physicians and more than 95% of the public. Reproduced with permission from Schucker, et al.[4]

TABLE 1-3. *"At What Level of Serum Cholesterol Do You Usually Initiate Drug Therapy, If at All?"* Reproduced with permission from National Heart, Lung, and Blood Institute.[4]

		% Responding				
Specialty†	N	≤6.72‡ mmol/L (≤260 mg/dL)	6.75-7.21 mmol/L (261-279 mg/dL)	7.24-8.77 mmol/L (280-339 mg/dL)	≥8.79 mmol/L (≥340 mg/dL)	Never
General/family practice						
1983	787	8§		20	38	33
1986	631	20	3	33	28	16
1990	805	74	5	13	1	2
Internal medicine						
1983	377	8		24	41	27
1986	318	22	3	43	20	11
1990	399	72	7	14	1	2
Cardiology						
1983	412	10		32	37	20
1986	312	34	9	34	15	8
1990	400	75	5	13	1	2

*In responding, physicians were asked to consider 40- to 60-year-old men without evidence of cardiovascular disease or diabetes. Rounding may result in rows adding to slightly more or less than 100%. In 1990, approximately 4% of respondents did not cite a treatment level in terms of total cholesterol.
†For general/family practice, the SEs of all percents are less than 1.9. Moreover, for percents less than or equal to 8 or greater than or equal to 90, the SEs are less than 1.0. For internal medicine and cardiology, the SEs of all percents are less than 3.0; for percents less than or equal to 10, the SEs are less than or equal to 1.5.
‡In 1990, drug therapy was initiated at levels between 6.21 mmol/L (240 mg/dL) and 6.70 mmol/L (259 mg/dL) by 46% of general/family practitioners, 45% of internists, and 47% of cardiologists. Approximately 13% of each specialty reported a level below 6.21 mmol/L (240 mg/dL).
§Because of the way interviewers coded responses in 1983, data cannot be categorized by these two specific levels.

awareness and use of the recommendations from the Report of the National Cholesterol Education Program Expert Panel on Detection, Evaluation, and Treatment of High Blood Cholesterol in Adults, and the public reported marked increases in awareness of dietary methods to lower serum cholesterol. These changes suggest educational gains; the data also suggest areas for continued cholesterol educational initiatives.

Trends in levels

Burke and associates[5] from Winston-Salem, North Carolina, and Minneapolis, Minnesota, assessed community trends in the awareness, treatment, and control of hypercholesterolemia (serum total cholesterol 6.21 mmol/L [240 mg/dL]) during the 1980s in the Minneapolis-St. Paul metropolitan area. Twin Cities residents 25 to 74 years old participated in independent, cross-sectional, population-based surveys of risk factors for cardiovascular disease in 1980–1982 (n = 3365) and 1985–1987 (n = 4545). Mean serum total cholesterol levels, as adjusted for age, decreased significantly from 1980–1982 to 1985–1987 in men (from 5.30 mmol/L [205 mg per dL]) and women (from 5.19 mmol/L [201 mg/dl] to 5.04 mmol/L [195 mg/dL]) (Figure 1-4). The prevalence of hypercholesterolemia as adjusted for age decreased significantly in men (18 to 15%) and women (17 to 14%) (Figure 1-5) (Table 1-4). The ratio of total cholesterol to HDL

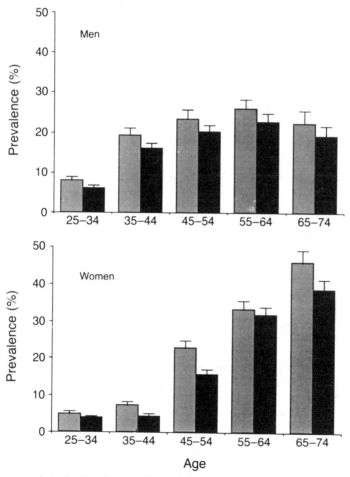

Fig. 1-4. Trends in the Prevalence of Hypercholestrolemia in Survey Participants in 1980–1982 and 1985–1987. Hatched bars indicate levels in 1980–1982, and solid bars levels in 1985–1987. T bars indicate the standard error of the mean. Hypercholestrolemia was defined as a serum cholesterol level ≥6.21 mmol per liter (240 mg per deciliter). In men, the age adjusted prevalence was 17.8 percent in 1980–1982 and 15.1 percent in 1985–1987 (P<0.05). In women, the age adjusted prevalence was 17.1 percent in 1980–1982 and 13.6 percent in 1985–1987 (P<0.05). Reproduced with permission from Burke et al.[5]

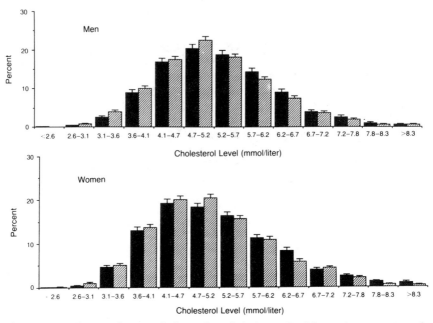

Fig. 1-5. Distribution of Serum Cholesterol Levels in Survey Participants in 1980–1982 and 1985–1987. Solid bars indicate levels in 1980–1982 and hatched bars levels in 1985–1987. T bars indicate the standard error of the mean. Reproduced with permission from Burke, et al.[5]

cholesterol was unchanged during this period, because of a concurrent decline in the level of HDL cholesterol. Participants with hypercholesterolemia in the 1985–1987 survey were more likely than those in the 1980–1982 survey to be aware of their condition (33% vs 25%), to be treated with lipid-lowering agents (4.3 vs 1.9%), and to have their condition controlled (1.9 vs 0.3%). Among those who reported treatment by a physician for hyperlipidemia, changes were observed in the type of treatment recommended. A significant increase was noted from 1980–1982 to 1985–1987 in the percentage of men being treated for hyperlipidemia with lipid-lowering medication (5.2 vs 11.6%) and with exercise programs (10.3 vs 20.1%). In women being treated for hyperlipidemia, a nonsignificant increase was noted in the use of lipid-lowering medication (8.2 vs 13.9%), and a significant increase was observed in the number of exercise prescriptions (4.1 vs 12.0%). The authors found a substantial decline in the prevalence of hypercholesterolemia in the Twin Cities between 1980–1982 and 1985–1987 that may be attributed to changes in lifestyle, such as diet and exercise, and to a lesser extent to more aggressive intervention with lipid-lowering drugs by physicians.

Levels in a Minnesota city

As part of a large cross-sectional investigation—the Rochester Family Heart Study—Kottke and associates[6] from Rochester, Minnesota, measured plasma levels of lipids, lipoproteins, and apolipoproteins in a sample from the general population of male and female subjects aged 5 to 90 years. Polyclonal radioimmunoassays developed at the Mayo Clinic were used for measurement of apolipoproteins A-I, A-II, C-II, C-III, and E, whereas a monoclonal enzyme-linked immunosorbent assay was used

TABLE 1-4. *Mean serum total cholesterol and HDL cholesterol levels in residents of the twin cities in the Minnesota Heart Survey, according to age, sex, and year. Reproduced with permission from Burke, et al.[5]*

Variable/Age (Yr)*	Men		Women	
	1980–1982	1985–1987	1980–1982	1985–1987
	millimoles per liter (milligrams per deciliter)			
Total cholesterol				
25–34	4.84 (187.1)	4.73 (182.9)	4.57 (176.8)	4.51 (174.4)
35–44	5.38 (208.2)	5.23 (202.2)	4.88 (188.6)	4.72 (182.6)
45–54	5.56 (215.0)	5.42 (209.5)	5.56 (215.0)	5.29 (204.5)
55–64	5.65 (218.4)	5.53 (213.7)	5.87 (226.8)	5.82 (225.2)
65–74	5.51 (213.1)	5.29 (204.6)	6.15 (238.0)	5.90 (228.3)
Age-adjusted	5.30 (204.8)	5.16 (199.6)[†]	5.19 (200.6)	5.04 (194.8)[†]
95% CI	5.25–5.35	5.12–5.20	5.14–5.23	5.00–5.08
HDL cholesterol				
25–34	1.14 (44.1)	1.10 (42.5)	1.40 (54.3)	1.36 (52.5)
35–44	1.10 (42.6)	1.07 (41.3)	1.39 (53.6)	1.40 (54.1)
45–54	1.11 (42.8)	1.07 (41.4)	1.44 (55.8)	1.42 (54.9)
55–64	1.09 (42.2)	1.05 (40.5)	1.46 (56.6)	1.39 (53.6)
65–74	1.17 (45.3)	1.08 (41.9)	1.35 (52.3)	1.32 (50.9)
Age-adjusted	1.12 (43.2)	1.08 (41.6)[†]	1.41 (54.7)	1.39 (53.8)
95% CI	1.10–1.13	1.06–1.09	1.40–1.43	1.38–1.41
Total:HDL cholesterol ratio				
25–34	3.90	4.00	3.03	2.96
35–44	4.57	4.50	3.15	3.07
45–54	4.77	4.72	3.65	3.49
55–64	4.78	4.86	3.68	3.76
65–74	4.21	4.41	4.16	4.06
Age-adjusted	4.37	4.41	3.35	3.27
95% CI	4.01–4.80	4.10–4.77	3.13–3.61	3.08–3.47

*CI denotes confidence interval.

†P<0.05 for the comparison with 1980–1982 values.

for apolipoprotein B. On the basis of 984 subjects who reported that they were fasting, were not pregnant, had never smoked, and were taking no medications thought to influence lipid levels, the authors determined age- and gender-specific percentiles for plasma levels of cholesterol, triglycerides, HDL cholesterol, and 6 apolipoproteins. These percentiles will facilitate identification of persons who are in the highest and lowest percentiles for their age and gender. The levels of the apolipoproteins varied for both age and gender. This is the first study to provide a reference sample for plasma levels of these apolipoproteins for male and female subjects 5 to 90 years of age selected from the general population.

In endurance athletes compared to sedentary men

Endurance athletes have higher HDL concentrations than sedentary controls. To examine the mechanism for this effect, Thompson and colleagues[7] in Providence, Rhode Island, compared HDL apoprotein metabolism in 10 endurance athletes aged 34 years and 10 sedentary men aged 36 years. Subjects were maintained on controlled diets for 4 weeks, and metabolic studies using autologously labeled ^{125}I HDL were performed during the final 2 weeks. Lipids and lipoproteins were measured daily during these 2 weeks, and the average of 14 values was used in the analysis. HDL cholesterol (58 vs 41 mg/dl), HDL$_2$ cholesterol (26 vs 12 mg/dl), and apolipoprotein A-I (144 vs 115 mg/dl) were higher in the athletes, whereas triglyceride concentrations (60 vs 110 mg/dl) were lower. Postheparin lipoprotein lipase activity was not different, but hepatic triglyceride lipase activity was 27% lower in the athletes. The athletes' mean clearance rate of triglycerides after an infusion of Travamulsion was nearly 2-fold that of the inactive men. There was no difference in HDL apoprotein synthetic rates, whereas the catabolic rates of both apo A-I and apolipoprotein A-II were reduced in the trained men. Apo A-I and apo A-II half lives correlated with HDL cholesterol in each group but not consistently with lipase activities or fat clearance rates. This relation between apoprotein catabolism and HDL cholesterol was strongest at HDL cholesterol concentrations of less than 60 mg/dl. The investigators concluded that higher HDL levels in active men are associated with increased HDL protein survival.

Cholesterol screening

Several previous studies that looked at the effects of labeling individuals as hypertensive found increases in psychosocial distress, diminished feelings of well-being, or absenteeism. Other studies found no such effects. Thus far, similar studies relating to labeling for high blood cholesterol levels have not been published. The results of the Massachusetts Model Systems for Blood Cholesterol Screening Project reported by Havas and associates[8] from Baltimore, Maryland, and Boston, Massachusetts, investigated whether labeling effects occurred as a result of the community-based screening, education, and referral programs it conducted in Worcester and Lowell, Massachusetts. Nine questions concerning perceptions of physical and psychological well-being were asked on a questionnaire given to screening participants. The same questions were asked as part of a follow-up questionnaire given to all individuals identified as having high blood cholesterol levels at one of the screenings. Comparison of the baseline and follow-up results did not demonstrate significant overall negative effects among any age, sex, racial, income, or educational groups. On the contrary, responses to many of the questions revealed small but statistically significant improvements in perceptions of physical and psychological well-being. The absence of negative labeling effects may be attributable to the positive, supportive approach to participant counseling taken by the project.

To predict the consequences of cholesterol screening among elderly Americans who do not have symptoms of heart disease, Garber and associates[9] from Stanford and Palo Alto, California, Hanover, New Hampshire, and Washington, D.C., explored the cost implications of a cholesterol screening program, evaluated evidence linking hypercholesterolemia to CAD and mortality in the elderly, and describe the likely effects of therapy of hypercholesterolemia. According to their calculations, if all Americans 65 years of age and older adhered to a cholesterol screening program similar to the one proposed by the National Cholesterol Education Program, minimum annual expenditures for screening and treatment would be between $1.6 billion and $16.8 billion, depending on the effectiveness of diet and the cost of the medications used to treat hypercholesterolemia.

The National Cholesterol Education Program has provided guidelines for identification of persons at high risk of CAD because of lipid abnormalities. These recommendations are based on total cholesterol as the initial screening tool and have become the stimulus for clinic- and community-based screen programs nationwide. However, the use of the guidelines may be problematic because individuals may have total cholesterol levels in the desirable range but low LDL or high HDL levels considered at high risk. Bush and Riedel[10] in Baltimore, Maryland evaluated the ability of the screening recommendations to identify correctly persons at high risk of CAD because of lipid abnormalities.

Using the National Cholesterol Education Program guidelines, the investigators simulated a population-based screening program with data from visits 1 and 2 of the Lipid Research Clinics Program Prevalence Study. Individuals were considered to be at high risk of CAD if they had LDL levels >160 mg/dl or HDL levels <36 mg/dl. Following the guideline process, 21% of those with high LDL concentrations and 66% of those with low HDL concentrations would not be routinely referred for immediate treatment. Overall, 41% of those at high risk of CAD would not be promptly evaluated. The sensitivity of the guidelines for promptly identifying individuals with lipoprotein abnormalities is 59%. This relatively low sensitivity of total cholesterol as a screening tool should be the impetus for rethinking the screening guidelines. Specifically, the cost-benefit ratio of routine screening for lipoproteins, particularly HDL cholesterol, needs to be carefully considered.

To examine how insurance companies assess proposals for life insurance from applicants with raised total cholesterol concentrations and to determine the excess mortality rating applied, Neil and Mant[11] surveyed 49 companies underwriting life insurance in the UK. Four fictional men aged 30 seeking 20-year term policies paying benefit only on death were analyzed. Two had total cholesterol concentrations of 6.4 and 8.1 mmol/l but no other cardiovascular risk factors; 1 was overweight, hypertensive, smoked 20 cigarettes daily, and had a total cholesterol concentration of 8.1 mmol/l; and 1 had possible familial hypercholesterolemia and a total cholesterol concentration of 10.7 mmol/l after treatment. All companies used explicit criteria to assess the mortality risk associated with hyperlipidemias, and 47 companies applied the same criteria to men and women. No excess mortality rating was imposed on an applicant with a total cholesterol concentration of 6.4 mmol/l, but a small excess was applied to an applicant with a concentration of 8.1 mmol/l (median excess 50%, range 0.75%). When multiple cardiovascular risk factors were present the same concentration of 8.1 mmol/l resulted in a substantial excess (median 125%, range 50–200%). A smaller but more variable excess was applied to an applicant with possible familial hypercholesterolemia (median 75%, range 0–200%). Despite considerable differences among companies in the excess mortality ratings applied, increases in term life insurance premiums are likely to be restricted to patients with severe hypercholesterolemia, in particular those with familial hypercholesterolemia. In the absence of other cardiovascular risk factors milder hypercholesterolemia is unlikely to result in higher premiums.

To evaluate the accuracy and reliability of lipoprotein cholesterol measurements obtained during screening, Bachorik and associates[12] from Baltimore, Maryland, analyzed split venous samples from fasting participants for total cholesterol, triglyceride, and HDL cholesterol with screening and standardized laboratory methods. LDL cholesterol levels were calculated using the Friedewals equation. Split venous samples from nonfasting participants were analyzed for total cholesterol. Capillary blood samples were analyzed for total cholesterol with the screening method. Total cholesterol measurements in screening venous blood samples were 5.4% and 3.8% lower than the laboratory values in samples from fasting and nonfasting participants, respectively. Triglyceride and HDL-cholesterol values in venous samples obtained from fasting participants were, on average, 9.8% and 11.2% lower than the respective laboratory measurements. Screening HDL-cholesterol values varied, differing from the laboratory values by as much as 40% in 95% of participants. In fasting participants, total cholesterol in capillary samples averaged 5.5% higher than in venous samples; in nonfasting participants the capillary samples were 3.1% higher. Screening for either total cholesterol or LDL cholesterol identified 93% of the persons with LDL-cholesterol values of 3.36 mmol/L (130 mg/dL) or higher. Total cholesterol can be reliably measured in samples from fasting or nonfasting persons. The values in capillary blood samples were slightly higher than those in venous samples. Screening HDL-cholesterol values were too variable to establish the HDL-cholesterol level reliably. Participants with high LDL-cholesterol levels were identified as accurately by measuring total cholesterol only when compared with calculating the LDL-cholesterol level from total cholesterol, triglyceride, and HDL-cholesterol concentrations.

Accuracy of measurements

Christenson and associates[13] from Durham and Chapel Hill, North Carolina, compared 4 testing strategies for assessing total and HDL cholesterol in a homogeneous group of male outpatients at increased risk for cardiovascular disease: (1) a single measurement at 1 occasion; (2) the mean of duplicate measurements at one occasion; (3) the mean of single measurements in specimens collected 1 week apart; and (4) the overall mean of duplicate measurements at 2 occasions 1 week apart. Results of strategy 1 were comparatively less reliable as demonstrated by lower intraclass correlation coefficients and higher within-subject variance components. Use of strategy 3 decreased within-subject variance by 50% and improved the 95% confidence interval by 30% for both total and HDL cholesterol, compared with strategy 1. Duplicate testing on either 1 or 2 occasions resulted in a nominal improvement in reliability and confidence. Calculating the mean of single measurements in specimens collected 1 week apart is clinically useful because: (1) it reduces the risk of misclassification, (2) it improves intervention monitoring, (3) it supports the National Cholesterol Education Program guidelines for total cholesterol, and (4) it improves the use of HDL as an independent risk factor.

To evaluate laboratory performance, McQueen and associates[14] from several medical centers in Canada sent 8 to 13 samples of fresh human serum from volunteers to 250 laboratories in the Canadian province of Ontario licensed to perform lipid analysis. Fresh human specimens were used because of potential matrix effects with processed materials. The authors showed that on all survey samples, 71% (range 63–82%) of participating laboratories were within ± 5% of the target cholesterol value and that 93% were within ± 10%. The goal of the National Cholesterol Education Program for 1992 is total error of no more than ± 9 for 95% of results. The unblanked triglycerides results show that on all samples 40% (14% to 59%) of participants are within ± 5% and 68% (range, 31%

to 86%) are within ± 10% of the target value. For triglycerides results from 0.9 to 2.0 mmol/L, 80% or more are within ± 0.2 mmol/L. Between 2.0 and 3.0 mmol/L, 90% are within ± 0.3 mmol/L of the target values. For HDL cholesterol, for all samples 35% (range, 24% to 50%) of laboratories are within ± 5% and 68% (range, 55% to 88%) are within ± 10%. A range of 80% to 95% of participants are within ± 0.2 mmol/L of the target values. For calculated LDL cholesterol, 51% and 62% of the laboratories surveyed are within ± 5%, with 83% and 89% within ± 10% of the target values. The authors concluded that the laboratory measurement of lipids is approaching the degree of accuracy and precision required for clinical purposes, and that the use of fresh human serum samples is a viable approach to their proficiency testing.

Estimating the true level

An individual's blood cholesterol measurement may differ from the true level because of short-term biological and technical measurement variability. Using data on the within-individual and population variance of serum total cholesterol, Irwig and associates[15] from Sydney, Australia, addressed the following concerns: Given a cholesterol measurement, what is the individual's likely true level? The confidence interval for the true level is wide and asymmetrical around extreme measurements because of regression to the mean (Figure 1-6). Of particular concern is the misclassification of people with a screening measurement below 5.2 mmol/L who may be advised that their cholesterol level is "desirable" when their true level warrants further action. To what extent does blood cholesterol change in response to an intervention? In general, confidence intervals are too wide to allow decision making and patient feedback about an individual's cholesterol response to a dietary intervention, even with multiple measurements. If no change is observed in an individual's cholesterol value based on 3 measurements before and 3 after dietary intervention, the 80% confidence interval ranges from a true increase of 4% to a true decrease of 9%.

Population strategies for reducing levels

The Expert Panel on Population Strategies for Blood Cholesterol Reduction, a part of the National Cholesterol Education Program, provided an executive summary of 16 recommendations regarding ways to have a healthier American population in regard to prevention of CAD[16]. The full report of this expert panel appeared in the June 1991 issue of Circulation.

Effects of diets

Using a 1-page bar-coded food frequency questionnaire, Selzer and associates[17] from Los Angeles and Pasadena, California, analyzed the food habits of 996 adults who participated in diet screening at the annual meetings of the American Heart Association (1989) and the American College of Cardiologists (1990) for sex, age, and regional differences. Estimated nutrient intakes were also compared with those from the Department of Agriculture's 1985 and 1986 Continuing Survey of Food Intake of Individuals. The average diet reported in this study satisfied National Cholesterol Education Program guidelines for cholesterol intake, but was higher than that recommended for total and saturated fats. In addition, dietary fat intake was influenced by sex, age and geographic region. Re-

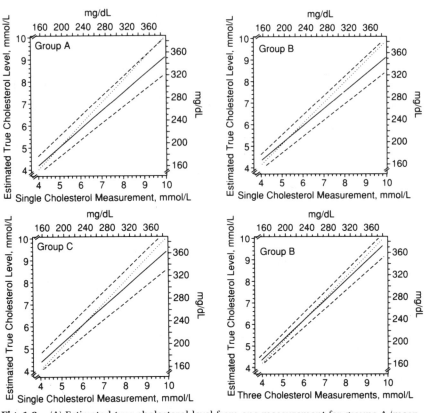

Fig. 1-6. (A) Estimated true cholesterol level from one measurement for groups A (mean 5.2 mmol/L; men less than 35 and women less than 45 years old) and C (mean 6.4 mmol/L; women 55 years and older). Solid line indicates the estimated true level; dashed lines, 80% confidence intervals. The faint diagonal line is an equivalence line. (B) Estimated true cholesterol level for one or three measurements for group B (mean, 5.8 mmol/L; men 35 years and older and women 45 through 54 years). Solid line indicates the estimated true level; dashed lines, 80% confidence intervals. The faint diagonal line is an equivalence line. Reproduced with permission from Irwig, et al.[15]

duction in total and saturated fat intake was confined to men >35 years of age; intake of these nutrients was highest among young, Midwestern women. These results suggest the need for diet intervention programs, targeted specifically to young adults with additional consideration given to regional variation. Repeated surveys of cardiac care givers might be used as an early indicator of the nationwide effectiveness of dietary intervention programs.

Major new public health problems occur in developing countries as they become more affluent and change their traditional dietary patterns. To study this phenomenon in microcosm, McMurry and associates[18] from Portland, Oregon, substituted an "affluent" diet for the traditional diet of a group of Tarahumara Indians, a Mexican people known to consume a low-fat, high-fiber diet and to have a very low frequency of risk factors for CAD. Thirteen Tarahumara Indians (5 women and 8 men) consumed their traditional diet (2700 kcal per day) for 1 week and were then fed a diet typical of affluent societies, which contained excessive calories (4100 kcal per day), total fat, saturated fat, and cholesterol, for five weeks. After 5 weeks of consuming the affluent diet, the subjects' mean (±SE) plasma cholesterol level increased by 31%, from 121 ± 5 to 159 ± 6 mg per deciliter (3.13 ± 0.13 to 4.11 ± 0.16 mmol/L). The increase in the plasma cholesterol level was primarily in the LDL fraction, which rose 39%, from 72 ± 3 to 100 ± 4 mg/dl (1.86 ± 0.08 to 2.59 ± 0.10 mmol/L). HDL cholesterol, usually low in this population, increased by 31%, from 32 ± 2 to 42 ± 3 mg per deciliter (0.83 ± 0.05 to 1.09 ± 0.08 mmol/L). Consequently, the ratio of LDL to HDL levels changed little (2.25 with the base-line diet and 2.38 with the affluent diet). Plasma triglyceride levels increased by 18%, from 91 ± 8 to 108 ± 11 mg/dl (1.03 ± 0.09 to 1.22 ± 0.12 mmol/L), with a significant increase in the very LDL triglyceride fraction. All the subjects gained weight, with a mean increase of 3.8 kg (7%). When Tarahumara Indians from a population with virtually no CAD risk factors consumed for a short time a hypercaloric diet typical of a more affluent society, they had dramatic increases in plasma lipid and lipoprotein levels and body weight.

Usefulness in predicting coronary artery disease

To assess the relation of serum lipid levels to angiographic CAD, Romm and associates[19] from Washington, D.C., obtained lipid profiles on 125 men and 72 women undergoing diagnostic coronary angiography. CAD, defined as ≥25% diameter narrowing in a major coronary artery, was present in 106 men (85%) and 54 women (75%). Multiple regression analyses revealed that only HDL cholesterol level in men, and age and total/HDL cholesterol ratio in women, were independently associated with the presence of CAD after adjustment for other risk factors (Table 1-5). HDL cholesterol level and age were significantly correlated with both extent (number of diseased vessels) and severity (percent maximum stenosis) of CAD in men. In women, age was the only independent variable related to severity, whereas age and total/HDL cholesterol ratio were related to extent. Of 71 patients with total cholesterol <200 mg/dl, 79% had CAD. With multiple regression analyses, HDL cholesterol was the only variable independently related to the presence and severity of CAD in these patients after adjustment for age and gender; extent was significantly associated with age and male gender, and was unrelated to any of the lipid parameters. With use of multiple logistic and linear regression analyses of the group of 197 patients, HDL cholesterol was the most powerful independent variable associated with the presence and severity of CAD after adjustment for age and gender. HDL cholesterol was also an independent predictor of extent. Age was independently associated with each of the end points examined, and was the variable most significantly related to extent. These data add to the growing body of in-

TABLE 1-5. *Age, plasma lipids and lipoproteins in men and women with and without coronary artery disease. Reproduced with permission from Romm, et al.*[19]

	Men		Women	
	CAD Absent	CAD Present	CAD Absent	CAD Present
No. of patients (%)	19 (15)	106 (85)	18 (25)	54 (75)
Age (years)	57 ± 60	60 ± 1	56 ± 4	67 ± 2†
Total cholesterol (mg/dl)	215 ± 9	213 ± 4	217 ± 9	228 ± 7
LDL cholesterol (mg/dl)	145 ± 9	147 ± 4	140 ± 10	151 ± 6
Triglycerides (mg/dl)	137 ± 15	181 ± 11*	149 ± 22	155 ± 12
HDL cholesterol (mg/dl)	48 ± 3	39 ± 1†	53 ± 4	47 ± 2
Total:HDL cholesterol	4.8 ± 0.4	5.9 ± 0.2*	4.6 ± 0.4	5.6 ± 0.4*

* p <0.05; † p <0.01.
Values are mean ± standard error of the mean.
CAD = coronary artery disease; HDL = high-density lipoprotein; LDL = low-density lipoprotein.

formation demonstrating an important association between HDL and CAD.

Stemmermann and associates[20] from Honolulu, Hawaii, followed up for 18 or more years Hawaiian men of Japanese ancestry after a baseline examination showed a quadratic distribution of death rates at different levels of serum total cholesterol. Mortality from cancer progressively decreased and mortality from CAD progressively increased with rising levels of serum cholesterol. There was a positive association between baseline serum cholesterol levels and deaths from CAD at 0 to 6 years, 7 to 12 years, and 13 years and longer after examination. The inverse relationship between cancer and serum cholesterol levels was stronger in the first 6 years than in the next 6 years and, although still inverse, lost statistical significance after 13 years. Cancers of the colon and lung showed the strongest association with low baseline serum cholesterol levels, while gastric or rectal cancer failed to show this association. Organ specificity and persistence of the inverse association beyond 6 years suggest that the nutritional demands of cancers may not entirely explain the inverse association with some cancers. The quadratic distribution of deaths in this cohort remained after CAD, stroke, and cancer were removed from the analysis. For the entire period of observation, the lowest mortalities were found in men with serum cholesterol levels between 4.65 and 6.18 mmol/L (between 180 and 239 mg/dL).

Posner and associates[21] from Boston, Massachusetts, examined the relation between dietary lipids and the 16-year incidence of CAD mortality and morbidity in 2 male cohorts, aged 45 to 55 years (n = 420) and 56 to 65 years (n = 393) from the Framingham Study. Dietary lipids were assessed through a single 24-hour recall at the initiation of follow-up in 1966 to 1969. In the younger cohort, there were significant positive associations between the incidence of CAD and the proportion of dietary energy intake from total fat and monounsaturated fatty acids. The proportion of energy intake from saturated fatty acids had a marginally significant positive association with CAD. The associations remained even after adjustment for cardiovascular disease risk factors, including serum cholesterol level, suggesting that their effects are at least partially independent of other established risk factors. In contrast to the younger cohort, none of the dietary lipids were associated with CAD in the older cohort. Dietary intervention for the prevention of CAD in younger men is supported by these findings.

To explore the extent to which the relation between plasma total cholesterol concentration and risk of death from CAD in men persists into old age, Shipley and associates[22] from London, UK, performed an 18-year follow-up of male Whitehall civil servants. Plasma total cholesterol concentrations and other risk factors were determined at first examination in 1967–1969 when they were aged 40 to 69 years (Figure 1-7). Death of men up to 31 January 1987 were recorded. A total of 18,296 male civil servants were studied including 4,155 of whom had died during the follow-up. Of the latter number, 1,676 were men who died of CAD. The mean cholesterol concentration in these men was 0.32 mmol/l higher than that in all other men. This difference in cholesterol concentrations fell 0.15 mmol/l with every 10 years' increase in age at screening. The risk of raised cholesterol concentration fell with age at death. Compared with other men cholesterol concentration in those who died of CAD was 0.44 mmol/l higher in those who died aged <60 and 0.26 mmol/l higher in those aged 60–79. For a given age at death the longer the gap between cholesterol measurement and death the more predictive the cholesterol

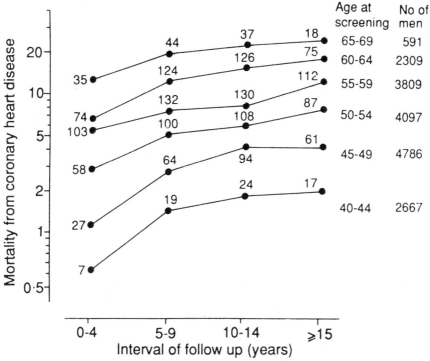

Fig. 1-7. Mortality from coronary heart disease (deaths/1000 person years) by age at screening and interval of follow up. (Observed number of deaths from coronary heart disease are given by each point). Reproduced with permission from Shipley, et al.[22]

concentration, both for CAD and all cause mortality. Reducing plasma cholesterol concentrations in middle age may influence the risk of death from CAD in old age.

To investigate the relation between lipids and angiographic CAD in women, Hong and associates[23] from Washington, D.C., obtained fasting lipid profiles on 108 women undergoing coronary angiography (group 1). CAD, defined as ≥25% luminal diameter narrowing in a major coronary artery, was present in 57 (53%). Neither serum total cholesterol nor triglyceride levels correlated with the presence of CAD. Mean total/HDL cholesterol ratio was higher among women with than without CAD (5.5 ± 0.3 vs 4.2 ± 0.2). Multiple regression analyses identified a higher total/HDL cholesterol ratio as the variable most predictive of the presence, extent (number of narrowed arteries), and severity (% maximum stenosis) of CAD. Age and lack of estrogen use were also independently associated with the presence of CAD, age and low-density lipoprotein cholesterol level were additional indicators of extent, and age was the only other discriminator of severity of CAD. In 56 women with total cholesterol <200 mg/dl (group II), mean total/HDL cholesterol ratio was higher in women with (n = 24) than without CAD (4.3 ± 0.2 vs 3.5 ± 0.2). Higher total/HDL cholesterol ratio was the variable most predictive of the presence of CAD, and the lone variable associated with severity after adjustment for other risk factors. Age was independently associated with presence and extent, and hypertension was also independently related to extent. Thus, among these women, total/HDL cholesterol ratio is the best indicator of the presence, severity and extent of CAD in general, and is the best predictor of presence and severity in patients with total cholesterol <200 mg/dl.

The National Cholesterol Education Program guidelines for treatment of high cholesterol levels especially target patients who have multiple risk factors for CAD. Veterans have an increased prevalence of cigarette smoking, are predominantly male, and may have higher rates of other risk factors than other groups. To assess the prevalence of cardiac risk factors, current cholesterol screening practices, and the potential impact of the National Cholesterol Education Program guidelines on the Veterans Affairs health care system, Richlie and associates[24] from Denver, Colorado, reviewed 185 randomly selected charts of out-patients who were actively receiving follow-up at a Veterans Affairs Medical Center. The patients had an average age of 58.3 years and 99.5% were male. Of these patients, 60% had a serum cholesterol level checked within the last 999 days. Nearly all patients (84%) had 2 or more risk factors noted. The mean cholesterol level was 5.85 mmol/L (226 mg/dL), with 72% of patients having levels above 5.20 mmol/L (200 mg/dL) and 36.1% having levels above 6.20 mmol/L (240 mg/dL) and 36.1% having levels above 6.20 mmol/L (240 mg/ dL). Of patients who had their cholesterol level checked, 69% (77/111) would require lipoprotein analysis by National Cholesterol Education Program guidelines (cholesterol, ≥6.20 mmol/L [≥240 mg/dL] or 5.15 to 6.20 mmol/L [200 to 239 mg/dL] with 2 or more risk factors), yet only 16% (12/77) had lipoprotein analyses done. Extrapolating from these data, the Denver Veteran Affairs Medical Center, which cares for 28,000 patients, has more than 19,000 patients who would need lipoprotein analysis to meet current guidelines. Full evaluation and subsequent treatment of dyslipidemias in veterans would require tremendous financial and man-power commitments.

As marker of risk of acute myocardial infarction

Salonen and co-investigators[25] in Kuopio, Finland, investigated the association of cholesterol concentrations in serum HDL and its subfractions HDL_2 and HDL_3 with risk of AMI in 1,799 randomly selected men 4, 48, 54 or 60 years old. Baseline examinations in the Kuopio Ischemic Heart Disease Risk Factor Study were done during 1984–1987. In Cox multivariate survival models adjusted for age and examination year, serum HDL cholesterol of less than 42 mg/dl was associated with a 3.3 fold risk of AMI, serum HDL_2 cholesterol of than 25 mg/dl was associated with a 4.4-fold risk of AMI and serum HDL_3 cholesterol 15 mg/dl was associated with a 2.2-fold risk of AMI. Adjustments for obesity, ischemic heart disease, other cardiovascular disease, maximal oxygen uptake, systolic blood pressure, antihypertensive medication, serum LDL cholesterol, and triglyceride concentrations reduced the excess risk associated with serum HDL, HDL_2, and HDL_3 cholesterol in the lowest quartiles by 52%, 48%, and 41%, respectively. Additional adjustments for alcohol consumption, cigarettes smoked daily, smoking years, and leisure time energy expenditure reduced these excess risks associated with low HDL, HDL_2, and HDL_3 cholesterol levels by another 25%, 24% and 21%, respectively. These data confirm that both total HDL and HDL_2 levels have inverse associations with the risk of AMI and may thus be protective factors in CAD, whereas the role of HDL_3 remains equivocal.

The independent contributions of subfractions of HDL cholesterol (HDL_2 and HDL_3) and apolipoproteins in predicting the risk of AMI are unclear. Prospective data are sparse, but HDL_2 is widely believed to be a more important predictor than HDL_3. Stampfer and associates[26] from Boston, Massachusetts, collected blood samples at baseline from 14,916 men aged 40 to 84 years who were participating in the Physicians' Health Study. After 5 years of follow-up, plasma samples from 246 men with new AMI (case subjects) were analyzed together with specimens from 246 men matched to them for age and smoking status who had not had a myocardial infarction. The levels of total cholesterol and apolipoprotein B-100 were significantly associated with an increased risk of AMI (data on levels of LDL cholesterol were unavailable) (Figure 1-8). Both HDL cholesterol and HDL_2 levels were associated with a substantially decreased risk of myocardial infarction, but the HDL_3 level was the strongest predictor; the relative risk was 0.3 for those in the 5th of the group with the highest HDL_3 levels, as compared with the 5th with the lowest levels. The benefit of a higher HDL cholesterol level was most pronounced among those with lower total cholesterol levels. Levels of apolipoprotein A-I and apolipoprotein A-II were also associated with decreased risk. However, the levels of HDL subfractions and apolipoproteins did not add significantly to the value of a multivariate model that included the ratio of total to HDL cholesterol in predicting myocardial infarction, whereas that ratio remained a significant independent predictor of risk. After adjustment for other risk factors, a change of 1 unit in the ratio of total to HDL cholesterol was associated with a 53% change in risk. This study underscores the importance of HDL cholesterol in predicting the risk of myocardial infarction and demonstrates protective effects on both the HDL_3 and HDL_2 subfractions of HDL cholesterol. The authors found little or no predictive value for the levels of apolipoproteins A-I, and A-II, and

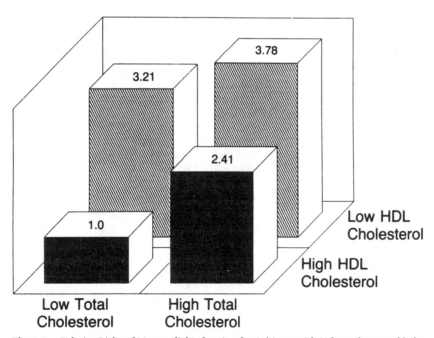

Fig. 1-8. Relative Risks of Myocardial Infarction for Subjects with Values above and below the Median for Total and HDL Cholesterol Levels. The median for total cholesterol was 5.49 mmol per liter, and that for HDL cholesterol 1.22 mmol per liter. The interaction of total cholesterol and HDL cholesterol was statistically significant in a model that also included total cholesterol and HDL cholesterol as separate terms (P = 0.01). Reproduced with permission from Stampfer, et al.[26]

B or HDL subfractions after conventional risk factors and the ratio of total to HDL cholesterol were considered.

Lipoprotein (a) in coronary artery disease

Lipoprotein (a) [Lp(a)] is composed of 1 LDL particle, to which 1 molecule of apolipoprotein (a) is covalently linked. Elevated levels of Lp(a) have been associated with CAD and Lp(a) has been shown to be highly heritable. Genest and associates[27] from Boston and Framingham, Massachusetts, and Elkton, Maryland, determined the prevalence of familial Lp (a) excess in patients with CAD. They determined plasma levels of Lp (a) in 180 patients (150 men and 30 women) with angiographically documented CAD before age 60 years, and in 459 control subjects (276 men and 183 women) clinically free of cardiovascular disease. In addition, Lp(a) levels were determined in families of 102 of the CAD probands (87 men and 15 women). No gender differences in Lp(a) levels were observed between men and women (patients or control subjects). Patients with CAD had higher Lp(a) levels than did control subjects (19 ± 21 vs 13 ± 15 mg/dl). The prevalence of Lp(a) excess (defined as >90th percentile of controls) was 17% in patients with CAD. Lp(a) levels were not correlated with cholesterol, LDL cholesterol, HDL cholesterol or apolipoproteins A-1 or B. There was a weak correlation between Lp(a) and triglycerides (r = 0.166) in patients and control subjects. Stepwise discriminant analysis revealed that Lp(a) was a risk factor for the presence of CAD in men, independent of smoking, hypertension, diabetes, LDL and HDL cholesterol, or apolipoprotein A-1 and B levels. Family studies revealed that Lp(a) levels are strongly genetically determined. Spearman rank correlations for Lp(a) levels between proband-spouse and midparent-midoffspring indicate that Lp(a) levels are largely genetically determined. The prevalence of familial Lp(a) excess was 16% (14 of 87) in men and 20% (6 of 30) in women. Our data indicate that Lp(a) is a common genetic disorder in patients with premature CAD and that it is highly heritable. In addition, Lp(a) levels are independent of other lipoprotein parameters.

Low levels in coronary artery disease

To examine the relation between serum total cholesterol concentration and mortality (from CAD and from other causes) below the range of cholesterol values generally seen in western populations, Chen and associates[28] from Shanghai, Peoples Republic of China, prospectively studied 9,021 Chinese men and women aged 35 to 64 years at baseline and followed them 8 to 13 years. The average serum cholesterol concentration was 4.2 mmol/l at baseline and only 43 (7%) of the deaths that occurred during the 8 to 13 year follow-up were attributed to CAD. There was a strongly positive and apparently independent relation between serum total cholesterol concentration and death from CAD, and within the range of usual serum total cholesterol concentration studied (3.8–4.7 mmol/l) there was no evidence of any threshold. After appropriate adjustment for the regression dilution bias, a 4% difference in usual cholesterol concentration was associated with a 21% difference in mortality from CAD. There was no significant relation between serum cholesterol concentration and death from stroke or all types of cancer. The 79 deaths due to liver cancer or other chronic liver disease were inversely related to cholesterol concentration at baseline. Blood cholesterol concentration was directly related to mortality from CAD even in those with what was, by Western standards, a "low" cholesterol concentration. There was no good evidence of an adverse effect of cholesterol on other causes of death.

Low high-density lipoprotein and "desirable" total cholesterol

Because the National Cholesterol Education Program guidelines suggest that levels of total serum cholesterol <5.17 mmol/liter (200 mg/dl) are "desirable," Ginsburg and associates[29] from Boston, Massachusetts, performed a retrospective observational analysis to determine the prevalence of CAD in patients with total cholesterol <200 mg/dl and the prevalence of total cholesterol <200 mg/dl in patients with CAD by angiography. Cholesterol levels <5.17 mmol/L (200 mg/dl) were found in 1,084 of 2,535 patients (42%) having cholesterol measured on hospital admission; 690 of these 1,084 (64%) had CAD (Table 1-6). These patients were mostly men, had a family history of premature CAD, and 60% (414

TABLE 1-6. *Hospitalized patients with total cholesterol ≤5.17 mmol/ liter (200 mg/dl): coronary artery disease as a function of high-density lipoprotein threshold of 0.90 mmol/liter (35 mg/dl). Reproduced with permission from Ginsburg, et al.*[29]

Part I: Coronary Artery Disease by Clinical Diagnosis

	Coronary Artery Disease	
	Present (n = 690)	Absent (n = 394)
HDL <0.90 mmol/liter (35 mg/dl)	414 (60%)	186 (47%)
HDL ≥0.90 mmol/liter (35 mg/dl)	192 (28%)	170 (48%)
Chi-square = 16.61; p <0.001		

Part II: Coronary Artery Disease by Angiography

	Coronary Artery Disease	
	Present (n = 424)	Absent (n = 86)
HDL <0.90 mmol/liter (35 mg/dl)	252 (59%)	41 (48%)
HDL ≥0.90 mmol/liter (35 mg/dl)	172 (41%)	45 (52%)
Chi-square = 4.04; p <0.05		

Part III: Elective Angiography

	Coronary Artery Disease	
	Present (n = 281)	Absent (n = 61)
HDL <0.90 mmol/liter (35 mg/dl)	180 (64%)	30 (49%)
HDL ≥0.90 mmol/liter (35 mg/dl)	101 (36%)	39 (51%)
Chi-square = 4.68; p <0.04		

HDL = high-density lipoprotein.

of 690) had HDL cholesterol <0.90 mmol/L (35 mg/dl). In a separate group of patients defined from the same admission population but having angiographically established CAD, 32% (424 of 1,197) had a total cholesterol <5.17 mmol/liter (200 mg/dl), 59% of whom (252 of 424) had HDL <0.90 mmol/L (35 mg/dl). An analysis of persons admitted electively for angiography (to exclude any effects of hospitalization per se on serum lipids) revealed a similar proportion of persons with total cholesterol 5.17 mmol/liter (200 mg/dl) (35%), CAD (82%), and HDL 0.90 mmol/liter (35 mg/dl). The authors' observations suggest that low serum cholesterol levels (<5.17 mmol/L [200 mg/dl]) are seen frequently in patients suspected of having or who have established CAD; moreover, a false sense of security may be established among physician and patient with the finding of a serum cholesterol level <5.17 mmol/liter (200 mg/dl)—men with a family history of premature CAD and low levels of HDL characterize persons with CAD in this low cholesterol group.

Normal levels in an 88-year-old man who eats 25 eggs a day

Kern[30] from Denver, Colorado, studied an 88-year-old man who lived in a retirement community who was entirely asymptomatic and healthy except for an extremely poor memory without other specific neurologic deficits. His general health had always been good. His weight had always been from 82 to 86 kg and his height was 1.87 meters. There was never evidence of myocardial ischemia, stroke, or renal disease. He had numerous serum total cholesterol levels taken over a period of some years and they ranged from 3.88–5.18 mmol/l (150–200 mg/dL). He never smoked cigarettes and he never drank alcohol excessively. His father died from unknown causes at age 40 and his mother died at age 76. One sister died at age 82 and another was alive at 86. He ate 20 to 30 eggs a day and he did this for at least 15 years and probably longer. He kept a careful record, egg by egg, of the number ingested each day. The patient's plasma total cholesterol was 5.18 mmol/l (200 mg/dL); LDL cholesterol 3.68 mmol/l (142 mg/dL); and HDL 1.17 mmol/l (45 mg/dL). The ratio of LDL to HDL cholesterol was 3.15. The mean amount of cholesterol absorbed was 55% in the subject on a low cholesterol diet (300 of the 567 μmol of cholesterol ingested per day) and 46% on the high cholesterol diet (1390 of the 2995 μmol in the daily diet). The patient absorbed only 18%. Thus, although he ingested approximately 12,953 μmol of cholesterol daily, he absorbed only 2331 μmol or 941 μmol per day more than the subjects on the high cholesterol diet. In the patient 967 μmol of cholic acid and 546 μmol of chenodeoxycholic acid were synthesized daily for a total rate of bile-acid synthesis of 1513 μmol daily—approximately twice the mean rate of synthesis in the normal volunteers (766 μmol daily on the low-cholesterol diet and 812 μmol daily on the high-cholesterol diet). Thus, the patient disposed of 701 μmol more cholesterol per day as bile acids than did the normal subjects on the high-cholesterol diet. The patient's fractional turnover rate was diminished somewhat. The bile-acid pool was greatly increased in the patient and was at least twice that of the normal subjects during the low- and high-cholesterol diets. The patient's total bile-acid pool was 10,751 μmol compared with 4,143 and 4,738 mmol in the normal subjects during the low- and high-cholesterol diets respectively. Although it would have been desirable to have studied this patient on a low-cholesterol diet as well as on his customary diet of 25 eggs per day, it was impossible to do so. His cholesterol metabolism, therefore, was compared with that of other subjects who were being studied by the same techniques. These results explain in dramatic fashion the apparent paradox of an enormous dietary cholesterol intake and longevity to the age of 88 without clinically important atherosclerosis. The patient had extremely efficient compensatory mechanisms—namely, a marked reduction in the efficiency of cholesterol absorption, greatly increased synthesis of bile acids, and apparently reduced cholesterol synthesis relative to his cholesterol absorption. The decrease in the efficiency of cholesterol absorption to only 18% of the unusually large intake played an important part in maintaining a normal plasma cholesterol level. Approximately 10,622 of the 12,953 μmol of cholesterol ingested each day passed through the patient's gastrointestinal tract to be excreted in the feces. Although he still absorbed 2331 μmol of cholesterol per day (2032 and 941 μmol per day more than the mean amount absorbed by the normal subjects during the low- and high-cholesterol diets, respectively), he compensated further, primarily by doubling the usual rate of bile-acid synthesis.

Triglycerides as a major atherosclerotic risk factor

Welin and associates[31] from Uppsala, Sweden, examined 2 cohorts of elderly men, 60 and 67 years old. The 2 cohorts overlapped to a large extent in terms of numbers but not in the follow-up periods. The men have been followed-up for 7 and 8 years respectively. Among the 748 60-year old men without prior AMI the 7-year incidence of CAD was 8%. The incidence was related to BP, smoking habits and serum triglycerides (but not serum cholesterol) both in univariate and multivariate analyses. The incidence of CAD increased 5-fold from the lowest to the highest quintile of triglycerides. Among the 595 67-year-old men without prior AMI the 8-year incidence of CAD was 11%. Both serum cholesterol and triglycerides were significant risk factors in univariate analyses but only triglycerides in multivariate analyses. The incidence of CAD increased almost 3-fold from the lowest to the highest quintile of triglycerides. Increased serum triglycerides is a major coronary risk factor in elderly men.

Primary hypercholesterolemia

Hypercholesterolemia is a well-established risk factor for CAD. However, the mechanisms underlying hypercholesterolemia, elevated LDL in particular, are not well understood. To determine these mechanisms, Vega and coworkers[32] in Dallas, Texas, studied LDL kinetics in a group of men with primary hypercholesterolemia. LDL kinetics in 134 middle-aged men with high-risk levels of LDL cholesterol (more than 160 mg/dl) were compared with kinetics in 16 men with borderline high-risk levels of LDL cholesterol (120–159 mg/dl) and 14 men with heterozygous familial hypercholesterolemia. Patients with primary hypercholesterolemia were further divided into moderate hypercholesterolemia and severe hypercholesterolemia groups. Four factors contributed to increasing LDL cholesterol concentrations above the borderline range to moderately elevated levels: 37 patients had no increase in LDL apolipoprotein B levels but had abnormally high LDL cholesterol-to-apo B ratios; 14 patients had very low fractional catabolic rates for LDL, similar to familial hypercholesterolemia patients; 35 patients had fractional clearing rates for LDL in the borderline range but high production for LDL; and 22 patients had a high flux of LDL (high production rates and high fractional clearing rates). In general, patients with severe hypercholesterolemia resembled those with moderate LDL elevations, except that their LDL particles were enriched with cholesterol. The data from this study reveal that there are several distinct patterns of LDL metabolism responsible for primary hypercholesterolemia.

To determine the excess mortality from all causes and from CAD in patients with familial hypercholesterolemia and to examine how useful various criteria for selective measurement of cholesterol concentration in cardiovascular screening programs are in identifying these patients, the Scientific Steering Committee on behalf of the Simon Broome Register Group[33] from multiple medical centers in the United Kingdom performed a prospective cohort study involving 11 hospital out-patient lipid clinics and included 282 men and 244 women aged 20–74 years with hetero-zygous familial hypercholesterolemia. The cohort was followed up for 2,234 person years during 1980–1989. Fifteen of the 24 deaths were due to CAD giving a standardized mortality ratio of 386. The excess mortality from this cause was highest at age 20–39 years (standardized mortality ratio 9,686; 3,670 to 21,800) and decreased significantly with age. The standardized mortality ratio for all causes was 183 and also was highest at age 20–39. There was no significant difference between men and women. Criteria for measurement of cholesterol concentration in cardiovascular screening programs (family history, presence of AMI, angina, stroke, cor-neal arcus, xanthelasma, obesity, hypertension, diabetes, or any of these) were present in 78% of patients. Familial hypercholesterolemia is asso-ciated with a substantial excess mortality from CAD in young adults but may not be associated with a substantial excess mortality in older patients.

Familial hyperchylomicronemia

Familial hypercholesterolemia (type 1 hyperlipoproteinemia) is a rare autosomal recessive disorder characterized by severe chylomicronemia secondary to a congenital deficiency of either lipoprotein lipase or apo-lipoprotein C-II. Familial hypercholesterolemia generally manifests itself in infancy and early childhood as repeated attacks of abdominal pain and as a creamy appearing (lipemic) plasma, both due to ingestion of dietary fats that have delayed clearance from the plasma. Complications due to hyperchylomicronemia include acute pancreatitis, eruptive xan-thomas, lipemia retinalis, and hepatosplenomegaly. Plasma triglyceride concentrations generally range from 1,500 to 4,500 mg/dl. The plasma total cholesterol generally ranges from 160 to 400 mg/dl. Both LDL cho-lesterol and HDL cholesterol are usually exceedingly low in the range of 20–40 mg/dl and 5–20 mg/dl, respectively. Little morphologic data have been reported on patients with familial hypercholesterolemia. Malekza-deh and associates[34] from Bethesda, Maryland, described at necropsy 4 patients aged 29 to 63 years who had familial hyperchylomicronemia. The unusual finding at necropsy was the absence of atherosclerotic plaques in the patients and the presence in each of the 4 patients of lipid deposits on the endocardium of left atrium. The mechanism of formation of the lipid deposits on LA endocardium was not determined.

Lipoprotein lipase hydrolyzes the triglyceride core of chylomicrons and VLDL and has a crucial role in regulating plasma lipoprotein levels. Deficiencies of lipoprotein lipase activity lead to aberrations in lipoprotein levels. Worldwide, the frequency of lipoprotein lipase deficiency is highest among French Canadians. Ma and associates[35] from Quebec and Mon-treal, Canada, and Seattle, Washington, sought to determine the molec-ular basis of the disorder in this population. The entire coding sequence of the lipoprotein lipase gene from one French Canadian patient was amplified by the polymerase chain reaction and sequenced. Exon 5 from 36 other French Canadian patients was amplified and analyzed by dot blot hybridization with allele-specific oligonucleotides. Sequence analysis revealed a missense substitution of leucine for proline at residue 207 in exon 5. This mutation was found on 54 of the 74 mutant alleles (73%) in the patients. Studies of site-directed in vitro mutagenesis have confirmed that this mutation generates inactive lipoprotein lipase and is the cause of lipoprotein lipase deficiency. The authors identified a missense mutation at residue 207 of the lipoprotein lipase gene that is the most common cause of lipoprotein lipase deficiency in French Canadians. This mutation can be easily detected by dot blot analysis, providing opportunity for definitive DNA diagnosis of the disorder and identification of heterozygous carriers.

Effects of obesity

Obesity is an important determinant of serum lipids and lipoproteins in adults. Since obesity begins early in life as a rule, Wattigney and associates[36] from New Orleans, Louisiana, and associates of the Bogalusa Heart Study examined the impact of obesity on serum lipid and lipoprotein levels in 3311 children and young adults (aged 5–26 years) from a totally biracial community. Study subjects were grouped according to race, sex, and age categories (5–10 years, 11–16 years, 17–22 years, and 23–26 years), excluding females using oral contraceptives or who-were pregnant. Overall, associations increased with age, being most prominently noted in white males. A negative association was noted between ponderosity and HDL cholesterol. Similar results were seen using subscapular skinfold thickness as a measure of central obesity. Overweight was defined as exceeding 20% above the National Health Anthropometric and Nutritional Examination Survey II survey 50th percentiles. The prevalence of overweight individuals increased with age, being most prominent in black females. The percent(s) of hypercholesterolemic cases, based on the National Cholesterol Education Program criteria, likewise increased with age. A marked proportion of older white males were classified as borderline high and high for LDL cholesterol. A regression model using subscapular skinfold to predict serum lipids and lipoproteins within each age group indicated a consistent increase in the adverse nature of the lipid profile. Intervention and education programs aimed at reducing obesity at younger ages are recommended to reduce serum lipid and lipoprotein levels developing in young adulthood.

Relation to systemic hypertension

High BP has been associated with elevated atherogenic blood lipid fractions, but epidemiological surveys often give inconsistent results across population subgroups. A better understanding of the relation between BP and blood lipids may provide insight into the mechanism(s) whereby hypertension is associated with increased risk of CAD. Bonna and Thelle[37] in Tromso, Norway, assessed the cross-sectional relations of serum total cholesterol, high HDL cholesterol, non-HDL cholesterol (total minus HDL cholesterol), and triglyceride levels with BP in a population of 8,081 men 20–54 years old and 7,663 women 20–49 years old. Stratified analyses and multivariable methods were used to control for potential confounding anthropometric and lifestyle variables. Total and non-HDL cholesterol levels increased significantly with increasing systolic or diastolic BP in both sexes (Figure 1-9). Men 20–29 years old had steeper regression slopes for BP by total cholesterol level than did women of similar age. In men, the association between BP and total cholesterol level decreased with age, whereas in women, it increased with age. Body mass index modified the relation, whereas smoking, physical activity, and alcohol consumption had little influence on the association. Triglyceride levels increased with BP, but this relation was weak in lean subjects. HDL cholesterol level correlated positively with blood pressure in population subgroups having a high alcohol consumption. These results support the hypothesis that there are biological interrelations between BP and blood lipids that may influence the mechanisms whereby BP is associated with risk of CAD.

Dyslipidemic hypertension

Selby and associates[38] from several medical centers identified 60 cases of dyslipidemic hypertension in the 1028 middle-aged, white, male twin participants in the first examination of the National Heart, Lung, and Blood Institute Twin Study (1969–1973). The prevalence of dyslipidemic hypertension was similar by zygosity but proband concordance was 3 times greater in monozygotic than dizygotic twins (0.44 [7 concordant and 18 discordant pairs] vs 0.14 [2 concordant and 24 discordant pairs]), suggesting a genetic effect on the condition. Low HDL cholesterol level was the most common lipid abnormality in concordant pairs. Mortality from ischemic heart disease was significantly higher in individuals with dyslipidemic hypertension. Obesity and glucose intolerance were closely associated with the syndrome. Moreover, within the 18 discordant monozygotic twin pairs, the twins with dyslipidemic hypertension had gained significantly more weight as adults and were significantly heavier than their unaffected cotwins. Thus, although genetic factors may influence

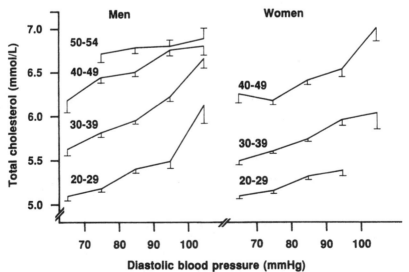

Fig. 1-9. Plot of mean concentrations of serum total cholesterol levels (mmol/l) by diastolic blood pressure in men 20–29, 30–39, 40–49, and 50–54 years old and in women 20–29, 30–39, and 40–49 years old. Cells with less than 20 observations were pooled with adjacent category. T bars are SEM. Reproduced with permission from Bonna, et al.[37]

development of dyslipidemic hypertension, nongenetic, potentially modifiable aspects of obesity are also closely related to expression of this clinically important syndrome.

Effects of stress

Niaura and associates[39] from Providence, Rhode Island, examined the effects of psychological stress on plasma lipid, lipoprotein, and apolipoprotein levels in 3 related studies. In the first study, tax accountants (n = 20) and a comparable control group (n = 20) were assessed during and after the tax season. In the second and third studies, first-year medical students (n = 24 and n = 16) were assessed at midsemester and immediately before the examinations. Across studies, the stressors induced significant psychological distress. There were no corresponding changes in lipid and lipoprotein levels. Mean stress-induced change in total cholesterol level was -0.04 mmol/L (-1.6 mg/dL) for the accountants and 0 mmol/L (0 mg/dL) and 0.10 mmol/L (4 mg/dL) for medical students in the second and third studies, respectively. In all studies, change in total cholesterol level correlated with change in total serum protein levels (r = .42 to .60). These results suggest that commonly occurring stressful situations do not produce significant changes in plasma lipid and lipoprotein levels.

Effects of anabolic steroids

Glazer[40] from Rochester, New York, reviewed the current body of published reports linking anabolic steroids to atherogenic alterations in serum lipid levels. Anabolic steroids cause marked HDL level depression (weighted average = 52%) and severe depression of HDL levels (weighted average = 78%) while raising LDL cholesterol levels an average of 36%.

Effects of acetylcholine-induced coronary vasoreactivity

Recent evidence suggests that HDL cholesterol has important vasoactive properties which may contribute to its beneficial effects on atherosclerotic CAD. The endothelium-dependent vasodilator acetylcholine has been used in a number of experimental studies to assess endothelial function. Kuhn and associates[41] from Washington, D.C. investigated the relation between serum lipoproteins and acetylcholine-induced coronary vasoreactivity in 27 patients undergoing elective coronary arteriography. Mean serum cholesterol, LDL cholesterol, HDL cholesterol and triglyceride levels were 189 ± 7 (4.84 ± 0.18 mmol/L), 134 ± 6 (3.47 ± 0.15 mmol/L), 41 ± 3 (1.06 ± 0.08 mmol/L) and 106 ± 30 mg/dl (1.20 ± 0.03 mmol/L), respectively. After a baseline arteriogram, acetylcholine was infused into the left main coronary artery and percent change from baseline dimension was determined in 27 angiographically smooth coronary artery segments and in 14 arterial segments with evidence of mild atherosclerotic disease. Intact vascular smooth muscle function was then confirmed in all segments by dilation to intracoronary nitroglycerin. Acetylcholine produced significant vasoconstriction of both angiographically smooth ($13 \pm 4\%$) and diseased ($19 \pm 4\%$) coronary segments. A positive correlation was observed between HDL cholesterol and normal acetylcholine-induced coronary vasoreactivity in both angiographically smooth and diseased coronary segments. No significant correlation was observed, however, between total and LDL cholesterol, or between total cholesterol to HDL ratio and the response of coronary artery diameter to acetylcholine infusion. These findings suggest that HDL cholesterol promotes normal endothelial cell function in both normal and atherosclerotic coronary segments. This beneficial effect may be related to a direct effect of HDL on release of endothelial-derived relaxing factor or may be secondary to its effects on endothelial cell proliferation. Thus, while HDL has important antiatherogenic properties, the clinical benefit of HDL elevation may be related, in part, to its effects on endothelial function and coronary vasoreactivity.

Effects of L-arginine on hypercholesterolemia-induced endothelial dysfunction

Hypercholesterolemia impairs endothelial function, possibly by interference with the intracellular formation of endothelium-derived relaxing factor from its precursor L-arginine. Whether L-arginine reverses hypercholesterolemia-induced endothelial dysfunction in the coronary circulation was investigated by Drexler and associates[42] from Freiburg, Germany. Epicardial artery cross-sectional area and coronary blood flow velocity were measured in 8 hypercholesterolemic patients (mean serum cholesterol 7.8 mmol/l) and 7 age-matched controls before and after graded intracoronary infusions of the endothelium-dependent agent acetylcholine (0.036, 0.36, 3.6 µg/min). The effect of intracoronary infusion of L-arginine (160 umol/min via the guiding catheter) on these measurements was then examined. In controls, acetylcholine induced a moderate dose-dependent constriction of the epicardial artery segment of the left anterior descending artery and increased coronary blood flow (by 239% at the highest dose). In patients with hypercholesterolemia, the vasoconstrictive effect of acetylcholine on epicardial segments was similar to that in controls, but the increase in coronary blood flow with acetylcholine was significantly attenuated (highest dose: 61% [19]). L-arginine restored the acetylcholine-induced increase in blood flow in patients with hypercholesterolemia (198% [61] vs baseline) but did not affect coronary blood flow in controls. The findings suggest that hypercholesterolemia impairs endothelium-dependent dilatation of the coronary microcirculation and that this impairment can be restored by short-term administration of L-arginine.

THERAPY OF HYPERLIPIDEMIA

Diet

The National Cholesterol Education Program recommends a diet containing less than 30% of calories in the form of fat, less than 10% in saturated fat, and less than 300 mg of cholesterol per day. Since Americans' diets generally exceed these recommendations, Small and associates[43] of Boston, Massachusetts, investigated an easy kitchen method to reduce substantially saturated fat and cholesterol in ground meat. Raw ground meat was heated in vegetable oil and rinsed with boiling water to extract fat and cholesterol. The fat-free broth was recombined with the meat to restore flavor. The amounts of total fat, saturated fat, and cholesterol in the meat after extraction were compared with the amounts in meat cooked as patties and in stir-fried, rinsed meat. When raw ground beef containing 9.6–20.8% fat was cooked as patties and the fat poured off, 6–17% of the fat and 1.3–4.3% of the cholesterol were lost. In stir-fried, rinsed ground beef, 23–59% of the fat and 9.0–18.8% of the cholesterol were lost. When vegetable oil was used to extract fat and cholesterol from beef containing 20.7% fat, a mean ($\pm$ SD) of 67.7 $\pm$ 1.6% of the fat and 39.2 $\pm$ 5.1% of the cholesterol were lost. The differences between conventionally cooked meat and meat prepared by the extraction of fat were significant. An average of 43% (range, 38–49) of cholesterol was extracted from a wide variety of ground meats. Although conventional cooking produced no change in fatty-acid composition as compared with raw meat, our extraction process greatly increased the ratio of unsaturated to saturated fat, from 1.32 in conventionally cooked meat to 2.92–4.56 in meat after extraction. Extraction resulted in the loss of 72–87% of saturated fat. This method produces a tasty meat product that is much lower in saturated fat and cholesterol than conventionally cooked meat, and that can be used in sauces, soups, and solid meat products.

In July 1991 the decennial revision of "Recommended Daily Amounts of Food Energy and Nutrients for Groups of People in the United Kingdom" published in 1979 appeared. The new book by the Panel on Dietary Reference Values Committee on Medical Aspects of Food Policy is entitled "Dietary Reference Values for Food Energy and Nutrients for the United Kingdom" (London: HMSO, 1991).[44] This version is a vast improvement on its predecessor. It is a volume of 210 pages (compared to 27 in 1979). It provides reference nutrient intakes (the renamed recommended daily amounts) for 35 nutrients instead of 10 and it also offers 2 more useful figures—the estimated average requirement and the lower reference nutrient intake, below which deficiency is probable. There are informative chapters about energy, fat, nonstarch polysaccharides (which had been called fiber) sugars, starches, and protein; 1 for each vitamin; and 1 each for calcium, magnesium, phosphorus, sodium, potassium, chloride, iron, zinc, copper, selenium, molybdenum, manganese, chromium, iodine, fluoride, and "other minerals." In general the estimated energy requirements are reduced, especially for women during pregnancy compared to the 1979 recommendations.

Americans consume an average of 37% of their energy intake as fat. Many authorities recommend restricting fat intake to 30% of energy intake to reduce the rates of CAD and perhaps of cancer of the breast, colon, and prostate gland. Based on the assumptions that underlie those recommendations, Browner and associates[45] from San Francisco, California, estimated the effect of this dietary change on mortality. If all Americans restricted their intake of dietary fat by reducing consumption of saturated fat and accompanying dietary cholesterol, the corresponding reductions in serum cholesterol levels could reduce CAD mortality rates by 5% to 20%, depending on age. If the relationship between dietary fat and cancer is as strong as has been observed in some studies, the proportional effects on mortality from fat-related cancers could be even greater, although the absolute effects—given the lower mortality rates—would be smaller. Overall, if the assumptions are correct, about 42,000 of the 2.3 million deaths that would have occurred in adults each year in the United States could be deferred. This 2% benefit, equivalent to an increase in average life expectancy of 3 to 4 months, would accrue chiefly to people over the age of 65 years.

Barnard[46] from Los Angeles, California, presented data from 4,587 adults who attended a 3-week residential, life-style modification program consisting of a high-complex-carbohydrate, high-fiber, low-fat, and low-cholesterol diet combined with daily aerobic exercise, primarily walking. Total cholesterol values were reduced by 23%, from 6.06 to 4.66 mmol/L (234 to 180 mg/dL). LDL cholesterol values were also reduced by 23%, from 3.9 to 3.0 mmol/L (151 to 116 mg/dL), with most of the change occurring during the first 2 weeks. Male subjects showed a greater reduction in total cholesterol (24.4% vs 20.8%) and LDL cholesterol (25% vs 19.4%) values compared with female subjects. Follow-up studies for 18 months on a small group showed that, in most cases, continued compliance with the program maintained total cholesterol values well below 5.18 mmol/L (200 mg/dL), the level recommended by the National Cholesterol Education Program. High density cholesterol was reduced by 16%, but the ratio of total cholesterol to HDL cholesterol was reduced by 11%. Female subjects showed a greater drop in HDL cholesterol values than did male subjects (19.4% vs 11.6%). Serum triglyceride values were reduced by 33%, from 2.29 to 1.54 mmol/L (200 to 135 mg/dL); again, male subjects showed a greater reduction than did the female subjects (37.9% vs 22.5%). Body weight was also significantly reduced, 5.5% for male subjects and 4.4% for female subjects. These results show that most adults can significantly reduce serum lipid values and the risk of atherosclerosis and its clinical sequelae through life-style modification consisting of diet and exercise.

The National Cholesterol Education Program (NCEP) recommends a low-saturated-fat, low-cholesterol diet, with weight loss if indicated, to correct elevated plasma cholesterol levels. Weight loss accomplished by simple caloric restriction or increased exercise typically increases the level of HDL cholesterol. Little is known about the effects on plasma lipoproteins of a hypocaloric NCEP diet with or without exercise in overweight people. Wood and associates[47] from Stanford, California, tested the hypothesis that exercise (walking or jogging) will increase HDL cholesterol levels in moderately overweight, sedentary people who adopt a hypocaloric NCEP diet. The authors randomly assigned 132 men and 132 women 25 to 49 years old to 1 of 3 groups: control, hypocaloric NCEP diet, or hypocaloric NCEP diet with exercise. One hundred nineteen of the men and 112 of the women returned for testing after 1 year. After 1 year, the subjects in both intervention groups had reached or closely approached NCEP Step 1 dietary goals and reduced their mean body fat significantly (range of reduction in mean fat weight, 4.0 to 7.8 kg) (Figure 1-10). Weight loss on the NCEP diet alone did not significantly change HDL cholesterol levels in either the men or the women as compared with the subjects in the control group. Plasma levels of HDL cholesterol increased significantly more in the men who exercised and dieted (mean [± SE] change, +13±13%) than in the men who only dieted (+2±3%) or the men who acted as controls (−4±2%). HDL cholesterol levels remained about the same in the women who exercised and dieted (+1 ± 2%); they were higher than in the women who only dieted (−10 ± 3%), but not higher than in the controls (−3 ± 3%). Regular exercise in overweight men and women enhances the improvement in plasma lipoprotein levels that results from the adoption of a low-saturated-fat, low-cholesterol diet.

To evaluate the long-term efficacy of diets in lowering serum cholesterol concentration Ramsay and associates[48] from Sheffield, United Kingdom, examined 16 published controlled trials of 6 months' duration or longer. To be included trials had to have been conducted in hospital clinics, or industry, or mental hospitals or institutions, or in general

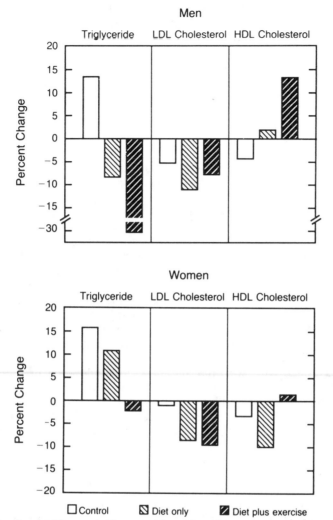

Fig. 1-10. Percent Changes in Plasma Triglyceride and Lipoprotein Cholesterol Concentrations in the Study Groups after One Year. The mean change for a group is expressed as a percentage of the base-line level for that group. Percent changes are calculated directly from Tables 1 and 2, which include standard deviations. Reproduced with permission from Wood, et al.[47]

populations. Trials had been conducted in high-risk subjects, in unselected healthy subjects, or for secondary prevention in patients with CAD. Women were included in only 4 of the 16 trials. Diets equivalent to the step 1 diet were employed in 8 trials with individual intervention by dietitian or occupational physicians or with population advice. Intensive trials which were more rigorous than the step 2 diet were employed in 8 trials. Net change in serum total cholesterol concentration in subjects receiving treatment with diet was compared with values in control subjects after 6 months to 10 years. In 5 trials with the step 1 diet as individual intervention the net reduction in serum cholesterol concentration ranged from 0% to 4% over 6 months to 6 years. In trials with population education reductions in cholesterol concentrations were 0.6–2.0% over 5 to 10 years. When population and individual dietary advice were combined changes in cholesterol concentration ranged from a fall of 2.1% to a rise of 1.0% over 4 to 10 years. Diets more intensive than the step 2 diet reduced serum cholesterol concentration by 13% over 5 years in selected high risk men in the population; by 6.5–15.1% over 2 to 5 years in hospital outpatients; and by 12.8–15.5% over 1 to 4 and ½ years in patients in institutions. The response to a step 1 diet is too small to have any value in the clinical management of adults with serum cholesterol concentrations above 6.5 mmol/l.

B-glucan in oatmeal

Oat cereals rich in water-soluble fiber B-glucan have been studied as a dietary therapy for hypocholesterolemia. To determine the hypocholesterolemic response of B-glucan in the diet, Davidson and associates[49] from Chicago, Illinois, randomized 156 adults with LDL cholesterol levels greater than 4.14 mmol/L (160 mg/dL) or between 3.37 and 4.14 mmol/L (130–160 mg/dL) with multiple risk factors to 1 of 7 groups. Six groups received either oatmeal or oat bran at doses (dry weight) of 28 g (1 oz), 56 g (1 oz), and 84 g (3 oz). A seventh group received 28 g of farina (B-glucan control). At week 6 of treatment, significant differences were found for both total cholesterol and LDL-cholesterol levels among the farina control and the treatment groups who were receiving 84 g of oatmeal, 56 g of oat bran, and 84 g of oat bran, with decreases in LDL-cholesterol levels of 10.1%, 15.9%, and 11.5%, respectively. Fifty-six grams of oat bran resulted in significantly greater reductions in LDL-cholesterol levels than 56 g of oatmeal. Nutrient analysis shows no difference in dietary fat content between these treatment groups; therefore, the higher B-glucan content of oat bran most likely explains the significantly greater LDL-cholesterol reductions. A dose-dependent reduction in LDL-cholesterol levels with oat cereals supports the independent hypocholesterolemic effects of B-glucan.

Guar gum

Spiller and associates[50] from Los Altos and Stanford, California, compared the hypolipidemic effect of guar gum (GG, 15 g/day) with that of an oat fiber source (OFS, 77 g/day). Both treatments supplied the same amount of total dietary fiber (11 g/day) and were taken with water 3 times a day for 3 weeks at mealtime. Thirteen free-living adult men and women participated in the study. Their total plasma cholesterol was 244 ± 21 mg/dl (mean ± SD), and plasma triglycerides were 149 ± 93 mg/dl before the intervention. Diets were monitored to ensure that no changes occurred other than the replacement of carbohydrate calories for the 200 kcal/day supplied by the oat fiber source. Combined averages for both of the crossover phases showed that guar gum induced a reduction in total cholesterol of 26 ± 10 mg/dl and in LDL cholesterol of 25 ± 9 mg/dl. The oat fiber source induced a reduction in total cholesterol of 9 ± 13 mg/dl and in LDL cholesterol of 11 ± 4 mg/dl. Although both treatments were effective in reducing elevated total cholesterol, guar gum at the levels fed was significantly more effective in reducing total cholesterol. Neither treatment induced significant changes in HDL cholesterol or very LDL cholesterol.

Marine oil capsules

Because marine oil capsules vary widely in their content of omega-3 fatty acids (Table 1-7), saturated fat, and cholesterol composition and biologic potency, Davidson and associates[51] from Chicago, Illinois, compared the lipid lowering effects of 3 preparations in patients with different forms of hyperlipidemia. The ester and triglyceride forms of marine oil both effectively lowered triglyceride, but the response of LDL cholesterol was variable; it declined modestly in patients with hypercholesterolemia and was either unchanged or increased in those with hypertriglyceridemia. The saturated fat and cholesterol content of the marine oil preparation appeared to influence the LDL cholesterol response. Therefore, marine oil capsules are useful for lowering levels of VLDL cholesterol, but the large dose required to achieve and sustain this effect (4.5 g of omega-3 fatty acids, or 9 to 18 capsules daily) may limit long-term compliance.

Estrogen replacements

Dupont and Page[52] from Nashville, Tennessee, conducted a meta-analysis concerning breast cancer and estrogen replacement therapy. The overall relative risk of breast cancer associated with this therapy was

TABLE 1-7.   *Omega-3 fatty acid content of selected fish, fish oils, and commercial marine oil preparations.* Reproduced with permission from Davidson, et al.[51]

Food Item	Total Fat, g	Total Saturated Fat, g	EPA, g	DHA, g	Cholesterol, mg
Cod (Pacific)	0.6	0.1	0.1	0.1	61
Mackerel (Atlantic)	13.9	3.6	0.9	1.6	80
Salmon (Chinook)	10.4	2.5	0.8	0.6	74
Cod liver oil	100.0	17.6	9.0	9.6	570
Salmon oil	100.0	23.8	8.8	11.1	485
Triglyceride MaxEPA†	100.0	25.4	17.8	11.6	600
New MaxEPA†	100.0	25.4	17.8	11.6	20
Promega‡	100.0	10.0	28.0	12.0	20
Ethyl ester Super-EPA§	100.0	8.0	32.0	20.0	20

*EPA indicates eicosapentaenoic acid; DHA, docosahexaenoic acid.
†MaxEPA, 30% omega-3 fatty acids, R.P. Scherer, Detroit, Mich.
‡Promega, 40% omega-3 fatty acids, Warner Lambert, Morris Plains, NJ.
§Contains 50% omega-3 fatty acids. Pharmacaps Inc, Elizabeth, NJ.

1.07. The variation of the estimated risks among the studies was far greater than could plausibly be explained by chance alone. To explain this variation, the authors looked at the effects of type, duration, and dosage of treatment. Overall, women who took 0.625 mg/d or less of conjugated estrogens had a risk of breast cancer that was 1.08 times that of women who did not receive this therapy. The relative risks from these individual studies of low-dosage therapy did not differ significantly from each other. Women who took 1.25 mg/d or more of conjugated estrogens had a breast cancer relative risk of 2.0 or less in all studies. However, the variation in observed risks at this higher dosage was significant. This implies that other risk factors varied among those studied, making it difficult to estimate the overall risk associated with this dosage. The relative risk of breast cancer associated with estrogen replacement therapy among women with a history of benign breast disease was 1.16. The combined results from multiple studies provide strong evidence that menopausal therapy consisting of 0.625 mg/d or less of conjugated estrogens does not increase breast cancer risk.

In a prospective study of 8,881 postmenopausal female residents of a retirement community in southern California, Henderson and associates[53] from Los Angeles, California, evaluated the relation between estrogen use and overall mortality. After 7½ years of follow-up, there had been 1,447 deaths. Women with a history of estrogen use had 20% lower age-adjusted, all-cause mortality than lifetime nonusers. Mortality decreased with increasing duration of use and was lower among current users than among women who used estrogens only in the distant past. Current users with more than 15 years of estrogen use had a 40% reduction in their overall mortality. Among oral estrogen users, relative risks of death could not be distinguished by specific dosages of the oral estrogen taken for the longest time. Women who had used estrogen replacement therapy had a reduced mortality from all categories of acute and chronic arteriosclerotic disease and cerebrovascular disease. This group of women had a reduced mortality from cancer, although this reduction was not statistically significant. The mortality from all remaining causes combined was the same in estrogen users and lifetime nonusers.

Barrett-Connor and Bush[54] from San Diego and LaJolla, California, and Baltimore, Maryland, reviewed the evidence that estrogen is protective against the development of cardiovascular disease in women. The authors pointed out that no studies in women have looked at endogenous estrogen levels as predictors of cardiovascular disease. Studies of surrogate measures of endogenous estrogen such as parity, age at menarche, and age at menopause have provided inconsistent results. Current use of oral contraceptives increases risk in older women who smoke cigarettes, but most studies of past use show no increased risk. Most, but not all, studies of hormone replacement therapy in postmenopausal women show around a 50% reduction in risk of a coronary event in women using unopposed oral estrogen. These important observations need to be confirmed in a double-blind, randomized clinical trial, since the protection is biologically plausible and the magnitude of the benefit would be quite large if selection factors can be excluded.

To study the influence of combined hormone replacement therapy on levels of serum lipids, lipoproteins, and apolipoproteins, Haarbo and associates[55] from Glostrup, Denmark, randomized 139 healthy early postmenopausal women selected by means of a questionnaire, a medical examination, and a laboratory screening procedure to be a representative sample of postmenopausal Danish women aged 45 to 55 years old to 4 treatment and 2 placebo groups. The 4 groups receiving hormone replacement therapy were given 2 mg estradiol valerate equivalents (E), either sequentially combined with 75 μg levonorgestrel (E/LNG), 10 mg medroxyprogesterone acetate (E/MPA), or 150 μg desogestrel (E/DG), or continuously combined with 1 mg cyproterone acetate (E/CPA). Serum lipids, lipoproteins, and apolipoproteins were measured before institution of hormone replacement therapy and at 9 well-defined times during the following 84 days. Total response and cyclical variations were calculated. All active treatment regimens reduced serum LDL cholesterol significantly: E/CPA, 6%; E/LNG, 10.9%; E/MPA, 14.4% (7.4% to 20.9%); E/DG, 10.7% (3.3% to 17.6%). The changes in serum total cholesterol and apolipoprotein B were similar but smaller than those in LDL cholesterol. None of these treatment regimens induced significant overall changes in serum HDL cholesterol or apolipoprotein A_1 (Apo A_1). The sequentially combined hormone treatments induced significant cyclical variations in HDL cholesterol, with an increase during estrogen therapy and a decrease during combined therapy: E/LNG, 13.3%; E/MPA, 6.9%; E/DG, 10.3%. No cyclical changes in HDL cholesterol were found in the group receiving continuously combined hormone replacement therapy (E/CPA). The changes in Apo A_1 parallel those in HDL cholesterol. All the treatment regimens produced changes in levels of serum lipids, lipoproteins, and apolipoproteins that may be considered favorable in terms of cardiovascular disease.

Postmenopausal estrogen replacement therapy may reduce the risk of cardiovascular disease, and this beneficial effect may be mediated in part by favorable changes in plasma lipid levels. The effects on plasma lipoprotein levels of postmenopausal estrogens in the low doses currently used have not been precisely quantified, and the mechanism of these effects is unknown. Walsh and associates[56] from Boston, Massachusetts, conducted 2 randomized, 2 double-blind crossover studies in healthy and postmenopausal women who had normal lipid values at baseline. In study 1, 31 women received placebo and conjugated estrogens at 2 doses (0.625 mg and 1.25 mg per day), each treatment for 3 months (Figure 1-11). In study 2, 9 women received placebo, oral micronized estradiol (2 mg per day), and transdermal estradiol (0.1 mg twice a week), each treatment for 6 weeks. The metabolism of VLDL and LDL was measured by endogenously labeling their protein component, apolipoprotein B. In study 1, the conjugated estrogens at doses of 0.625 mg per day and 1.25 mg per day decreased the mean LDL cholesterol level by 15% and 19%, respectively; increased the HDL cholesterol level by 16% and 18%, respectively; and increased VLDL triglyceride levels by 24% and 42%, respectively (Figure 1-11, Table 1-8). In study 2, oral estradiol increased the mean concentration of large VLDL apolipoprotein B by 30 ± 10% by increasing its production rate by 82 ± 18%. Most of this additional large VLDL was cleared directly from the circulation and was not converted to small VLDL or LDL. Oral estradiol reduced LDL cholesterol concentrations by 14 ± 3%, because LDL catabolism increased by 36 ± 7%. The oral estradiol increased the HDL cholesterol level by 15 ± 2%. Transdermal estradiol had no effect. The postmenopausal use of oral estrogens in low doses favorably alters LDL and HDL levels that may protect women against atherosclerosis, while minimizing potentially adverse effects on triglyceride levels. The decrease in LDL levels results from accelerated LDL catabolism; the increase in triglyceride levels results from increased production of large, triglyceride-rich VLDL.

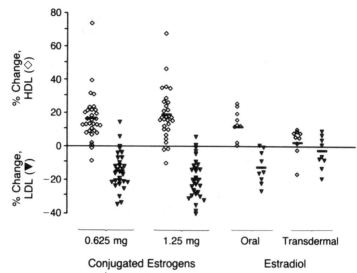

Fig. 1-11. Effect of Estrogen Treatments on Plasma LDL and HDL Cholesterol Concentrations. Each point represents the individual percentage change with estrogen as compared with placebo. The horizontal bar denotes the mean of the percentage changes. Reproduced with permission from Walsh, et al.[56]

Review of randomized trials

Yusuf and Garg[57] from Bethesda, Maryland, reviewed randomized trials to analyze the long-term effects of therapies on angiographic end points. These authors reviewed 6 randomized trials, comparing the effects of modulating lipid levels on angiographic coronary changes. This is a splendid review.

Lovastatin

In the Expanded Clinical Evaluation of Lovastatin (EXCEL) Study, a multicenter, double-blind, diet- and placebo-controlled trial, Bradford and associates[58] from multiple USA medical centers evaluated the efficacy and safety of lovastatin in 8,245 patients with moderate hypercholesterolemia. Patients were randomly assigned to receive placebo or lovastatin at a dosage of 20 mg once daily, 40 mg once daily, 20 mg twice daily, or 40 mg twice daily for 48 weeks. Lovastatin produced sustained, dose-related changes as follows (for dosages of 20 to 80 mg/d): decreased LDL-cholesterol level (24% to 40%), increased HDL-cholesterol level (6.6% to 9.5%), decreased total cholesterol level (17% to 29%), and decreased triglyceride level (10% to 19%) (Table 1-9). The National Cholesterol Education Program's LDL-cholesterol level goal of less than 4.14 mmol/L (160 mg/dL) was achieved by 80% to 96% of patients, while the <3.36 mmol/L (130 mg/dL) goal was achieved by 38% to 83% of patients. The difference between lovastatin and placebo in the incidence of clinical adverse experiences requiring discontinuation was small, ranging from 1.2% at 20 mg twice daily to 1.9% at 80 mg/d (Table 1-10). Successive transaminase level elevations >3 times the upper limit of normal were observed in 0.1% of patients receiving placebo and 20 mg/d of lovastatin, increasing to 0.9% in those receiving 40 mg/d and 1.5% in those receiving

TABLE 1-8. *Effect of conjugated estrogens on plasma VLDL, LDL, and HDL. Reproduced with permission from Walsh, et al.[56]*

Lipoprotein	Placebo	Conjugated Estrogens	
		0.625 mg	1.25 mg
	mean ±SD	% change from placebo value (95% CI)*	
VLDL			
Cholesterol — mmol/liter	0.24±0.05	+16 (−7 to 39)	+30 (7 to 53)†
(mg/dl)	(9.3±1.8)	(P = 0.14)	(P = 0.008)
Triglycerides — mmol/liter	0.49±0.07	+24 (8 to 40)	+42 (26 to 58)†
(mg/dl)	(43±6)	(P = 0.003)	(P<0.0001)
Apolipoprotein B — nmol/liter	38±31	+29 (5 to 53)	+22 (−2 to 46)
(mg/dl)	(2.1±1.7)	(P = 0.02)	(P = 0.08)
LDL			
Cholesterol — mmol/liter	3.6±0.7	−15 (−11 to −19)	−19 (−15 to −23)
(mg/dl)	(139±26)	(P<0.0001)	(P<0.0001)
Triglycerides — mmol/liter	0.24±0.11	+20 (10 to 30)	+30 (20 to 40)
(mg/dl)	(21±10)	(P<0.0001)	(P<0.0001)
Apolipoprotein B — nmol/liter	1560±530	−10 (−4 to −16)	−9 (−3 to −15)
(mg/dl)	(86±29)	(P = 0.0009)	(P = 0.005)
HDL			
Cholesterol — mmol/liter	1.67±0.3	+16 (12 to 20)	+18 (14 to 22)
(mg/dl)	(66±12)	(P<0.0001)	(P<0.0001)
Triglycerides — mmol/liter	0.21±0.06	+32 (26 to 38)	+43 (37 to 49)†
(mg/dl)	(19±5)	(P<0.0001)	(P<0.0001)
HDL$_2$			
Cholesterol — mmol/liter	0.36±0.19	+50 (36 to 64)	+59 (45 to 73)
(mg/dl)	(14±7)	(P<0.0001)	(P<0.0001)
Apolipoprotein A-I — nmol/liter	9280±4280	+46 (27 to 65)	+39 (20 to 58)
(mg/dl)	(26±12)	(P<0.0001)	(P<0.0001)
Apolipoprotein A-II — nmol/liter	2010±920	−6 (−23 to 11)	−3 (−20 to 14)
(mg/dl)	(3.5±1.6)	(P = 0.5)	(P = 0.5)
HDL$_3$			
Cholesterol — mmol/liter	1.34±0.23	+6 (3 to 10)	+6 (3 to 10)
(mg/dl)	(52±9)	(P = 0.0002)	(P = 0.0003)
Apolipoprotein A-I — nmol/liter	54,610±8210	+14 (8 to 20)	+22 (16 to 28)†
(mg/dl)	(153±23)	(P<0.0001)	(P<0.0001)
Apolipoprotein A-II — nmol/liter	17,800±2870	+10 (6 to 13)	+10 (6 to 13)
(mg/dl)	(31±5)	(P<0.0001)	(P<0.0001)
Total cholesterol —	5.71±0.90	−4 (−1 to −7)	−6 (−3 to −9)
mmol/liter (mg/dl)	(220±35)	(P = 0.003)	(P<0.0001)
Total triglycerides —	0.95±0.07	+24 (15 to 33)	+38 (29 to 47)†
mmol/liter (mg/dl)	(84±6)	(P<0.0001)	(P<0.0001)

*The effect of estrogen on each lipoprotein concentration is expressed as the mean change from the placebo concentration, with 95 percent confidence intervals (CI) calculated from the within-subject variation.

†P<0.05 for the comparison with the percentage change for 0.625 mg of estrogen.

TABLE 1-9. *Change from baseline in plasma lipid and lipoprotein levels.* *Reproduced with permission from Bradford, et al.[58]*

		Treatment Group			
		Lovastatin			
Variable	Placebo	20 mg qpm	40 mg qpm	20 mg bid	40 mg bid
LDL-cholesterol	+0.4 (11)	−24 (11)	−30 (11)	−34 (11)	−40 (11)
HDL-cholesterol	+2.0 (12)	+6.6 (13)	+7.2 (13)	+8.6 (13)	+9.5 (13)
Total cholesterol	+0.7 (8)	−17 (8)	−22 (8)	−24 (8)	−29 (9)
LDL-cholesterol/ HDL-cholesterol ratio	+0.2 (16)	−27 (14)	−34 (14)	−38 (13)	−44 (13)
Total cholesterol/ HDL-cholesterol ratio	+0.6 (13)	−21 (12)	−26 (12)	−29 (11)	−34 (11)
Triglycerides†	+3.6	−10	−14	−16	−19

*Values are percent change from baseline (SD). LDL indicates low-density lipoprotein; HDL, high-density lipoprotein. Statistically significant differences for all lipid/lipoprotein variables are as follows: placebo vs 20 mg once daily with the evening meal (qpm) (P<.001); 40 mg qpm vs 20 mg with the morning and evening meals (bid) (P<.017 or less); trend with increasing daily dose, 20 mg vs 40 mg (40 mg qpm and 20 mg bid combined) vs 80 mg (P<.001).

†Median triglyceride values are presented; all others are mean values. The first and third quartile values for triglycerides were, respectively (−13, +21) for placebo, (−23, +6) for 20 mg qpm, (−28, +1) for 40 mg qpm, (−28, −1) for 20 mg bid, and (−32, −5) for 40 mg bid.

TABLE 1-10. *Incidence of serum transaminase level elevations.* Reproduced with permission from Bradford, et al.[58]*

| | | Treatment Group, No. (%) | | | |
| | | | Lovastatin | | |
Elevation	Placebo	20 mg qpm	40 mg qpm	20 mg bid	40 mg bid
>3 times ULN					
Successive†	2 (0.1)	2 (0.1)	12 (0.9)	11 (0.9)	20 (1.5)
Single	15 (1.2)	10 (0.8)	22 (1.9)	21 (1.8)	42 (3.2)
>2 times ULN					
Successive	7 (0.5)	6 (0.5)	17 (1.3)	21 (1.7)	42 (3.0)
Single	28 (2.2)	28 (2.1)	44 (3.7)	54 (4.1)	81 (6.1)

*Incidence is calculated by life-table estimate of an elevation in either alanine aminotransferase or aspartate aminotransferase level at the specified level within 48 weeks of treatment. ULN indicates upper limit of normal (50 and 65 U/L for aspartate aminotransferase [ages <66 and ≥66 years, respectively] and 55 U/L for alanine aminotransferase). Successive elevations are those confirmed by repeated testing.
†$P<.001$ for trend with increasing daily doses of lovastatin; other levels of increase were not tested. Included are 10 patients with elevations not considered drug related by investigators: 20 mg once daily with the evening meal (qpm) (n = 1), 40 mg qpm (n = 5), 20 mg with the morning and evening meals (bid) (n = 3), and 40 mg bid (n = 1) (see text for explanation).

80 mg/d of lovastatin. Myopathy, defined as muscle symptoms with a creatine kinase elevation greater than 10 times the upper limit of normal, was found in only 1 patient (0.1%) receiving 40 mg once daily and 4 patients (0.2%) receiving 80 mg/d of lovastatin. Thus, lovastatin, when added after an adequate trial of a prudent diet, is a highly effective and generally well-tolerated treatment for patients with moderate hypercholesterolemia.

Laties and associates[59] from several medical centers assessed the crystalline lenses of hypercholesterolemic patients before and after 48 weeks of treatment with lovastatin or placebo to determine the effect of lovastatin on the human lens. Patients were given a blomicroscopic (slit-lamp) examination of the lens, and a previously validated, standardized classification system was used to describe the findings. A total of 8,245 patients were randomly assigned in equal numbers to treatment with placebo or lovastatin 20 or 40 mg once or twice daily in this double-blind, parallel-group study. Statistical analyses of the distribution of cortical, nuclear and subcapsular opacities at 48 weeks, adjusted for age and presence of an opacity at baseline, showed no significant differences between the placebo and lovastatin-treated groups. Visual acuity assessments at week 48 were also not found to have significantly different distributions among treatment groups. Moreover, no significant differences were found among the groups in the frequencies of ≥2-line worsening in visual acuity with concurrent progression in lenticular opacity, cataract extraction, or any spontaneously reported adverse ophthalmologic experience. No evidence was found for an effect of lovastatin on the human lens after 48 weeks of treatment.

Cobb and associates[60] from New York, New York, and East Lansing, Michigan, compared the effectiveness of lovastatin with both a high-fat versus low-fat diet. Hypercholesterolemic subjects were studied under metabolic ward conditions for diet periods of 3 weeks while receiving lovastatin (40 mg/d) or placebo. Multiple lipoprotein levels were measured during the final week of each diet period. Nineteen subjects completed the study on the high-fat (43% of kilojoules) diet and 16 on the low-fat (25% of kilojoules) diet. Lovastatin reduced total cholesterol by 23% and LDL cholesterol by 30%, compared with placebo on both diets, with no significant diet-drug interaction. HDL cholesterol was raised by 7% to 8% on the diet regimens. Addition of lovastatin to the low-fat diet permitted 80% of subjects on this diet, but less than 50% of those on the high-fat diet, to achieve current guidelines. Although lovastatin produces a comparable percentage reduction in lipoprotein profiles on either diet, the accompanying low-fat diet remains advisable for additional reduction of LDL cholesterol levels to specified goals.

Rubinstein and associates[61] from Tel Aviv, Israel, conducted a study in which only 10 mg of lovastatin was given to 28 subjects with plasma total cholesterol of 200–240 mg/dl (5.18–6.21 mmol/l) a day. Cholesterol plasma levels decreased in 19% and LDL cholesterol decreased by 24% from baseline levels after 20 weeks of treatment (Table 1-11). All 28 patients decreased their cholesterol values to <200 mg% (5.18 mmol/l), and only 1 had a LDL >130 mg% (3.36 mmol/l) at termination of the study. Achievement of desirable values of cholesterol with 10 mg of lovastatin was accompanied by less adverse effects and with significant financial saving. The calculated saving for lovastatin consumers in the USA could be an amount of $60,000,000. Thus, it is recommended that this drug be manufactured in 10 mg tablets.

Hay and associates[62] from Stanford, California, and Houston, Texas, considered the costs and benefits of cholesterol lowering in the primary prevention of CAD using lifetime lovastatin therapy as the intervention model for adults between 35 and 55 years of age. The analysis projected the benefits of CAD risk reduction using estimates from the Framingham Heart Study. The chosen analytic perspective was that of the patient. For average-risk men with total serum cholesterol levels between 5.69 and 9.83 mmol/liter (220 and 380 mg/dl), the cost per life-year saved ranged from $9,000 to $106,000, whereas for average-risk women, the cost ranged from $35,000 to $297,000 (1989 U.S. dollars). In high-risk men (with smoking habit and hypertension), the cost per life-year saved values ranged from $6,000 to $53,000, whereas in high-risk women the cost per life-year saved values ranged from $19,000 to $160,000. The results were more favorable than those found in previous studies of alternate medication therapies for hypercholesterolemia. Even using conservative parameter assumptions, at least 800,000 Americans aged 35 to 55 years are at sufficiently high risk for CAD, so that the net cost of lovastatin therapy can be favorably compared with other widely used medical interventions.

Pravastatin

Jones and associates[63] from multiple USA medical centers conducted a multicenter, double-blind, placebo-controlled study to evaluate dose response effects and safety of once-daily administration of pravastatin, a new inhibitor of 3-hydroxy-3-methylglutaryl coenzyme A (HMG-CoA) reductase. Pravastatin 5, 10, 20, 40 mg or placebo was administered at bedtime to 150 patients with primary hypercholesterolemia inadequately

TABLE 1-11. *Mean values of lipids and changes in percent from baseline levels. Reproduced with permission from Rubinstein, et al.[61]*

Lipids	0 Baseline Values (mg/dl)	% Change Caused by Lovastatin (weeks)			
		4	8	16	20
Total chol.	226 ± 18.6	−18.4	−18.1	−18.2	−19.2
LDL	163.2 ± 14.4	−23.7	−24.5	−22.5	−24.1
HDL	42.6 ± 5.3	+2.4	+4.4	+2.6	+4.0
Triglycerides	152 ± 16.6	−16.0	−14.8	−17.1	−19.6

p <0.01 from baseline.
chol. = cholesterol; HDL = high-density lipoprotein; LDL = low-density lipoprotein.

controlled on a low-fat, low cholesterol (American Heart Association Phase I) diet. After 8 weeks of treatment, pravastatin produced dose-dependent reductions in LDL cholesterol of 19.2 to 34.1% and reductions in total cholesterol of 14.3 to 25.1% (Figure 1-12). The relation between the $\log_e$ dose of pravastatin and decrease in LDL cholesterol was linear. HDL cholesterol increased up to 11.7% and triglycerides decreased by as much as 23.9%. Pravastatin was well tolerated; no patient withdrew from the study as a consequence of treatment-related adverse events. Despite its relatively short serum half-life of approximately 2 h, once-daily administration of pravastatin provides a safe and effective means of reducing elevated LDL and total cholesterol.

Rubenfire and associates[64] investigated the cholesterol-lowering properties of pravastatin in a double-blind, placebo-controlled, multi-center study with primary hypercholesterolemia. Following a 6- to 8-week dietary lead-in period, patients were randomized to twice-daily placebo or active drug for 16 weeks. Patients receiving 10 mg of pravastatin twice a day for 8 weeks experienced mean total cholesterol and LDL cholesterol level reductions of 20% (6.85 vs 5.48 mmol/L [265 vs 212 mg/dL]) and 28% (5.17 vs 3.75 mmol/L [200 vs 145 mg/dL]), respectively (Figure 1-13). At 20 mg twice a day for an additional 8 weeks, pravastatin reduced plasma total cholesterol, LDL cholesterol, and apolipoprotein B-100 levels by 23% (6.85 vs 5.30 mmol/L [265 vs 205 mg/dL]), 31% (5.17 vs 3.59 mmol/L [200 vs 139 mg/dL]), and 23% (118 vs 91 mg/dL), respectively. HDL cholesterol, HDL_b cholesterol, and apolipoprotein A-1 plasma concentrations increased by 11%, 60%, 7%, and 10%. Plasma triglyceride concentrations decreased in both the pravastatin- and placebo-treated patients. Pravastatin was generally well tolerated and an effective agent for the treatment of primary hypercholesterolemia.

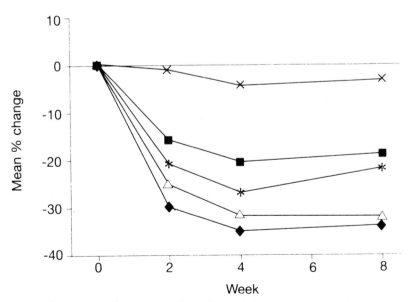

Fig. 1-12. Time- and dose-response effect of once-daily pravastatin and placebo on LDL cholesterol in patients with primary hypercholesterolemia. Key: placebo-x; pravastatin 5 mg ■: 10 mg -*-; 20 mg -△-; 40 mg -♦-. Percent change was significant (p≤.001) versus placebo and baseline at all time points. Reproduced with permission from Jones, et al.[63]

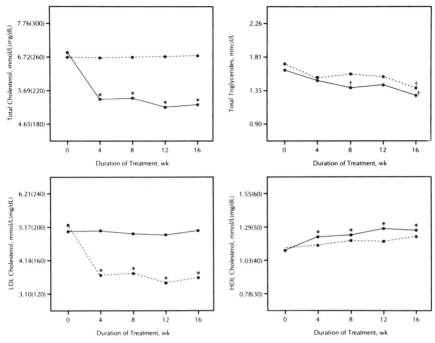

Fig. 1-13. Mean plasma lipid and lipoprotein cholesterol concentrations in patients treated with pravastatin (solid line) (n = 57) or placebo (broken line) (n = 25). LDL indicates low-density lipoprotein; HDL, high-density lipoprotein. At the end of week 8, the dosage of study medication was increased from one to two tablets twice a day (40 mg/d of active drug or placebo). Asterisk indicates P<.01; dagger P<.05. Reproduced with permission of Rubenfire, et al.[64]

Pravastatin versus gemfibrozil

Crepaldi and associates[65] for the Italian Multicenter Pravastatin Study I compared the efficacy and safety of pravastatin and gemfibrozil in the treatment of primary hypercholesterolemia. Three hundred eighty-five outpatients from 13 lipid clinics in Italy participated in this randomized double-blind study. Patients were assigned to receive either 40 mg once daily of pravastatin or 600 mg of gemfibrozil twice daily after an initial diet lead-in period. After 24 weeks, mean reductions from baseline values of plasma total and LDL cholesterol were, respectively, 23% and 30% with pravastatin and 14% and 17% with gemfibrozil. Significant lipid-lowering effects were noted within 4 weeks. Apolipoprotein B decrease was 21% with pravastatin and 13% with gemfibrozil. A statistically significant increase of HDL cholesterol of 5% was achieved with pravastatin compared with a 13% increase for gemfibrozil. Serum triglyceride values decreased 5% with pravastatin and 37% with gemfibrozil. Familial and polygenic hypercholesterolemic patients were also examined separately. Pravastatin effectiveness in reducing LDL cholesterol was greater by 6% in polygenic than in familial hypercholesterolemic patients. Treatment for 25 patients (8 treated with pravastatin and 17 treated with gemfibrozil) was discontinued during the study. The incidence of clinical symptoms and laboratory alterations was low for both treatment groups. Pravastatin and gemfibrozil were well tolerated, but pravastatin was significantly more effective in reducing total and LDL cholesterol levels in primary (either familial or polygenic) hypercholesterolemias than gemfibrozil.

Simvastatin

Simvastatin, a 3-hydroxy-3-methylglutaryl-coenzyme A reductase inhibitor, has been administered to approximately 2,400 patients with primary hypercholesterolemia with a mean follow-up of 1 year in controlled clinical studies and their open extensions. Approximately 10% of this population received simvastatin for a period of ≥2 years. Boccuzzi and associates[66] from Rohway, New Jersey, analyzed this population who had received the drug for >2 years. The mean age was 50 years, 62% were men and 27% had preexisting CAD. Simvastatin was titrated to the maximum dose of 40 mg each evening in 56% of the study population (last recorded dose). The most frequently reported drug-related clinical adverse experiences were constipation (2.5%), abdominal pain (2.2%), flatulence (2.9%) and headaches (1%). Persistent elevations of serum transaminase levels >3 times the upper limit of normal were observed in only 1% of this cohort with only 0.1% of the total population requiring discontinuation of therapy. There were no clinically apparent episodes of hepatitis. Discontinuation of therapy due to myopathy was extremely rare (0.08%). Only minimal increases in the frequency of lens opacities (1%) were observed from baseline to the last lens examination during follow-up, consistent with the expected increase in lens opacity development due to normal aging. Patients who were >65 years old had a clinical and laboratory safety profile comparable to the nonelderly population. An evaluation of long-term efficacy indicates that the magnitude of total and LDL cholesterol reduction and HDL lipoprotein cholesterol increases initially observed were maintained after 3 years of chronic treatment with simvastatin (Figure 1-14). Long-term clinical experience with simvastatin continues to indicate that it is an efficacious and well-tolerated lipid-lowering agent.

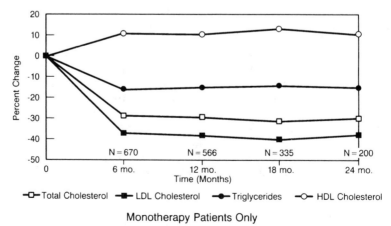

Monotherapy Patients Only

Fig. 1-14. Long-term lipid response to simvastatin 10 to 40 mg/day (mean change (%) over time). HDL = high-density lipoprotein; LDL = low-density lipoprotein. Reproduced with permission of Boccuzzi, et al.[66]

Niacin

Etchason and associates[67] from Rochester, Minnesota, described the development of hepatitis in 5 patients who were taking low dosages (3 grams per day or less) of time-release niacin. In 4 of the 5 patients, clinical symptoms of hepatitis developed after the medication had been taken for a relatively short time (2 days to 7 weeks). This manifestation of hepatotoxicity seems to differ from that previously reported in association with use of crystalline niacin, which occurred with high dosage and prolonged usage of the medication. In view of the recent increased frequency of prescribing niacin for the treatment of hyperlipidemia, physicians should be aware of the potential for hepatotoxicity with even low-dose and short-term use of time-release niacin.

Keenan and associates[68] from Minneapolis, Minnesota, performed a randomized, controlled, double-blind study using a new form of niacin (Enduracin), which employs a wax-matrix vehicle for sustained release, in 201 men and women aged 20 to 70 years with elevated LDL cholesterol values in the 75th to 95th percentiles. Four niacin treatment groups (daily doses of 2000, 1500, 1250, and 1000 mg) were compared with placebo- and diet-treated controls to determine side-effect profile and optimal range of efficacy. The groups given 2000 and 1500 mg demonstrated significant reductions in values of LDL cholesterol (-26% and -19.3%, respectively), total cholesterol (-18.4% and -13.3%), and total cholesterol-HDL cholesterol ratio (-20.4% and -19.4%) when compared with diet- and placebo-treated controls. Smaller improvements were seen in HDL cholesterol and triglyceride levels. Blood chemistry monitoring indicated that reduction in LDL cholesterol level strongly correlated with an increase in baseline levels of some enzymes for niacin-treated subjects. The improved side-effect profile of the wax-matrix form of niacin was particularly notable. The dropout rate due to side effects was only 3.4% and was coupled with good medication compliance.

To evaluate the efficacy and side effects of niacin therapy in dyslipidemic individuals, Henkin and associates[69] from Birmingham, Alabama, performed a retrospective analysis of all patients with dyslipidemia treated by niacin (n = 82) at their clinic during 1987 to 1990, including a subgroup of 17 dyslipidemic heart transplant recipients. Niacin was well tolerated in 83% of the nontransplant group (n = 65) at an average dose of 2.5 ± 0.9 g/day. Similar beneficial lipoprotein effects were found in the transplant and nontransplant patients. The HDL cholesterol response to niacin therapy was independent of the baseline HDL cholesterol level. In the transplant group, 11 patients (65%) discontinued treatment, primarily because of hyperglycemia; this was especially prominent in those patients with pretreatment diabetes mellitus. Of the 15 patients using sustained-release niacin, 8 cases of hepatitis were recorded, some during therapy with relatively low niacin doses. Several different sustained-release preparations were responsible for this phenomenon, suggesting that the cause was not a contaminant in the preparation. No cases of hepatitis were documented in the 67 patients using regular niacin. One case of hepatitis was recently observed in a patient who switched from 1 type of regular niacin to another; however, the authors have data to suggest that the substituted preparation was not an immediate-release niacin. A familial predisposition to hepatitis is suggested by the occurrence of this side effect in identical twin brothers and 2 sisters. A pharmacy survey disclosed that most pharmacists are unaware of the relationship of sustained-release niacin to hepatitis, have a negative impression of regular niacin, and do not stock this formulation. Finally, the authors found that in this small sample of patients, niacin used with lovastatin is a particularly effective drug combination and appears to have few side effects beyond those seen with niacin alone. The authors' experience supports the fact that regular niacin is a useful lipid-modifying drug. When used appropriately, patients can usually tolerate adequate doses for prolonged periods and achieve meaningful results. However, this requires a certain amount of physician skill and patient motivation. The use of sustained-release preparations to overcome this problem can lead to harmful consequences and should only be done under strict medical supervision. In the authors' opinion, the availability of sustained-release niacin as a non-prescription drug is unjustified and should be reexamined. Finally, the authors observed that reduction of VLDL cholesterol with niacin alone leads to an elevation in LDL cholesterol in many patients; this indicates to the authors that the mechanism whereby niacin lowers VLDL cholesterol and total cholesterol is not solely the result of a decreased synthesis of VLDL cholesterol.

Probucol

Oxidized LDL interacts with macrophages to induce intracellular cholesterol ester accumulation and foam cell formation. Probucol is a lipid-lowering drug with a well-known antioxidant action. The thiobarbituric acid (TBA)-reacting substances were measured by Masana and associates[70] from Barcelona, Spain, as an index of plasma and LDL lipid peroxidation in a group of hypercholesterolemic patients compared with a normolipidemic control group. The effect of probucol treatment on plasma and LDL lipid peroxidation in the hypercholesterolemic group was also evaluated. Twenty-five patients (10 men and 15 women) with total cholesterol levels >6.5 mmol/liter were given probucol for 24 weeks. Lipid and apoprotein measurements were obtained at 0, 12 and 24 weeks. TBA-reacting substances were given probucol for 24 weeks. Lipid and apoprotein measurements were obtained at 0, 12 and 24 weeks. TBA-reacting substances were also measured in plasma and the LDL fraction. Twenty-five normolipidemic subjects matched for sex, age and body mass index underwent complete blood analysis for purposes of comparison at week 0. Plasma, LDL and HDL cholesterol, and plasma apoproteins A-1 and B significantly decreased after 12 and 24 weeks of probucol treatment. Hypercholesterolemic subjects (men and women) had significantly higher TBA-reacting substances in plasma and LDL than control subjects had. The amount of TBA-reacting substances in plasma and LDL showed a very significant decrease after probucol treatment (40 and 44%, respectively, after 24 weeks). This reduction was not related to age, sex or body mass index, and was greater than the decrease in lipids. These results support a potential role for probucol as a coadjuvant drug in any lipid-lowering antiatherogenic therapy.

Cholestyramine bar vs powder

In a prospective, randomized trial, Sweeney and associates[71] from Atlanta, Georgia, and Palo Alto, California, compared the powder and the bar forms of cholestyramine in 83 healthy men and women with LDL cholesterol or total cholesterol levels greater than the 90th percentile. Patients were randomly assigned to receive either cholestyramine powder, 2 packets (8 g), twice daily, or cholestyramine confectionery bar, in maple or mint flavors, 2 bars (8 g), twice daily. Fasting serum total cholesterol, LDL cholesterol, HDL cholesterol, and triglycerides were measured at baseline, after 6 to 8 weeks of following the American Heart Association Step I diet alone, and after 8 weeks of taking either the cholestyramine bar or powder. Total cholesterol decreased significantly by 16% in the bar group and 17% in the powder group. LDL cholesterol decreased by 28% and 29% in the bar and powder groups, respectively. There was no significant change in HDL cholesterol. Triglycerides increased in both groups, by 29% in the bar group and by 25% in the powder group. There was no difference between bar and powder in the effect on blood lipids. The majority of the lipid-lowering effect was seen within 14 days. Mean patient endpoint compliance with the therapy was 91.8 ± 3.6% in the bar group and 94.8 ± 2.1% in the powder group. There was no difference between groups. The cholestyramine confectionery bar is as effective as cholestyramine powder in the treatment of hyperlipidemia. The majority of the lipid-lowering effect is seen within 14 days of therapy. Although patient compliance is comparable between the 2 forms, gastrointestinal side effects were slightly greater with the bar form. Therefore, although the bar offers an alternative form of therapy, there appears to be no advantage with regard to patient compliance or palatability.

Filicol vs gemfibrozil

Ros and associates[72] from Barcelona, Spain, treated 50 patients with primary hypercholesterolemia (including 18 with familial hypercholesterolemia) and stable LDL cholesterol levels >3.90 mmol/L (>150 mg/dL) (6.10 ± 1.30 mmol/L; 236 ± 50 mg/dL) while on a hypolipidemic diet and treated for 12 weeks with either 9 g/d of filicol, a microporous cholestyramine analogue, or 1.2 g/d of gemfibrozil in a randomized clinical trial. Tolerance was good with both drugs. Filicol and gemfibrozil caused similar decrements of total cholesterol (14% for both), LDL cholesterol (20% and 18%, respectively), and apolipoprotein B (16% and 21%, respectively). Close to 40% of the patients had decreases of greater than 25% in LDL cholesterol levels with both drugs. Gemfibrozil, but not filicol, significantly increased plasma HDL cholesterol (16%) and apolipoprotein A-1 (17%) levels and reduced triglyceride levels (35%). No loss of efficacy was observed with either drug in subsets of patients who had a good 12-week response rate and had extended therapy for up to 12 months. This study demonstrates that gemfibrozil may have a beneficial effect on all aspects of the plasma lipid profile in patients with severe hypercholesterolemia, a clinical situation where it can be used with potential advantages over standard doses of anion-exchange resins.

Antacid containing aluminum hydroxide

To evaluate the efficacy, safety, and hypocholesterolemic effect of an aluminum hydroxide-containing antacid in hypercholesterolemic individuals, Sperber and associates[73] from Beer-Sheva, Israel, prospectively randomized in a double-masked, placebo-controlled phase of 2 months' duration, followed by an open-design treatment phase of 2 months' duration and a washout phase of 2 months' duration 56 men and women with hypocholesterolemia (total cholesterol greater than 6.2 mmol/L). Fifty individuals completed the study. After 2 months of dietary modification (low-fat, low-cholesterol diet), the participants were randomized into 2 matched groups. Group 1 (28 participants) was treated for 2 months with a chewable antacid tablet containing simethicone, magnesium hydroxide, and 113 mg of aluminum hydroxide per tablet, at a dose of 2 tablets 4 times daily. Group 2 (22 participants) was given a similar number of placebo tablets for 2 months. During the following 2 months, both groups received the antacid at the above dose. Lipoprotein levels were evaluated at baseline and every 2 months thereafter for 6 months. Compared with pretreatment levels, Group 1 experienced a decrease in LDL cholesterol of 9.8% after 2 months and 18.5% after 4 months. Compared with Group 2, the decrease in LDL cholesterol in Group 1 was 6.2% at the end of the 2-month double-masked, placebo phase. Although the HDL cholesterol was also reduced in Group 1 at the end of 4 months of therapy (10.2%), the HDL cholesterol/LDL cholesterol ratio increased by 13% during the same interval. The treatment was well tolerated, with minimal side effects. An aluminum hydroxide-containing antacid reduces LDL cholesterol in hypercholesterolemic individuals. Although HDL cholesterol was also reduced to a lesser extent, the overall atherogenic index was improved.

Chromium supplementation

To determine the efficacy of glucose tolerance factor (GTF) chromium for increasing serum levels of HDL cholesterol in patients taking beta-blockers, Roeback and associates[74] from Chapel Hill and Durham, North Carolina, entered 72 men into a randomized, double-blind, placebo-controlled trial and 63 patients (88%) completed the study. Current medications, including beta blockers were continued. During the 8-week treatment phase, patients in the chromium group received a total daily dose of 600 μg of biologically active chromium divided into 3 equal doses; control patients received a placebo of identical appearance and taste. Mean baseline levels of ADL and total cholesterol were 0.93 ± 0.28 mmol/L and 6.0 ± 1.0 mmol/L (36 ± 11.1 mg/dL and 232 ± 38.5 mg/dL), respectively. The difference between groups in adjusted mean change in HDL cholesterol levels, accounting for baseline HDL cholesterol levels, age, weight, change, and baseline total cholesterol levels, was 0.15 mmol/L (5.8 mg/dL) with a 95% confidence interval showing that the treatment effect was $> +0.04$ mmol/L ($+ 1.4$ mg/dL). Mean total cholesterol, triglycerides and body weight did not change significantly during treatment for either group. Compliance as measured by pill count was 85%, and few side effects were reported. Two months after the end of treatment, the between-group difference in adjusted mean change from baseline to end of post-treatment follow-up was -0.003 mmol/L (-0.1 mg/dL). Two months of chromium supplementation resulted in a clinically useful increase in HDL cholesterol levels in men taking beta-blockers.

CIGARETTE SMOKING

As a risk factor for a coronary event

Although cigarette smoking is the leading avoidable cause of premature death in middle age in the USA, some have claimed that no association is present among older persons. LaCroix and associates[75] from Boston, Massachusetts, Iowa City, Iowa, and New Haven, Connecticut, prospectively examined the relation of cigarette smoking habits with mortality from all causes, cardiovascular causes, and cancer among 7,178 persons aged 65 years or older without a history of AMI, stroke, or cancer who lived in 1 of 3 communities: East Boston, Massachusetts; Iowa and Washington Counties, Iowa; and New Haven, Connecticut. At the time of the initial interview, prevalence rates of smoking in the 3 communities ranged from 5.2 to 17.8% among women and from 14.2 to 25.8% among men. During 5 years of follow-up there were 1,442 deaths, 729 due to cardiovascular disease and 316 due to cancer. In both sexes, rates of total mortality among current smokers were twice what they were among participants who had never smoked. Relative risks, as adjusted for age and community, were 2.1 among the men and 1.8 among the women. Current smokers had higher rates of cardiovascular mortality than those who had never smoked (as adjusted for age and community, the relative risk was 2.0 among the men and 1.6 among the women), as well as increased rates of cancer mortality (relative risk, 2.4 among the men and 2.4 among the women). In both sexes, former smokers had rates of cardiovascular mortality similar to those of the participants who had never smoked, regardless of age at cessation, whereas the rates for all cancers, as well as smoking-related cancers, remained elevated among men who had once smoked. The prospective findings indicate that the mortality hazards of smoking extend well into later life, and suggest that cessation will continue to improve life expectancy in older people.

When analyzing risk factors for first AMI in the Copenhagen City Heart Study, a large prospective population study of 20,000 men and women, smoking was found to influence risk significantly in a dose-dependent manner, the risk increasing 2% to 3% for each gram of tobacco smoked daily in a report by Nyboe and associates[76] from Copenhagen, Denmark. Risk was particularly associated with inhalation, the risk for inhalers being almost twice that of noninhalers. No difference in risk could be demonstrated between various types of tobacco (pipe, cigar, or plain and filtered cigarettes). The risk seemed associated with current smoking only, inasmuch as the duration of the smoking habit was not important. Ex-smokers had the same risk as those who had never smoked regardless of duration of smoking and time elapsed since quitting. Relative excess risk was significantly higher in female smokers than in male smokers, and daily alcohol intake appeared to have some protective effect on the risk of first AMI among heavy smokers.

Relation of smoking cessation to weight gain

Many believe that the prospect of weight gain discourages smokers from quitting. Accurate estimates of the weight gain related to the cessation of smoking in the general population are not available. Williamson and associates[77] from Atlanta, Georgia, and Hyattsville, Maryland, related changes in body weight to changes in smoking status in adults 25 to 74 years of age who were weighed in the first National Health and Nutrition Examination Survey (NHANES I, 1971 to 1975) and then weighed a second time in the NHANES I Epidemiologic Follow-up Study (1982–1984). The cohort included continuing smokers (748 men and 1,137 women) and those who had quit smoking for a year or more (409 men and 359 women). The mean weight gain attributable to the cessation of smoking, as adjusted for age, race, level of education, alcohol use, illnesses related to change in weight, base-line weight, and physical activity, was 2.8 kg in men and 3.8 kg in women. Major weight gain (>13 kg) occurred in 9.8% of the men and 13.4% of the women who quit smoking. The relative risk of major weight gain in those who quit smoking (as compared with those who continued to smoke) was 8.1 in men and 5.8 in women, and it remained high regardless of the duration of cessation. For both sexes, blacks, people under the age of 55, and people who smoked 15 cigarettes or more per day were at higher risk of major weight gain after quitting smoking. Although at base line the smokers weighed less than those who had never smoked, they weighed nearly the same at follow-up. Major weight gain is strongly related to smoking cessation, but it occurs in only a minority of those who stop smoking. Weight gain is not likely to negate the health benefits of smoking cessation, but its cosmetic effects may interfere with attempts to quit. Effective methods of weight control are therefore needed for smokers trying to quit.

Transdermal nicotine patch

The use of nicotine chewing gum combined with psychological support improves the success rate in quitting smoking. Tonnesen and associates[78] from Copenhagen, Denmark, studied the safety and efficacy of a transdermal nicotine patch in cigarette smoking cessation. The authors conducted a double-blind, randomized study comparing the effects of a 16-hour nicotine patch (15 ± 3.5 mg of nicotine in 16 hours) with those of a placebo patch. Of the 289 smokers (207 women and 82 men) enrolled in the study, 145 were treated with nicotine patches and 144 with placebo patches for 16 weeks. Rates of sustained abstinence were significantly better with active treatment than with placebo: 53, 41, 24, and 17% of those in the nicotine-patch group were abstinent after 6, 12, 26, and 52 weeks, respectively, as compared with 17, 10, 5, and 4% of those in the placebo-patch group. Only 2 subjects with the nicotine patch and 1 with the placebo patch had to withdraw from the study because of side effects. The nicotine skin patch proved to be safe and effective, as demonstrated by a higher rate of abstinence than with placebo. However, the absolute rate of abstinence after 1 year was only 17%, which is lower than the rate in studies that have combined the use of nicotine chewing gum with behavioral therapy.

BODY WEIGHT AND OBESITY

Waist-to-hip ratio

A "male" distribution of adipose tissue in women (excess of fat in the abdomen compared with that in the hips; i.e., elevated waist/hip ratio) has been related to symptomatic cardiovascular disease. An elevated waist/hip ratio has also been related to symptomatic cardiovascular disease and cerebral vascular diseases in men, as well as to risk factors for these diseases and various metabolic conditions. To determine whether adipose distribution was related to coronary atherosclerosis, Thompson and associates[79] from Chapel Hill and Winston-Salem, North Carolina, performed a case-controlled study in patients with angiographically documented CAD and an angiographically normal hospital and neighborhood controls. The data show that distribution of adiposity as assessed by waist/hip ratio is significantly related to coronary atherosclerosis in both females and males. Waist/hip ratio is significantly greater in female cases compared with either control group; in males, waist/hip ratio is significantly greater in cases compared with asymptomatic neighborhood controls but not compared with patients with normal coronary arteries. These results persist after control for age, plasma concentrations of lipids and lipoproteins, body mass index, history of hypertension, history of diabetes, and smoking status. The connection between the male adipose distribution in females and coronary atherosclerosis partly explains the greater likelihood of symptomatic cardiovascular disease in them. Males with excess deposition of fat in the abdominal region are also likely to experience increased risk.

Wing and associates[80] from Pittsburgh, Pennsylvania, measured waist/hip ratio in 487 middle-aged women participating in the Healthy Women Study. Upper body fat distribution was found to be associated with numerous behaviors that affect cardiovascular risk, including smoking, low exercise levels, weight gain during adulthood, and higher caloric intake. Moreover, waist/hip ratio was also associated with higher levels of anger, anxiety, and depression and lower levels of perceived social support. Women with upper body fat obesity had higher systolic BP, total cholesterol, LDL cholesterol, triglycerides, and apolipoprotein B and lower levels of HDL and the HDL subfractions 2 and 3. These associations remained significant after adjusting for body mass index. Among 108 women who had repeat measurements of waist/hip ratio, changes in waist/hip ratio over a 3-year period were significantly correlated with changes in activity and with decreases in HDL_2. Thus, waist/hip ratio appears to be an integral component of the cardiovascular risk profile. Waist/hip ratio is related to those behaviors and psychosocial attributes that influence cardiovascular risk.

Relation to insulin resistance and prevalence of diabetes

McKeigue and associates[81] from London, UK, tested the hypothesis that the high mortality from CAD in South Asians (Indian, Pakistani, and Bangladeshi) living in London, United Kingdom, compared with Europeans in London was due to metabolic disturbances related to insulin resistance in a population survey of 3,193 men and 561 women aged 40–69 years living in London, UK. The sample was assembled from industrial work forces and general practitioners' lists. In comparison with the European group, the South Asian group had a higher prevalence of diabetes (19% vs 4%), higher BP, higher fasting and post-glucose serum insulin concentrations, higher plasma triglyceride, and lower HDL cholesterol concentrations. Mean waist-hip girth ratios and trunk skinfolds were higher in the South Asian than in the European group. Within each ethnic group waist-hip ratio was correlated with glucose intolerance, insulin, BP, and triglyceride. These results confirm the existence of an insulin resistance syndrome, prevalent in South Asian populations and associated with a pronounced tendency to central obesity in this group. Control of obesity and greater physical activity offer the best chances for prevention of diabetes and CHD in South Asian people.

Impact on left ventricular mass

To determine the relation of varying degrees of obesity with LV mass and geometry, Lauer and associates[82] from Boston and Framingham, Massachusetts, obtained M-mode echocardiograms in 3,922 healthy participants of the Framingham Heart Study. Measured height and weight were used to calculate body-mass index, a measure of obesity. Body-mass index was strongly correlated with LV mass. After adjusting for age and BP, body-mass index remained a strong independent predictor of LV mass, LV wall thickness, and LV internal dimension. Body-mass index was associated with prevalence of echocardiographic LV hypertrophy, particularly in subjects with a body-mass index exceeding 30 kg/m². Obesity is significantly correlated with LV mass, even after controlling for age and BP. The increase in LV mass associated with increasing adiposity reflects increases in both LV wall thickness and LV internal dimension.

Variability as a health factor

Fluctuation in body weight is a common phenomenon, due in part to the high prevalence of dieting. Lissner and associates[83] from several medical centers examined the associations between variability and body weight and health end points in subjects participating in the Framingham Heart Study which involves follow-up examinations every 2 years after entry. The degree of variability of body weight was expressed as the coefficient of variation of each subject's measured body-mass-index values at the first 8 biennial examinations during the study and on their recalled weight at 25 years of age. Using the 32-year follow-up data, the authors analyzed total mortality, mortality from CAD, and morbidity due to CAD and cancer in relation to intraindividual variation in body weight, including only end points that occurred after the 10th biennial examination. The authors used age-adjusted proportional-hazards regression for the data analysis. Subjects with highly variable body weights had increased total mortality, mortality from CAD, and morbidity due to CAD. Using a multivariate analysis that also controlled for obesity, trends in weight over time, and 5 indicators of cardiovascular risk, the authors found that the positive associations between fluctuations in body weight and end points related to mortality and CAD could not be attributed to these potential confounding factors. The relative risks of these end points in subjects whose weight varied substantially, as compared with those whose weight was relatively stable, ranged from 1.27 to 1.93. Fluctuations in body weight may have negative health consequences, independent of obesity and the trend of body weight over time.

EXERCISE

Duncan and associates[84] from Dallas, Texas, studied whether the quality and quantity of walking necessary to decrease the risk of cardiovascular disease among women differed substantially from that required to improve cardiorespiratory fitness. They performed a randomized, controlled, dose-response clinical trial with a follow-up of 24 weeks. One hundred and two sedentary premenopausal women aged 20 to 40 years were randomized to 1 of 4 treatment groups: 59 completed the study (16 aerobic walkers [8 km/h group], 12 brisk walkers [6.4 km/h group], 18 strollers [4.8 km/h group], and 13 sedentary controls). Intervention groups walked 4.8 km/day, 5 days per week at 8.0 km/h, 6.4 km/h, or 4.8 km/h on a tartan-surfaced, 1.6 km track for 24 weeks. As compared with controls, maximal oxygen uptake increased significantly in a dose response manner (aerobic walkers > brisk > walkers > strollers). In contrast, HDL cholesterol concentrations were not dose related and increased significantly and to the same extent among women who experienced considerable improvements in their physical fitness and those who had only minimal improvements in fitness (4.8 km/h group, +0.08 mmol/L). HDL cholesterol also increased among the 6.4 km/h group, but did not attain statistical significance (+0.06 mmol/L). Dietary patterns revealed no significant differences among groups. Thus, the authors concluded that vigorous exercise is not necessary for women to obtain meaningful improvements in their lipoprotein profile. Walking at intensities that do not have a major impact on cardiorespiratory fitness may nonetheless produce equally favorable changes in the cardiovascular risk profile.

DIABETES MELLITUS, HYPERGLYCEMIA, AND HYPERINSULINEMIA

Barrett-Connor and associates[85] from San Diego, La Jolla, and Berkeley, California, reported the 14-year sex-specific effect of non-insulin-dependent diabetes mellitus on the risk of fatal CAD in a geographically defined population of men and women aged 40 through 79 years. There were 207 men and 127 women who had diabetes at baseline based on medical history or fasting hyperglycemia. They were compared with 2,137 adults who had fasting euglycemia and a negative personal and family history of diabetes. The relative hazard of ischemic heart disease death in diabetics vs nondiabetics was 1.8 in men and 3.3 in women, after adjusting for age, and 1.9 and 3.3, respectively, after adjusting for age, systolic BP, cholesterol, body mass index, and cigarette smoking using the Cox regression model. The sex difference in the independent contribution of diabetes to fatal heart disease was largely explained by the persistently more favorable survival rate of women (than men) without diabetes.

In a report by Wilson and associates[86] from Framingham and Boston, Massachusetts, the association of nonfasting blood glucose levels with cardiovascular disease incidence was determined prospectively in 1382 men and 2094 women aged 45 to 84 years participating in the Framingham Heart Study. For this study, all patients were classified in 1970 as diabetic or nondiabetic. Every 2 years they were examined, categorized according to casual blood glucose samples obtained at the clinic visit, reclassified for development of cardiovascular disease and diabetes mellitus, and followed 10 years for cardiovascular disease. During the follow-up period, 350 men and 369 women developed cardiovascular disease. Age-adjusted cardiovascular disease rates were positively associated with glucose levels in nondiabetic women who did not develop diabetes during follow-up. No such associations were seen in men. Multivariate analyses confirmed the independent association of blood glucose levels with later cardiovascular disease in nondiabetic women. This study shows that hyperglycemia in the original Framingham cohort is an independent risk factor for cardiovascular disease in nondiabetic women, but not among men.

Manson and associates[87] from Boston and Cambridge, Massachusetts, examined the relation of maturity-onset clinical diabetes mellitus with the subsequent incidence of CAD, stroke, total cardiovascular mortality, and all-cause mortality in a cohort of 116,177 US women aged 30–55 years and free of known CAD, stroke, and cancer in 1976. During 8 years of follow-up (889,255 person-years), the authors identified 338 nonfatal AMIs, 111 coronary deaths, 259 strokes, 238 cardiovascular deaths, and 1,349 deaths from all causes. Diabetes was associated with a markedly increased risk of nonfatal AMI and fatal CAD, ischemic stroke, total cardiovascular mortality, and all-cause mortality. A major independent effect of diabetes persisted in multivariate analyses after simultaneous control for other known coronary risk factors (for these end points, [95% CI] = 3.1, 3.0, 3.0, and 1.9, respectively). The absolute excess coronary risk due to diabetes was greater in the presence of other risk factors, including cigarette smoking, hypertension, and obesity. These prospective data indicate that maturity-onset clinical diabetes is a strong determinant of CAD, ischemic stroke, and cardiovascular mortality among middle-aged women. The adverse effect of diabetes is amplified in the presence of other cardiovascular risk factors, many of which are modifiable.

Physical activity is recommended by physicians to patients with non-insulin-dependent diabetes mellitus (NIDDM) because it increases sensitivity to insulin. Whether physical activity is effective in preventing this disease is not known. Helmrich and associates[88] from Stanford, Connecticut, used questionnaires to examine patterns of physical activity and other personal characteristics in relation to the subsequent development of NIDDM in 5,990 male alumni of the University of Pennsylvania. The disease developed in a total of 202 men during 98,524 man-years of follow-up from 1962 to 1976. Leisure-time physical activity, expressed in kilocalories expended per week in walking, stair climbing, and sports, was inversely related to the development of NIDDM. The incidence rates declined as energy expenditure increased from less than 500 kcal to 3500 kcal. For each 500-kcal increment in energy expenditure, the age-adjusted risk of NIDDM was reduced by 6% (relative risk, 0.94; 95% confidence interval, 0.90 to 0.98). This association remained the same when the data were adjusted for obesity, hypertension, and a parental history of diabetes. The association was weaker when the authors considered weight gain between the time of college attendance and 1962 (relative risk, 0.95; 95% confidence interval, 0.90 to 1.00). The protective effect of physical activity was strongest in persons at highest risk for NIDDM, defined as those with a high body-mass index, a history of hypertension, or a parental history of diabetes. These factors, in addition to weight gain since college, were also independent predictors of the disease. Increased physical activity is effective in preventing NIDDM, and the protective benefit is especially pronounced in persons at the highest risk for the disease.

The possibility that hyperinsulinemia may be involved in the etiology of atherosclerotic cardiovascular disease was first suggested 20 years ago. During the last decade, this possibility has received support from 3 large prospective studies. The association between cardiovascular disease, glucose intolerance, obesity, and hypertension and hyperinsulinemia was examined cross-sectionally by Modan and co-investigators[89] in Tel Hashomer, Israel in a representative sample of the adult Jewish population aged 40–70 years. Previously known diabetics were excluded. Cardiovascular disease comprising clinical or electrocardiographic evidence of CAD, as well as clinical evidence of cerebrovascular or peripheral vascular disease, was identified in 97 men and 39 women. A significant hyperinsulinemia-sex interaction was found for CVD rate, with adjusted risk ratios, relative to the rate in 298 normoinsulinemic women, being 1.15 in 328 normoinsulinemic men, 0.85 in 277 hyperinsulinemic women, and 2.27 in 360 hyperinsulinemic men. Age-adjusted cardiovascular disease rates in men versus women were: a) similar and low among all normoinsulinemic normotensives and hyperinsulinemics free of any of the glucose, obesity and hypertension conditions; b) similar and high among normoinsulinemic hypertensives; c) significantly higher in men among hyperinsulinemic normotensives with glucose intolerance and/or obesity and all hyperinsulinemic hypertensives. These trends remained significant after adjusting for age, ethnic group, and blood lipids. Therefore, hyperinsulinemia was associated with excess cardiovascular disease risk in men but not in women, and all excess cardiovascular disease risk in men was confined to hyperinsulinemic individuals in the presence of glucose intolerance, obesity, or hypertension.

PARENTAL HISTORY

Coldtiz and associates[90] from Boston, Massachusetts, examined the relation between parental history of AMI and risk of CAD prospectively among 45,317 U.S. male health professionals who were free of diagnosed CAD, 40 to 75 years of age in 1986 and followed for 2 years. These men provided details of parental history of AMI, including their parents' age at the first event, their personal history of hypertension, hypercholesterolemia and diabetes mellitus, and a detailed dietary assessment completed at baseline. During 72,454 person-years of follow-up, 181 non-fatal AMIs were documented, 49 men died from AMI or sudden death, and 140 underwent coronary artery surgery or angioplasty. Compared with men without any history of parental AMI, those whose mothers or fathers had had an AMI at 70 years of age had a substantially elevated risk of AMI (relative risk = 2.2, 95% confidence interval, 1.2 to 3.8 for maternal history; relative risk = 1.7, 95% confidence interval 1.2 to 2.3 for paternal history). Risk of AMI increased with decreasing age at parental AMI. Paternal but not maternal history of AMI was related to increased risk of coronary artery surgery. These associations were not appreciably altered by controlling for diet or established risk factors, either individually or in multivariate models. These prospective data indicate that a history of AMI in either parent is associated with an increased risk of CAD among men.

ALCOHOL CONSUMPTION

To investigate the hypothesis that the apparent protective effect of habitual alcohol consumption on CAD is due to drinkers at high risk of CAD becoming non-drinkers, Jackson and associates[91] from Auckland, New Zealand, performed a case-controlled population study where data was obtained from interviews with patients with non-fatal AMI and their controls and with the next of kin of those who had died of CAD and their controls. Two groups of cases were studied. The first comprised 227 men and 72 women with non-fatal AMI identified from a population based surveillance program for CAD; controls were 525 men and 341 women randomly selected from the same population group and matched for age and sex. The second group comprised 128 men and 30 women who had died of CAD and had been identified from the surveillance program; controls were a sample of the previous control group and comprised 330 men and 214 women matched for age and sex. All participants were aged 25 to 64 years and without diagnosed CAD. Regular alcohol consumption; HDL cholesterol and LDL concentrations were the main outcome measures. Men with AMI and men who had died of CAD were more likely to have been never drinkers (had never drunk more than once a month) than controls (18% vs 12% and 23% vs 13% respectively). After possible confounding factors had been controlled for, people in all categories of drinking (up to more than 56 drinks per week) had at least a 40% reduction in risk of fatal and non-fatal CAD compared with never drinkers. Former drinkers also had a lower risk of non-fatal AMI than never drinkers (relative risks 0.41 and 0.10 in men and women respectively) but a similar risk of death from CAD. The reduction in risk was consistently greater in women than in men in all drinking categories but there was no clear dose-response effect in either sex. The results support the hypothesis that light and moderate alcohol consumption reduces the risk of CAD. This protective effect in this population was not due to the misclassification of former drinkers with a high risk of CAD as non-drinkers.

Although an inverse association between alcohol consumption and risk of CAD has been consistently found in several studies, some have argued that the association is due at least in part to the inclusion in the non-drinking reference group of men who abstain because of pre-existing disease. Rimm and associates[92] from Boston, Massachusetts, studied the association between self-reported alcohol intake and CAD prospectively among 51,529 male health professionals. In 1986 the participants completed questionnaires about food and alcohol intake and medical history, CAD risk factors, and dietary changes in the previous 10 years. Follow-up questionnaires in 1988 sought information about newly diagnosed CAD. Three hundred fifty confirmed cases of CAD occurred. After adjustment for coronary risk factors, including dietary intake of cholesterol, fat, and dietary fiber, increasing alcohol intake was inversely related to CAD incidence (Figure 1-15). Exclusion of 10,302 current non-drinkers or 16,342 men with disorders potentially related to CAD (e.g., hypertension, diabetes, and gout) which might have led men to reduce their alcohol intake, did not substantially affect the relative risks. These findings support the hypothesis that the inverse relation between alcohol consumption and risk of CAD is causal.

BLOOD PLATELETS

Experimental animal and clinical studies indicate that blood platelets have an important role in atherosclerosis and formation of thrombi. Prospective studies presenting evidence of an association between blood platelet count and cardiovascular mortality have not been performed. Thaulow and co-workers[93] in Oslow, Norway studied healthy middle-aged men with blood platelets counted, and their responsiveness to aggregating agents from 1973 to 1975. The aim was to assess the possible association between these variables and CAD. At 14 years of follow-up a significantly higher CAD mortality was observed among the 25% of subjects with the highest platelet counts. Platelet aggregation performed in a random subsample (150 of the 487 men), revealed that the 50% with the most rapid aggregation response after ADP stimulation had significantly increased CAD mortality compared with the others. These associations could not be explained by differences in age, lipids, blood pressure, or smoking habits. The present study is the first to present conclusive, prospective evidence of an association between platelet concentration and aggregability and long-term incidence of fatal CAD in a population of apparently healthy middle-aged men.

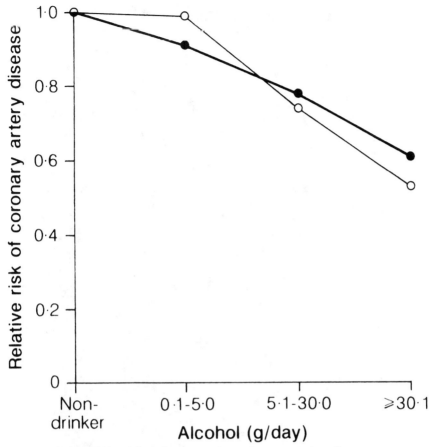

Fig. 1-15. Relative risks of alcohol consumption and coronary artery disease among men from the Health Professionals Follow-up Study. ○ = 44059 men free of myocardial infarction, angina, CABG or PCTA, stroke, and cancer (except non-melanoma skin cancer). ● = Cohort without 16242 men who at baseline, reported myocardial infarction, angina, CABG, PCTA, stroke, cancer (except non-melanoma skin cancer), gout, diabetes, high cholesterol, high triglycerides hypertension, tachycardia, heart rhythm disturbances, or other heart disturbances. Reproduced with permission of Rimm et al.[92]

HYPERHOMOCYSTEINEMIA

Hyperhomocysteinemia arising from impaired methionine metabolism, probably usually due to a deficiency of cystathionine B-synthase, is associated with premature cerebral, peripheral, and possibly coronary arterial disease. Both the strength of this association and its independence of other risk factors for cardiovascular disease are uncertain. Clarke and associates[94] from Dublin and Manchester, UK, studied the extent to which the association could be explained by heterozygous cystathionine B-synthase deficiency. They first established a diagnostic criterion for hyperhomocysteinemia by comparing peak serum levels of homocysteine after a standard methionine-loading test in 25 obligate heterozygotes with respect to cystathionine B-synthase deficiency (whose children were known to be homozygous for homocystinuria due to this enzyme defect) with the levels in 27 unrelated age- and sex-matched normal subjects. A

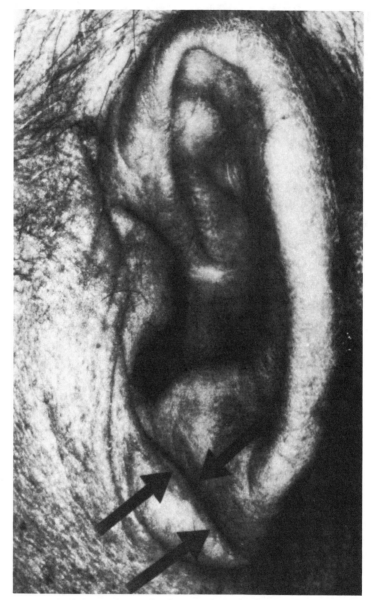

Fig. 1-16. A typical diagonal ELC. The three arrows make the prominent crease even more obvious. Reproduced with permission of Elliott, et al.[95]

level of 24.0 μmol per liter or more was 92% sensitive and 100% specific in distinguishing the 2 groups. The peak serum homocysteine levels in these normal subjects were then compared with those in 123 patients whose vascular disease had been diagnosed before they were 55 years of age. Hyperhomocysteinemia was detected in 16 of 38 patients with cerebrovascular disease (42%), 7 of 25 with peripheral vascular disease (28%), and 18 of 60 with coronary vascular disease (30%), but in none of the 27 normal subjects. After adjustment for the effects of conventional risk factors, the lower 95% confidence limit for the odds ratio for vascular disease among the patients with hyperhomocysteinemia, as compared with the normal subjects, was 3.2. The geometric-mean peak serum homocysteine level was 1.33 times higher in the patients with vascular disease than in the normal subjects. The presence of cystathionine B-synthase deficiency was confirmed in 18 of 23 patients with vascular disease who had hyperhomocysteinemia. Hyperhomocysteinemia is an independent risk factor for vascular disease, including coronary disease, and in most instances is probably due to cystathionine B-synthase deficiency.

DIAGONAL EARLOBE CREASE

To ascertain whether the diagonal earlobe crease (Figure 1-16) is associated prospectively with future death or cardiac events over 8 years of follow-up in 2 sets of patients, those with known CAD and those without, Elliott and Karrison[95] performed a prospective, observational study of 108 patients in 4 cohorts (each matched for age, sex, and race, but differing in the presence or absence of both a diagonal earlobe crease and CAD). Follow-up information was gathered by telephone interviews, and dates and causes of death were determined by reference to death certificates (n = 48), hospital records (n = 9), or attending physician statements (n = 1). During 8 to 10 years of follow-up, 58 of the patients had died. Patients with earlobe creases had poorer survival rates than those without creases, by stratified log-rank test. Cardiac death rates (due to AMI, "sudden cardiac death," or heart failure) were also higher for patients with earlobe creases: 8.0 versus 0.9 cardiac deaths per 100 patient-years in patients without CAD at entry, and 11.7 versus 3.7 cardiac deaths per 100 patient-years in patients with CAD in 1979 to 1982. Cardiac event rates (cardiac death, nonfatal AMI, or CABG) were also higher in those with earlobe creases: 10.4 versus 1.4 events per 100 patient-years for those without known CAD, and 15.8 vs 5.7 events per 100 patient-years for those with CAD. These results suggest that a diagonal earlobe crease is associated with increased all-cause and cardiac morbidity and mortality. Patients with earlobe creases may be at higher risk for coronary events, and might be especially cautioned to control or reduce other cardiac risk factors, even if currently without diagnostic evidence of CAD.

References

1. Bostick RM, Luipker RV, Kofron PM, Pirie PL: Changes in physician practice for the prevention of cardiovascular disease. Arch Intern Med 1991 (Mar);151:478–484.
2. Genest JJ, McNamara JR, Salem DN, Schaefer EJ: Prevalence of risk factors in men with premature coronary artery disease. Am J Cardiol 1991 (June 1);67:1185–1189.
3. Homer D, Ingall TJ, Baker HL Jr, O'Fallon WM, Kottke BA, Whisnant JP: Serum lipids and lipoproteins are less powerful predictors of extracranial carotid artery atherosclerosis than are cigarette smoking and hypertension. Mayo Clin Proc 1991 (Mar);66:259–267.
4. National Heart, Lung, and Blood Institute: Change in cholesterol awareness and action: Results from national physician and public surveys. Arch Intern Med 1991 (Apr);151:666–673.
5. Burke GL, Sprafka JM, Folsom AR, Hahn LP, Luepker RV, Blackburn H: Trends in serum cholesterol levels from 1980 to 1987: The Minnesota Heart Survey. N Engl J Med 1991 (Apr 4);324:941–946.

6. Kottke BA, Moll PP, Michels VV, Weidman WH: Levels of lipids, lipoproteins, and apolipoproteins in a defined population. Mayo Clin Proc 1991 (Dec);66:1198–1208.

7. Thompson PD, Cullinane EM, Sady SP, Flynn MM, Chenevert CB, Herbert PN: High Density Lipoprotein Metabolism in Endurance Athletes and Sedentary Men. Circulation 1991 (July);84:140–152.

8. Havas S, Reisman J, Koumjian L: Does cholesterol screening result in negative labeling effects? Results of the Massachusetts model systems for blood cholesterol screening project. Arch Intern Med 1991 (Jan);151:113–119.

9. Garber AM, Littenberg B, Sox HC, Wagner JL, Gluck M: Costs and health consequences of cholesterol screening for asymptomatic older Americans. Arch Intern Med 1991 (June);151:1089–1095.

10. Bush TL, Riedel D: Screening for Total Cholesterol—Do the National Cholesterol Education Program's Recommendations Detect Individuals at High Risk of Coronary Heart Disease? Circulation 1991 (April);83:1287–1293.

11. Neil HAW, Mant D: Cholesterol screening and life assurance. Br Med J 1991 (Apr 13);302:891–893.

12. Bachorik PS, Cloey TA, Finney CA, Lowry DR, Becker DM: Lipoprotein-cholesterol analysis during screening: Accuracy and reliability. An Intern Med 1991 (May 1);114:741–747.

13. Christenson RH, Roeback JR Jr, Watson TE, Hla KM: Improving the reliability of total and high-density lipoprotein cholesterol measurements. Arch Pathol Lab Med 1991 (Dec);115:1212–1216.

14. McQueen MJ, Henderson AR, Patten RL, Krishnan S, Wood DE, Webb S: Results of a province-wide quality assurance program assessing the accuracy of cholesterol, triglycerides, and high-density lipoprotein cholesterol measurements and calculated low-density lipoprotein cholesterol in Ontario, using fresh human serum. Arch Pathol Lab Med 1991 (Dec);115:1217–1222.

15. Irwig L, Glasziou P, Wilson A, Macaskill P: Estimating an individual's true cholesterol level and response to intervention. JAMA 1991 (Sept 25);266:1678–1685.

16. National Heart, Lung, and Blood Institute, National Institutes of Health, US Department of Health and Human Services: National cholesterol education program: Report of the expert panel on population strategies for blood cholesterol reduction: Executive summary. Arch Intern Med 1991 (June);151:1071–1084.

17. Selzer RH, Dubois-Blowers L, Darnall CJ, Azen SP, Blankenhorn DH: Fat and cholesterol intake of attendees at two national USA cardiovascular annual meetings. Am J Cardiol 1991 (May 15);67:1090–1096.

18. McMurry MP, Cerqueira T, Connor SL, Connor WE: Changes in lipid and lipoprotein levels and body weight in Tarahumara Indians after consumption of an affluent diet. N Engl J Med 1991 (Dec 12);325:1704–1708.

19. Romm PA, Green CE, Reagan K, Rackley CE: Relation of serum lipoprotein cholesterol levels to presence and severity of angiographic coronary artery disease. Am J Cardiol 1991 (Mar 1);67:479–483.

20. Stemmermann GN, Chyou PH, Kagan A, Nomura AMY, Yano K: Serum cholesterol and mortality among Japanese-American men: The Honolulu (Hawaii) heart program. Arch Intern Med 1991 (May);151:969–972.

21. Posner BM, Cobb JL, Belanger AJ, Cupples A, D'Agostino RB, Stokes J III: Dietary lipid predictors of coronary heart disease in men: The Framingham Study. Arch Intern Med 1991 (June);151:1181–1187.

22. Shipley MJ, Pocock SJ, Marmor: Does plasma cholesterol concentration predict mortality from coronary heart disease in elderly people? 18 year follow up in Whitehall study. Br Med J 1991 (July 13);303:89–92.

23. Hong MK, Romm PA, Reagan K, Green CE, Rackley CE: Usefulness of the total cholesterol to high-density lipoprotein cholesterol ratio in predicting angiographic coronary artery disease in women. Am J Cardiol 1991 (Dec 15);68:1646–1650.

24. Richlie DG, Winters S, Prochazka AV: Dyslipidemia in veterans: Multiple risk factors may break the bank. Arch Intern Med 1991 (July);151:1433–1436.

25. Salonen JT, Salonen R, Seppanen K, Rauramaa R, Tuomilehto J: HDL, HDL_2, and HDL_3, Subfractions, and the Risk of Acute Myocardial Infarction—A Prospective Population Study in Eastern Finnish Men. Circulation 1991 (July);84:129–139.

26. Stampfer MJ, Sacks FM, Salvini S, Willett WC, Hennekens CH: A prospective study of cholesterol, apolipoproteins, and the risk of myocardial infarction. N Engl J Med 1991 (Aug 8);325:373–381.

27. Genest J Jr, Jenner JL, McNamara JR, Ordovas JM, Silberman SR, Wilson PWF, Schaefer EJ: Prevalence of lipoprotein (a) [Lp(a)] excess in coronary artery disease. Am J Cardiol 1991 (May 15);67:1039–1045.

28. Chen Z, Peto R, Collins R, MacMahon S, Lu J, Li W: Serum cholesterol concentration and coronary heart disease in population with low cholesterol concentrations. Br Med J 1991 (Aug 3);303:276–282.

29. Ginsburg GS, Safran C, Pasternak RC: Frequency of low serum high-density lipoprotein cholesterol levels in hospitalized patients with "desirable" total cholesterol levels. Am J Cardiol 1991 (July 15);68:187–192.

30. Kern F Jr: Normal plasma cholesterol in an 88-year-old man who eats 25 eggs a day: Mechanisms of adaptation. N Engl J Med 1991 (Mar 28);324:896–899.

31. Welin L, Eriksson H, Ohlson LO, Svardsudd K, Tibblin G, Wilhelmsen L: Triglycerides, a major coronary risk factor in elderly men: A study of men born in 1913. European Heart Journal 1991 (June);12:700–704.

32. Vega GL, Denke MA, and Grundy SM: Metabolic Basis of Primary Hypercholesterolemia. Circulation 1991 (July);84:118–128.

33. Scientific Steering Committee on Behalf of the Simon Broome Register Group: Risk of fatal coronary heart disease in familial hypercholesterolemia. Br Med J 1991 (Oct 12);303:893–896.

34. Malekzadeh S, Dressler FA, Hoeg JM, Brewer HB Jr, Roberts WC: Left atrial endocardial lipid deposits and absent to minimal arterial lipid deposits in familial hyperchylomic-ronemia. Am J Cardiol 1991 (June 15);67:1431–1434.

35. Ma Y, Henderson HE, Ven Murthy MR, Roederer G, Monsalve MV, Clarke LA, Normand T, Julien P, Gagne C, Lambert M, Davignon J, Lupien PJ, Brunzell J, Hayden MR: A mutation in the human lipoprotein lipase gene as the most common cause of familial chylomicronemia in French Canadians. NEJM 1991 (June 20);324:1761–1766.

36. Wattigney WA, Harsha DW, Srinivasan SR, Webber LS, Berenson GS: Increasing impact of obesity on serum lipids and lipoproteins in young adults: The Bogalusa Heart Study. Arch Intern Med 1991 (Oct);151:2017–2022.

37. Bonna KH, Thelle DS: Association Between Blood Pressure and Serum Lipids in a Population—The Tromsø Study. Circulation 1991 (April);83:1305–1314.

38. Selby JV, Newman B, Quiroga J, Christian JC, Austin MA, Fabsitz RR: Concordance for dyslipidemic hypertension in male twins. JAMA 1991 (Apr 24);265:2079–2084.

39. Niaura R, Herbert PN, Saritelli AL, Goldstein MG, Flynn MM, Follick MJ, Gorkin L, Ahern DK: Lipid and lipoprotein responses to episodic occupational and academic stress. Arch Intern Med 1991 (Nov);151:2172–2179.

40. Glazer G: Atherogenic effects of anabolic steroids on serum lipid levels: A literature review. Arch Intern Med 1991 (Oct);151:1925–1933.

41. Kuhn FE, Mohler ER, Satler LF, Reagan K, Lu DY, Rackley CE: Effects of high-density lipoprotein on acetylcholine-induced coronary vasoreactivity. Am J Cardiol 1991 (Dec 1);68:1425–1430.

42. Drexler H, Zeiher AM, Meinzer K, Just H: Correction of endothelial dysfunction in coronary microcirculation of hypercholesterolemic patients by L-arginine. Lancet 1991 (Dec 21/28);338:1546–1550.

43. Small DM, Oliva C, Tercyak A: Chemistry in the kitchen: Making ground meat more healthful. N Engl J Med 1991 (Jan 10);324:73–77.

44. Garrow: New dietary reference values: With an exemplary literature review thrown in. Br Med J 1991 (July 20);303:148.

45. Browner WS, Westenhouse J, Tice JA: What if Americans ate less fat? A quantitative estimate of the effect on mortality. JAMA 1991 (June 26);265:3285–3291.

46. Barnard RJ: Effects of life-style modification on serum lipids. Arch Intern Med 1991 (July);151:1389–1394.

47. Wood PD, Stefanick ML, Williams PT, Haskell WL: The effects on plasma lipoproteins of a prudent weight-reducing diet, with or without exercise, in overweight men and women. N Engl J Med 1991 (Aug 15);325:461–466.

48. Ramsay LE, Yeo WW, Jackson PR: Dietary reduction of serum cholesterol concentration: Time to think again. Br Med J 1991 (Oct 19);303:953–957.

49. Davidson MH, Dugan LD, Burns JH, Bova J, Story K, Drennan KB: The hypocholesterolemic effects of B-glucan in oatmeal and oat bran: A dose-controlled study. JAMA 1991 (Apr 10);265:1833–1839.

50. Spiller GA, Farquhar JW, Gates JE, Nichols SF: Guar gum and plasma cholesterol: Effect of guar gum and an oat fiber source on plasma lipoproteins and cholesterol in hypercholesterolemic adults. Arteriosclerosis and Thrombosis 1991 (Sept/Oct);11:1204–1208.

51. Davidson MH, Burns JH, Subbaiah PV, Conn ME, Drennan KB: Marine oil capsule therapy for the treatment of hyperlipidemia. Arch Intern Med 1991 (Sept);151:1732–1740.

52. Dupont WD, Page DL: Menopausal estrogen replacement therapy and breast cancer. Arch Intern Med 1991 (Jan);151:67–72.

53. Henderson BE, Paganini-Hill A, Ross RK: Decreased mortality in users of estrogen replacement therapy. Arch Intern Med 1991 (Jan);151:75–78.

54. Barrett-Connor E, Bush TL: Estrogen and coronary heart disease in women. JAMA 1991 (Apr 10);265:1861–1867.

55. Haarbo J, Hassager C, Jensen SB, Riis BJ, Christiansen C: Serum lipids, lipoproteins, and apolipoproteins during postmenopausal estrogen replacement therapy combined with either 19-nortestosterone derivatives or 17-hydroxyprogesterone derivatives. Am J Med 1991 (May);90:584–589.

56. Walsh BW, Schiff I, Rosner B, Greenberg L, Ravnikar V, Sacks FM: Effects of postmenopausal estrogen replacement on the concentrations and metabolism of plasma lipoproteins. N Engl J Med 1991 (Oct 24);325:1196–1204.

57. Yusuf S, Garg R: Randomized trials to assess the long-term effects of therapies on angiographic end points. Chest 1991 (May 5);99:1243–1247.

58. Bradford RH, Shear CL, Chremos AN, Dujovne C, Downton M, Franklin FA, Gould AL, Hesney M, Higgins J, Hurley DP, Langendorfer A, Nash DT, Pool JL, Schnaper H: Expanded clinical evaluation of lovastatin (EXCEL) study results: I. Efficacy in modifying plasma lipoproteins and adverse event profile in 8245 patients with moderate hypercholesterolemia. Arch Intern Med 1991 (Jan);151:43–49.

59. Laties AM, Shear CL, Lippa EA, Gould AL, Taylor HR, Hurley DP, Stephenson WP, Keates EU, Tupy-Visich MA, Chremos AN: Expanded clinical evaluation of lovastatin (Excel) study results II. Assessment of the human lens after 48 weeks of treatment with lovastatin. Am J Cardiol 1991 (Mar 1);67:447–453.

60. Cobb MM, Teitelbaum HS, Breslow JL: Lovastatin efficacy in reducing low-density lipoprotein cholesterol levels on high- vs low-fat diets. JAMA 1991 (Feb 27);265:997–1001.

61. Rubinstein A, Lurie Y, Groskop I, Weintrob M: Cholesterol-lowering effects of a 10 mg daily dose of lovastatin in patients with initial total cholesterol levels 200 to 240 mg/dl (5.18 to 6.21 mmol/liter). Am J Cardiol 1991 (Nov 1);68:1123–1126.

62. Hay JW, Wittels EH, Gotto AM Jr: An economic evaluation of lovastatin for cholesterol lowering and coronary artery disease reduction. Am J Cardiol 1990 (Apr 15);67:789–796.

63. Jones PH, Farmer JA, Cressman MD, McKenney JM, Wright JT, Proctor JD, Berkson DM, Farnham DJ, Wolfson PM, Colfer HT, Rackley CE, Sigmund WR, Schlant RC, Arensberg D, McGovern ME: Once-daily pravastatin in patients with primary hypercholesterolemia: A dose-response study. Clin Cardiol 1991 (Feb);14:146–151.

64. Rubenfire M, Maciejko JJ, Blevins RD, Orringer C, Kobylak L, Rosman H, Southeastern Michigan Collaborative Group: The effect of pravastatin on plasma lipoprotein and apolipoprotein levels in primary hypercholesterolemia. Arch Intern Med 1991 (Nov);151:2234–2240.

65. Crepaldi G, Baggio G, Area M, Avellone G, Avogaro P, Bon B, Bompiani GD, Capurso A, Cattin L, D'Alo G, Descovich GC, Feruglio FS, Gaddi A, Gnasso A, Liberatore S, Lupattelli G, Mancini M, Miccoli R, Muggeo M, Muntoni S, Navalesi R, Patrizi GF, Pintus F, Querena M, Resta F, Ricci G, Segato T, Sirtori R, Sirtori M, Ventura A: Pravastatin vs gemfibrozil in the treatment of primary hypercholesterolemia: The Italian Multicenter Pravastatin Study I. Arch Intern Med 1991 (Jan);151:146–152.

66. Boccuzzi SJ, Bocanegra TS, Walker JF, Shapiro DR, Keegan ME: Long-term safety and efficacy profile of simvastatin. Am J Cardiol 1991 (Nov 1);68:1127–1131.

67. Etchason JA, Miller TD, Squires RW, Allison TG, Gau GT, Marttila JK, Kottke BA: Niacin-induced hepatitis: A potential side effect with low-dose time-release niacin. Mayo Clin Proc 1991 (Jan);66:23–28.

68. Keenan JM, Fontaine PL, Wenz JB, Myers S, Huang Z, Ripsin CM: Niacin revisited: A randomized, controlled trial of wax-matrix sustained-release niacin in hypercholesterolemia. Arch Intern Med 1991 (July);151:1424–1432.

69. Henkin Y, Oberman A, Hurst DC, Segrest JP: Niacin revisited: Clinical observations on an important but underutilized drug. Am J Med 1991 (Sept);91:239–246.

70. Masana L, Bargallo T, Plana N, Laville A, Casals I, Sola R: Effectiveness of probucol in reducing plasma low-density lipoprotein cholesterol oxidation in hypercholesterolemia. Am J Cardiol 1991 (Oct 1);68:863–867.

71. Sweeney ME, Fletcher BJ, Rice CR, Berra KA, Rudd CM, Fletcher GF, Superko RS: Efficacy and compliance with cholestyramine bar versus powder in the treatment of hyperlipidemia. Am J Med 1991 (Apr);90:469–473.

72. Ros E, Zambon D, Bertomeu A, Cuso E, Sanllehy C, Casals E: Comparative study of a microporous cholestyramine analogue (Filicol) and gemfibrozil for treatment of severe primary hypercholesterolemia. Arch Intern Med 1991 (Feb);151:301–305.

73. Sperber AD, Henkin Y, Zuili I, Bearman JE, Shany S: The hypocholesterolemic effect of an antacid containing aluminum hydroxide. Am J Med 1991 (Dec);91:597–604.

74. Roeback JR Jr, Hla KM, Chambless LE, Fletcher RH: Effects of chromium supplementation on serum high-density lipoprotein cholesterol levels in men taking beta-blockers: A randomized, controlled trial. An Intern Med 1991 (Dec 15);115:917–924.

75. Lacroix AZ, Lang J, Scherr P, Wallace RB, Cornoni-Huntley J, Berkman L, Curb JD, Evans D, Hennekens CH: Smoking and mortality among older men and women in three communities. N Engl J Med 1991 (June 6);324:1619–1625.

76. Nyboe J, Jensen G, Appleyard M, Schnohr P: Smoking and the risk of first acute myocardial infarction. Am Heart J 1991 (August);122:438–447.

77. Williamson DF, Madans J, Anda RF, Kleinman JC, Giovino GA, Byers T: Smoking cessation and severity of weight gain in a national cohort. N Engl J Med 1991 (Mar 14);324:739–745.

78. Tonnesen P, Norregaard J, Simonsen K, Sawe U: A double-blind trial of a 16-hour transdermal nicotine patch in smoking cessation. N Engl J Med 1991 (Aug 1);325:311–315.

79. Thompson CJ, Ryu JE, Craven TE, Kahl FR, Crouse JR III: Central adipose distribution is related to coronary atherosclerosis. Arteriosclerosis and Thrombosis 1991 (Mar/Apr);1991:327–333.

80. Wing RR, Matthews KA, Kuller LH, Meilahn EN, Plantings P: Waist to hip ratio in middle-aged women: Associations with behavioral and psychosocial factors and with changes in cardiovascular risk factors. Arteriosclerosis and Thrombosis 1991 (Sept/Oct);11:1250–1257.

81. McKeigue PM, Shah B, Mermot MG: Relation of central obesity and insulin resistance with high diabetes prevalence and cardiovascular risk in South Asians. Lancet 1991 (Feb 16);337:382–386.

82. Lauer MS, Anderson KM, Kannel WB, Levy D: The impact of obesity on left ventricular mass and geometry: The Framingham heart study. JAMA 1991 (July 10);266:231–236.

83. Lissner L, Odell PM, D'Agostino RB, Stokes J III, Kreger BE, Belanger AJ, Brownell KD: Variability of body weight and health outcomes in the Framingham population. NEJM 1991 (June 27);324:1839–1844.

84. Duncan JJ, Gordon NF, Scott CB: Women walking for health and fitness: How much is enough? JAMA 1991 (Dec 18);266:3295–3299.

85. Barrett-Connor EL, Cohn BA, Wingard DL, Edelstein SL: Why is diabetes mellitus a stronger risk factor for fatal ischemic heart disease in women than in men? The Rancho Bernardo Study. JAMA 1991 (Feb 6);265:627–631.

86. Wilson PWF, Cupples A, Kannel WB: Is hyperglycemia associated with cardiovascular disease? The Framingham Study. Am Heart J 1991 (February);121:586–590.

87. Manson JE, Colditz GA, Stampfer MJ, Willett WC, Krolewski AS, Rosner B, Arky RA, Speizer FE, Hennekens CH: A prospective study of maturity-onset diabetes mellitus and risk of coronary heart disease and stroke in women. Arch Intern Med 1991 (June);151:1141–1147.

88. Helmrich SP, Ragland DR, Leung RW, Paffenbarger RS Jr: Physical activity and reduced occurrence of non-insulin-dependent diabetes mellitus. NEJM 1991 (July 18);325:147–152.

89. Modan M, Or J, Karasik A, Drory Y, Fuchs Z, Lusky A, Chetrit A, Halkin H: Hyperinsulinemia, Sex, and Risk of Atherosclerotic Cardiovascular Disease. Circulation 1991 (September);84:1165–1175.

90. Colditz GA, Rimm EB, Giovannucci E, Stampfer MJ, Rosner B, Willett WC: A prospective study of parental history of myocardial infarction and coronary artery disease in men. Am J Cardiol 1991 (May 1);67:933–938.

91. Jackson R, Scragg R, Beaglehole R: Alcohol consumption and risk of coronary heart disease. Br Med J 1991 (July 27);303:211–216.

92. Rimm EB, Giovannucci EL, Willett WC, Colditz GA, Ascherio A, Rosner B, Stampfer MJ: Prospective study of alcohol consumption and risk of coronary disease in men. Lancet 1991 (Aug 24);338:464–468.

93. Thaulow E, Erikssen J, Sandvik L, Stormorken H, Cohn PF: Blood Platelet Count and Function Are Related to Total and Cardiovascular Death in Apparently Healthy Men. Circulation 1991 (August);84:613–617.

94. Clarke R, Daly L, Robinson K, Naughten E, Cahalane S, Fowler B, Graham I: Hyperhomocysteinemia: An independent risk factor for vascular disease. N Engl J Med 1991 (Apr 25);324:1149–1155.

95. Elliott WJ, Karrison T: Increased all-cause and cardiac morbidity and mortality associated with the diagonal earlobe crease: A prospective cohort study. Am J Med 1991 (Sept);91:247–254.

2

Coronary Artery Disease

Coronary deaths in the USA

In 1988, 2,167,999 deaths were registered in the USA—a total of 44,676 more deaths than in 1987 and the largest annual final number ever recorded.[1] As in the previous years, three fourths of deaths were caused by the first 4 leading causes of death—heart disease, cancer, stroke, and unintentional injury. The mortality data was compiled by CDC's National Center for Health Statistics (NCHS) for 1988. The national death statistics are based on information contained on death certificates that have been filed in state vital statistics offices as required by state law and compiled by NCHS into a national data base for monitoring the nation's health and for research. The data is based on the underlying cause of death (the disease or injury which initiated the train of morbid events leading directly to death or the circumstances of the accidents or violence which produced the fatal injury).

Angioscopy in acute coronary events

To investigate the pathogenesis of acute coronary disorders and to clarify what type of plaque precedes these disorders, Mizuno and associates[2] from Japan, performed percutaneous transluminal coronary angioscopy by means of a new angioscope during catheterization in 100 consecutive patients. The quality of the angioscopic image was good enough for analysis in 84 patients (14 with AMI [within 8 hours of onset], 16 with recent AMI [3 days-2 months since onset], 24 with old AMI, 10 with unstable angina, and 20 with stable angina). Thrombi were observed in most patients with acute coronary disorders (all 14 with AMI, 9 of 10 with unstable angina). Occlusive thrombi were more common in patients with AMI than in those with unstable angina (11 [79%] vs 1 [10%]), whereas mural (non-occlusive) thrombi were more common in the unstable angina than in the AMI group (8 [80%] vs 3 [21%]). Xanthomatous ulcerated plaques or ragged irregular surfaces were seen in patients with acute coronary disorders and in those with recent AMI. Xanthomatous plaques were more common in patients with acute coronary disorders (50%) than in those with stable angina (15%) or old AMI (8%). By contrast white and smooth plaques were seen in cases of stable angina and old myocardial infarction. Angioscopy could display the intracoronary lumen more precisely than could coronary arteriography. This angioscopic study suggested that although a thrombus overlying a rupture in the lining of the plaque was common in both unstable angina and AMI, the character of the thrombus may differ between these disorders, and lipid-rich xanthomatous plaque may precede rupture.

Frequency of acute lesions in acute coronary events

Kragel and associates[3] in Bethesda, Maryland, studied the frequency and type of acute lesions in the 4 major epicardial coronary arteries at necropsy in 14 patients with unstable angina, 21 patients with sudden cardiac death and 32 patients with a first fatal AMI. None of the 67 patients had a grossly visible LV scar and only the group with AMI had LV myocardial necrosis. Although the frequency of intraluminal thrombus was similar in patients with unstable angina (29%) and sudden death (29%) and significantly lower than in those with AMI (69%), the thrombus in the patients with unstable angina and sudden death consisted almost entirely of platelets and was nonocclusive, whereas the thrombus in the group with AMI consisted almost entirely of fibrin and was occlusive. The frequency of plaque rupture was not different in the patient with unstable angina (36%), and sudden death (19%) and was significantly lower than in the group with AMI (75%). The frequency of plaque hemorrhage was not different in the groups with unstable angina (64%) and sudden death (38%) and was significantly lower than in the group with AMI (90%) (Table 2-1). The frequency of atherosclerotic plaques containing multiluminal channels was similar in patients with unstable angina, sudden death and AMI, but the percent of 5 mm long segments of the four major coronary arteries containing multiluminal channels was greatest in the unstable angina patients. Therefore, the frequency of thrombus, plaque rupture and plaque hemorrhage in the coronary arteries among patients with unstable angina and sudden coronary death was similar

TABLE 2-1. *Frequency of acute coronary lesions and multiluminal channels at necropsy in patients with unstable angina pectoris, sudden coronary death and acute myocardial infarction. Reproduced with permission from Kragel.*[3]

| | | Coronary Arteries | | | |
Coronary Subset	No. of Patients	Thrombus	Plaque Rupture	Plaque Hemorrhage	Multiluminal Channels
Unstable angina pectoris	14	4 (29%)*	5 (36%)*	3 (21%)*	14 (100%)
Sudden coronary death	21	6 (29%)*	4 (19%)*	4 (19%)*	17 (81%)
Acute myocardial infarction	32	22 (69%)†	24 (75%)†	20 (63%)†	29 (90%)
Total	67	32 (48%)	33 (49%)	27 (40%)	60 (90%)

* versus † in same vertical column = p < 0.02.

and less than in patients with AMI. The type of thrombus and the amount of lumen obstructed by thrombus were similar in the groups with unstable angina and sudden coronary death and quite different from those in the group with AMI.

Coronary plaque composition

Dollar and associates[4] from Bethesda, Maryland, analyzed the composition of atherosclerotic plaques in the 4 major epicardial coronary arteries in 8 women <40 years of age (mean 34) with fatal CAD and compared these data to previous studies of 37 adults >45 years of age (mean 59) with fatal CAD. Histologic sections were taken at 5-mm intervals from the entire lengths of the right left main, left anterior descending and left circumflex coronary arteries. With the use of a computerized morphometry system, analysis of the 4 major epicardial coronary arteries showed the major component of plaque to be a combination of cellular (mean percent total plaque area = 65%, standard error = 6%) and dense (19%, standard error = 6%) fibrous tissue (Figure 2-1). Arterial segments narrowed >75% in cross-sectional areas from these young women were compared with similarly narrowed arteries from 37 older patients (32 men [86%]) with fatal CAD previously reported by this laboratory, and showed significantly more cellular fibrous tissue and lipid-rich foam cells, and lesser amounts of dense fibrous and heavily calcified tissue (Figure 2-2). The large amount of lipid-containing foam cells and relative lack of acellular scar tissue in coronary plaques in these young women suggests a greater potential for reversibility of these plaques in this subset of patients with CAD.

Gertz and associates[5] from Bethesda, Maryland, determined the composition of atherosclerotic plaques in 733 5-mm segments of the 4 major (LM, LAD, LC and right) epicardial coronary arteries of 18 patients ≥90 years of age by a computerized planimetric analysis. By analysis of all coronary segments of all patients >90, the plaques consisted primarily of fibrous tissue (87 ± 8%) with calcific deposits (7 ± 6%, pultaceous debris (5 ± 4%) and foam cells (1 ± 1%) occupying a much smaller percentage of plaque area. Analysis of composition according to the 4

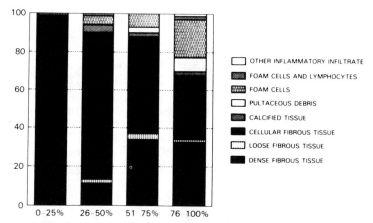

Fig. 2-1. Graph showing the plaque composition (mean percentage) in each of the 4 categories of cross-sectional area narrowing. Reproduced with permission of Dollar, et al.[4]

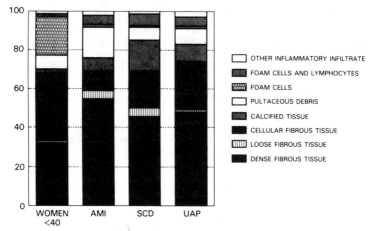

Fig. 2-2. Graph comparing plaque composition (mean percentage) in sections narrowed >75% in cross-sectional area in the present study and in older patients with a fatal acute myocardial infarct (AMI), sudden coronary death (SCD) and unstable angina pectoris (UAP). Reproduced with permission of Dollar, et al.[4]

degrees of luminal cross-sectional area narrowing revealed marked step-wise increases in pultaceous debris (from $0 \pm 0\%$ at 0 to 25% narrowing to $18 \pm 22\%$ at 76 to 100% narrowing) and calcific deposits (from 0 ± 0 to $10 \pm 15\%$), and decreases in fibrous tissue (from 99 ± 3 to $71 \pm 23\%$) and area occupied by the media (from 35 ± 8 to $16 \pm 8\%$). When the analysis was restricted to sections narrowed >75%, no significant differences were found in plaque components or medial area between patients with and without myocardial infarcts at necropsy.

Acute pulmonary edema vs chest pain at presentation

Graham and Vetrovec[6] from Richmond, Virginia, retrospectively reviewed 119 patients admitted to the coronary care unit with pulmonary edema and compared them with 119 patients admitted to the coronary care unit with chest pain. Cardiac catheterization in 71 patients with pulmonary edema and 93 with chest pain showed left main and 3-vessel coronary artery diseases to be equally common in both groups, although anginal pain was infrequent in patients with pulmonary edema (n = 28, 24%). LV function was reduced in the patients with pulmonary edema compared with those with chest pain (mean EF 42 vs 59%). More patients with pulmonary edema were black, and had diabetes and preexisting hypertension than those with chest pain. The results of cardiac catheterization were the same for black and white patients with pulmonary edema. In conclusion, patients with pulmonary edema have a high incidence of cardiac disease, and pulmonary edema may be 1 manifestation of silent myocardial ischemia. Important demographic differences exist between patients admitted with pulmonary edema and those who present with chest pain.

Disease severity in diabetes mellitus

Cardiovascular events remain a leading cause of morbidity and mortality in patients with juvenile-onset, insulin-dependent diabetes mellitus. In an investigation performed by Valsania and associates[7] from Boston, Massachusetts, to examine the extent and severity of the atherosclerotic lesions underlying this excess morbidity and mortality, clinical and angiographic findings were examined in 32 patients with insulin-dependent diabetes and in 31 nondiabetic patients, matched for age and symptoms, undergoing elective cardiac catheterization for evaluation of CAD. With respect to the individuals without diabetes, patients with insulin-dependent diabetes were significantly more likely to have severe narrowings, to have them in all 3 major coronary arteries, and to have them in distal segments. Severe narrowing of multiple vessels was significantly more common in men than in women and in individuals with hypercholesterolemia. It was concluded that the high risk of cardiovascular events observed in young patients with insulin-dependent diabetes is secondary to advanced atherosclerotic lesions in coronary arteries. Involvement of distal segments of coronary arteries make these patients frequently unsuitable for bypass grafts.

Saturated fat intake and insulin resistance

To determine whether there is an association between diet and plasma insulin concentration that is independent of obesity, Maron and co-workers[8] in Stanford, California, studied the relation of dietary composition and caloric intake to obesity and plasma insulin concentrations in 215 nondiabetic men aged 32–74 years with angiographically proven CAD. After adjusting for age, the intake of saturated fats and cholesterol were positively correlated with body mass, waist-to-hip circumference ratio, and fasting insulin. Carbohydrate intake was negatively correlated with body mass index, waist-to-hip ratio, and fasting insulin. Intake of mono-unsaturated fatty acids did not correlate significantly with body mass index or waist-to-hip circumference ratio but did correlate positively with fasting insulin. Intake of dietary calories was negatively correlated with body mass index. In multivariate analysis, intake of saturated fatty acids was significantly related to elevated fasting insulin concentration independently of body mass index. These cross-sectional findings in non-diabetic men with coronary artery disease suggest that increased consumption of saturated fatty acids is associated independently with higher fasting insulin concentrations.

Cocaine

Isner and Chokshi[9] from Boston, Massachusetts, reviewed cardiovascular complications of cocaine. They discussed the association between cocaine use and acute myocardial infarction and other complications including aortic rupture, infective endocarditis, arrhythmias and conduction disturbances and pneumopericardium.

Kolodgie and colleagues[10] in Washington, D.C., Columbus, Ohio, and Baltimore, Maryland, evaluated mechanisms of myocardial ischemia and sudden death in cocaine abusers by obtaining autopsy records in 5,871 patients from the medical examiners' files at Baltimore, Maryland, and northern Virginia. Four hundred and ninety five persons (8.4%) were identified by positive toxicologic findings for cocaine. Of these, six subjects (1.2%) had total thrombotic occlusions, involving primarily the LAD. The mean number of adventitial mass cells per coronary segment and the degree of atherosclerosis were determined. These observations were compared with findings in age- and gender-matched subjects who died from cocaine overdose and in patients who had sudden cardiac death without a history of drug abuse. There was significantly more mast cells in subjects with cocaine-associated thrombosis than in the other groups (Figure 2-3). The number of mast cells showed a significant correlation with the degree of cross-sectional narrowing in subjects with cocaine-associated thrombosis, but not in subjects with sudden death due to thrombosis. Subjects with cocaine-associated thrombosis had significant coronary atherosclerosis without plaque hemorrhage. These findings suggest that adventitial mast cells may potentiate atherosclerosis and vasospasm, thrombosis, and premature sudden death in long-term cocaine abusers.

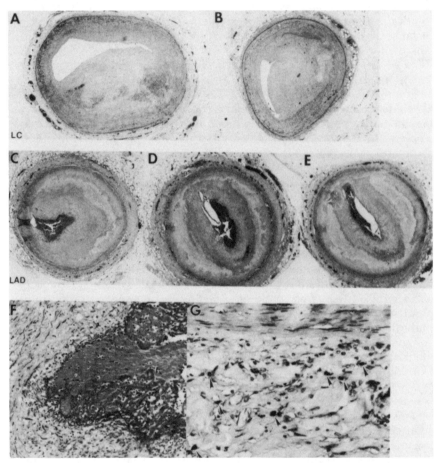

Fig. 2-3. Patient 1 A and B Sections from the left circumflex (LC) coronary artery with B showing 90% luminal narrowing. Note the absence of a thrombus C, D and E. Consecutive sections of the left anterior descending (LAD) coronary artery with 90% to 95% cross sectional area luminal narrowing by atherosclerotic plaque with superimposed total obstruction by platelet thrombus. F. Close-up view of the area of intima in C in contact with the platelet thrombus which contains a few entrapped inflammators cells. G. Toluidine blue strain demonstrating the presence of a large number of mast cells (arrowheads) in the adventia of the left anterior descending coronary artery. (Movat stain A and B magnification 20: hematoxylin and eosin C D and E magnification 15: F magnification × 150 toluidine blue G magnification 3000. Reproduced with permission of Kolodgie, et al.[10]

Relation of coronary spasm to atherosclerotic progression

Nobuyoshi and colleagues[11] in Kitakyushu, Japan, studied 239 patients undergoing serial coronary angiography with a concomitant ergonovine provocation test between July 1974, and June, 1987. The progression of CAD was studied in relation to risk factors, especially coronary artery spasm. Patients were classified into 3 groups: (1) new AMI (39 patients); (2) progression without AMI (90 patients); and (3) nonprogression group (110 patients). To assess how risk factors and coronary spasm are related to the occurrence of new AMI and progression without infarction, 11 variables in the 3 groups were examined: age, gender, the time interval between the studies, fasting blood sugar, systolic blood pressure, diastolic BP, smoking, serum cholesterol, triglycerides, uric acid, and a positive response to the ergonovine provocation test. Multiple regression analysis selected three independent predictors of progression without AMI: cholesterol, systolic BP, and a positive response to the ergonovine provocation test. Multiple regression analysis also selected 3 independent predictors of the occurrence of new AMI: fasting blood sugar, systolic BP, and a positive response to the ergonovine provocation test. The positive response to the ergonovine provocation test was the strongest factor for occurrence of both new AMI and progression without AMI. Both new AMI and progression without AMI frequently occurred in the proximal segments of the right coronary artery, the proximal and middle segments of the LAD, and the middle segments of the circumflex coronary artery. Although occurrence of both new AMI and progression without AMI were often evident in coronary artery segments with severe narrowing, >50% of new AMIs occurred in relation to segments narrowed <50%. Thus, this study suggests that coronary spasm may play a significant role in progression of CAD and that usual risk factors are closely related to the disease progression. This study also demonstrates that patients with AMI often show a marked increase in stenosis severity in which a minimal coronary stenosis progresses to total obstruction.

Vasomotor response of coronary arteries to mental illness

Mental stress can cause angina in patients with CAD, but its effects on coronary vasomotion and blood flow are poorly understood. Because atherosclerosis affects the reactivity of coronary arteries to various stimuli, such as exercise, Yeung and associates[12] from Boston, Massachusetts, postulated that atherosclerosis might also influence the vasomotor response of coronary arteries to mental stress. The investigators studied 26 patients who performed mental arithmetic under stressful conditions during cardiac catheterization. (An additional 4 patients who did not perform the mental arithmetic served as controls.) Coronary segments were classified on the basis of angiographic findings as smooth, irregular, or stenosed. In 15 of the patients without focal stenoses in the left anterior descending artery, acetylcholine (10^{-8} to 10^{-6} mol/L) was infused into the artery to test endothelium-dependent vasodilation. Changes in coronary blood flow were measured with an intracoronary Doppler catheter in these 15 patients. The response of the coronary arteries to mental stress varied from 38% constriction to 29% dilation, whereas the change in coronary blood flow varied from a decrease of 48% to an increase of 42%. The direction and magnitude of the change in the coronary diameter were not predicted by the changes in the heart rate, BP, or plasma norepinephrine level. Segments with stenoses (n = 7) were constricted by a mean ($\pm$ SE) of 24 $\pm$ 48%, and irregular segments (n = 20) by 9 $\pm$ 3%, whereas smooth segments (n = 25) did not change significantly (dilation, 3 $\pm$ 3%). Coronary blood flow increased by 10 $\pm$ 10% in smooth vessels, whereas the flow in irregular vessels decreased by 27 $\pm$ 5%. The degree of constriction or dilation during mental stress correlated with the response to the infusions of acetylcholine. Atherosclerosis disturbs the normal vasomotor response (no change or dilation) of large coronary arteries to mental stress; in patients with atherosclerosis paradoxical constriction occurs during mental stress, particularly at points of stenosis. This vasomotor response correlates with the extent of atherosclerosis in the artery and with the endothelium-dependent response to an infusion of acetylcholine. These data suggest that in atherosclerosis unopposed constriction caused by a local failure of endothelium-dependent dilation causes the coronary arteries to respond abnormally to mental stress.

Panic disorder and normal coronary arteries

Patients with normal coronary angiograms who have chest pains simulating that of ischemic heart disease often have substantial social, health, and work disabilities. Beitman and associates[13] from Columbia, Missouri, hypothesized that the diagnosis of panic disorder would mark those for whom continuing disability is most likely. They interviewed 72 such patients at the time of their normal coronary angiogram and then again an average of 38 months later. The 36 with panic disorder demonstrated significantly more disability at follow-up than did the other study patients (Table 2-2). The authors concluded that those patients with normal coronary angiograms who have panic disorder are more disabled than those who do not have panic disorder. The authors emphasized that panic disorder in psychiatric samples has been shown to be highly treatable.

Procedural use and management in men vs women

Previous studies at individual hospitals have reported differences in the use of major diagnostic and therapeutic procedures for women and men with CAD. To assess whether these differences can be generalized, Ayanian and Epstein[14] from Boston, Massachusetts, performed a retrospective analysis of coronary angiography and revascularization (CABG or PTCA) in women and men hospitalized for CAD in 1987, using abstract data on 49,623 discharges in Massachusetts and 33,159 discharges in Maryland. The authors used multiple logistic regression to estimate the adjusted odds of the use of procedure, controlling for principal diagnosis, age, secondary diagnosis of congestive heart failure or diabetes mellitus, race, and insurance status. The adjusted odds of undergoing angiography were 28% and 15% higher for men than for women in Massachusetts and Maryland, respectively. The respective adjusted odds of undergoing revascularization were 45% and 27% higher for men than for women. Because these differences could be related to differing thresholds for hospital admission, the authors performed a second analysis limited to patients with diagnosed AMI (11,865 discharges in Massachusetts and 6,894 discharges in Maryland), a group in which all patients would be expected to receive hospital care. The male-to-female odds ratios in both states remained similar in magnitude and were statistically significant for angiography and revascularization. These findings demonstrate that women who are hospitalized for CAD undergo fewer major diagnostic

TABLE 2-2. *Functional status at follow-up for those with and without panic disorder (measures of disability).* Reproduced with permission from Beitman, et al.*[13]

Measure of Disability	Panic Disorder, % (n = 36)	No Panic Disorder, % (n = 36)	χ^2
Chest pain			
In the past week	71.9	33.3	9.24†
During rest	66.7	23.3	11.89‡
During sleep	30.0	0.0	10.81‡
Worse since catheterization	21.9	7.4	5.31
View of own health and vigor			
Health worse since catheterization	31.3	3.3	8.75†
Ability to perform physical activity worse since catheterization	27.3	3.3	9.62†
Moderate to strong belief that they are suffering from heart disease	30.6	8.3	5.68§
Difficulty doing tasks ranging from ordinary activities to nearly everything	47.2	19.4	6.25†
Other psychiatric disorders			
Depression (since catheterization)	22.2	8.3	2.68
Alcohol abuse (since catheterization)	22.2	6.3	3.23
Medication use			
Cardiologic	58.3	38.9	2.72
Psychiatric	33.3	15.6	2.75
Type of treatment sought since catheterization			
Psychiatric	21.9	4.8	1.61
Medical (any)	93.9	93.3	0.01
Hospitalization	42.4	26.7	1.72
Work status since catheterization			
Changed work situation due to health	20.6	6.7	2.56
Unemployed (nonhomemaker)	39.4	33.3	0.69
Total No. of workdays missed last year due to panic disorder symptoms	16.2	2.0	4.25§

*We employed a conservative α level of .01 to control for experimentwise error due to multiple comparisons. The measure of disability "Total No. of workdays missed last year due to panic disorder symptoms" is expressed as a mean value, and the statistic used is an F test.
†$P < .01$.
‡$P < .001$.
§$P < .05$.

and therapeutic procedures than men. These differences may represent appropriate levels of care for men and women, but it is also possible that they reflect underuse in women or overuse in men. Further study should assess the cause of these differences and their effect on patients' outcomes.

Despite the fact that CAD is the leading cause of death among women in the western world, previous studies have suggested that physicians are less likely to pursue an aggressive approach to CAD in women than in men. To define this issue further, Steingart and associates[15] from multiple North American medical centers compared the care previously received by men and women who were enrolled in a large post-infarction intervention trial. The authors assessed the nature and severity of anginal symptoms and the use of antianginal and anti-ischemic interventions before enrollment in the 1,842 men and 389 women with LVEF ≤40% after an AMI who were randomized in the Survival and Ventricular Enlargement trial. Before their index infarction, women were as likely as men to have had angina and to have been treated with antianginal drugs. However, despite reports by women of symptoms consistent with greater functional disability from angina, fewer women had undergone cardiac catheterization (15.4% of women vs 27.3% of men) or CABG (5.9% of women vs 12.7% of men). When these differences were adjusted for important covariates, men were still twice as likely to undergo an invasive cardiac procedure as women, but CABG was performed with equal frequency among the men and women who did undergo cardiac catheterization. Physicians pursue a less aggressive management approach to CAD in women than in men, despite greater cardiac disability in women.

Hypomagnesemia with chest pain

To evaluate the frequency of low blood levels of total and ultrafilterable magnesium (total and ultrafilterable hypomagnesemia) in patients with chest pain in the emergency department, and to determine if hypomagnesemia is associated with other clinically important diagnostic and outcome variables in cardiac care, Salem and associates[16] from Baltimore, Maryland, and Boston, Massachusetts, prospectively studied extracellular magnesium homeostasis in patients with chest pain in the emergency department and a cohort of patients without chest pain with a clinical indication for blood sampling. During a 4-month period, 147 patients presenting to the emergency department were studied: 67 patients (mean ± SD age, 61 ± 13 years) with a chief complaint of chest pain (study group) and 80 patients (55.6 ± 19 years) with other diagnoses (control group). Total and ultrafilterable hypomagnesemia occurred more frequently in patients with chest pain (20/67 [30%] and 9/67 [13%]) than in the control group (12/80 [15%] and 3/80 [4%]). Patients with a chief complaint of chest pain who were receiving diuretic medications were hypomagnesemic more frequently (9/16 [56%]) than patients not receiving diuretics (12/51 [23%]). In patients with chest pain admitted to the hospital with a diagnosis of "rule out" AMI, the frequency of hypokalemia was greater among hypomagnesemic patients (6/14 [43%]) than normomagnesemic patients (3/31 [10%]). A similar frequency of hypomagnesemia was noted in patients with a final diagnosis of AMI (4/15 [27%]) when compared with other patients admitted with chest pain (10/31 [32%]) in whom AMI was excluded. No association was noted among hypomagnesemia and length of hospital stay or the occurrence of hypotension or dysrhythmias. Total and ultrafilterable hypomagnesemia are frequent occurrences in patients with and without chest pain in the emergency department. Diuretic use is associated with hypomagnesemia in patients presenting with chest pain in the emergency department. These results support the concept that hypomagnesemia is common in patients with chest pain in the emergency department and is associated with hypokalemia but is not predictive of whether the patient with chest pain has had an AMI.

DETECTION

By clinical characteristics

To determine which clinical characteristics obtained by a physician during an initial clinical examination are important for estimating the likelihood of severe CAD and to determine whether estimates based on these characteristics remain valid when applied prospectively and in different patient groups, Pryor and associates[17] from Durham, North Carolina, examined clinical characteristics predictive of severe CAD in 6,435 consecutive symptomatic patients referred for suspected CAD between 1969 and 1983 (Figure 2-4). Eleven of 23 characteristics were important for estimating the likelihood of severe CAD. A model using these characteristics accurately estimated the likelihood of severe disease in an independent sample of 2,342 patients referred since 1983. The model also accurately estimated the prevalence of severe disease in large series of patients reported in the literature. These findings suggest that the clinician's initial evaluation can identify patients at high or low risk of anatomically severe CAD. Cost-conscious quality care is encouraged by identifying patients at higher risk for severe CAD who are most likely to benefit from further evaluation.

Signal-averaged electrocardiogram

In an investigation by Solomon and Tracy[18] from Washington, D.C., the ability to noninvasively detect CAD in patients undergoing diagnostic cardiac catheterization was studied using a signal-averaged electrocardiogram. An initial study of 13 patients revealed that a QRS duration ≥100 msec, a root mean square voltage in the terminal 40 msec of the QRS <50 μV, and a low amplitude signal duration >28 msec were suggestive of CAD. These parameters were then used prospectively to examine 40 consecutive patients with chest pain of undetermined etiology referred for cardiac catheterization. Patients with CAD had significantly longer filtered QRS and low amplitude signal durations and lower root mean square voltages compared with patients without CAD. The sensitivity, specificity, and positive predictive value of a single parameter ranged from 62% to 76%, 74% to 89%, and 75% to 87%, respectively. Thus, the

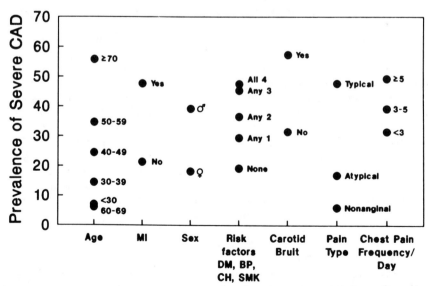

Fig. 2-4. Prevalence of severe coronary artery disease (CAD) (in patients with significant disease) by patient characteristics. DM = diabetes mellitus; BP = hypertension; CH = history of hyperlipidemia or hypercholesterolemia; MI = myocardial infarction; SMK = smoking. Reproduced with permission of Pryor, et al.[17]

signal-averaged electrocardiogram may be a useful tool in evaluating patients for the presence of CAD.

Echocardiography in the emergency room

Sabia and co-workers[19] in Charlottesville, Virginia, designed a prospective study to test the hypothesis that the assessment of LV systolic function at the time of emergency room presentation provides valuable diagnostic and prognostic information in patients with cardiac-related symptoms. The study is based on a 2-year follow-up of 171 consecutive patients evaluated in the emergency room for such symptoms. In the course of follow-up, one third of the patients suffered a major cardiac event. For those with LV systolic dysfunction, the age-adjusted rate of early events (occurring within 48 hours of presentation) was more than eight times higher than for those without LV systolic dysfunction. For events occurring after 48 hours of emergency room presentation, LV systolic dysfunction was associated with a nearly fourfold excess of cardiac events. Other than advanced age, the most important confounder for early events included an abnormal electrocardiogram diagnostic for AMI. Confounders for late events included advanced age and a history of hypertension. LV systolic dysfunction on two-dimensional echocardiography was the only finding associated with early and late events after controlling for other risk factors. In addition, the prediction of these events derived from the combination of historical, clinical, electrocardiographic, and two-dimensional echocardiographic findings was significantly improved when accounting for the presence or absence of LV systolic dysfunction. The investigators concluded that the two-dimensional echocardiographic assessment of LV systolic function provides valuable diagnostic and prognostic information in subjects presenting to the emergency room with cardiac-related symptoms.

Echocardiography during exercise

To evaluate the accuracy of exercise 2-dimensional echocardiography for the recognition of CAD, 53 patients (46 men and 7 women, age range 35 to 69 years) without either previous AMI or resting wall motion abnormalities, were studied by Galanti and associates[20] from Florence, Italy. According to coronary angiography 26 had normal coronary arteries, 14 had 1-vessel, 7 had 2-vessel, and 6 had 3-vessel disease. After withdrawal of any therapy, all patients underwent a single exercise stress test with a stress table during which cine-loop digitized echocardiography was acquired and thallium-201 was injected. Echocardiographic images were evaluated at rest and at peak exercise. Three-view planar scintigraphic images were collected immediately after exercise and 4 hours later. For the overall recognition of CAD, exercise electrocardiography had 78% sensitivity and 65% specification; myocardial scintigraphy had 100% sensitivity and 92% specificity; and exercise echocardiography had 93% sensitivity and 96% specificity. Global accuracy was 72% for exercise electrocardiography, 94% for stress echocardiography, and 96% for myocardial scintigraphy. For the classification of the individual involved coronary arteries, the sensitivity of myocardial scintigraphy was 85% and that of exercise echocardiography was 63%; the related specificities were 98% and 98%, respectively. It was concluded that exercise echocardiography is highly accurate for the recognition of CAD, whereas it appears less sensitive in the identification of the involved vessels, particularly in patients with multivessel disease.

Dobutamine echocardiography

Two-dimensional echocardiography performed during dobutamine infusion has been proposed as a potentially useful method for detecting CAD. However, the safety and diagnostic value of dobutamine stress echocardiography has not been established. Sawada and co-workers[21] in Indianapolis, Indiana, recorded echocardiograms during step-wise infusion of dobutamine to a maximum dose of 30 micro grams/kg/min in 103 patients who also underwent quantitative coronary angiography. The echocardiograms were digitally stored and displayed in a format that allowed simultaneous analysis of rest and stress images. Development of a new abnormality in regional function was used as an early end point for the dobutamine infusion. No patient had a symptomatic arrhythmia or complications from stress-induced ischemia. Significant CAD ($\geq$50% diameter stenosis) was present in 35 of 55 patients who had normal echocardiograms at rest. The sensitivity and specificity of dobutamine-induced wall motion abnormalities for CAD was 89% and 85% respectively. The sensitivity was 81% in those with one-vessel disease and 100% in those with multivessel or left main disease. Forty-one of 48 patients with abnormal echocardiograms at baseline had localized rest wall motion abnormalities. Fifteen had CAD confined to regions that had abnormal rest wall motion, and 26 had disease remote from these regions. Thirteen of 15 patients without remote disease did not develop remote stress-induced abnormalities, and 21 of 26 who had remote disease developed corresponding abnormalities. Echocardiography combined with dobutamine infusion is a safe and accurate method for detecting CAD and for predicting the extent of disease in those who have localized rest wall motion.

To assess the value of dobutamine echocardiography for detecting CAD, Cohen and associates[22] from East Orange and Newark, New Jersey, prospectively studied 70 men (mean age 62 $\pm$ 8 years) presenting for coronary angiography. Dobutamine (2.5 to 40 μg/kg/min) was infused in 3-minute stages. Digital echocardiograms were recorded on-line at baseline, during low- and high-dose dobutamine infusion, and at recovery. An echocardiogram positive for CAD was defined as one showing a new wall motion abnormality induced by dobutamine. Compared with coronary angiography, the overall sensitivity of dobutamine echocardiography for detecting CAD was 86%, specificity 95% and accuracy 89%. The sensitivity for detecting 3-vessel CAD was 100%, 89% for 2-vessel and 69% for 1-vessel CAD. The accuracy of predicting multivessel disease by 2 methods was 71 and 84%, respectively. Heart rate at the echocardiographic ischemic threshold was lower in patients with 3- and 2-vessel CAD versus 1-vessel CAD (89 $\pm$ 17, 95 $\pm$ 18 and 118 $\pm$ 18 beats/min, respectively); rate-pressure product was also lower in patients with 3- and 2-vessel CAD versus 1-vessel CAD (12.7 $\pm$ 3.6, 13.7 $\pm$ 2.8 and 18.9 $\pm$ 44 $\times$ 10^3 beats/min $\times$ mm Hg, respectively). Heart rate was the most important physiologic determinant of ischemia induced by dobutamine. There were no major complications during the study. Thus, dobutamine digital echocardiography is an excellent test for identifying CAD and should be beneficial in patients unable to exercise.

Transesophageal stress echocardiography

Zabalgoitia and associates[23] from San Antonio, Texas, and Chicago, Illinois, examined a new nonexercise test to detect significant CAD prospectively evaluating 36 patients with chest pain syndrome and normal LV contractility. Transesophageal atrial pacing was used to provoke ischemia during monitoring of LV contractility by transesophageal echocardiography. A 12-lead electrocardiogram was recorded. A transesophageal stress echocardiogram was abnormal if new segmental wall motion abnormalities developed. On the basis of the transesophageal stress echocardiographic results, patients were separated into normal (group 1, n = 16) and abnormal response (group 2, n = 20). Arteriography revealed significant CAD in 21 patients, 19 from group 2 and 2 from group 1. Sensitivity and specificity of the transesophageal stress echocardiogram were 90% and 93%, respectively, and those for pacing electrocardiogram were 43% and 100%, respectively. In addition, the transesophageal stress echocardiogram accurately predicted the coronary artery perfusion bed involved. In 10 patients, Wenckebach AV block developed during pacing and resolved immediately by the administration of atropine sulfate. No serious complications were seen. Thus the transesophageal stress echocardiogram is a highly sensitive and specific novel technique to detect significant CAD in patients with chest pain syndrome and normal resting LV contractility.

Intravascular ultrasound

Siegel and colleagues[24] in Los Angeles, California, studied 70 postmortem human arterial segments in vitro to establish a histopathologic basis for angioscopic and ultrasound image interpretation. The investigators used 7- to 9-French fiber-optic angioscopes and 20- to 30-MH^z intravascular ultrasound imaging catheters. Three observers assigned an angioscopic and ultrasound image classification to each vessel segment. The image and histological classification categories were then compared. The sensitivity, specificity, and accuracy of both methods separately or in combination for normal vessels were each greater than or equal to 95%. The predictive value was better for angioscopy than for ultrasound due to incorrect ultrasound interpretations of normal anatomy in the presence of thrombus. For stable atheroma the sensitivity, specificity, and accuracy of the individual methods were each greater than 90%. However, both angioscopy and ultrasound had classification errors in that disrupted atheroma was identified and classified as stable atheroma. Consequently, the predictive value was 74% for angioscopy and 78% for ultrasound. For disrupted atheroma the sensitivities for angioscopy and ultrasound were only moderate, whereas the specificity, accuracy, and predictive value were each high. For thrombus detection, the specificity, accuracy, and predictive value were high for each method. The sensitivity of angioscopy was 100%. However, sensitivity was lower for ultrasound due to false-negative interpretation of laminar clots in normal vessels and an inability to distinguish disrupted or stable atheroma from intraluminal thrombus. Contingency analyses showed that each imaging method alone or combined had significant agreement with the results obtained from histology. When assessing all cases in which angioscopy and ultrasound were concordant, there was a 92% agreement with the histological classification.

Necropsy studies demonstrate that CAD is frequently complex and eccentric. However, angiography provides only a silhouette of the vessel lumen. Intravascular ultrasound is a new tomographic imaging method for evaluation of coronary dimensions and wall morphology. Nissen and co-investigators[25] in Lexington, Kentucky, used a multielement 5.5F, 20-MHz ultrasound catheter to examine 8 normal subjects and 43 patients with CAD. The investigators assessed the safety of coronary ultrasound and the effect of vessel eccentricity on comparison of minimum luminal diameter by angiography and ultrasound. Normal and atherosclerotic wall morphology and stenosis severity were also evaluated by intravascular ultrasound (Figure 2-5). The only untoward effect was transient coronary spasm in 5 patients. At 33 sites in normal subjects, the lumen was nearly circular, yielding a close correlation between angiographic and ultrasonic minimum diameter. At 90 sites in patients with CAD, ultrasound demonstrated a concentric cross section; correlation was also close. However, at 72 eccentric sites, correlation was not as close. For 41 stenoses, correlation between angiography and ultrasound for area reduction was moderate. In normal subjects, wall morphology revealed a thin intimal leading edge and subadjacent sonolucent zone. Patients with CAD exhibited increased thickness and echogenicity of the leading edge, thickened sonolucent zones and/or attenuation of ultrasound transmission. These data establish that intravascular ultrasound is feasible and safe and yield luminal measurements that correlate generally with angiography. Differences between angiographic and ultrasonic measures of lumen size in eccentric vessels probably reflect the dissimilar perspectives of tomographic and silhouette imaging techniques. Intravascular ultrasound provides detailed images of normal and abnormal wall morphology not previously possible in vivo.

Catheter-based ultrasound is a new imaging modality to examine endovascular detail in the coronary circulation. This technique requires

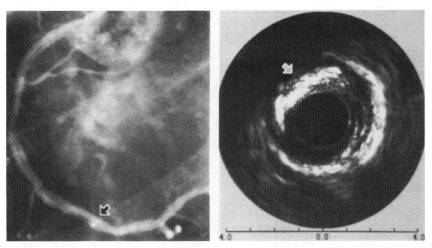

Fig. 2-5. Representative cineangiographic and intravascular ultrasound images. Left panel: arrow indicates location of ultrasound transducer in angiographically normal segment of right coronary artery. Right panel: central circular dark structure is ultrasound catheter. Arrow points to area of increased echogenicity with marked attenuation of ultrasound transmission. Scale at bottom of image shows distance in millimeters. Reproduced with permission of Nissen, et al.[25]

direct placement of the catheter in the arterial segment of interest. Sudhir and coworkers[26] in San Francisco, California, examined the feasibility of a less invasive approach by imaging the coronary arterial circulation by using a 5F (30 MHz) imaging catheter placed in the cardiac venous system. Using simultaneous fluoroscopy, the investigators studied anesthetized closed-chest dogs (n = 6) and human subjects undergoing right sided heart catheterization (n = 11). After cannulation of the coronary sinus, the LC coronary artery was visualized from the great cardiac vein and on advancing the catheter into the anterior interventricular vein, the LAD artery was identified. Where artery and vein were parallel to each other, circular cross-sectional images of the coronary artery were outlined, whereas oblique and transverse orientation of artery to vein produced ellipsoid images or long-axis images. In the dogs, ultrasound-determined cross-sectional area of the coronary arteries correlated closely with angiography. In humans, the LC artery was readily visualized from the great cardiac vein in all subjects but because of anatomic variability, the LAD artery was consistently from the anterior interventricular vein. There was significant correlation between ultrasound-determined cross-sectional areas of the coronary arteries with those from angiography in humans. In all subjects, the ultrasound transducer could be safely advanced into the anterior interventricular vein to the cardiac apex. Limitations of the technique include ultrasonic penetration problems, caused in part by the large size of the human coronary veins and variability in artery-vein relations. The investigators concluded that transvenous imaging of coronary arteries with intravascular ultrasound is a less invasive, promising new approach to the study of structure and morphology in the coronary vasculature.

Symptom-limited exercise testing

Fragasso and associates[27] in Milan, Italy, evaluated the possibility that maximal exercise testing might induce prolonged impairment of LV function in 15 patients with angiographically proved CAD and 9 age-matched controls with atypical chest pain and normal coronary arteries. LVEF, peak filling and peak emptying rates, and LV wall motion were analyzed. All control subjects had a normal exercise test at maximal work loads and improved LV function during exercise. Patients developed 1 mm ST depression at 217 ± 161 seconds at a work load of 70 ± 30 W and a rate-pressure produce of 18,530 ± 4,465 mm Hg × beats/min. Exercise was discontinued when angina or equivalent symptoms occurred and diagnostic ST depression developed much earlier than symptoms. At peak exercise, patients showed a decreased LVEF and peak emptying and filling rates. LVEF and peak emptying rate normalized within the recovery period, whereas peak filling rate remained depressed throughout recovery and was still reduced 2 days after exercise. Thus, in patients with severe impairment of coronary flow reserve, maximal exercise may cause sustained impairment of diastolic function. Exercise testing in these patients should be performed with caution, and a more conservative diagnostic approach based on the development of ST changes rather than occurrence of symptoms should be used.

Raised exercise diastolic blood pressure

Akhras and Jackson[28] from London, UK, found a rise in diastolic BP of more than 15 mm Hg during a symptom-limited treadmill exercise test in 91 (17%) of 541 consecutive patients investigated for chest pain or after recent uncomplicated AMI. Of the 91 patients, 63 also had electrocardiographic evidence of myocardial ischemia, but 28 did not have 1 mm ST segment depression, of whom 24 had angiographic evidence of >70% diameter stenosis of ≥2 major coronary arteries. Fifty-five of these 91 patients underwent CABG; repeat angiography in 22 at 12 months showed an improved LVEF in 18 who had a normal postoperative diastolic BP response, but no change in EF in the 4 who still had an abnormal rise in diastolic BP on exercise. Exercise-induced ischemia may cause a reversible fall in cardiac output that sometimes leads to reflex vasoconstriction and a rise in diastolic BP before a fall in systolic BP or electrocardiographic evidence of ST segment depression. An abnormal diastolic BP response to exercise may identify some patients at high risk of myocardial infarction who might otherwise have false-negative exercise tests.

Angiography

To establish and compare the characteristics of patients older and younger than 70 years of age with chest pain selected to undergo coronary angiography and to assess the value of coronary angiography in older patients with chest pain, Elder and associates[29] from Edinburgh, UK, performed a retrospective analysis of clinical case notes and coronary angiography reports in 134 consecutive patients with chest pain aged 70 years or older investigated by coronary angiography between 1978 and 1988 and in 134 randomly selected patients aged <70 over the same period. Clinical angiographic features at the time of angiography and management after angiography were the main outcome measures. Older patients represented a small, but increasing, proportion of those investigated. Older patients had more severe symptoms at the time of angiography, were taking more antianginal drugs, and had had their symptoms for longer than younger patients. At angiography more older patients had triple vessel CAD, LM stem stenosis, or LV impairment. After angiography similar proportions of older and younger patients underwent CABG, with more elderly patients requiring urgent operation; although operative mortality was higher for elderly patients, symptomatic benefit was similar to that in younger patients. Older patients with angina selected to undergo coronary angiography and subsequent coronary surgery have more severe symptoms and underlying cardiac disease. Earlier referral and investigation might yield a population with lower operative risk. Selection of patients for coronary angiography and coronary artery surgery should be based on the potential for benefit and should avoid "agism."

Isolated left main narrowing

In an investigation by Topaz and colleagues[30] from Richmond, Virginia, among 21,545 adult patients who underwent consecutive coronary angiography, 16 (0.07%) were found during their coronary arteriography to have a significant isolated stenotic lesion (luminal diameter narrowing ≥50%) located at the LM. The remaining major epicardial coronary arteries and their branches were free of disease. A strong predilection for the isolated lesion to occur at the ostium of the LM was found (12 patients). The most common presenting symptom was angina of <4 weeks duration, although one-third of the patients were asymptomatic. Resting electrocardiograms were normal in 12 patients, while 3 patients had T wave inversion and another had nonspecific ST-T changes. Eleven patients exhibited severe stenosis, with 8 having 70% to 89% stenosis and 3 having 90% to 95% stenosis. Five patients had 50% to 69% stenosis. No significant differences were found between patients with angina and patients without angina with respect to age, LV end-diastolic pressure, LVEF, and mean percent stenosis of the obstructive lesion. Despite the severity and the crucial location of the obstructive lesion, most patients with an isolated significant LM stenosis appear to have a preserved LVEF, normal wall motion, and no significant alteration of the LV end-diastolic pressure.

Thallium-201 scintigraphy

Garber and colleagues[31] in Pawtucket and Providence, Rhode Island, and Storrs, Connecticut, evaluated the effects of varying exercise intensity on the ischemic threshold in 33 patients with CAD and provokable myocardial ischemia documented by thallium-201 myocardial scintigraphy. These patients underwent two exercise tests 2 to 7 days apart. Symptom-limited incremental treadmill exercise test was followed by a 20 minute submaximal treadmill test at an intensity approximating 70% of the peak heart rate attained during the incremental test. During the incremental exercise test, angina developed in 16 patients and 17 patients were asymptomatic. At least 0.1 mV of ST segment depression developed in all subjects during the incremental exercise test at a mean exercise duration of 5 ± 3 minutes, a rate-pressure product of 19,130 ± 5,735 and oxygen uptake of 20 ± 7 ml/kg per min. During the submaximal exercise test, 28 (85%) of the 33 patients had significant ST segment depression. Among these patients, 24 (86%) were asymptomatic, including 10 patients who had previously reported angina during the incremental test. The average time to onset of 0.1 mV ST segment depression during the submaximal test was 8 ± 5 minutes. These changes occurred at a rate-pressure product of 15,250 ± 3,705 and an oxygen uptake of 14 ± 6 ml/kg per min, and they were significantly lower than values obtained during the graded exercise. Six of the 33 patients had angina during both tests, although 2 patients had no accompanying ST segment depression during the submaximal test. These data indicate that myocardial ischemia, whether or not accompanied by angina, may occur at a lower rate-pressure product and oxygen uptake during submaximal, steady state exercise compared with symptom-limited incremental exercise. The ischemic threshold varies under different exercise conditions.

Thallium reinjection

Thallium reinjection immediately after conventional stress-redistribution imaging improves the detection of viable myocardium, as many myocardial regions with apparently irreversible thallium defects on standard 3–4 hour redistribution images manifest enhanced thallium uptake after reinjection. Because the 10-minute period between reinjection and imaging may be too short, Dilsizian and co-investigators[32] in Bethesda, Maryland, designed a study to determine whether 24-hour imaging after thallium reinjection improves additional information regarding myocardial viability beyond that obtained by imaging shortly after reinjection. The investigators studied 50 patients with chronic stable CAD undergoing exercise thallium tomography, radionuclide angiography, and coronary arteriography. Immediately after the 3–4 hour redistribution images were obtained, 1 mCi thallium was injected at rest, and images were reacquired at 10 minutes and 24 hours after reinjection. The stress, redistribution, reinjection, and 24-hour images were then analyzed qualitatively and quantitatively. Of the 127 abnormal myocardial regions on the stress images, 55 had persistent defects on redistribution images by qualitative analysis, of which 25 demonstrated improved thallium uptake after reinjection (Figure 2-6). At the 24-hour study, 23 of the 25 regions with previously improved thallium uptake by reinjection showed no further improvement. Similarly, of the 30 regions determined to have irreversible defects after reinjection, 29 remained irreversible on 24-hour images. These findings were confirmed by the quantitative analysis. The mean normalized thallium activity in regions with enhanced thallium activity after reinjection increased from 57% on redistribution studies to 70% after reinjection but did not change at 24 hours. In regions with

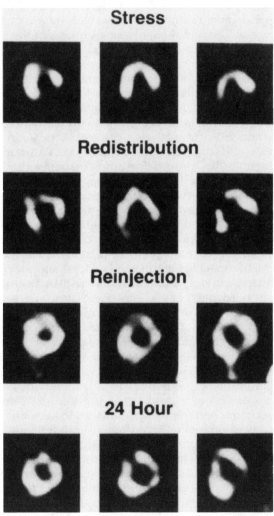

Fig. 2-6. Stress, redistribution, reinjection, and 24-hour short axis thallium tomogram images are shown for a patient with coronary artery disease. Tomogram are sections 4 pixels thick from apex (left) to base (right). An apparently irreversible inferior defect on redistribution images improves after reinjection and does not change further after 24 hours. Reproduction with permission of Dilsizian, et al.[32]

irreversible defects that were unaltered by reinjection, mean regional thallium activity did not differ from the reinjection to the 24-hour studies. Twenty-four-hour imaging after reinjection showed improvement in only four of 35 irreversible regions. These data indicate that thallium reinjection at rest after 3–4 hours of redistribution provides most of the clinically relevant information pertaining to myocardial viability in regions with apparently irreversible thallium defects. Hence, thallium reinjection may be used instead of 24 hour imaging in most patients in whom a persistent thallium defect is observed on conventional redistribution images.

Dipyridamole thallium-201 imaging

To investigate the significance and mechanism of dilatation of the LV cavity on dipyridamole thallium-201 imaging, Takeishi and associates[33] from Yamagata, Japan, performed both dipyridamole thallium-201 imaging and dipyridamole radionuclide angiography on 83 patients with known angiograms. The dipyridamole/delayed ratio of the LV dimension from the thallium-201 image was defined as the LV dilatation ratio. An LV dilatation ratio greater than the mean $+2$ standard deviations in patients without CAD was defined as abnormal. Twenty-two of 83 patients showed an abnormal LV dilatation ratio, and 18 of the 22 patients (82%) had triple-vessel CAD. By defect and without analysis, the sensitivity and specificity for correctly identifying the patients as having triple-vessel CAD was 72% and 76%, respectively, whereas LV dilatation ratio had a sensitivity of 72% and a specificity of 93%. When LV dilatation ratio was used in combination with the defect and washout criteria, sensitivity increased to 84% without a loss of specificity. In those 22 patients with abnormal LV dilatation ratios, end-diastolic volume measured by radionuclide angiography did not change after dipyridamole infusion. Dilatation of the LV cavity on dipyridamole thallium-201 imaging reflected relative subendocardial hypoperfusion induced by dipyridamole rather than actual chamber enlargement. The LV dilatation ratio was moderately sensitive and highly specific for triple-vessel CAD and provided complementary information to dipyridamole thallium-201 imaging.

Watters and colleagues[34] in San Francisco, California, evaluated myocardium at potential risk using preoperative dipyridamole perfusion scintigraphy with manifest ischemia on intraoperative transesophageal echocardiography in 26 patients at increased risk of a coronary event undergoing noncardiac surgery. Clinical outcome was assessed. Induced intraoperative wall motion abnormalities were more common in patients and myocardial segments with than in those without a preoperative reversible perfusion defect (Figure 2-7). A preoperative reversible perfusion defect was more common in patients and segments with than in those without a new intraoperative wall motion abnormality. Six patients, including five with a reversible scintigraphic defect but only three with a new wall motion abnormality had a recognized perioperative ischemic event. Events occurred more often among patients with than in those without a reversible perioperative scintigraphic defect, but this difference did not reach statistical significance. Intraoperative wall motion abnormalities were reversible and did not differentiate between risk groups. These data support the known relation between reversible scintigraphic defects and perioperative events, and they identify another manifestation of ischemic risk in the relation between reversible scintigraphic defects and induced intraoperative wall motion abnormalities.

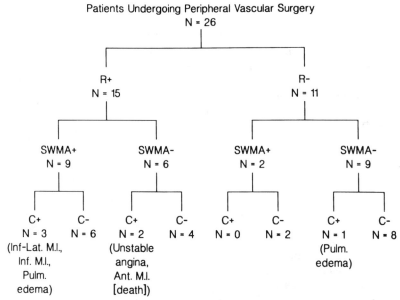

Patients Undergoing Peripheral Vascular Surgery
N = 26

R+ N = 15   R- N = 11

SWMA+ N = 9   SWMA- N = 6   SWMA+ N = 2   SWMA- N = 9

C+ N = 3 (Inf-Lat. M.I., Inf. M.I., Pulm. edema)   C- N = 6   C+ N = 2 (Unstable angina, Ant. M.I. [death])   C- N = 4   C+ N = 0   C- N = 2   C+ N = 1 (Pulm. edema)   C- N = 8

Fig. 2-7. Comparison of results of preoperative thallium perfusion scintigraphy, intra-operative two-dimensional transesophageal echocardiography and clinical outcome in 26 patients undergoing peripheral vascular surgery. Ant. = anterior; C+ and C− = presence and absence, respectively, of cardiac complication; Inf. = inferior; Lat. = lateral; M.I. = myocardial infarction; Pulm. = pulmonary; R+ and R− = presence and absence, respectively, of a reversible perfusion defect; SWMA+ and SWMA− = presence and absence, respectively, of a segmental wall motion abnormality. Reproduced with permission of Watters, et al.[34]

Dobutamine thallium myocardial perfusion tomography

Pennell and colleagues[35] in London, UK, evaluated the efficacy of dobutamine infusion for thallium myocardial perfusion tomography in 50 patients with exertional chest pain undergoing coronary arteriography. Dobutamine was infused in 5 minute stages at incremental rates from 5 to 20 μg/kg per min or until limited by symptoms. The myocardium was divided into nine segments for analysis of perfusion. Thirty-nine of 40 patients with CAD had a reversible perfusion defect demonstrated by dobutamine thallium tomography (sensitivity 97%) and 8 of 10 patients with normal coronary arteries had normal myocardial perfusion (specificity 80%). These values were significantly better than the sensitivity and specificity of exercise ECG (78% and 44%, respectively). There was a significant relation between the mean number of segments with abnormal perfusion and the number of disease coronary vessels. There was also a significant relation between the maximal tolerated dose of dobutamine and the treadmill exercise time, but a wide range of exercise times was achieved in the 15 and 20 μg/kg per min groups. Dobutamine infusion was well tolerated in all patients. There were no significant arrhythmias or limiting symptoms other than chest pain. Dobutamine thallium myocardial perfusion tomography is a useful technique for the detection, localization and assessment of ischemia, especially when exercise potential is limited.

Thallium-201 with adenosine

Coyne and associates[36] from the Lackland Air Force Base, Texas, used adenosine to determine whether thallium-201 scintigraphy with adenosine might have comparable diagnostic value to that obtained with standard exercise thallium-201 testing. One hundred subjects were studied with exercise thallium-201 and thallium imaging after adenosine, including 47 with angiographically proven CAD and 53 controls. Overall sensitivity of the thallium-201 procedures was 81% for the exercise study and 83% for the adenosine study. The specificity was 74% for the exercise study and 75% for the adenosine study. The diagnostic accuracy of the exercise study was 77% and that of the adenosine study was 79%. Ninety-four percent of the patients had an adverse effect due to the adenosine infusion, but most of these were mild and well tolerated. All adverse effects disappeared within 30 to 45 seconds of the termination of the study. Therefore, thallium-201 scintigraphy after intravenous infusion of adenosine has a diagnostic value similar to that of exercise thallium-201 testing in the detection of CAD. Adenosine thallium-201 testing may be particularly useful in evaluating patients unable to perform exercise test.

Abreau and associates[37] in Houston, Texas, used adenosine thallium-201 myocardial scintigraphy with adenosine infusion in 607 patients undergoing this test because of suspected CAD or for low risk stratification early after AMI. Adenosine increased the heart rate from 75 ± 14 to 92 ± 16 beats/min and decreased systolic blood pressure from 138 to 121 mm Hg. Side effects were frequent and similar in both groups. Flushing occurred in 35%, chest pain in 34%, headache in 21% and dyspnea in 19% of patients. Only 36% of Group I patients with chest pain during adenosine had concomitant transient perfusion abnormalities compared with 61% of Group II patients. First and second-degree AV block occurred in 10% and 4% of patients, respectively, and ischemic ST changes in 13% of cases. Concomitant chest pain and ischemic ST segment depression were uncommon, but when present, predicted perfusion abnormalities in 73% of patients. Most side effects disappeared rapidly after stopping adenosine. The side effects were severe in only 2% of patients and in only six patients (1%) was it necessary to discontinue the infusion. No severe adverse reactions such as AMI or death occurred. These data indicate the excellent safety of adenosine infusion as an adjunct to thallium-201 scintigraphy in humans even a few days after AMI.

Nishimura and associates[38] in Houston, Texas, evaluated the diagnostic efficacy of maximal pharmacologic coronary vasodilation with intravenously administered adenosine in combination with thallium-201 single-photon emission computed tomography for detection of CAD in 101 consecutive patients with concomitant CAD. Tomographic images were assessed visually and from computer-quantified polar maps of the thallium-201 distribution. Significant CAD defined as >50% luminal diameter stenosis was present in 70 patients. The sensitivity for detecting patients with CAD using quantitative analysis was 87% in the total group, 82% in patients without AMI and 96% in those with prior AMI. The specificity was 90%. The sensitivity for diagnosing CAD in patients without AMI was single, double and triple vessel disease was 76%, 86% and 90%, respectively. All individual stenoses were identified in 68% of patients with double-vessel and in 65% of those with triple-vessel CAD. The extent of perfusion defects was directly related to the extent of CAD. Thus, quantitative thallium-201 single-photon emission computed tomography during adenosine infusion has high sensitivity and specificity for diagnosing CAD.

Technetium-99m teboroxime and MIBI tomography

Fleming and associates[39] in Houston, Texas, used technetium-99m teboroxime in 30 patients who underwent single photon emission computed tomography imaging at peak exercise and again 60 minutes later at rest. All patients had a thallium-201 stress test (n = 26) or automated quantitative coronary arteriography (n = 25) or both, without intervening CABG or AMI. Images were reviewed by two investigators who had no knowledge of clinical data. Coronary lesions with ≥50% diameter narrowing by quantitative coronary arteriography were considered significant. Both thallium-201 and Tc-99m teboroxime detected disease in all patients with two or three vessel CAD. One vessel CAD was detected with Tc-99m teboroxime in 9 of 10 patients and with thallium-201 in 8 of 10. In patients without angiographically significant disease, Tc-99m teboroxime demonstrated normal perfusion in six of eight patients and thallium-201 in three of five. The presence or absence of CAD detected by Tc-99m teboroxime or thallium-201 was compared with quantitative coronary arteriography, there was no difference between Tc-99m teboroxime and thallium-201. These results suggest that Tc-99m teboroxime provides results comparable to thallium as an imaging agent. The rapid biologic half-life of 5.3 minutes allows studies to be completed in 60 to 90 minutes.

Kettunen and associates[40] from Oulu, Finland, examined 42 patients with known stable CAD, referred for coronary angiography, with technetium-99m-hexakis-2-methoxy-2-methyl-propyl-isonitrile (MIBI) tomography combined with a high-dose dipyridamole infusion (0.7 mg/kg) and handgrip stress. MIBI tomography was unable to show CAD only in 2 patients, thus yielding a sensitivity figure of 95%. MIBI tomography correctly identified 27 (82%) of 33 stenotic lesions (≥50% diameter stenosis) of the left anterior descending artery, 17 (61%) of 28 of those of the left circumflex artery, and 28 (90%) of 31 of those of the right coronary artery. The overall vessel sensitivity was 78%. The computed lumen diameter stenoses were more advanced in cases detected than in those not detected with MIBI tomography: 87 ± 14 vs 76 ± 14%. The 50 to 69% stenoses did not show any tendency to produce less positive findings than those with ≥70% stenoses. In the subgroup of 21 patients who also presented for thallium scintigraphy, the overall diseased vessel identification rate was 76% for thallium tomography and 83% for MIBI tomography. Minor noncardiac side effects related to the dipyridamole-handgrip test occurred only in 5% of 63 study sessions. A high-dose dipyridamole combined with isometric exercise is a safe stress method, and when used during scintigraphy, MIBI tomography is at least as efficient a tool as thallium tomography in detecting diseased vessel territories in patients in CAD.

Rubidium-82 positron emission tomography

Stewart and associates[41] from Ann Arbor, Michigan, investigated in 81 patients the diagnostic performance of rubidium-82 (Rb-82) positron emission tomography (PET) and thallium-201 (Tl-201) single proton emission-computed tomography (SPECT) for detecting CAD. PET studies using 60 mCi of Rb-82 were performed at baseline and after intravenous infusion of 0.56 mg/kg dipyridamole in conjunction with handgrip stress. TI-201 SPECT was performed after dipyridamole-handgrip stress and, in a subset of patients, after treadmill exercise. Sensitivity, specificity and overall diagnostic accuracy were assessed using both visually and quantitatively interpreted coronary angiograms. The overall sensitivity, specificity and accuracy of PET for detection of CAD (50% diameter stenosis) were 84, 88 and 85%, respectively. In comparison, the performance of SPECT revealed a sensitivity of 84%, specificity of 53% and accuracy of 79%. Similar results were obtained using either visual or quantitative angiographic criteria for severity of CAD. In 43 patients without prior AMI, the sensitivity for detection of disease was 71 and 73%, respectively, similar for both PET and SPECT. There was no significant difference in diagnostic performance between imaging modalities when 2 different modes of stress (exercise treadmill vs intravenous dipyridamole plus handgrip) were used with SPECT imaging. Thus, Rb-82 PET provides improved specificity compared with TI-201 SPECT for identifying CAD, most likely due to the higher photon energy of Rb-82 and attenuation correction provided by PET. However, post-test referral cannot be entirely excluded as a potential explanation for the lower specificity of TI-201 SPECT.

Intravenous adenosine and intracoronary papaverine

Kern and associates[42] in St. Louis, Missouri, assessed the use of adenosine as an alternative agent for determining coronary vasodilator reserve at rest and during peak hyperemic response to continuous intravenous adenosine and intracoronary papaverine in 34 patients, including 17 without and 17 with significant left CAD and in 17 patients, 11 without and 6 with, significant LAD after low dose intravenous adenosine. The maximal adenosine dose did not change mean arterial pressure, but increased the heart rate. For continuous adenosine infusions, mean coronary blood flow velocity increased 64 ± 104%, 122 ± 94% and 198 ± 59% and 15 ± 51%, 110 ± 95% and 109 ± 86% in groups 1 and 2, respectively for each of the three doses. Mean coronary flow velocity increased significantly after 100 and 150 μg/kg of adenosine and 10 mg of intracoronary papaverine. The mean coronary vasodilator reserve ratio for adenosine and papaverine was 2.94 ± 1.50 and 2.94 ± 1, respectively, in group 1 patients and was significantly and similarly reduced in group 2 patients. Low dose bolus injection of adenosine increased mean coronary flow velocity equivalently to that after continuous infusion of 100 μg/kg, but less than after papaverine. There was a strong correlation between adenosine infusion and papaverine for both mean coronary flow velocity and coronary vasodilator reserve ratio. No patient had significant arrhythmias or prolongation of the corrected QT interval with adenosine, but papaverine increased the QT interval and produced nonsustained VT in one patient. These data indicate that intravenous adenosine in doses >100 μg/kg for most patients is nearly equivalent to intracoronary papaverine without producing QT prolongation making this agent a potentially superior and safe alternative to intracoronary papaverine for determination of coronary vasodilator reserve.

Ultrafast computed tomography

Coronary artery calcium indicates atherosclerosis. Ultrafast computed tomography (CT) can noninvasively visualize and quantify coronary calcium, permitting the natural history of calcified plaque to be studied.

Janowitz and associates[43] from Miami Beach, Florida, evaluated the ability of ultrafast CT to follow the progression of calcified plaque within the coronary arteries in patients with and without obstructive CAD. Twenty-five subjects had serial ultrafast CT scans of the coronary arteries a mean of 406 days apart. Changes in the number of calcific deposits, calcified plaque area and volume, calcium density and total calcium score were measured. In the 20 patients with calcium on the first study, there were statistically significant increases in mean peak CT number, total calcified plaque volume, total calcified plaque area and total calcium score. Subjects with proved obstructive CAD (n = 10) on angiography had a 48% increase in calcified plaque volume compared with 22% in asymptomatic subjects (n = 10). Comparison of serial studies showed that smaller calcific deposits often coalesced into single larger calcific deposits. Ninety-eight percent (235 of 241) of deposits identified on the first study were accounted for on the second study. Patients with obstructive CAD had a higher number of new calcific deposits than did those in the asymptomatic group (55 vs 18). Serial ultrafast CT accurately tracks the progression of coronary artery calcium. It is a useful technique for assessing changes in calcified plaque formation in both asymptomatic subjects and in patients with obstructive CAD. It may be useful for studying the natural history of CAD and the effects of intervention on the course of CAD.

PROGNOSTIC INDICES

ST-segment changes in the emergency room

To determine the reliability of the admission electrocardiogram in predicting outcome in patients hospitalized for chest pain at rest, Cohen and associates[44] from New York, New York, randomized 90 patients into a trial of aspirin versus heparin in unstable angina or non-Q-wave AMI and prospectively followed them for 3 months. The emergency room admission electrocardiogram was analyzed for ST-segment deviation ≥1 mm/lead and T-wave changes. Unfavorable outcomes were recurrent ischemic pain, AMI, and coronary revascularization with angioplasty or CABG. In patients who underwent coronary arteriography, a myocardium in jeopardy score ranging from 0 to 10 was assigned, based on the number of vessels with a diameter stenosis ≥70% and the location of the stenoses. Considering all 90 patients, an admission electrocardiogram with ST-segment deviation in ≥2 leads had a positive predictive value for adverse clinical events of 79% and a negative predictive value of 64%. In the subset of patients without LV hypertrophy and whose admission electrocardiograms were recorded during chest pain (62 of 90), the positive predictive value of ST deviation in ≥2 leads improved to 89% and the negative value to 72%. Of the 62 patients, 53 underwent coronary arteriography. There was a positive linear correlation between the total number of leads with ST-segment deviation and the myocardium in jeopardy score. In patients with unstable angina or non-Q-wave myocardial infarction, an admission electrocardiogram recorded during pain and revealing ST-segment changes in ≥2 leads is by itself a reliable predictor of major clinical events. The total number of leads with ST changes predicts the extent of myocardium in jeopardy.

ST-T wave abnormalities

Crenshaw and colleagues[45] in Memphis, Tennessee, studied the clinical, hemodynamic, and angiographic correlates of the prognostic importance of electrocardiogram ST-T wave abnormalities in patients with chronic CAD. Data from 9,731 patients undergoing cardiac catheterization from 1976 through 1986 were analyzed. Five thousand five hundred and thirty-one had severe obstruction of at least one major coronary artery, 1,706 had mild obstruction, and 2,494 had no significant obstructions. Of the patients with severe obstructions, 2,536 were treated medically and 2,995 were treated by surgery. Patients with an ST-T abnormality had more clinical risk factors, including older age and greater prevalence of diabetes, hypertension, and prior AMI and greater LV dysfunction, including higher end-diastolic pressure and greater prevalence of contraction abnormality than did those patients without these electrocardiogram patterns. Survival time was significantly reduced in those patients with ST-T wave abnormalities and with severe or mild CAD; in those patients without CAD, ST-T wave changes did not correlate with reduced survival. Stepwise regression analysis was applied to each group to determine the independent predictors of 5-year survival. In patients with severe CAD or no disease, an ST-T wave abnormality was not chosen as an independent predictor of 5-year survival. However in the group with mild disease, ST-T wave changes were an independent predictor of reduced survival. Thus, the independent impact of an ST-T wave abnormality on survival is dependent on the severity of underlying CAD (Figure 2-8).

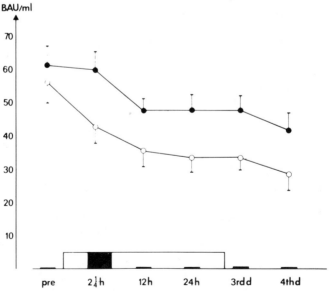

Fig. 2-8. Mean and 1 SD (vertical bars) of factor XII-dependent fibrinolytic activity in two groups of patients with acute myocardial infarction treated with recombinant tissue-type plasminogen activator (rt-PA). Eight patients had myocardial reinfarction during the study period (open circles) in contrast to the remaining 12 patients (closed circles). Activity levels were measured before treatment (pre) and 2¼ h, 12 h and 24 h after initiation of treatment and on the morning of the 3rd (3rd d) and 4th (4th d) days after admission. The solid bars indicate rt-PA treatment period and open bars indicate heparin infusion. BAU = blood activating units. Reproduced with permission of Crenshaw, et al.[45]

Treadmill exercise score

The treadmill exercise test identifies patients with different degrees of risk of death from cardiovascular events. Mark and associates[46] from Durham, North Carolina, devised a prognostic score, based on the results of treadmill exercise testing, that accurately predicts outcome among inpatients referred for cardiac catheterization. This study was designed to determine whether this score could also accurately predict prognosis in unselected outpatients. The authors prospectively studied 613 consecutive outpatients with suspected CAD who were referred for exercise testing between 1983 and 1985. Follow-up was 98% complete at 4 years. The treadmill score was calculated as follows: duration of exercise in minutes—(5 × the maximal ST-segment deviation during or after exercise, in mm)—(4 × the treadmill angina index) (Figure 2-9). The numerical treadmill angina index was 0 for no angina, 1 for nonlimiting angina, and 2 for exercise-limiting angina. Treadmill scores ranged from −25 (indicating the highest risk) to +15 (indicating the lowest risk). Predicted outcomes for the outpatients, based on their treadmill scores, agreed closely with the observed outcomes. The score accurately separated patients who subsequently died from those who lived for 4 years (area under the receiver-operating-characteristic curve = 0.849). The treadmill score

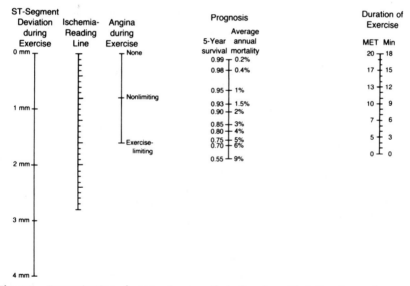

Fig. 2-9. Determination of prognosis proceeds in five steps. First, the observed amount of exercise-induced ST-segment deviation (the largest elevation or depression after resting changes have been subtracted) is marked on the line for ST-segment deviation during exercise. Second, the observed degree of angina during exercise is marked on the line for angina. Third, the marks for ST-segment deviation and degree of angina are connected with a straight edge. The point where this line intersects the ischemia-reading line is noted. Fourth, the total number of minutes of exercise in treadmill testing according to the Bruce protocol (or the equivalent in multiples of resting oxygen consumption (METs) from an alternative protocol) is marked on the exercise-duration line. Fifth, the mark for ischemia is connected with that for exercise duration. The point at which this line intersects the line for prognosis indicates the five-year survival rate and average annual mortality for patients with these characteristics. Reproduced with permission of Mark, et al.[46]

was a better discriminator than the clinical data and was even more useful for outpatients than it had been for inpatients. Approximately two thirds of the outpatients had treadmill scores indicating low risk ($\geq +5$), reflecting longer exercise times and little or no ST-segment deviation, and their 4-year survival rate was 99% (average annual mortality rate, 0.25%). Four percent of the outpatients had scores indicating high risk (< -10), reflecting shorter exercise times and more severe ST-segment deviation; their four-year survival rate was 79% (average annual mortality rate, 5%). The treadmill score is a useful and valid tool that can help clinicians determine prognosis and decide whether to refer outpatients with suspected CAD for cardiac catheterization. In this study, it was a better predictor of outcome than the clinical assessment.

Supine echocardiography vs exercise radionuclide angiography

The ability of supine exercise electrocardiography and exercise radionuclide angiography to predict time to subsequent cardiac events (cardiac death, nonfatal AMI or late CABG or PTCA) were compared by Simari and associates[47] in 265 patients with normal resting electrocardiograms who were not taking digoxin. All patients had undergone coronary catheterization and were initially treated medically. Follow-up study was performed at a median of 51 months. Separate logistic regression models, which had been previously developed to predict 3-vessel or left main CAD, were compared using a Cox regression analysis to predict time to a subsequent cardiac event. The exercise electrocardiography model, consisting of the magnitude of ST depression, exercise heart rate and patient gender, was a powerful predictor of subsequent events. The exercise radionuclide angiography model, which included the exercise response of the pressure-volume ratio in addition to the exercise electrocardiography variables, had similar prognostic power. In a separate analysis considering only cardiac death and nonfatal AMI, the exercise electrocardiography model remained a significant predictor of events. None of the radionuclide angiography variables added significantly to the prognostic power of the exercise electrocardiography model. Thus, in patients with a normal resting electrocardiogram who are not taking digoxin, the supine exercise electrocardiography model that predicts 3-vessel or left main CAD also predicts future cardiac events. Exercise radionuclide angiography does not provide any additional prognostic information in such patients.

Radionuclide angiography

Johnson and associates[48] from Durham, North Carolina, examined the prognostic value of radionuclide angiography in patients with suspected CAD. Nine hundred and eight patients who underwent rest and exercise radionuclide angiocardiography without subsequent cardiac catheterization were followed for a median of 4.6 years. Fifty-two cardiovascular deaths and 28 nonfatal myocardial infarctions occurred during the follow-up period. Thirty-nine radionuclide angiocardiographic and clinical variables were analyzed in association with the end points of cardiovascular death, total cardiac events and death from all causes using the Cox proportional hazards model and Kaplan-Meier survival estimates. Univariable analysis identified the exercise EF as the best predictor of cardiovascular death (chi-square = 82), total cardiac events (chi-square

= 84) and death from all causes (chi-square = 66). A small subset of patients (n = 45) with an exercise EF <0.35 were at high risk for future cardiac events, whereas most patients (n = 776) had an exercise EF ≥0.50 and a low probability of a subsequent event. Three variables—the exercise EF, the exercise change in heart rate, and gender—contained independent prognostic information determined by multivariable analysis. The exercise EF was the strongest independent predictor for every end point. The measurement of ventricular function during exercise provides important independent prognostic information in patients with suspected CAD. Radionuclide angiocardiography successfully identifies patients requiring invasive assessment, and the low probability of cardiac events in patients with good exercise ventricular function obviates the need for interventional therapy.

With isolated left anterior descending occlusion

The purpose of this study by Van Lierde and associates[49] from Leuven, Belgium, was to determine the long-term prognosis of patients with an isolated total occlusion of the LAD. A total of 173 male patients with a chronic LAD occlusion and <50% narrowing of the other coronary arteries (group I) was compared with a group of 177 male patients with only insignificant CAD and normal LV function (group II). Baseline characteristics of both groups were comparable except for the inclusion of 54 patients (31%) with moderately or markedly reduced LV systolic function in group I. During an 8-year follow-up period there was a greater number of patients with cardiac events in group I when compared with group II: cardiac death 11% versus 0.6%, myocardial infarction 13% versus 3.4%, and myocardial revascularization procedures 12% versus 3.4%. Stepwise discriminant analysis showed that a reduced EF and a family history of CAD were the best predictors for these adverse cardiac events.

UNSTABLE ANGINA PECTORIS

Outcome during regular aspirin use

Cohen and associates[50] in New York, New York, evaluated 93 patients admitted within 48 hours of chest pain with unstable angina at rest or non-Q wave AMI. On admission, 29 patients (31%) were taking daily aspirin and 64 (68%) were receiving no antiplatelet agent. After enrollment in the study, all patients received antithrombotic therapy with either aspirin or heparin according to protocol. The 2 groups of users versus nonusers of aspirin prior to randomization were similar with regard to age, gender, coronary risk factors, prior antianginal medication, duration of symptomatic coronary disease, presentation with non-Q wave AMI and extent of electrocardiogram changes on admission. Quantitative analysis of coronary arteriograms showed similar myocardium-in-jeopardy scores. Follow-up events, including recurrent ischemia, AMI and need for CABG or PTCA were 27%, 33% for the development of myocardial ischemia in patients with and without prior aspirin use; 3% and 5% for AMI in patients with and without prior aspirin use, respectively; and 44% and 51% for revascularization in patients with and without prior aspirin use, respectively. Thus, patients who use aspirin but develop rest angina are similar to other patients with rest angina. The "resistant to aspirin" group does not constitute a subgroup at higher risk for cardiac events or need for revascularization.

Lipoprotein (a) levels

Lipoprotein (a) [Lp(a)] appears to be involved in atherogenesis and in vitro studies have suggested that it may interfere with thrombolysis. Qiu and associates[51] from Montreal, Canada, determined Lp(a) serum levels by radioimmunoassay inn 124 patients with CAD. Of these, 47 had acute myocardial infarction, 13 had unstable angina, and 64 were age-matched patients with stable angina. Of the 60 patients with acute CAD, 34 received thrombolysis and 26 did not. In addition to Lp(a), serum plasminogen, a_2 antiplasmin, fibrinogen, and D-dimer (cross-linked fibrin degradation products) levels were measured. These tests were repeated after 6 hours in patients with myocardial infarction and unstable angina. No significant difference was found for admission Lp(a) levels among patients with myocardial infarction (0.324 ± 0.047 g/L), unstable angina (0.435 ± 0.123 g/L) and stable angina (0.431 ± 0.023 g/L), between patients with myocardial infarction with or without thrombolytic treatment, nor between late and early measurements in patients with unstable angina and AMI. Plasminogen, a_2 antiplasmin and fibrinogen values decreased significantly after thrombolytic treatment. The size of this decrease correlated positively with higher Lp(a) blood levels. Patients with Lp(a) >0.25 g/liter had a 66% decrease in fibrinogen and a 53% decrease in antiplasmin, compared with 35 and 32% respectively, in patients with Lp(a) level ≤0.25 g/L. Plasminogen levels revealed a similar trend, with a 61% decrease for the higher values and a 45% decrease for the lower values. These data indicate that serum Lp(a) levels are not increased in AMI and unstable angina, and are not influenced by thrombolytic treatment. In addition, no evidence was found that higher levels reduced systemic fibrinolytic activity, as assessed by the usual diagnostic tests.

Reversible ST-segment shifts and thrombosis

Eisenberg and associates[52] in St. Louis, Missouri, studied patients with unstable angina to determine whether specific electrocardiogram abnormalities associated with ischemia, the presence of coronary lesions consistent with thrombus on angiography or recurrent myocardial ischemia are associated with increases in thrombin activity as manifest by increased plasma concentrations of fibrinopeptide A. The concentration of fibrinopeptide A in plasma was increased to 6.7 ± 3.1 nM for the group as a whole (n = 29). Increases were greater in the 17 patients who exhibited reversible ST segment shifts than in the 12 patients exhibiting reversible T wave abnormalities alone (Figure 2-10). Nine of the 17 patients with reversible ST segment shifts who underwent coronary angiography had lesions with morphologic characteristics consistent with atherosclerotic plaque complicated by thrombosis compared with only 2 of 9 patients with T wave changes. Plasma concentrations of fibrinopeptide A were markedly elevated in 7 of the 11 patients in whom complex lesions were noted on angiographic examination. Therefore, the occurrence of reversible ST segment shifts identifies a group of patients with unstable angina in whom ongoing thrombosis is likely and who may be particularly likely to benefit from antithrombotic therapy.

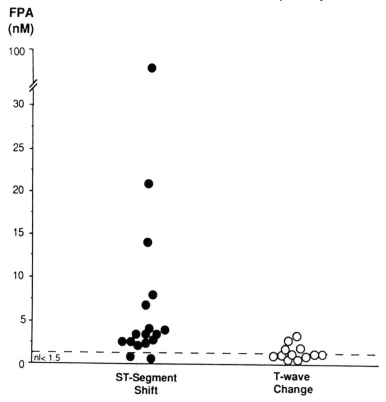

Fig. 2-10. Comparison of plasma concentrations of fibrinopeptide A (FPA) in 29 patients with unstable angina: 17 patients who exhibited ST segment shifts on the admission electrocardiogram (ECG) (black circles) and 12 patients with T wave changes only on the admission ECG (gray circles). Concentrations of fibrinopeptide A in plasma of healthy nonhospitalized volunteers (nl) are <1.5 nM. Fibrinopeptide A was elevated to a significantly greater extent in patients who exhibited ST segment shifts than in those with T wave changes (p<0.01). Reproduced with permission of Eisenberg, et al.[52]

Fibrinolytic activity

Zalewski and co-workers[53] in Philadelphia, Pennsylvania evaluated the role of the fibrinolytic system in patients with unstable angina at rest associated with transient electrocardiographic changes. Tissue plasminogen activator activity in plasma was comparable among patients with unstable angina, patients with stable exertional angina, and control patients with normal coronary arteriograms. In contrast, plasminogen activator inhibitor-1 activity in plasma was elevated in the unstable angina group as compared with either the stable angina group or the controls. Coronary angiography performed within 24 hours after the last anginal episode showed a similar extent of CAD in the unstable and stable angina groups. Intracoronary thrombi were observed in 8 patients in the stable angina group while no thrombus was noted in the stable angina group. These investigators concluded that patients with unstable angina at rest have a reduced fibrinolytic activity and an increased incidence of intracoronary thrombi.

Predischarge exercise test

Wilcox and colleagues[54] in Sydney, Australia, studied the prognostic significance of exercise testing compared with clinical and electrocardiogram variables in a prospective study of 107 patients with unstable angina discharged from the hospital on medical therapy. During a follow-up period of 13 ± 1 months, 10 patients had a nonfatal AMI or died and 22 were readmitted with recurrent unstable angina. The relation between 20 clinical, electrocardiogram and exercise test variables and the risk of adverse outcome, including death, nonfatal AMI or recurrent unstable angina was analyzed using both univariate and multivariate logistic regression analysis. Univariate predictors of adverse outcome included diabetes mellitus, evolutionary T wave changes, T wave changes on the preexercise electrocardiogram, and low maximal rate-pressure product during exercise. Independent predictors of adverse outcome in multivariate analysis included diabetes mellitus, evolutionary T wave changes after admission, rest pain during hospitalization, ST depression during exercise and low maximal rate-pressure product (Figure 2-11). A predictive model constructed using the regression equation and all independent predictors stratified patients into high and low risk groups. The

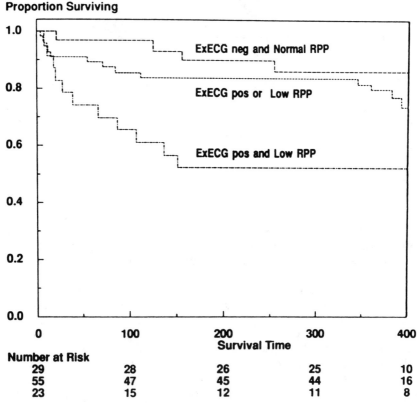

Fig. 2-11. Event-free survival (in days). Effect of abnormal exercise test responses on the cumulative probability of death, nonfatal myocardial infarction or recurrent unstable angina in 107 patients (log-rank 8.4, p<0.02). ExECG = exercise electrocardiogram; neg = negative; pos = positive; RPP = rate-pressure product. Reproduced with permission of Wilcox, et al.[54]

results of a predischarge exercise test add independent prognostic information to clinical and electrocardiogram data in medically treated patients with unstable angina and may be used in combination with clinical and electrocardiogram data to identify patients at risk of adverse events.

Thallium-201 imaging

Brown[55] in Burlington, Vermont, assessed the prognostic value of thallium-201 imaging in 52 consecutive patients admitted with unstable angina who responded to medical therapy and underwent stress thallium-201 imaging within 1 week of discharge. Patients were followed up for 39 ± 11 months. Cardiac events included cardiac death (n = 3), nonfatal AMI (n = 4) and admission for unstable angina or revascularization (n = 17). The ability of thallium-201 data, including redistribution, fixed defects, and normal results to predict future cardiac events was compared with clinical data and cardiac catheterization data using logistic regression. Thallium-201 redistribution was the only significant predictor of cardiac death or nonfatal AMI. The number of myocardial segments with thallium-201 redistribution and a history prior AMI were the only significant predictors of all cardiac events. Cardiac death or nonfatal AMI occurred more frequently in patients with thallium-201 redistribution (6 of 23) than in those without redistribution (1 of 29). Total cardiac events developed more frequently in patients with thallium-201 redistribution. Thus, stress thallium-201 imaging has important prognostic value in patients admitted with unstable angina who respond to medical therapy and may identify subgroups at high versus low risk for future cardiac events.

Dipyridamole perfusion scintigraphy

Zhu and colleagues[56] from San Francisco, California, evaluated the safety, accuracy, and potential clinical utility of intravenous dipyridamole perfusion scintigraphy with thallium-201 in 170 patients, 78 with suspected and 92 with known unstable angina. All had coronary angiography. Noncardiac side effects (26%), induced chest discomfort (44%), and ST segment changes (12%) were similar in the 2 groups. No significant arrhythmias occurred. Two patients had prolonged chest pain, both with extensive reversible image abnormalities and associated creatinine kinase-MB release; both had elective CABG. Twenty-eight patients had normal coronary arteries, and 35 had single-vessel disease. Scintigraphic per patient sensitivity and specificity were 91% and 79% with a per vessel sensitivity of 74% and a per vessel specificity of 78% without between-group differences. During a brief follow-up period, 62 patients with image abnormalities had coronary revascularization, and there were 7 deaths without intergroup differences. In a similar patient group that did not have angiography, scintigraphic defects were less frequent and less extensive, revascularization was not performed, and subsequent deaths occurred less often. Dipyridamole perfusion scintigraphy is an accurate alternative to exercise testing in the evaluation of patients with unstable angina pectoris. Although not without risk, the method appears relatively safe and should be considered as a guide to diagnosis, and probably to prognosis and management.

Technetium-99m sestamibi tomography

Bilodeau and associates[57] in Montreal, Canada, studied the sensitivity and specificity of technetium-99m hexakis-2-methoxy-2-isobutyl-isonitrile (sestamibi) single-photon emission computed tomography imaging for diagnosing CAD in 45 patients admitted to the hospital with a clinical suspicion of unstable angina. Only patients without prior AMI were included and all patients had technetium-99m sestamibi injections and 12-lead electrocardiograms during and ≤4 hours after chest pain. Coronary angiography during hospitalization showed significant CAD (≥50% luminal diameter reduction) in 26 of the 45 patients. The imaging studies obtained after injection of technetium-99m sestamibi during an episode of spontaneous chest pain had a sensitivity of 96% for the detection of CAD. 12-lead electrocardiograms at the time of injections had a sensitivity of 35%. With the patient in the pain-free state, respective sensitivity values were 65% and 38%. Specificity for the radionuclide study was 79% during pain and 84% in the pain-free state. For the electrocardiogram, it was 74% both during and between episodes of pain. The site of the perfusion defect corresponded to the most severe CAD in 88% of patients. The severity of the perfusion defect correlated with the extent of CAD. Persistence of the perfusion defect in the pain-free state was associated with a larger initial defect and with involvement of the LAD. This study demonstrates a high accuracy of technetium-99m sestamibi studies for the detection of CAD and for the identification of the involved coronary arteries in patients with spontaneous chest pain.

Angiographic morphology

Complex coronary stenosis morphology frequently occurs in patients with unstable angina pectoris. Its relation to transient myocardial ischemia and hospital outcome, however, has not been asserted. To address this issue, Bugiardini and associates[58] from Bologna, Italy, studied 88 patients with significant (≥50% diameter narrowing) CAD presenting with angina—new onset (n = 38), worsening (n = 20) or at rest (n = 30). Patients with LM CAD, normal coronary arteries, or occlusion of the ischemia-related arteries were not included in the study. Continuous electrocardiographic recordings were obtained during the first 24 hours. Angiography was performed within 1 week from admission. Complex morphology was defined as any stenosis with irregular borders, overhanging edges or intracoronary thrombus. Only data referring to the in-hospital outcome were considered in this study. Adverse end points were sudden death, AMI and emergency revascularization. Analysis of the angiograms revealed a complex morphology in 58 patients (group 1). The remaining 30 patients served as control subjects (group 2). Thirty-two of the 58 group 1 patients had an unfavorable clinical outcome (positive predictive value, 55%). A similar outcome occurred in only 2 of the 30 group 2 patients (negative predictive value, 93%). Of the 32 group 1 patients who had an unfavorable clinical outcome, 29 had a cumulative duration of transient myocardial ischemia of >60 minutes per 24 hours. A similar duration of ischemia, however, was observed in another 6 group 1 and in 8 group 2 patients. Thus, association of complex coronary morphology with sustained (≥60 minutes per 24 hours) myocardial ischemia is highly predictive of subsequent coronary events (positive and negative predictive value, 83 and 91% respectively), compared with the absence of 1 or both findings.

STABLE ANGINA PECTORIS

Plasma concentrations of vitamins A, C, and E and carotene

Riemersma and associates[59] from Edinburgh, UK, and Berne, Switzerland, examined the relation between risk of angina pectoris and plasma concentrations of vitamins A, C, and E and carotene in a population case-control study of 110 patients with angina pectoris, identified by the Chest Pain Questionnaire, and 394 controls selected from a sample of 6000 men aged 35–54 years. Plasma concentrations of vitamins C and E and carotene were significantly inversely related to the risk of angina. There was no significant relation with vitamin A. Smoking was a confounding factor. The inverse relation between angina and low plasma carotene disappeared and that with plasma vitamin C was substantially reduced after adjustment for smoking. Vitamin E remained independently and inversely related to the risk of angina after adjustment for age, smoking habit, BP, lipids, and relative weight. The adjusted odds ratio for angina between the lowest and highest quintiles of vitamin E concentrations was 2.68. These findings suggest that some populations with a high incidence of CAD may benefit from eating diets rich in natural antioxidants, particularly vitamin E.

Vasomotor responses

Kaski and colleagues[60] in London, UK, studied the vasomotor responses of eccentric and concentric coronary artery stenoses to ergonovine given as 20 μg intracoronarily or 300 μg intravenously and isosorbide dinitrate given as 1 mg by the intracoronary route in 51 patients with chronic stable angina. The diameter of the reference segments by angiography and that of eccentric and concentric coronary stenoses that ranged from 50% to 90% luminal diameter reduction were measured by computerized quantitative coronary arteriography before and after ergonovine and isosorbide dinitrate. Ergonovine reduced stenosis diameter by ≥10% in 80% of the eccentric stenoses and 42% of concentric stenoses. Mean diameter reduction with ergonovine was 19 ± 3% and 9.5 ±2% for eccentric and concentric stenoses, respectively. Isosorbide dinitrate increased coronary diameter in 70% of eccentric and 43% of concentric stenoses. Mean diameter of eccentric stenoses increased from 1.15 ± 0.05 to 1.35 ± 0.06 mm after the nitrates, whereas the diameter of concentric stenoses increased from 1.05 ± 0.05 to 1.14 ± 0.05 mm. Average dilation of reference segments with the administration of isosorbide dinitrate and constriction with ergonovine were not significantly different in patients with concentric and eccentric stenoses. Therefore, in patients with chronic stable angina, both eccentric and concentric stenoses have the potential for dynamic changes of caliber in response to vasoactive intervention. However, more eccentric stenoses exhibit these responses.

To assess whether vasoreactivity of significant coronary stenosis (>50% intraluminal diameter reduction) and that of angiographically normal coronary segments differs in proximal and distal locations, Tousoulis and associates[61] from London, UK, studied 53 patients (43 men, 13 women, mean age 55 ± 11 years) with chronic stable angina and angiographically documented CAD. While abstaining from antianginal therapy, all 53 patients underwent coronary arteriography before and after 1 mg of intracoronary isosorbide dinitrate and 21 of the 53 also before and after 20 to 30 μg intracoronary ergonovine. Computerized quantitative angiography was used to assess changes in the intraluminal diameter of 126 normal coronary segments (63 proximal, 63 distal) and 43 significant coronary stenoses. Nitrates dilated proximal normal coronary segments by 7.4 ± 1.2% and distal normal coronary segments by 15 ± 1.7%. Significant proximal coronary stenoses dilated by 11 ± 2.5% and distal stenoses by 23 ± 2.8% after nitrates. Ergonovine reduced the diameter of proximal normal coronary segments by 9.3 ± 1.7% and that of normal distal segments by 15.5 ± 1.4%, prosimal stenoses by 11 ± 2.2% and distal stenoses by 18.4 ± 2.8%. Analysis of segments showed that nitrates dilated 19 of 63 (30%) proximal normal segments (by ≥10%), 31 of 63 (49%) distal and 21 of 43 (49%) stenoses. Ergonovine constricted (by ≥10%) 15 of 37 (41%) proximal normal segments, 27 of 37 (73%) distal and 13 of 22 (59%) significant stenoses. These findings indicate that distal normal coronary segments have greater reactivity to nitrates and to ergonovine than proximal segments. Stenosis reactivity parallels that of angiographically normal segments.

Thallium-201 scintigraphy

Heller and associates[62] from Pawtucket and Providence, Rhode Island, performed a study to evaluate the presence of angina pectoris, electrocardiographic changes and reversible thallium-201 defects resulting from 2 different levels of exercise in 19 patients with known CAD and evidence of exercise-induced ischemia. The exercise protocols consisted of a symptom-limited incremental exercise test (Bruce protocol) followed within 3 to 14 days by a submaximal, steady-state exercise test performed at 70% of the maximal heart rate achieved during the Bruce protocol. The presence and time of onset of angina and electrocardiographic changes (≥0.1 mV ST-segment depression) as well as oxygen uptake, exercise duration and pressure-rate product were recorded. Thallium-201 (25 to 3.0 mCi) was injected during the last minute of exercise during both protocols, and the images were analyzed using both computer-assisted quantitation and visual interpretations. Incremental exercise resulted in anginal symptoms in 84% of patients, and electrocardiographic changes and reversible thallium-201 defects in all patients. In contrast, submaximal exercise produced anginal symptoms in only 26% and electrocardiographic changes in only 47%, but resulted in thallium-201 defects in 89% of patients. The locations of the thallium-201 defects, when present, were not different between the 2 exercise protocols. These findings confirm the sequence of the ischemic cascade using 2 levels of exercise and demonstrate that the cascade theory is applicable during varying ischemic intensities in the same patient.

Technetium-99m sestamibi scintigraphy

Parodi and colleagues[63] in Pisa, Italy, studied the feasibility, safety, and accuracy of technetium-99m hexakis 2-methoxy-2-isobutyl isonitrile (Sestamibi) scintigraphy associated with intravenous high dose dipyridamole in 101 patients with effort chest pain and no prior myocardial infarction. Planar myocardial perfusion images were obtained at rest and after dipyridamole. High dose dipyridamole was used when typical chest pain or electrocardiogram signs of ischemia, or both did not occur during or after the standard dose of dipyridamole. With high dose dipyridamole,

34 patients had pain or electrocardiogram signs of myocardial ischemia or both, whereas the remaining 28 patients had Sestamibi injection in the absence of symptoms or electrocardiogram changes. All patients underwent coronary angiography: 81 had significant CAD ($\geq$50% reduction of luminal diameter) and 20 patients had normal coronary arteries. The overall sensitivity, specificity and predictive accuracy of Sestamibi scintigraphy were 81%, 90%, and 83%, respectively. No significant hypotension, ventricular arrhythmias or other serious adverse reactions occurred in any of the patients tested with high dose dipyridamole. Minor side effects occurred in 52% and 57% of patients at standard and high dose dipyridamole, respectively, but these were well tolerated. These data suggest that Sestamibi scintigraphy associated with high dose dipyridamole is an accurate method of evaluating suspected CAD in patients. It did not cause an increased number of side effects as compared with those associated with the standard dose protocol.

SILENT MYOCARDIAL ISCHEMIA

Mangano and colleagues[64] in San Francisco, California, determined the incidence and characteristics of perioperative myocardial ischemia during a 4 day perioperative period in 100 patients with or at risk for coronary heart disease undergoing noncardiac surgery. Continuous two channel electrocardiogram monitoring which helped to determine the frequency and severity of electrocardiogram ischemic episodes defined by ST segment depression $\geq$1 mm or elevation $\geq$2 mm during the perioperative (up to 2 days), intraoperative and early postoperative periods (first 2 days). Preoperatively, 28 patients (28%) exhibited 105 episodes of ischemia. Intraoperatively, 27 patients had 39 episodes and postoperatively, 42 patients had 187 episodes. There was no difference between the pre- and intraoperative episode characteristics. However, postoperative ischemic episodes were the most severe. The mean ST change was 1.5, 2 and 2.6 mm for pre-, intra- and postoperative episodes, respectively. The duration of ischemic episodes was 69, 45 and 207 min, respectively. Ninety-four percent of all postoperative ischemic episodes were silent. Eighty percent of all episodes occurred without acute changes in heart rate and 77% of intraoperative episodes occurred without acute changes in blood pressure. However, postoperative heart rates were chronically higher. Patients with coronary heart disease versus those with risk factors alone were equally likely to develop ischemia during any period and 11 of 13 adverse cardiac outcomes were preceded by postoperative ischemia. Thus, in noncardiac surgical patients with or at risk for coronary heart disease the following conclusions appear justified: (1) preoperative ischemia is relatively common occurring equally in patients with documented and potential coronary heart disease; (2) anesthesia and surgery are not associated with an increased incidence or severity of ischemia; (3) ischemia is most frequent and severe during the postoperative period; and (4) postoperative ischemia is silent and may be related to chronically elevated heart rates in some patients.

Previous studies have shown that little if any increase in heart rate occurs 1 minute before the onset of ischemia in ambulant patients with CAD. McLeanchan and co-workers[65] in Boston, Massachusetts tested the hypothesis that there are characteristic relations between heart rate and ischemia in ambulatory patients with CAD. Twenty-one patients with proven CAD demonstrated 212 episodes of ischemia during 504 hours of continuous monitoring of the electrocardiogram. An important increase in heart rate from 74 to 94 beats/min occurred between 5 and 30 minutes (not 1 minute) before the onset of ischemia. A significantly higher heart rate at onset of ischemia was seen during Bruce protocol exercise testing than during daily life (117 vs 95 beats/min). However, when a less-strenuous, but more prolonged, exercise protocol was used in a subgroup of patients, ischemia occurred at a heart rate that was significantly lower than during the Bruce protocol (88 vs 103 beats/min.) and was not significantly different from the threshold heart rate at onset of ischemia during daily life (88 vs 84 beats/min.). As part of 2 placebo controlled trials, treatment with both propranolol and nitroglycerin altered the distribution of ischemic events by heart rate but in opposite directions. Although propranolol largely eliminated events occurring at high (>100 beats/min) and moderate (80–100 beats/min) heart rates, the number of events at low (<80 beats/min) heart rates was increased. In contrast, nitroglycerin reduced episodes at low and moderate heart rates only. Important increases in heart rate occur before the onset of ischemia during daily life, but this increase occurs much earlier than has been reported. Duration of heart rate increase appears to influence the heart rate threshold for ischemia, and this may contribute to the occurrence of ischemia at lower heart rates during daily life than during standard exercise testing. Last, different classes of drugs appear to have characteristic effects on ischemia occurring at different heart rates that may be useful in planning therapy.

Ischemia on ambulatory electrocardiographic monitoring has been shown to adversely affect short-term prognoses in patients with unstable angina, after AMI and with chronic stable angina. In a long-term study, Yeung and collaborators[66] in Boston, Massachusetts followed 138 patients with chronic stable angina and positive exercise tests for cardiac events (e.g., death, myocardial AMI, PTCA or CABG). In 105 patients ambulatory electrocardiographic monitoring was performed after all antianginal medication was withheld for 48 hours. In 26 patients, the diagnostic tests were repeated while on their usual medication. In addition to the 105 patients, 33 patients had their monitoring performed only while on their usual medication. During 37 months of follow-up, there were nine deaths, nine AMIs and 35 CABG procedures. In patients monitored off medication, Cox survival analysis showed that the occurrence of ischemia on electrocardiographic monitoring was the most significant predictor of death and AMI in the subsequent 2 years and of all adverse events for 5 years. Patients who were monitored on medication and did not have ischemia appeared to have more adverse events than patients who had no ischemia while being monitored off medication. Asymptomatic ischemia on ambulatory electrocardiographic monitoring in patients with stable angina predicts death and AMI for 2 years and all adverse events for 5 years. Monitoring performed while on medication may show no ischemia; however, this may not indicate low risk of future coronary events.

A diurnal pattern of changes in transient myocardial ischemia has been well documented in patients with CAD with an increase in the early morning hours. To further investigate potential triggers of myocardial ischemia, Barry and associates[67] from Boston, Massachusetts, and Sheffield, UK, examined certain defined and distinct episodes of waking and rising during the nighttime. Of 113 patients who underwent ambulatory monitoring of the electrocardiogram, 466 episodes of ischemia lasting 3,926 minutes were detected in 67 of the patients. In 20 patients who had ischemia at night, 21 reported 36 occasions of waking and rising, and 67% of these events were associated with ST-segment depression. Frequency and duration of ischemia were similar in the nocturnal episodes versus the early morning episodes of ischemia as were the increases in heart rate at 30, 10, 5 and 1 minute before the onset. Even before waking, there was an increase in heart rate beginning approximately 30 minutes before the onset of ischemia. This increase became significant 5 minutes before onset both in the early morning and on rising at night. Patients with nocturnal ischemia had significantly worse clinical signs of CAD. This study shows that rising at night is often associated with episodes of myocardial ischemia and, like the morning events on rising, is likely an important trigger of ischemia in patients with CAD.

Hinderliter and colleagues[68] in Chapel Hill, North Carolina, evaluated 50 patients with CAD and exercise-induced ST segment depression to determine the role of increased myocardial oxygen demand in the pathophysiology of myocardial ischemia occurring during daily activities. Each patient underwent ambulatory electrocardiogram monitoring for ST segment shifts during normal daily activities and symptom-limited bicycle exercise testing with continuous electrocardiogram monitoring. All 50 patients had ST segment depression ≥0.01 mV during exercise. A total of 241 episodes of ST depression were noted in the ambulatory setting in 31 patients. Only 6% of these were accompanied by angina. Significant (0.1 mV) ST depression during ambulatory monitoring was preceded by a mean increase in heart rate of 27 ± 12 beats/min. Patients with ischemia during daily activities developed ST segment depression earlier during exercise and tended to have significant electrocardiogram changes at a lower exercise heart rate and rate-pressure product than did those without ST segment depression during ambulatory monitoring. In the 31 patients with ischemia during daily activities, the mean heart rate associated with ST segment depression was closely correlated with the heart rate precipitating electrocardiogram changes during exercise testing. These data suggest an important role for increased oxygen demand in the pathophysiology of ischemia during daily activities and they indicate that 1) most episodes of ischemia during daily activity are associated with significant increases in heart rate; 2) patients with ischemia during daily activities developed ST segment depression earlier during exercise and tended to develop electrocardiogram changes at a lower exercise heart rate and rate-pressure product than those without ST segment shifts in the ambulatory setting; and 3) patients with a relatively high exercise ischemic threshold developed ST depression in association with high heart rates during daily activities.

To evaluate the significance of ischemic ST depression without anginal chest pain during exercise testing among patients with diabetes mellitus, Weiner and associates[69] from several Coronary Artery Surgery Study registry centers analyzed data on 45 such patients. These patients (group 1, silent ischemia) were compared with 37 diabetic patients with both ischemic ST depression and chest pain (group 2, symptomatic ischemia), with 31 diabetic patients without ischemic ST depression or chest pain (group 3, no ischemia), and with 429 patients without diabetes who had silent ischemia during exercise testing (Figure 2-12). All patients had documented CAD (>70% diameter narrowing). The 6-year survival among patients with silent ischemia was worse in diabetic than nondiabetic

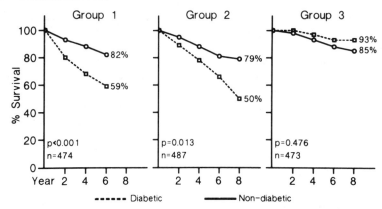

Fig. 2-12. Cumulative survival for diabetic and nondiabetic patients. Survival was worse in diabetic patients with silent (group 1) or symptomatic (group 2) ischemia, but was similar in nondiabetic patients without ischemia (group 3). Reproduced with permission of Weiner, et al.[69]

patients (59 vs 82%, respectively). By contrast, the 6-year survival among patients without ischemia was similar among diabetic and nondiabetic patients (93 vs 85%, respectively). Among diabetic patients, survival at 6 years with medical treatment was 59% for group 1, 66% for group 2 and 93% for group 3. Survival among subsets of patients with diabetes and silent ischemia (group 1) based on the extent of CAD and LV function ranged from 100 to 32%. The survival of the 45 patients with diabetes mellitus and silent ischemia (group 1) treated medically was compared with that of 28 patients receiving CABG. Survival at 6 years was enhanced by surgery compared with medical treatment among group 1 diabetic patients with 3-vessel CAD and either preserved LV (85 vs 52%, respectively) or impaired LV function (100 vs 32%, respectively). These data suggest that, among patients with diabetes and CAD, silent myocardial ischemia during exercise testing adversely affects survival, and that CABG surgery improves the survival of diabetic patients with silent myocardial ischemia and 3-vessel CAD.

Silent ischemia has been shown to be predictive of postoperative cardiac events in vascular surgery patients. However, no controlled data regarding its predictive value in nonvascular surgery patients are available. Fleisher and colleagues[70] from New Haven, Connecticut, studied 67 vascular surgery and 79 nonvascular surgery patients, all of whom had increased risk for cardiac disease, to determine whether the occurrence of preoperative silent myocardial ischemia is predictive of morbid postoperative cardiac events in a diverse surgical group. The presence of preoperative silent ischemia in both nonvascular and vascular surgical patients had similar predictive value (0.38 and 0.38, respectively) for postoperative morbid cardiac events. The absence of preoperative silent ischemia predicted an excellent outcome in patients undergoing nonvascular surgery (0.99), but was a less robust predictor in the vascular patients (0.86). These data suggest that the functional status of the coronary circulation is one of the most important determinants of outcome.

Deedwania and Carbajal[71] from San Francisco, California, prospectively evaluated and compared the prognostic significance of ambulatory silent ischemia detected by Holter monitoring during daily life with several exercise test parameters in 86 patients with stable angina and positive exercise tests. Forty-seven patients (group 1) had no evidence of ischemia and 39 (group 2) had 1 or more episodes of silent ischemia during the monitoring period. During mean follow-up of 24 ± 8 months there were only 2 cardiac deaths (nonsudden) in group 1 (4% mortality) compared with 9 (3 sudden and 6 nonsudden) in group 2 (23% mortality). Kaplan-Meier actuarial analysis revealed worse survival for patients in group 2. The Cox regression analysis of clinical variables, electrocardiographic and exercise parameters, angiographic data and Holter monitoring results revealed silent ischemia during daily life as the most powerful predictor of cardiac mortality. These results demonstrate that in patients with chronic stable angina and abnormal exercise tests, ambulatory ischemia detected by Holter monitoring provides significant additional prognostic information to that derived from evaluation of exercise test parameters alone.

Resting ST segment depression has been identified as a marker for adverse cardiac events in patients with and without known CAD. To correlate this with exercise testing, coronary angiography, and how it impacts on long-term prognosis, a retrospective study was performed by Miranda and associates[72] from Long Beach and Irvine, California, on 476 patients, of whom 223 had no clinical or electrocardiographic evidence of prior AMI while 253 were survivors of AMI. All patients performed a standard exercise test and underwent diagnostic coronary angiography within an average of 32 days of their exercise test (range 0 to 90 days). Exclusions were women, those with left BBB, LV hypertrophy, use of digoxin, previous revascularization procedures, or significant valvular or congenital heart disease. Long-term follow-up was carried out for an average of 45 months (± 17). Of the patients without prior AMI, 23 (10%) had persistent resting ST segment depression, and of those with a prior history of AMI, 37 (15%) also had resting ST segment depression. Patients with resting ST segment depression and no prior AMI had a higher prevalence of severe CAD (3-vessel and/or LM) (30%) than those without resting ST segment depression (16%). The criterion of ≥2 mm of additional exercise-induced ST segment depression was a particularly useful marker in these patients for the diagnosis of any CAD. Patients with resting ST segment depression and a prior AMI had a 2.5 times higher prevalence of severe CAD compared with patients without resting ST segment depression and also had larger left ventricles postinfarction. To identify severe CAD in post-infarction patients with persistent resting ST segment depression, the criteria of ≥2 mm of additional exercise-induced ST segment depression or having the additional exercise-induced ST segment depression persist ≥4 minutes into recovery were better markers than the standard criterion of ≥1 mm of additional ST segment depression. Receiver operating characteristics curve analysis revealed that additional exercise-induced ST segment depression continued to discriminate between those with or those without any, or severe, CAD despite having baseline ST segment depression at rest. After a cumulative follow-up of 4.4 years, patients with resting ST segment depression, with or without prior AMI, had a lower infarct-free survival rate than those without it. Resting ST segment depression (not due to LV hypertrophy, conduction defects, or drug effect) is a marker for a higher prevalence of severe CAD with a poor prognosis, and standard exercise testing continues to be diagnostically useful in these patients.

VARIANT ANGINA PECTORIS AND CORONARY SPASM

Okumura and colleagues[73] in Kumamoto, Japan evaluated the influence of histamine on coronary artery spasm in 21 patients with variant angina after blockage of the H_2 receptor with cimetidine. Intracoronary injection of acetylcholine was also performed in 19 of the 21 patients. Ergonovine was intravenously administered in one patient. Coronary artery diameter was measured with cinevideodensitometry analysis. A mean plasma histamine concentration in the coronary sinus increased from 4×10^{-9} to 7×10^{-8} M 5 minutes after histamine infusion into the left coronary artery. Coronary spasm was induced in 6 patients (29%) with histamine and 18 (95%) with acetylcholine and in 1 with ergonovine. The effect of histamine on the luminal diameter was analyzed at the site of spasm in the 26 coronary arteries in which spasm was induced by acetylcholine or ergonovine. Among the 20 coronary arteries with a normal arteriogram or a fixed stenosis, histamine decreased the diameter in 4, increased it in 14 and caused no change in 2. Among the 6 coronary arteries with a fixed stenosis $\geq 75\%$, histamine decreased the diameter in 5 and increased it in 1 (Figure 2-13).

To evaluate the efficacy of slow-release nifedipine (a single dose of 20 mg given at 10 P.M. or 2 doses of 20 mg at 10 P.M. and 6 A.M.) on ischemic episodes in patients with variant angina, Morikami and associates[74] performed a single-blind crossover study with ambulatory electrocardiographic monitoring in 15 patients (13 men and 2 women, mean age 63 years). In all there were 646 ischemic episodes detected with ambulatory electrocardiographic monitoring during the study period, and 618 episodes of them occurred during placebo periods with a circadian variation. Sixty-nine percent of the episodes in placebo periods were asymptomatic. The number of anginal attacks, nitroglycerin tablets taken, ST-segment elevation and the total ischemic duration significantly decreased during nifedipine therapy compared with results after the placebo therapy period, respectively. Twenty-eight ischemic episodes occurred during nifedipine therapy when the plasma level of nifedipine was low. Thus, asymptomatic ischemic episodes and the administration of slow-release nifedipine is highly effective in suppressing not only symptomatic but also asymptomatic myocardial ischemia in patients with variant angina. The timing of the administration of slow-release nifedipine is an important factor in suppressing ischemic episodes.

Motz and associates[75] from Dusseldorf and Freiburg, Federal Republic of Germany, performed a study to determine whether an impaired endothelium-mediated vasodilation in coronary resistance vessels exists in patients with *micro-vascular angina*. In 23 patients with clinically suspected CAD and smooth coronary arteries in the angiogram, coronary flow in response to an endothelium-related (acetylcholine) and endothelium-unrelated (dipyridamole) vasodilation was measured. Coronary flow was determined by the gaschromatographic argon method (1) before, (2) with intracoronary acetylcholine infusion, and (3) after dipyridamole administered intravenously. In 8 patients, acetylcholine did not significantly increase coronary flow (from 91 ± 28 to 118 ± 37 m./min · 100 g), whereas flow was greatly increased after administration of dipyridamole (258 ± 97 ml/min · 100 g), indicating an endothelium-related vasodilator defect. In 6 patients, neither acetylcholine nor dipyridamole caused a significant increase in coronary flow, indicating an impaired coronary vasodilation on the vascular site. In 6 patients, coronary flow increased

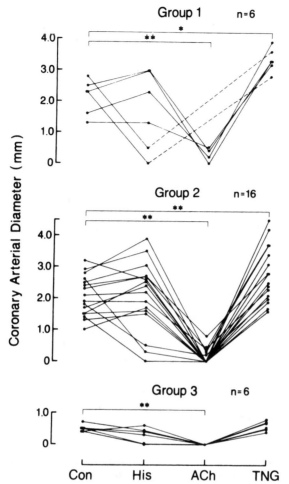

Fig. 2-13. Changes in luminal diameter at the site of coronary spasm in 21 patients (28 arteries) after administration of histamine (His), acetylcholine (ACh) and nitroglycerin (TNG). Data are shown for each group. In two group 1 patients, acetylcholine was not administered after histamine infusion, which resulted in coronary spasm (top panel, broken lines). Reproduced with permission of Okumura, et al.[73]

markedly after administration of both acetylcholine and dipyridamole (from 81 ± 26 to 191 ± 68 and 234 ± 87 ml/min · 100 g). In 3 patients given acetylcholine, coronary artery constriction occurred. No significant correlation was found between the response to acetylcholine and that to dipyridamole (4 = 0.40). The results indicate that in a subgroup of patients with smooth coronary arteries angina can be caused by an abnormality of the endothelial function in the micro-circulation.

Ardissino and associates[76] from Pavia and Zingonia, Italy, compared in 30 consecutive patients with Prinzmetal's angina pectoris, the antiischemic effect of felodipine, a new long-acting vasoselective calcium antagonist, administered at doses of 10 and 20 mg once daily with that of the well-established therapeutic regimen of nifedipine administered at a dose of 20 mg 4 times daily. Twenty-four-hour Holter monitoring was performed during a 2-day placebo run-in and at the end of each of 3 consecutive 6-day periods during which the 3 active treatments were administered in randomized sequence. Three patients withdrew, whereas 27 completed the study. The therapeutic regimens tested proved to be similarly effective; primary end points (ischemic episodes recorded by Holter monitoring, and anginal attacks reported on diary cards) occurred in 5 patients (19%) during nifedipine treatment, and in 7 (26%) and 3 (11%) during felodipine treatment with 10 and 20 mg, respectively. The distribution of residual ischemic episodes demonstrated that treatment with felodipine once daily provides 24-hour antiischemic protection. Twenty-six patients were followed up with 20 mg of felodipine once daily for a mean of 6 ± 5 months, and 21 of them (81%) remained free of symptoms and Holter-recorded ischemic attacks. It is concluded that for Prinzmetal's angina pectoris, 24-hour antiischemic protection may be achieved with administration of felodipine once daily. The availability of a simplified therapeutic approach may constitute a real advantage in terms of patient compliance and improving the quality of life.

MICROVASCULAR ANGINA

Dean and associates[77] compared glucose and insulin responses to a glucose load in 11 patients with angina pectoris attributed to microvascular coronary dysfunction with those in 11 healthy subjects matched for age, sex, and body mass. Stimulated hyperinsulinemia was demonstrated in the microvascular angina group. The findings suggest a role for increased concentrations of insulin in coronary microvascular dysfunction.

Kaski and colleagues[78] in London, UK, evaluated vasomotor responses of proximal and distal angiographically normal coronary artery segments in 12 patients with syndrome X, 17 age- and gender-matched patients with chronic stable angina and 10 control subjects with atypical chest pain and a normal coronary arteriogram. Ergonovine and isosorbide dinitrate were administered to all patients; ergonovine 300 μg was given by intravenous injection and isosorbide dinitrate 1 mg by intracoronary injection. Computerized coronary artery diameter measurement was performed before and after the administration of ergonovine and nitrate. Baseline intraluminal diameters of proximal and distal coronary segments were not significantly different in controls and patients with syndrome X or coronary artery disease. With ergonovine, proximal segments constricted by 10 ± 2%, 7 ± 2% and 11 ± 3% and distal segments by 12 ± 3%, 14 ± 3% and 14 ± 2% in controls and patients with syndrome X or CAD. With isosorbide dinitrate, responses of proximal and distal coronary arteries in controls and patients with syndrome X or coronary disease were again similar. These data indicate that coronary diameters and the vasomotor responses to ergonovine and isosorbide dinitrate of angiographically normal coronary artery segments at rest are not different in patients with noncardiac chest pain, syndrome X or CAD. Although coronary flow reserve is decreased in patients with syndrome X, reactivity of large epicardial vessels to nitrates and ergonovine is within the physiologic range.

Nihoyannopoulos and colleagues[79] in London, UK, obtained stress two-dimensional echo studies in 18 patients with angina, a positive exercise test, and normal coronary arteries by angiography; this group of patients has been referred to as having syndrome X. Rest and immediate posttreadmill exercise two-dimensional echos were performed with a digitized cine loop and side by side visual analysis in all patients. In 16 of these patients, right atrial pacing up to 160 beats/min was also performed and percent systolic wall thickening was calculated at five equally spaced segments around the LV, each corresponding to an anterior, lateral and inferior wall and the posterior and anterior ventricular septum. Measurements of percent systolic wall thickening were established in 10 age- and gender-matched normal persons for comparison. ST segment depression occurred in all patients during exercise and persisted for 42 seconds into the recovery period. Immediate post exercise echos were obtained within 20 ± 5 seconds and completed in 54 ± 11 seconds. No regional wall motion abnormalities were seen on two-dimensional imaging of any myocardial segment. Thirteen patients (72%) reported reproduction of their usual chest pain, which led to termination of the test. During rapid right atrial pacing, nine patients (56%) developed ST segment depression associated with angina in seven. In all 16 patients, percent systolic wall thickening increased over values at rest in each myocardial segment. Percent systolic wall thickening averaged 47 ± 6% at rest and increased to 74 ± 8% during right atrial pacing. Therefore, patients with syndrome X have normal systolic function at rest and immediately after exercise, despite ST segment depression resembling that seen during ischemia.

DRUGS FOR MYOCARDIAL ISCHEMIA

Aspirin

To evaluate the efficacy of low-dose (325 mg) aspirin in the primary prevention of AMI among patients with chronic stable angina pectoris, Ridker and associates[80] from Boston, Massachusetts, in a randomized, double-blind, trial studied 333 men with baseline chronic stable angina but no previous history of AMI, stroke, or transient ischemic attack. The patients had been enrolled in the physicians health study, a trial of aspirin among 22,071 male physicians. The patients were randomly assigned to receive alternate day aspirin therapy or placebo and were followed an average of 60 months for the occurrence of AMI, stroke, or cardiovascular death. During follow-up, 27 patients had confirmed AMI; 7 were among the 178 patients with chronic stable angina who received aspirin therapy and 20 were among the 155 patients who received placebo (relative risk, 0.30). While simultaneously controlling for other cardiovascular risk factors in a proportional hazards model, an overall 87% risk reduction was calculated (relative risk, 0.13). For the subgroup of patients with chronic stable angina but no previous CABG or coronary angioplasty, an almost identical reduction in the risk for AMI was found (relative risk, 0.14). Of 13 strokes, 11 occurred in the aspirin group and 2 in the placebo group (relative risk, 5.4). No stroke was fatal, but 4 produced some long-term impairment of function. One stroke, in the aspirin group, was hemorrhagic. The data indicated that alternate-day aspirin therapy greatly reduced the risk for first myocardial infarction among patients with chronic stable angina, a group of patients at high risk for cardiovascular death. Although our results for stroke were based on small numbers, they suggested an apparent increase in frequency of stroke with aspirin therapy;

this finding requires confirmation in randomized trials of adequate sample size.

Manson and associates[81] from Boston, Massachusetts, examined prospectively the association between regular aspirin use and the risk of a first AMI and other cardiovascular events in women in a prospective cohort study including 6 years of follow-up. US registered nurses (n = 87,678) aged 34–65 years and free of diagnosed CAD, stroke, and cancer at baseline were studied in 11 US states. Follow-up was 97% of total potential person-years. During 475,265 person-years of follow-up, the authors documented 240 non-fatal AMIs, 146 non-fatal strokes and 130 deaths due to cardiovascular disease. Among women who reported taking 1 through 6 aspirin per week, the age-adjusted relative risk of a first AMI was 0.68, as compared with those women who took no aspirin. After simultaneous adjustment for risk factors for CAD, the relative risk was 0.75. For women aged 50 years and older, the age-adjusted relative risk was 0.61 and the multivariate relative risk was 0.68. The authors observed no alteration in the risk of stroke. The multivariate relative risk of cardiovascular death was 0.89 and of important vascular events was 0.85. When examined separately, the results were nearly identical for the subgroups who took 1 through 3 and 4 through 6 aspirin per week. Among women who took seven or more aspirin per week, there were no apparent reductions in risk. The use of 1 through 6 aspirin per week appears to be associated with a reduced risk of a first AMI among women. A randomized trial in women is necessary, however, to provide conclusive data on the role of aspirin in the primary prevention of cardiovascular disease in women.

Low-dose aspirin has been postulated to decrease risks of cardiovascular disease by affecting atherosclerotic progression as well as acute thrombosis. In the Physicians' Health Study, a randomized double-blind placebo-controlled trial of alternate day aspirin (325 mg), 22,071 apparently healthy male physicians were treated and followed over a period of 5 years for the occurrence of AMI and of new angina pectoris. In an analysis of the cumulative incidence and cumulative relative risks of these end points, Ridker and associates[82] from Boston, Massachusetts, found that the full protective effect of aspirin in reducing the risk of AMI is apparent soon after initiation of therapy and does not change over time. In contrast, long-term aspirin therapy has no apparent role in decreasing the risk of developing future angina pectoris. Taken together, these clinical observations support the hypothesis that the primary effect of prophylactic low-dose aspirin therapy is to inhibit acute thrombosis, but do not support the hypothesis that long-term platelet inhibition for a duration of up to 5 years slows the initiation and progression of atherosclerosis.

Wallentin and colleagues[83] in Linkoping, Sweden, evaluated 796 men with unstable CAD, including patients with unstable angina or non-Q wave AMI who were randomized to double-blind placebo-controlled treatment with aspirin 75 mg/day. Long-term efficacy was judged from the occurrence of myocardial infarction or death or severe angina requiring referral for coronary angiography. The risk of AMI or death was reduced during aspirin treatment (Figure 2-14). Severe angina requiring referral for coronary angiography was less common during aspirin therapy. The combined event rate of AMI death and referral to coronary angiography was also reduced in the aspirin treated patients. The 75 mg aspirin dose was well tolerated. Treatment with aspirin 75 mg/day appears to be a reasonable recommendation to make for men following

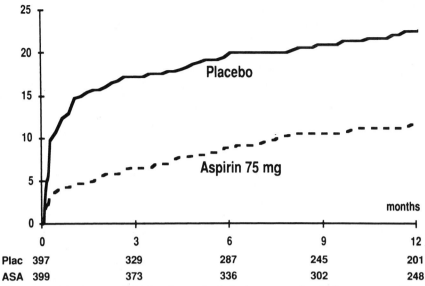

Fig. 2-14. Risk of myocardial infarction or death during 12 months of follow-up according to allocation to 75 mg/day of aspirin (ASA) or placebo (Plac). The graph is a life-table depiction of the cumulative risk and time for the occurrence of an outcome event. The numbers of patients at risk in each group are noted below the graph. Reproduced with permission of Wallentin, et al.[83]

their having unstable CAD. A dose of 75 mg/day of aspirin can usually be safely continued long-term.

The purpose of a study by Force and co-investigators[84] of Boston, Massachusetts was to determine the effects of the combination of aspirin and fish oil, which is rich in n-3 polyunsaturated fatty acids, on the eicosanoid profile of patients with CAD. Specifically, the investigators wanted to determine whether the aspirin-induced reduction in prostacyclin production is due to inhibition of endothelial cell cyclooxygenase or to reduced endoperoxide shift from platelets and whether aspirin negates the potential beneficial effects of fish oil on the eicosanoid profile. Fourteen patients with clinically stable but advanced CAD received 12 grams or 16 grams of fish oil concentrate containing 6 or 8 grams of n-3 fatty acids for 6 weeks. In addition to the fish oil, patients received increasing daily dose of aspirin from 50 to 1,300 mg. Each dose was taken for 2 weeks. With fish oil supplementation, red blood cell phospholipid fatty acid content of arachidonic acid decreased and eicosapentaenoic acid increased so that eicosapentaenoic acid as a percent of arachidonic acid increased from 20–26%. Serum thromboxane B_2, which represents the production of thromboxane A_2 by maximally stimulated platelets, was suppressed by 38% on fish oil alone and by 97% or greater on all doses of aspirin. Excretion of PGI_2-M, the main urinary metabolite of PGI_1, fell from 50ng/g of creatinine to 42 ng/g on fish oil alone. On 50 mg of aspirin per day, PGI_2-M excretion was 26 ng/g of creatinine, while on 100 mg and 325 mg of aspirin per day, PGI_2-M, was 24 ng/g and 27 ng/g, respectively. In contrast with the marked aspirin-induced decline in PGI_2-M, PGI_3-M excretion was not affected by the addition of aspirin, even at the higher doses. Thus, moderate dose aspirin at 325 mg per day or less taken once daily has no effect on PGI_3 despite significantly reducing PGI_2 production. This suggests that endothelial cell cyclooxygenase is minimally inhibited by such doses of aspirin and that a large percent of the PGI_2 produced in patients with advanced CAD derives from the transfer of prostaglandin endoperoxides from activated platelets to endothelial cells. The loss of these substrates accounts for the decrease in PGI_2 with moderate-dose aspirin. Thus, the aspirin-induced decrease in PGI_2 may in large part be an unavoidable consequence of aspirin-induced platelet cyclooxygenase inhibition. Aspirin does not negate the potentially beneficial effects of n-3 fatty acids on the eicosanoid profile.

Phenacetin abuse is known to produce kidney disease; salicylate use is supposed to prevent cardiovascular disease. Dubach and associates[85] from Basel, Switzerland, and Boston, Massachusetts, conducted a prospective, longitudinal epidemiologic study to examine the effects of these two drugs on cause-specific mortality and on cardiovascular mortality. In 1968 the authors evaluated a study group of 623 healthy women, 30 to 49 years old who had evidence of a regular intake of phenacetin and a matched control group of 621 women. Salicylate excretion also was measured. All subjects were examined over 20 years. Life-table analyses of mortality during the 20 years, with adjustment for the year of birth, cigarette smoking, and length of follow-up, revealed significant differences between the groups in overall mortality (study group vs. control group, 74 vs. 27 deaths; relative risk, 2.2), deaths due to urologic or renal disease (relative risk, 16.1), deaths due to cancer (relative risk, 1.9), and deaths due to cardiovascular disease (relative risk, 2.9). The relative risk of cardiovascular disease (fatal or nonfatal AMI, CHF, or stroke) was 1.8. The odds ratio for the incidence of hypertension was 1.6. The effects of phenacetin on morbidity and mortality, with adjustment for base-line salicylate excretion, were similar. In contrast, salicylate use had no effect on either mortality or morbidity. Regular use of analgesic drugs containing phenacetin is associated with an increased risk of hypertension and mortality and morbidity due to cardiovascular disease, as well as an increased risk of mortality due to cancer and urologic or renal disease. The use of salicylates carries no such risk.

Lipid-lowering agents

Although specific guidelines for the treatment of hypercholesterolemia have been published, it is not known whether physicians treating patients likely to have lipid disorders have adopted the recommendations. Cohen and colleagues[86] in Bronx, New York, assessed the approach of cardiologists to the treatment of hypercholesterolemia in a metropolitan teaching hospital by interviewing patients with chest pain who were admitted for coronary angiography in 1988–1989 and by measuring fasting blood lipid profiles. At one month and again 12–24 months later, patients were contacted by telephone to determine if there had been any changes in treatment. Of 95 patients evaluated, 81 had CAD. Only 17% of those with high levels of total cholesterol and/or LDL cholesterol were being actively treated with diet and/or drugs. In the remaining patients, either lipid studies had not been done or abnormal results had not been addressed. There was little change in treatment approach during the month after the diagnostic procedure. Furthermore, the experience was similar in those patients subjected to CABG. One to 2 years after the initial intervention, 69 of the original study group could be contacted again. Although active dietary or pharmacological therapy was initiated in some individuals during this interval, it was stopped in others. Thirty-five percent of hypercholesterolemic patients were receiving targeted therapy.

Thus, only a small proportion of patients with documented CAD and hypercholesterolemia were being actively treated for their lipid disorder, suggesting that the published treatment guidelines have not yet been fully accepted.

To study the effects of fenofibrate, a lipid-lowering medication, on patients with CAD, Hahmann and associates[87] from Homburg, Federal Republic of Germany, analyzed 191 minor coronary narrowings in 42 patients with CAD by quantitative coronary angiography using computer-assisted contour detection. Computed parameters were percent diameter reduction and percent plaque area. A prospectively formed intervention group of 21 patients treated with special diet and fenofibrate (200 to 400 mg/day) was checked every 6 weeks with regard to risk factors. After a mean interval of 21 months, coronary angiography was repeated, using the same x-ray system and nearly identical projections. The intervention group was angiographically compared at follow-up with an untreated comparison group, also comprising 21 patients. Both groups had high initial serum cholesterol (mean 311 mg/dl) and LDL cholesterol levels (mean 235 mg/dl). Only among the treated patients did lipid levels change significantly: cholesterol, −19%; LDL cholesterol, −20%; HDL cholesterol, +19%; and triglycerides, −30%. At angiographic follow-up, the changes in percent diameter reduction and percent plaque area correlated positively with the mean serum and LDL cholesterol levels of the intervention group. Significant differences were found in the change in percent plaque area between both groups. The intervention subgroup with angiographic regressions (11 patients) had significantly lower serum and LDL cholesterol levels than the intervention subgroup with angiographic progressions (10 patients). These results indicate the beneficial effect of fenofibrate on minor coronary narrowings. Because of its high reproducibility in measuring minor narrowings, quantitative coronary angiography proved to be a suitable method for angiographic follow-up.

Nitroglycerin

A superb review of nitrate tolerance, its clinical relevance, and strategies for its prevention was provided by Elkayam[88] from Los Angeles, California.

To assess efficacy of transdermal nitrate use, de Milliano and associates[89] from 4 cities in The Netherlands, conducted a randomized, placebo-controlled trial of continuous and intermittent use of nitroglycerin patches (10 mg/24 hours) in 127 patients with stable angina pectoris who discontinued exercise testing within 9 minutes because of angina. After a placebo run-in week, baseline (day 0) symptom-limited exercise testing was performed and repeated on day 1 and 14 before and after the administration of 0.5 mg of sublingual nitroglycerin. On day 0, total exercise duration was the same (within narrow limits) in all 3 groups and remained unchanged in the placebo group. On day 1, total exercise duration increased from 406 ± 115 to 469 ± 158 seconds in the continuously treated group and from 396 ± 105 to 475 ± 171 seconds in the intermittently treated group. In the intermittent group, exercise duration increased slightly to 483 ± 140 seconds on day 14, and in the continuous group exercise duration decreased to 447 ± 144 seconds. However, this decrease was not statistically significant. Similar treatment effects were seen for time to 1-mm ST depression. Sublingual nitroglycerin remained effective in all 3 groups and on all days. Eleven actively treated patients and 1 patient taking placebo discontinued the study because of headache.

It is concluded that continuous use of transdermal nitroglycerin remains partially effective and intermittent therapy remains fully effective in improving long-term exercise capacity with acceptable adverse effects in patients with stable angina pectoris.

To resolve the controversy surrounding the antianginal use of chronic, continuous 24-hour transdermal nitroglycerin therapy, the Steering Committee of the Transdermal Nitroglycerin Cooperative Study[90] performed a double-blind, placebo controlled, randomized, parallel group study. Eligible patients had chronic angina pectoris with symptom-limited, reproducible treadmill tests and were responsive to sublingual nitroglycerin (n = 562). Patients were randomly assigned to placebo or 1 of 7 doses of active treatment (15, 30, 45, 60, 75, 90 and 105 mg/24 hours). In the active drug groups, treatment was initiated with 15 mg/24 hours during the first week of double-blind dosing with subsequent weekly increases until the assigned dose was reached, after which the dose was held constant. Treadmill tests were performed 0, 4 and 24 hours after the initial double-blind patches were applied, after each titration step and after 8 weeks. At the end of double-blind therapy, a sublingual nitroglycerin exercise challenge was repeated. Exercise tolerance in patients using the active patch increased 34 seconds over patients taking placebo 4 hours after the initial application of double-blind therapy, but there was no statistically significant difference in exercise time between placebo and active drug groups by 24 hours after the first application or for the remaining 8 weeks of the trial. Increasing the dose did not overcome the loss of effect. A partial attenuation of the response to a sublingual nitroglycerin challenge seen on exercise tolerance testing also occurred, with patients who received the highest dose showing the greatest attenuation. There were no differences in angina frequency among the groups, although in a post hoc analysis, patients with >7 attacks per week had a reduction in anginal frequency of 6 to 7 attacks per week with active treatment versus 2 attacks per week with placebo. The study showed that (1) tolerance to the exercise effects of continuous transdermal nitroglycerin develops within 24 hours after application; and (2) increasing the dose does not overcome this tolerance. The observation that symptomatic improvement may occur in the absence of increases in exercise tolerance seems deserving of further study.

Vasodilator therapy may be associated with reflex counter-regulatory responses, and these responses may play a role in the development of tolerance to nitroglycerin. Parker and coworkers[91] in Boston, Massachusetts studied standing systolic BP, body weight, urinary sodium, and hormonal responses to continuous and intermittent transdermal nitroglycerin administration in normal volunteers. There was rapid attenuation of the hypotensive response to transdermal nitroglycerin therapy in the continuous but not in the intermittent therapy group. Significant weight gain and sodium retention occurred during continuous but not during intermittent nitroglycerin therapy. This was accompanied by a greater decrease in hematocrit in the continuous group, a finding that suggests that plasma volume expansion occurred during continuous nitroglycerin therapy. Continuous nitroglycerin therapy was associated with increases in plasma norepinephrine, atrial natriuretic peptide, arginine, vasopressin, and plasma renin activity. A different pattern of neurohormonal response was seen during intermittent therapy, with values tending to return to baseline levels after the nitrate-free interval. Continuous transdermal nitroglycerin therapy leads to counter-regulatory responses associated with sodium retention and probable plasma volume expansion. By contrast, intermittent transdermal nitroglycerin therapy is associated with a different pattern of hormonal response, the lack of sodium retention and no evidence of plasma volume expansion. It is likely that these counter-regulatory responses play an important role in the attenuation of nitrate effects.

Isosorbide dinitrate and diltiazem

Lehmann and associates[92] from Munich, Federal Republic of Germany, compared in 14 patients with documented CAD the extent and duration of antiischemic, antianginal and hemodynamic effects of monotherapies with 120 mg of sustained-release isosorbide dinitrate and diltiazem. Their combined therapy administered once daily in the morning with diltiazem given again in the evening also were compared according to a randomized, double-blind, crossover, placebo-controlled protocol including exercise testing for assessment of ST-segment depression (ST ↓) at an identical work load, exercise capacity and determination of plasma concentrations of both substances. Comparison of individual substances revealed more marked and sustained effects of isosorbide dinitrate (ST ↓ at 2 hours, −66%; at 6 hours, −50%), remaining statistically significant up to 12 hours (−24%) than of diltiazem (2 hours, −30%; 6 hours, −16%). Combined therapy resulted in increased effects (ST ↓ at 2 hours, −80%; 6 hours, −76%; 12 hours, −30%) as opposed to individual substances for a period of up to 12 hours. However, therapeutic coverage over 24 hours could not be demonstrated, even with renewed administration of sustained-release diltiazem in the evening. Plasma concentrations of isosorbide-5-mononitrate were >250 ng/ml for 12 hours on days when isosorbide dinitrate was given, decreasing to <100 ng/ml at 24 hours. On days when diltiazem was given, plasma levels >50 ng/ml were detected at 2 and at 6 hours, and at 24 hours only after a second tablet was given.

Esmolol

To assess the efficacy and safety of the ultra short-acting β-blocking agent, *esmolol*, in acute unstable angina, Barth and colleagues[93] from St. Louis, Missouri, administered esmolol to 21 patients who had persistent angina despite conventional medical therapy. Following a baseline Doppler echocardiographic examination, esmolol was titrated to reduce the rate-pressure product by at least 20%. Once the patients had been receiving a maintenance dosage for 30 minutes, Doppler echocardiographic studies were repeated. Mean esmolol dose at target response was 17 ± 16 mg/min, with the dosage range of 8 to 24 mg/min. Esmolol was effective in alleviating anginal chest pain in 18 of the 21 patients. Seven patients eventually underwent PTCA and 8 had CABG. The remainder were discharged receiving medical therapy including oral β-blockade. During esmolol therapy, heart rate and BP decreased significantly (86 ± 14 to 68 ± 12 beats/min and 125 ± 16 to 103 ± 20 mm Hg). Cardiac output decreased from 5.4 ± 1.3 to 4.5 ± 1.1 L/min secondary to a decrease in heart rate as stroke volume remained unchanged. LVEF increased from 47 ± 12 to 49 ± 13 with esmolol therapy, although this change was not statistically significant. Both the one-third filling fraction as well as the ratio of early-to-late diastolic filling velocities increased with esmolol therapy (35 ± 8% to 38 ± 8% and 0.73 ± 0.2 to 0.85 ± 0.23), indicating improvement in LV diastolic function. Other than transient hypotension, which quickly resolved upon downward titration of the infusion, there were no significant side effects related to the administration of esmolol. Thus the use of ultra short-acting β-blockade as add-on therapy in patients with acute unstable angina appears to be both safe and effective. It should be considered early as a treatment option in these patients.

Esmolol is a new cardioselective B blocker with unique pharmacokinetic properties resulting in a half-life of only 9 minutes. Hohnloser and associates[94] from Freiburg, Germany, and other members of the European Esmolol Study Group in a multicenter, randomized, placebo controlled study examined the hemodynamic and antiischemic effects of esmolol given as an adjunctive to conventional medical therapy in 113 patients with unstable angina. Fifty-nine patients received esmolol and 54 received matching placebo infusions. Esmolol was titrated in a step-wise manner at dosages of 2 to 24 mg/min until a 25% reduction in the double product was achieved; thereafter, esmolol was continuously infused for up to 72 hours. Esmolol caused a significant and persistent decline in heart rate and blood pressure throughout the entire study period. Clinical events, such as development of AMI or the need for urgent revascularization, occurred in 3 esmolol compared with 9 placebo patients. There was also a trend toward reduction of silent ischemia as judged by Holter monitoring (mean [± standard deviation] duration/patient/24 hours, 21 ± 81 minutes in the esmolol and 35 ± 128 minutes in the placebo groups). Esmolol-related adverse effects were mostly cardiovascular in origin and could be managed promptly by downward dose titration or cessation of drug infusion. Thus, esmolol appears to be a safe and effective drug for patients with unstable angina because it permits a large degree of flexibility in adapting the desired level of B blockade to the patient's changing clinical presentation.

Celiprolol vs propranolol

Frishman and associates[95] for the Celiprolol International Study Group assessed the comparative antianginal effects and safety of propranolol and celiprolol, a highly B_1-selective adrenoceptor blocker with selective partial B_2-adrenoceptor agonist activity in an international multicenter, placebo run-in, active control, double-blind, randomized, titration-to-effect study of 140 patients with stable, exercise-induced angina pectoris. At baseline, all patients received placebo for 2 weeks, then titrated doses of once-daily celiprolol (200, 400, 600 mg) or twice-daily propranolol (total daily dose 80, 160, 320 mg) over 4 weeks, followed by a 2-week maintenance period. Heart rate and BP, at rest and with exercise, weekly anginal attack frequency, nitroglycerin consumption and symptom-limited treadmill exercise times (modified Bruce protocol) were assessed. Compared with their respective baselines, both celiprolol and propranolol reduced anginal attack and nitroglycerin consumption rates to a comparable degree, while improving exercise tolerance. Treatment with propranolol compared with celiprolol, however, was associated with a significantly lower heart rate at rest. The double-product at the conclusion of exercise testing was significantly reduced by both drugs. Celiprolol and propranolol had similar effects on blood pressure, and were well tolerated. More symptomatic bradycardia occurred with propranolol. Despite the differences in their hemodynamic actions, once-daily celiprolol is as effective as twice-daily propranolol in the treatment of patients with stable angina pectoris.

Atenolol ± nifedipine

Hill and associates[96] from Gainesville, Florida, investigated the effects of atenolol (100 mg/day) and nifedipine (20 mg 3 times daily) and their combination on ambulant myocardial ischemia using a randomized, double-blind, placebo-controlled, crossover trial. Eighteen men with symptomatic CAD, exercise-induced ischemia and minimal symptoms, underwent 4 blinded treatment periods of 2 weeks' duration (2 placebo, 1 atenolol, 1 nifedipine). Those that did not have ischemia eliminated by monotherapy received combination therapy with both drugs. Forty-eight-hour ambulatory electrocardiographic monitoring was used to quantitate ischemic parameters at the end of each period. Both nifedipine and atenolol as monotherapy reduced the number of ischemic episodes and the average duration of each episode compared with placebo. Compared with placebo, nifedipine reduced the total duration of ischemia but the effect of atenolol on ischemia duration was of borderline significance. There were no differences in reduction of ischemic parameters when atenolol was compared with nifedipine (difference not significant). In the 9 patients who continued to have ischemia with monotherapy, combination therapy eliminated it in 2 and reduced the duration by >50% in the remaining patients compared with placebo. In conclusion, monotherapy with nifedipine or atenolol is similarly effective in eliminating or reducing ambulant ischemia. Combination therapy can provide additional benefit in those with continued ischemia.

Metoprolol vs nifedipine

Ardissino and associates[97] from Italy, Denmark, and Sweden classified the clinical characteristics of 65 patients with mixed angina pectoris by means of (1) a questionnaire investigating the proportion of symptoms occurring at rest and on effort, (2) an exercise stress test, (3) 24-hour ambulatory Holter monitoring, and (4) coronary angiography. According to the questionnaire, the proportion of effort-induced anginal episodes ranged from 1 to 99%. The ischemic threshold during exercise testing ranged from 110×10^2 to 350×10^2 mm Hg $\times$ beats/min. At least 1 episode of St-segment depression was observed in 29 of the 65 patients during Holter monitoring. Ischemic episodes during Holter monitoring were more frequent in patients reporting 50% of anginal attacks on effort, with moderate to severe limitation of exercise capacity and with multivessel CAD. The effect on ambulatory ischemia of a 6-week treatment with a B blocker (metoprolol CR, 200 mg once daily) or a dihydropyridine calcium antagonist (nifedipine retard 20 mg twice daily) were then compared according to a double-blind, parallel group design. Metoprolol significantly reduced the number and duration of the ischemic episodes during daily life irrespective of the patients' clinical characteristics. Nifedipine was ineffective, particularly in patients with angina predominantly on effort and with a moderate to severe reduction in exercise tolerance. It is concluded that in patients with mixed angina, ischemic episodes during daily life are more likely to occur in patients with a clinical presentation suggesting poor coronary reserve. The administration of a B blocker is highly effective in reducing ambulatory ischemia and should be considered as initial antiischemic treatment for mixed angina.

Diltiazem

Silent myocardial ischemia is an adverse prognostic marker in patients with CAD; however, controlled data on the effect of treatment are sparse and contradictory, and the relations among the occurrence of ST segment depression, drug, efficacy, and heart rate are unclear. Theroux and coworkers[98] in Montreal, Canada, assessed sixty patients with stable CAD, a positive treadmill exercise test and asymptomatic ST segment depression on ambulatory electrocardiographic record in a multicenter, double-blind, placebo-controlled, cross-over trial. Treadmill exercise tests and 72-hour electrocardiographic recordings were obtained at the end of two 2-week treatment periods with sustained-release diltiazem b.i.d. or equivalent placebo. Episodes of asymptomatic ST depression decreased by 50% or more in 70% of the patients from a median number of 4.5 to 1.5; their cumulative duration also decreased from 78.5 to 24.5 minutes (Figure 2-15). No circadian variation was found in the efficacy of diltiazem. The occurrence of ischemic type ST segment depression was modulated by changes in heart rate rather than by absolute heart rate. Diltiazem also improved exercise test end points but to a lesser extent. Time to ST segment depression increased to 341 from 296 seconds. Although less frequent with diltiazem administration, exercise-induced ST depression was more often asymptomatic. The investigators concluded that diltiazem reduces the frequency and severity of ischemic type ST depression in patients with stable CAD.

Diperdipine

The acute hemodynamic effects of a new dihydropyridine calcium channel blocker, diperdipine, which is suitable for intravenous administration, were studied by right and left cardiac catheterization in 16 patients with CAD by Di Donato and colleagues[99] from Florence, Italy, and Berlin, West Germany. Diperdipine markedly reduced systemic vascular resistance and improved stroke index and LVEF. Mean PA and PA wedge pressures were slightly increased as a possible consequence of enhanced venous return, whereas RA and LV end-diastolic pressures were not significantly changed. Nevertheless, an increase in preload was clearly indicated by an augmented LV end-diastolic index after administration of diperdipine. LV contractility, which was estimated by the end-systolic pressure-volume ratio and by maximal rate of LV systolic pressure rise was not significantly changed, though analysis of individual data suggests a minimally negative inotropic effect. However, such a minor effect on LV contractility was largely counterbalanced by the marked reduction of afterload, which produced a sharp improvement of stroke index. Enhancement of LVEF and reduction in systemic vascular resistance were inversely and directly correlated to control values. Overall, diperdipine was well tolerated, but 1 patient had a major untoward reaction that consisted of an ischemic episode that was possibly related to drug administration. In conclusion, intravenous diperdipine appears to be a potent arteriolar dilating agent that does not affect LV contractility.

Bepridil vs diltiazem

Singh[100] for the Bepridil Collaborative Study Group evaluated the efficacy and safety of bepridil hydrochloride (200–400 mg/day) in patients with chronic stable angina refractory to maximal tolerated doses of dil-

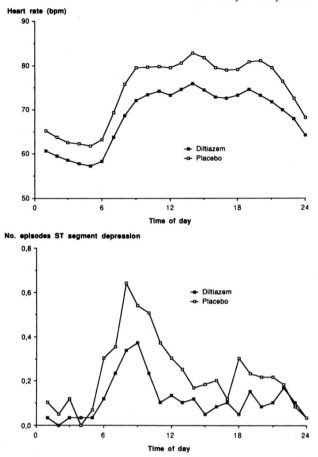

Fig. 2-15. Plots of heart rate (top panel) and distribution of episodes of ST depression (bottom panel) during 24 hours with placebo and diltiazem treatment. Diltiazem reduced both variables evenly during 24 hours except for a slightly greater effect on episodes of ST segment depression when the heart rate was faster and when episodes of ST depression were more frequent. The occurrence of ST depression correlated much better with heart rate changes than with absolute heart rates. Accelerating heart rate observed between 6:00 and 9:00 am is accompanied by an increasing incidence of episodes and the slowing from 8:00 pm to midnight by a decreasing incidence. At other times, when heart rate is more constant, episodes of ST segment depression are fewer with less variation in frequency. Reproduced with permission of Theroux, et al.[98]

tiazem (median 360 mg/day) in a randomized, multicenter, double-blind, parallel study. Baseline diltiazem data were obtained during a 2-week period, after which 86 patients were randomized to bepridil (n = 46) or diltiazem (n = 40). Angina frequency, nitroglycerin consumption and ischemic manifestations induced by exercise treadmill testing were evaluated over 8 weeks. Bepridil significantly increased time to angina onset, time to 1 and 2 mm of ST-segment depression, total exercise time and total work over baseline values. Changes in time to angina onset and time to 1 mm of ST-segment depression were significantly greater for bepridil than for diltiazem. Angina frequency and nitroglycerin consumption did not differ significantly between groups. Compared with baseline, bepridil significantly decreased heart rate (mean 4 beats/min) and prolonged QTc (mean 35 ms). The most frequent adverse effects in both groups were nausea, asthenia, dizziness, headache and diarrhea. Four patients taking bepridil and 1 taking diltiazem withdrew from the study because of adverse reactions. No sudden deaths, AMI or instances of sustained VT or torsades de pointes occurred in either group. The data indicate that bepridil provided safe and effective antianginal and antiischemic therapy in patients with chronic stable angina who exhibited less than optimal response to maximal tolerated doses of diltiazem.

Felodipine

To investigate the antiischemic efficacy and duration of action of the dihydropyridine calcium antagonist felodipine, Santoro and associates[101] from Piza, Italy, enrolled 15 patients with stable exertional angina in a double-blind, cross-over study comparing 2 doses (5 and 10 mg) of felodipine extended release (ER) and placebo given once daily for 1 week. Bicycle exercise tests were repeated at the end of each treatment period 4 and 24 hours after dosing. Four hours after dosing with both felodipine doses, only 5 patients discontinued the exercise test because of 2 mm of ST-segment depression, whereas 10 continued until exhaustion. Compared with placebo, total exercise time was increased by 19%, with no difference between doses. After 24 hours, exercise duration was prolonged up to physical exhaustion in 6 patients taking felodipine 10 mg; moreover, 11 patients taking 10 mg and 5 taking 5 mg increased time to 1 mm of ST depression 15% compared with exercise time during the placebo test. Mean time to 1 mm of ST depression at 24 hours was increased by 8% with 5 mg and by 18% with 10 mg. Total exercise time at 24 hours was increased with both doses with greater efficacy with the 10-mg dose. This increased exercise tolerance may be attributed to a reduced afterload and increased myocardial oxygen supply: systolic BP at rest was reduced, and rate-pressure product at 1 mm of ST depression was increased. In conclusion, a once-daily administration of felodipine ER provides antiischemic activity for 24 hours; the 5- and 10-mg doses are equally effective 4 hours after dosing, whereas the 10-mg dose is more efficacious at 24 hours. Because no differences in tolerability were observed, the 10-mg dose should be preferred for the once-daily treatment of chronic stable angina.

Nifedipine

Nesto and associates[102] from Boston, Massachusetts, assessed the effect of nifedipine versus placebo on total myocardial ischemic activity and circadian distribution of ischemic episodes in a randomized, double-blind, cross-over study involving 10 patients. After baseline exercise treadmill testing and 48-hour ambulatory electrocardiographic ST-segment monitoring, patients received either nifedipine (mean dose, 80 mg/day) or placebo administered 4 times per day, with the initial dose taken immediately upon arising in the morning. Patients were maintained on a stable dose of each study drug for 7 days, after which they underwent repeat exercise treadmill testing and 48-hour ambulatory electrocardiography. During exercise treadmill testing, greater exercise duration was achieved by patients receiving nifedipine than by those receiving placebo (421 ± 121 vs 353 ± 155 seconds, respectively). Time to >1 mm ST depression was significantly greater with nifedipine (282 ± 146 seconds) than at baseline (130 ± 72 seconds) and with placebo (150 ± 98 seconds). During ambulatory electrocardiographic monitoring, nifedipine reduced both the total number of ischemic episodes (18 vs 54 at baseline and 63 with placebo) and the total duration of ischemia (260 vs 874 at baseline and 927 minutes with placebo). The surge of ischemia between 06:00 and 12:00 noted at baseline and during placebo therapy was nearly abolished during nifedipine treatment. Nifedipine at this dosage, administered in this manner, is effective in reducing total ischemic activity and may prevent morning surges of ischemic episodes.

Nifedipine ± metoprolol

Melandri and associates[103] from Bologna, Italy, tested the usefulness of a sustained intravenous infusion of nifedipine and a combination of nifedipine and metoprolol in the early management of 14 patients with unstable angina pectoris. After a 24-hour run-in period, nifedipine was titrated in a stepwise fashion (mean dose 27 ± 7 µg/min). After nifedipine treatment coronary blood flow increased from 150 ± 66 to 183 ± 74 ml/min, whereas double product, myocardial oxygen consumption, and both arterial and coronary sinus norepinephrine levels were unchanged. Myocardial lactate uptake increased from 3.4 ± 26 to 31 ± 27 µmol/min and free fatty acid uptake from 7.2 ± 22 to 35 ± 34 µmol/min. A small nonsignificant improvement in amino acid metabolism was observed. Metoprolol was added in 7 patients and led to a decrease in double product and myocardial oxygen consumption. The lactate uptake/oxygen uptake ratio increased by 18% after metoprolol. The number of episodes of chest pain decreased from 2.4 ± 1.1/24 hours to 0.1 ± 0.2 in the nifedipine group and from 2.9 ± 1.1/24 hours to 0.3 ± 0.5 in the nifedipine plus metoprolol group. It was concluded that in the acute phase of unstable angina, intravenous nifedipine can be carefully titrated to improve coronary blood flow and oxidative metabolism. The addition of metoprolol is also associated with a reduction in myocardial oxygen demand. This treatment results in significant hemodynamic stability.

In an investigation performed by Egstrup[104] from Odense, Denmark, the circadian variation of total ischemic activity was examined during 3289 hours of ambulatory electrocardiographic monitoring in 101 patients with stable angina pectoris and proved CAD, who were not receiving any prophylactic antianginal therapy. The 101 patients displayed 411 episodes of ischemia, 312 (76%) of which were silent; a circadian rhythm was noted for the occurrence of total and silent ischemia. Thirty-eight percent of the ischemic episodes occurred between 6 A.M. and 12 noon, and total and silent ischemia were significantly more frequent during this period compared with the other 3 6-hour periods; a lesser peak was noted in the evening. The effects of metoprolol and combined therapy with metoprolol and nifedipine on the circadian variation of ischemic activity were studied in 2 subgroups of patients in a random, double-blind study design (31 patients receiving metoprolol and 42 receiving combined therapy). During therapy with metoprolol the morning increase in ischemic activity was attenuated, and the highest frequency of ischemia was then noted in the evening (6 A.M. to 12 noon compared with 6 P.M. to 12 midnight). Combined therapy abolished the morning peak as did metoprolol monotherapy, but even the evening increase in ischemic activity was attenuated. The diurnal distribution of the mean heart rate at the onset of ischemia, when patients were off therapy, showed a morning increase similar to the increase in ischemic activity but no second peak in the evening. A significant and equal reduction in the mean heart rate at the onset of ischemia was noted during therapy with metoprolol and combined therapy. This decrease in the heart rate at the onset of ischemia indicates that the main antiischemic effect of metoprolol is mediated through a reduction in myocardial oxygen demand with the most pronounced effect in the morning hours when the sympathetic tone is highest. However, attenuation of both the morning and evening peaks of ischemic activity during combined therapy suggests that a decrease in the myocardial oxygen supply may be more detrimental in the evening. This may have clinical relevance in regard to the use of various antiischemic drugs and the time of administration.

Nisoldipine

Tzivoni and associates[105] from Jerusalem, Israel, assessed the antiischemic properties of nisoldipine, a dihydropyridine calcium antagonist, in a multicenter, double-blind, placebo-controlled trial by repeated exercise testing and 72-hour ambulatory electrocardiographic monitoring in 82 patients with CAD. Patients with positive treadmill stress test results and ≥2 ischemic episodes per 24 hours were included in this study. Administration of all chronic antiischemic medications except B blockers were discontinued. During the first week all patients received placebo twice daily. During the second and third weeks, 41 patients received nisoldipine 10 mg and 41 patients received placebo twice daily. In the placebo group there were no changes in exercise parameters or in ambulatory electrocardiographic parameters. In the nisoldipine group, exercise duration increased from 403 to 448 seconds, time to 1 mm of ST depression increased from 224 to 298 seconds, time to pain increased from 241 to 321 seconds, and maximal ST depression was reduced from 2.6 to 2.3 mm. Among the ambulatory electrocardiographic parameters in the nisoldipine group, only the number of episodes was reduced, from 14.4 to 11.6 per patient. There was no significant reduction in total ischemic time (132 vs 120 minutes per patient). No significant side effects were observed. This is the largest clinical trial to date on the effects of nisoldipine on myocardial ischemia. The results indicate the nisoldipine was effective in improving all exercise parameters and only partially effective in suppressing ischemia during daily activity.

Frishman and associates[106] of the Nisoldipine Multicenter Angina Study Group assessed the duration and extent of antianginal effects of nisoldipine, a dihydropyridine calcium antagonist, in 178 patients with chronic stable angina pectoris. Using a placebo run-in, placebo-controlled, randomized, parallel study design, patients received placebo twice daily for 2 to 3 weeks and were then randomized to receive either placebo (n = 42), nisoldipine 10 mg once daily (n = 44), nisoldipine 10 mg twice daily (n = 47) or nisoldipine 20 mg once daily (n = 45) for 5 weeks. Frequency of angina and nitroglycerine consumption were assessed by weekly patient diaries. Exercise tolerance time was assessed at baseline and at weeks 1, 3 and 5 in the double-blind phase. Peak effects after 5 weeks of double-blind medication showed significant or nearly significant improvements with nisoldipine over placebo in time to termination of exercise, time to onset of angina, and time to onset of 1 mm ST-segment depression. There were no significant improvements in trough effects with nisoldipine. Also, placebo was not significantly different from nisoldipine in either the number of anginal attacks or nitroglycerin consumed. Although significantly more drug-related, adverse effects were observed with the nisoldipine regimen, 20 mg once daily, compared with placebo, nisoldipine appears to be an effective and well-tolerated antianginal drug. However, its duration of antianginal action, as measured by exercise stress testing, is relatively short. The drug needs to be examined using shorter dosing intervals and higher daily doses, or in a longer-acting sustained-release formulation.

Enalapril or captopril

Activation of neurohumoral hormones or sulfhydryl group depletion may contribute to the development of nitroglycerin tolerance. In an attempt to prevent nitrate tolerance, Katz and co-investigators[107] in Washington, D.C., evaluated the interaction of nitroglycerin with angiotensin converting enzyme inhibitors with and without a sulfhydryl group. Thirty-four subjects were randomized to a 7-day regimen of enalapril 10 mg twice a day, captopril 25 mg three times a day, or placebo. Venodilator response to nitroglycerin was assessed with forearm plethysmography by measuring the change in venous volume after administration of 0.4 mg sublingual nitroglycerin. Plethysmographic measurements were obtained serially (1) at baseline, (2) after 4 days angiotensin converting enzyme inhibition or placebo, (3) 2 hours after application of a 10 mg/24 hr nitroglycerin patch, and (4) 74 hours after continuous nitropatch application. Angiotensin converting enzyme inhibition alone caused no significant change in the response to sublingual nitroglycerin. Nitrate response remained unchanged after 2 hours of nitropatch exposure in all three groups. After 74 hours of continuous nitropatch application, the venodilator response to sublingual nitroglycerin was reduced by 40% in the placebo group, 10% in the enalapril group, and 2% in the captopril group. This attenuation was significant only in the placebo group. Pairwise comparison of nitrate response between groups was significantly different between the captopril and placebo groups and between the placebo and enalapril groups. Plasma rein levels increased equally in the enalapril and captopril groups. Body weight increased only in the placebo group suggesting prevention of nitrate-induced volume expansion in the angiotensin converting enzyme inhibitor groups. This study demonstrates that angiotensin converting enzyme inhibitors may prevent nitrate tolerance to long-term nitrate therapy.

Serotonin

Golino and colleagues[108] from Naples, Italy, and Houston, Texas, measured the cross-sectional area of the coronary artery by quantitative angiography and coronary blood flow with an intracoronary Doppler catheter. Measurements were obtained at baseline and during intracoronary infusions of serotonin (0.1, 1, and 10 µg per kilogram of body weight per minute for 2 minutes). The measurements of cross-sectional area of the coronary artery were repeated after an infusion of ketanserin, an antagonist of serotonin receptors thought to block the effect of serotonin on receptors in the arterial wall but not in the endothelium. In patients with normal coronary arteries, the highest dose of serotonin increased cross-sectional area by 52% and blood flow by 58%. This effect was significantly potentiated by the administration of ketanserin. In patients with coronary-artery atherosclerosis, serotonin reduced cross-sectional area by 64% and blood flow by 59%. Ketanserin prevented this effect. Therefore, serotonin has a vasodilating effect on normal human coronary arteries. However, when the endothelium is damaged, as in coronary artery disease, serotonin has a direct, unopposed vasoconstricting effect that may be blocked by serotonin receptor antagonists. These data are consistent with the hypothesis that platelet-derived substances, such as serotonin, may have a role in certain acute CAD syndromes.

Serotonin, a major product of platelet activation, has potent vasoactive effects in nonhuman animals, but its role in humans remains largely speculative. Using quantitative coronary angiography, McFadden and associates[109] from London, UK, compared the effects of intracoronary infusion of graded concentrations of serotonin on coronary arteries in 2 groups of patients with different clinical presentations of CAD (9 with stable angina and 5 with variant angina), with the effects in a control group of 8 subjects with normal arteries on angiogram. Normal coronary arteries had a biphasic response to intracoronary serotonin; dilation at concentrations up to 10^{-5} mol/L, but constriction at £0^{-4} mol per liter. Arteries in patients with stable angina constricted at all concentrations, with mean (± SEM) maximal decreases in diameter of 23.9 ± 3.6, 33.1 ± 3.9 and 41.7 ± 3.1% from base line in proximal, middle, and distal segments at a serotonin concentration of 10^{-4} mol per liter. Smooth segments constricted more than irregular segments (42 ± 5 vs 21 ± 2%). Four patients with stable angina had a marked reduction in collateral filling. All the patients with stable angina had angina during the intracoronary infusion of serotonin, and electrocardiographic changes were noted in 6. All the patients with variant angina had angina, electrocardiographic changes, and localized occlusive epicardial coronary-artery spasm at concentrations of 10^{-6} (n = 2) or 10^{-5} (n = 3) mol per liter. Patients with stable CAD do not have the normal vasodilator response to intracoronary serotonin, but rather have progressive constriction, which is particularly intense in small distal and collateral vessels. Patients with variant angina have occlusive coronary-artery spasm at a dose that dilates normal vessels and causes only slight constriction in vessels from patients with stable angina. These findings suggest that serotonin, released after the intracoronary activation of platelets, may contribute to or cause myocardial ischemia in patients with CAD.

PERCUTANEOUS TRANSLUMINAL CORONARY ANGIOPLASTY

With coronary angiography

If PTCA can be safely performed at the time of the initial diagnostic catheterization, it may result in shorter hospitalization stays and lower overall costs. Combined coronary angiography and PTCA were performed electively on 733 patients between January 1, 1984, and September 1, 1988 in a study by O'Keefe and associates[110] from Kansas City, Missouri. These patients were divided into 3 major subgroups based upon their indications for angioplasty: 444 (61%) procedures were performed for restenosis; 190 (26%) procedures were performed for unstable angina; and 99 (13%) procedures were performed in patients without unstable angina or previous PTCA. A subset of 219 patients from this study who underwent elective combined coronary angiography and PTCA during 1986 were compared with a matched population of 191 patients from the same year who had elective PTCA utilizing a traditional staged approach (coronary angiography and PTCA as separate procedures). The success and complication rates were similar for both of these groups. Patients who underwent the combined procedure were hospitalized for a mean of 4.6 days with average total charges of $11,128 compared with 8.0 days and $13,160 for patients undergoing separate procedures. Significant savings were also realized with respect to total contrast dose, fluoroscopic time, and total procedure time. Thus in informed patients with suitable coronary anatomy, the strategy of combined angiography and PTCA may present an opportunity for decreasing hospitalization stay, reducing total charges for revascularization, and reducing radiation exposure without compromising the safety or effectiveness of the procedure.

In angina pectoris

In a cohort of 1,720 consecutive patients from the National Heart, Lung, and Blood Institute, PTCA Registry (August 1985–May 1986), Bentivoglio and associates[111] from several USA medical centers compared 768 patients (45%) with stable angina and 952 patients (55%) with unstable angina. Unstable angina patients exhibited at least 1 of the following characteristics: new onset angina, rapidly progressing angina, angina at rest, angina refractory to medication, variant angina, acute coronary insufficiency, or angina recurring shortly after an AMI. The distribution of single- and multi-vessel disease was similar among stable and unstable angina patients; multi-vessel disease predominated. Average severity of stenosis and incidence of tubular and diffuse stenosis morphology were higher among patients with unstable angina. Patient success rates were similar in stable and unstable patients. However, on a per lesion basis, overall angiographic success rate and average reduction of severity of stenosis in successfully dilated lesions were significantly higher among patients with unstable angina. Incidence of major patient complications and of emergency CABG were also higher in patients with unstable angina but consistent with their more precarious clinical condition and stenosis morphology. During a 2-year follow-up, the cumulative distributions of death, AMI, repeat PTCA, and CABG were not significantly different in patients with stable angina compared to patients with unstable angina. Comparison of the current PTCA Registry cohort with the cases reported in the 1979–1982 Registry revealed a 19% higher success rate for both stable and unstable angina patients. Major complication rates decreased between time periods for stable but not for unstable angina patients. Incidence of emergency bypass surgery decreased more for stable than for unstable angina patients. Coronary angioplasty is indicated in properly selected patients with unstable angina and both single- and multi-vessel CAD.

In older patients

Between 1981 and 1990 Bedotto and associates[112] from Kansas City, Missouri, performed PTCA in 1,373 patients ≥65 years of age (mean 71 ± 5). These patients underwent 1,640 multivessel PTCA procedures. Of them, 224 patients (14%) had LVEF ≤40%, 412 (25%) had prior CABG and 48 (3%) had LM coronary dilatation. Of the 1,640 PTCA procedures, 697 were patients with 2-vessel disease and 943 were in patients with 3-vessel disease. A mean 3.5 lesions were dilated per patient, with an overall angiographic success rate of 96%. Complete revascularization was achieved in 857 (52%). A total of 52 patients (3%) had a major in-hospital complication: 27 patients (2%) died, 24 (1%) had a Q-wave myocardial infarction, and 14 (0.8%) underwent emergent CABG. Stepwise logistic regression analysis identified EF ≤40%, 3-vessel disease, female gender, and PTCA between 1981 and 1985 as independent predictors of mortality. Of the 1,373 patients, 1,023 have been followed for ≥1 year (mean follow-up 32.5 ± 21.3 months). There were 156 (15%) late deaths, 81 (8%) recurrent myocardial infarctions, and 162 (16%) CABGs. Actuarial survival, computed from the time of hospital discharge, was 92% at 1 year, 86% at 3 years and 78% at 5 years. Repeat PTCA was required in 371 patients (36.3%). Survival was better in those with 2- versus 3-vessel disease and in those with complete versus partial revascularization. These data indicate that multivessel PTCA is an effective and safe alternative to CABG in older patients with symptomatic coronary artery disease.

Thompson and associates[113] in Jacksonville, Florida, and Rochester, Minnesota, evaluated the immediate and long-term efficacy of PTCA in the elderly by studying 752 patients ≥65 years old and comparing patients ≥75 years old with those 65 to 74 years of age. The older patients were more highly symptomatic, they were more likely to have CHF, they were more likely to have multivessel CAD, and they were more likely to have multivessel PTCA. The immediate success rate of PTCA was higher in the oldest patients (93% vs 82%). The hospital mortality rate was also higher (6% vs 2%). Long-term overall survival was high. However, long-term event-free survival was lowest in the oldest patients, and recurrent severe angina was particularly common. Therefore, in elderly patients, PTCA is usually successful, but long-term relief from angina is less common than in younger patients.

In an investigation carried out by Little and associates[114] from Washington, D.C., results of multilesion PTCA were compared in 210 elderly patients (70 to 92 years, [group I]) and 210 younger patients (40 to 69 years, [group II]). The elderly patients included more women (43% vs 24%) and patients with unstable angina (73% vs 55%). PTCA was successful in 87% of lesions in group I and in 94% in group II. Only LC dilatation was less successful in group I (78% versus 91%). PTCA was successful in all lesions of ≥1 vessel in 89% of group I patients and in 94% of group II patients. Successful dilatation of all lesions was achieved in 77% of group I and in 85% of group II patients. Complication rates were similar for both groups. These data demonstrate a high rate of success and safety in elderly patients undergoing multilesion PTCA despite the presence of several risk factors (advanced age, female sex, unstable angina). The lower PTCA success rate in these patients compared with young subjects is almost entirely attributable to reduced success for LC lesions.

Mick and associates[115] from Cleveland, Ohio, evaluated early and late results for octogenarians undergoing first revascularization with PTCA or CABG. The study group consisted of 142 patients with CABG and 53 with PTCA. The groups with PTCA and CABG differed with respect to number of patients with angina class III to IV (92 and 67%, respectively), number with 3-vessel CAD (34 and 77%, respectively), presence of LM CAD (2 and 24%, respectively), and number with normal or mildly impaired LV function (82 and 65%, respectively). The groups with PTCA and CABG had similar procedural complications, including AMI (6 and 4%, respectively) and stroke (0 and 4%, respectively). Hospital mortality was low (6% with CABG and 2% with PTCA). Three-year survival, excluding hospital mortality, was 87% in patients with CABG and 81% in those with PTCA (Figure 2-16). Octogenarians underwent revascularization procedures with relatively low morbidity and mortality. In regard to the excellent long-term

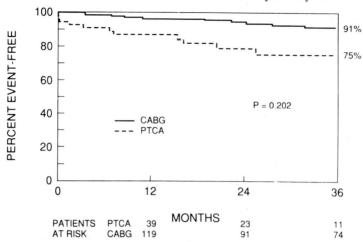

Fig. 2-16. Survival of octogenarians after coronary revascularization (free of cardiac death, myocardial infarction or coronary artery bypass grafting (CABG) (excluding hospital mortality). PTCA = percutaneous transluminal coronary angioplasty. Reproduced with permission of Mick et al.[115]

survival, "very" elderly patients with severe coronary artery disease should be considered for revascularization despite advanced age.

For total occlusions

PTCA of single total, subacute, or chronic coronary occlusions was performed in 90 patients in an investigation by Jost and colleagues[116] from Hannover, Germany. It was successful in 54 occlusions (60%), in 77% of those <6 weeks old, and in 44% of those >6 weeks duration. All procedures were uneventful. Control angiography was performed in 53 (98%) patients with successful angioplasty after an average interval of 97 ± 53 days. Stenosis had recurred in 16 patients (30%). During a follow-up period of 36 ± 13 months, 3 patients died, 5 patients underwent CABG, and 10 had repeat PTCA. Despite an additional late angiographic recurrence of stenosis in 7 patients, 36 patients revealed angiographic long-term success. In the 46 nonoperated patients, angina pectoris and exercise stress tests were substantially improved. Thus, PTCA of subacute and chronic total coronary occlusions is an uneventful procedure, the success rate depending on the duration of the occlusions. Despite a high angiographic recurrence rate, the angiographic and clinical long-term results are favorable.

The incidence of major complications after PTCA of a totally occluded artery was assessed retrospectively by Plante and colleagues[117] from Rotterdam, The Netherlands. A total of 1649 PTCA procedures were analyzed. After exclusion of procedures for AMI or total occlusion that resulted from restenosis, 90 patients were selected. Forty-four patients (49%) had stable angina and 46 (51%) had unstable angina. The estimated duration of occlusion was 87 ± 78 days in patients with stable angina, as compared with 10 ± 8 days in patients with unstable angina. Abrupt vessel closure during PTCA occurred only in patients with unstable angina (0% vs 17%). The major complication rate was 2.5% in the stable angina group, and 20% in unstable angina group. This rate was also significantly higher than the complication rate of 8% observed in 442 procedures that were performed during the same period in patients with unstable angina and nonocclusive stenosis. Patients with unstable angina who undergo PTCA of a totally occluded artery represent a subset at high risk for major complications.

Of left coronary artery with total occlusion of right coronary artery

In a study by De Bruyne and associates[118] from Brussels, Belgium, the safety and therapeutic benefits of PTCA of the LAD, the LC or both were assessed in 61 patients with chronic (>3 months) occlusion of the right coronary artery. Recanalization of the right coronary artery was not performed before dilatation of left coronary artery lesions. All lesions could be dilated without an acute ischemic event in the catheterization laboratory. However, 3 patients underwent CABG within the first 8 days after PTCA. There were no in-hospital deaths. Of the remaining 58 patients, 51 (88%) had repeat PTCA at a mean of 5.2 ± 2.5 months. Patients were divided into 2 groups according to the presence (n = 17) or absence (n = 34) of restenosis defined as ≥50% diameter stenosis at the dilated site. Baseline characteristics were comparable. The mean value for angina functional class at follow-up was significantly better in the group without than in the group with restenosis (0.4 ± 0.6 vs 2.1 ± 1.1). Sixty-five percent of the patients without restenosis were asymptomatic at follow-up. Seventy-five percent of the predicted maximal physical capacity was reached by 76% of the patients without restenosis compared with 33% in the group with restenosis. Results of exercise stress tests were clinically positive in 62% of patients with restenosis compared with 12% of patients without restenosis and ST-T depression was encountered more frequently in the former (75%) than in the latter group (21%). Among patients without restenosis, ST-T depression was often found during exercise when regional systolic function was normal or near normal in the myocardial segments depending on the right coronary artery. LVEF improved significantly in patients without restenosis at follow-up compared with the baseline value (55 ± 12% before PTCA vs 60 ± 12% at repeat angiography). Thus, in selected patients with chronic occlusion of the right coronary artery, PTCA of the left coronary artery results in a marked symptomatic improvement in the absence of restenosis, although the procedure provides incomplete anatomic revascularization by design.

Associated with left ventricular dysfunction

Stevens and associates[119] from Kansas City, Missouri, examined the risks and long-term outcome after 845 elective PTCA procedures in patients with LV dysfunction (EF ≤40%). Procedural results were compared with 8,117 consecutive procedures in patients with EF >40%. The patients with LV dysfunction were older (63 vs 60 years), had a greater incidence of prior myocardial infarction (84 vs 45%), prior bypass surgery (39 vs 21%), 3-vessel disease (62 vs 33%), and class IV angina (48 vs 41%) than the control group. Angiographic success was lower (93 vs 95%), and overall procedural mortality was increased (4 vs 1%) in the study group. Emergency surgery rates were identical (2%). No significant difference was found in rates of nonfatal Q-wave AMI (2 vs 1%). At mean follow-up of 33.5 months, 15% of the patients with LV dysfunction required late bypass surgery, 27% underwent repeat PTCA, and 59% were angina free. Actuarial survival at 1 and 4 years was 87 and 69%, respectively. Cox regression analysis identified 3-vessel disease, age ≥70 years, class IV angina and incomplete revascularization as correlates of long-term mortality. These data suggest that PTCA may be an effective treatment for CAD in patients with LV dysfunction.

Determinants of success

Savage and associates[120] in Philadelphia, Pennsylvania, used clinical and anatomic determinants of the initial success of PTCA in 826 patients enrolled in the Multi-Hospital Eastern Atlantic Restenosis Trial. The 639 men and 187 women ranged in age from 31 to 85 years. Successful PTCA was achieved in 886 (88.6%) of 1,000 lesions. Success rates were uniform among the eight individual centers. Outcome was not influenced by gender, age, or other clinical factors, including severity and duration of angina, prior AMI, rest pain, transient ST segment elevation, history of smoking or diabetes. In contrast, procedural outcome was significantly associated with lesion-specific angiographic factors. Stenoses 60% to 74%, 75% to 89%, 90% to 99%, and 100% were associated with success rates of 96%, 90%, 84%, and 69%, respectively. PTCA was less successful in calcified than in noncalcified lesions, in thrombotic than in nonthrombotic lesions, and in lesions in the right coronary artery than in other vessels. By multivariate logistic regression, preangioplasty percent stenosis, right coronary artery location, and lesion calcification were significant independent predictors of PTCA success. These results suggest that attempted PTCA is no longer adversely affected by previously important clinical features, including female gender or anatomic factors. Stenosis severity, calcium, thrombus, and right coronary artery location were the principal determinants of PTCA outcome.

Determinants of results in multivessel disease

Vandormael and associates[121] from St. Louis, Missouri, analyzed the predictors of 5-year cardiac survival in patients with multi-vessel CAD undergoing PTCA. The average age of the 637 patients was 59 ± 11 years in 472 men and in 165 women. Diabetes mellitus, previous myocardial infarction and unstable angina were present in 119 (19%), 261 (41%) and 305 (47%) patients, respectively. Angiographically, 460 patients had 2-vessel and 177 patients had 3-vessel CAD. The LV contraction score was ≥12 in 55 patients. Angiographic success (<50% residual stenosis) was achieved in 85% of the 1,343 narrowings and clinical success was obtained in 526 (83%) of the 637 patients. Complete revascularization was obtained in 177 (34%) of 526 successful patients. Procedure-related complications resulted in death in 9 patients (1.4%), in Q-wave myocardial infarction only in 6 patients (0.9%) and in emergency bypass surgery in 44 patients (6.9%) (of whom 10 had Q-wave myocardial infarction). Follow-up for ≥1 year and up to 6 years after PTCA was obtained in 608 (95%) of the 637 patients. To determine the predictors of 5-year cardiac survival, 28 clinical, angiographic and procedural variables were analyzed by Cox proportional-hazards regression. The estimated 5-year survival after PTCA was 88 ± 2% in successful patients and 77 ± 5% in patients in whom PTCA was unsuccessful (Figure 2-17). When clinical success was forced into the Cox regression, the LV contraction score of ≥12, diabetes mellitus and age ≥65 years showed additional adverse effects on survival. When analysis was limited to 503 patients with clinical success and ≥1 year

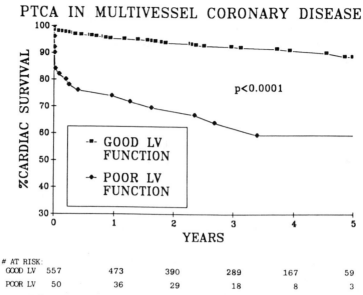

Fig. 2-17. Kaplan-Meier 5-year survival curves for patients with multivessel coronary artery disease with left ventricular (LV) contraction score ≥12 (poor LV function) and <12 (good LV function). The numbers of patients at risk in each group at each time interval are given at the bottom of the figure. The left ventriculogram was missing in 1 patient. Reproduced with permission of Vandormael, et al.[121]

complete follow-up, the only independent predictor of cardiac mortality was the LV score of ≥12. In conclusion, LV function was the most important determinant of cardiac survival in patients with multivessel CAD undergoing PTCA, independent of the clinical success of the procedure. Advanced age and diabetes mellitus were associated with additional risk in the overall group, but not in the successfully treated group. In patients with multivessel CAD, 5-year survival after PTCA is excellent in the absence of these adverse prognostic factors.

To assess the likelihood of intermediate-term event-free survival (freedom from death, CABG, and AMI) in patients with multivessel CAD undergoing PTCA, Ellis and colleagues[122] in Ann Arbor, Michigan evaluated and followed 350 consecutive patients from four clinical sites for 22 months. Eight clinical variables were evaluated at the clinical sites, and 23 angiographic variables describing the number, morphology, and topography of coronary stenoses were evaluated at a core angiographic laboratory. Most patients had Canadian Cardiovascular Society class II or IV angina, 2-vessel disease, and well-preserved LV function (mean EF, 58%). Follow-up was completed in 99% of patients. At 2 years, event-free survival was 72%, overall survival was 96%, freedom from CABG was 82%, and freedom from nonfatal AMI without surgery was 96%. Sequential Cox proportional hazards regression analyses allowing stepwise entry of variables prospectively coded as simple, as of intermediate complexity, or as complex found event-free survival to be independently predicted by low Canadian Cardiovascular Society angina class, no diabetes, no proximal LAD stenoses, and the sum of stenosis simplified risk-territory scores of ≤15. In the absence of class IV angina and these risk factors, 2-year event-free survival was 87% and overall survival was 100%. In the presence of ≥2 of these risk factors, event-free survival was <50%. Recognition of risk factors for poor long-term outcome in this setting may improve clinical decision making and provide a framework on which to base meaningful subgroup analyses in randomized trials assessing the efficacy of PTCA.

For "diffuse" narrowing

In this report by Goudreau and colleagues[123] from Richmond, Virginia, from January 1983 through December 1987, 98 patients underwent PTCA of ≥1 diffusely diseased coronary artery. Diffuse CAD was described as: group I, narrowing ≥50% that involved the entire vessel (40 patients); group II, long lesions ≥2 cm in length (39 patients); group III, ≥3 lesions in the same vessel (19 patients). There were 65 men and 33 women, with a mean age of 60 years; 64 patients (65%) had unstable angina, 23 patients (23%) were diabetic, 31 (32%) had prior myocardial infarctions, and 12 had prior CABG. Multivessel disease was present in 89% of patients. PTCA of only the diffusely diseased vessel was performed in 41 patients and additional vessels were dilated in 57 patients. Overall, of 396 lesions (4/patient) and 197 vessels (2/patient) attempted, success was achieved in 382 lesions (96%) and 187 vessels (95%); angiographic success was achieved in 112 of 120 diffusely diseased vessels (93%). Clinical success was achieved in 91 patients (93%). The overall complication rate (death, AMI, urgent CABG) was 8% (8 of 98); 6 patients (6%) had AMI (1 Q wave, 5 non-Q wave), 1 patient (1%) had urgent CABG, and 2 patients (2%) died (1 during CABG). The majority of complications (7 of 8 or 87%), including the 2 deaths, occurred in group I patients, with an 18% rate, versus 2.5% in group II and 0% in group III. Late follow-up data were available for 86 of 91 (95%) of successfully treated patients and ranged from 12 to 69 months (mean 29 months). Clinical recurrence occurred in 27 patients (31%): restenosis of the diffusely diseased vessel was present in 24 patients, and 3 patients had restenosis of another vessel. Restenosis was treated by repeat PTCA in 22 of 27 (81%) patients. Late myocardial infarction occurred in 4 patients (5%), and 4 patients (4.4%) died of cardiac causes during the follow-up period. Clinical recurrence and follow-up events were comparable for the 3 groups. Including those who had repeat PTCA, 72 patients (84%) maintained clinical improvement without AMI or CABG during the follow-up period. Actuarial survival was 93% at 36 months, and event-free survival (free of AMI and CABG) was 82% at 3 years after PTCA. Thus PTCA of diffuse CAD is safe and effective in selected patients. Immediate success and clinical recurrence rates are similar to results reported with PTCA for discrete lesions. However, the complication rate is higher and appears to be more frequent in the subgroup of patients with disease that involves the whole length of the vessel (group I).

Outcome after proven 4–12 month patency

The introduction of PTCA has changed the pattern of intervention in CAD. However, the long-term results in patients undergoing successful, elective, native-vessel PTCA are not yet fully characterized. Because the healing and subsequent proliferative response after angioplasty are time related, Weintraub and co-investigators[124] in Atlanta, Georgia, designed a study to determine the long-term outcome in patients whose dilated arteries have been demonstrated to be patent 4–12 months after successful, uncomplicated PTCA. The patients were grouped on the basis of 4–12 month catheterization into those whose vessels were angiographically "normal" or had luminal irregularities only at the PTCA sites, those whose vessels had luminal irregularities elsewhere with or without PTCA site luminal irregularities and those with significant obstructive disease at sites other than the PTCA sites. Of 1,502 such patients, long-term follow-up, was available in 1,491. At the time of the original angioplasty, the normal patients had a 2% incidence of multivessel disease; luminal irregularity patients, 9%; and obstructive disease patients, 59%. At angiographic restudy, 16% of the obstructive disease patients continued to have multivessel disease. The patients were followed for the events of death, AMI, CABG and repeat PTCA. The 6-year survival rate was 95%; cardiac survival, 96% and freedom from all events, 65%. The strongest correlate of events during follow-up was the angiographic status of the undilated segments. At 6 years, freedom from cardiac events was noted in 77% of the normal group, 61% of the luminal irregularity group, and 55% of the obstructive disease group. Diabetes and hypertension were also independent correlates of events (Figure 2-18). Results from the study show that associated disease in undilated segments is a strong predictor of late events in patients after successful, uncomplicated, restenosis-free PTCA. The need for further revascularization was frequent even in patients without obstructive disease. Completeness of revascularization is appropriate when possible, and limiting progression of CAD at sites remote from those dilated should improve on these late results.

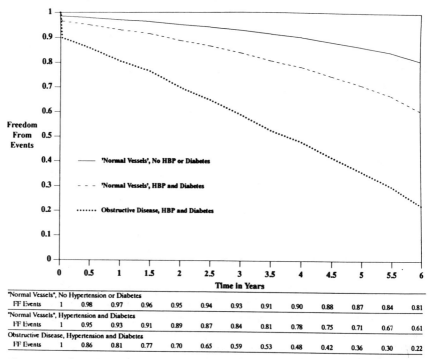

'Normal Vessels', No Hypertension or Diabetes												
FF Events 1	0.98	0.97	0.96	0.95	0.94	0.93	0.91	0.90	0.88	0.87	0.84	0.81
'Normal Vessels', Hypertension and Diabetes												
FF Events 1	0.95	0.93	0.91	0.89	0.87	0.84	0.81	0.78	0.75	0.71	0.67	0.61
Obstructive Disease, Hypertension and Diabetes												
FF Events 1	0.86	0.81	0.77	0.70	0.65	0.59	0.53	0.48	0.42	0.36	0.30	0.22

Fig. 2-18. Plots of predicted 6-year freedom from (FF) events in three patient profiles defined by Cox model. Profiles are patients who are angiographically normal without diabetes or hypertension (HBP), who are angiographically normal with diabetes and HBP, and who have obstructive disease and HBP. Reproduced with permission of Weintraub, et al.[124]

Late angiographic follow-up

In an investigation by Reeves and associates[125] from Montreal, Canada, 57 patients underwent PTCA of venous coronary bypass grafts from April 1981 to June 1987 and had a minimal follow-up of 18 months. The procedure was elective for 28 patients, urgent for 19, and was considered as an emergency for 10. A total of 64 grafts were dilated that had been bypassed 58 ± 48 months previously (range 2 to 184 months); lesions were located on the aortic anastomosis in 12 grafts, on the body in 38, and on the coronary anastomosis in 14. Technical success was 95% (61 of 64) per lesion; clinical success was 84% (54 of 64) per lesions and 83% (47 of 57) per patient. Thrombotic complications with images of a lacunar defect occurred in 11 grafts (17%). Predictive factors for these complications were: age of grafts (39% for >60 month grafts versus 2.6% for <60 month grafts); site of lesion (body lesion 29% versus anastomosis none); type of lesion (concentric and short 6% versus other 29%); and recent fibrinolysis (66% versus 11%). Long-term follow-up was available in the 47 successful patients and the 3 limited non-Q wave myocardial infarction patients. Two patients died at 13 and 17 months. Long-term angiographic follow-up was available in 45 of 48 patients (94%). At the end of the study, 35 of 57 (61%) venous bypass grafts in 32 patients (64%) were patent after ≥1 PTCAs. Ten patients (20%) had a second surgical procedure for restenosis and 6 (12%) had an occluded graft. Overall rate of restenosis including late sudden deaths was 56% (32 of 57 lesions), with a final patency rate after eventual repeat PTCA of 93% (13 of 14) for coronary anastomosis, 64% (7 of 11) for aortic anastomosis, and only 47% (15 of 32) for body graft lesions. In conclusion, PTCA of a venous bypass graft is a valuable procedure for recurrent angina in operated patients; careful selection and close follow-up improve its long-term success.

For aorto-coronary saphenous vein grafts

Plokker and associates[126] from 3 cities in The Netherlands analyzed data in 454 patients among their 19,994 patients who had angioplasty of one or more saphenous vein bypass grafts. In 46% of patients single graft angioplasty was attempted, and in 54% of patients sequential graft angioplasty was attempted. The clinical primary success rate was 90%. In-hospital mortality was 0.7%, 2.8% of patients sustained a procedural myocardial infarction, and 1.3% of patients underwent emergency bypass surgery. After a follow-up period of 5 years, 75% of patients were alive, and 26% were alive and event-free (no myocardial infarction, no repeat bypass surgery or repeat angioplasty). In patients in whom the initial angioplasty attempt was unsuccessful, only 3% were event-free at 5 years, versus 27% of successfully dilated patients. The time interval between the angioplasty attempt and previous surgery was a significant predictor for 5-year event-free survival. The event-free survival rates for patients who had bypass surgery 1 year before, between 1 and 5 years, and 5 years before angioplasty, were 45, 25 and 19%, respectively. Less than one-third of patients with previous bypass surgery who had angioplasty of the graft remained event-free after 5 years. In patients needing angioplasty within 1 year after CABG, better long-term results were achieved.

Jost and associates[127] from Hanover, Germany, investigated the influence of morphologic parameters on the recurrence of stenosis after PTCA of 49 stenoses in aortocoronary venous bypass grafts of 41 patients. Vessel dimensions were measured quantitatively. Angioplasty was successful in

46 stenoses (94%) of 38 patients (93%). In 35 patients (92% of successfully treated patients) with 42 stenoses, control angiography was performed after a mean interval of 189 ± 186 days. In 9 patients (26%), 9 stenoses (21%) had recurred. The diameter of the grafted coronary artery distal to the anastomosis was significantly smaller in grafted arteries with than without recurrent stenoses (1.92 ± 0.52 vs 2.45 ± 0.50 mm). Recurrence also correlated with the ratio between graft diameter and coronary artery diameter >1.35 and with the stenosis length >10 mm before angioplasty. Graft age, graft diameter and stenosis location in the graft had no significant influence on recurrence. Thus, the diameter of the grafted coronary artery and the length of the critical stenosis are parameters for recurrence after angioplasty of graft stenoses and should be considered in the selection of patients for this intervention.

For internal mammary arterial grafts

With the increasing use of the internal mammary artery as the conduit of choice in CABG, it is anticipated than an expanding patient population will have stenosis, usually at the site of internal mammary-to-coronary artery anastomosis. In a report by Dimas and colleagues[128] from Cleveland, Ohio, 31 patients underwent dilatation at either the site of anastomosis (24), the native coronary artery beyond the anastomosis (4), or both (3) with no mortality, AMI, or need for emergency CABG. Angiographic and clinical success was achieved in 28 patients (90%). There were 2 internal mammary artery dissections with both patients requiring elective CABG. Of the patients in whom dilatation was successful, 22 (79%) have been followed for >6 months and 19 (86%) have had sustained functional improvement at a mean of 35 months after angioplasty. No patient has had a myocardial infarction or died during follow-up. Although PTCA of the internal mammary artery has inherent difficulties because of the anatomic characteristics of the vessel, it can be performed with a high degree of primary success and a low incidence of complications and can provide long-term clinical improvement.

For acute re-occlusion

The sensitivity of the surface 12-lead electrocardiogram and that of standard (limb-lead) monitoring for the detection of ischemia during PTCA were compared in 115 patients in a study carried out by Bush and colleagues[129] from Houston, Texas. The purpose was to identify the electrocardiographic leads that provide the most sensitive indicators of coronary ischemia during PTCA and to evaluate the "ischemic fingerprint" that is obtained with 12-lead electrocardiogram during balloon inflation as a predictor of abrupt reocclusion after successful PTCA procedures. During balloon inflations of 30 seconds, ischemia was detected in 61 of 145 vessels (42%) by limb-lead monitoring alone versus 130 of 145 vessels (90%) by 12-lead electrocardiography. In the 9 patients (7.8%) who experienced abrupt reocclusion within 24 hours, the electrocardiogram during chest pain after PTCA was identical to that obtained during PTCA ("ischemic fingerprint"). None of the 6 patients who had chest pain after PTCA without evidence of abrupt reocclusion reproduced their ischemic fingerprint. The suggested optimal leads for monitoring ischemia are as follows: LAD, V_2 and V_3; LC, V_2 and V_3; and right coronary artery, III and aVF.

Intracoronary thrombosis

Experimental studies have demonstrated that intracoronary platelet aggregation and thrombus formation may induce marked vasoconstriction of epicardial arteries with endothelial injury. To examine the effects of intracoronary thrombus formation on coronary vasomotor tone of human epicardial arteries in vivo, Zeiher and co-workers[130] in Freiburg, Germany, studied 15 patients who developed intracoronary thrombi adherent to the guide wire during balloon dilatation. Epicardial artery luminal area was evaluated by quantitative coronary angiography proximal and distal to the site of intracoronary thrombus formation and in a reference vessel before and after thrombus formation as well as after intracoronary injection of nitroglycerin. All artery segments distal to the site of thrombus formation showed vasoconstriction with a luminal area reduction of -27%, whereas proximal vessel segments and reference vessels not manipulated during percutaneous transluminal coronary angioplasty did not demonstrate any significant luminal area changes during thrombus formation. Angiographic measurements after advancing the guide wire with the adherent thrombus revealed in all patients that vasoconstriction did develop at a new site distal to the thrombus with persistence of the initial vasoconstriction now residing proximal to the thrombus (Figure 2-19). Thus, there was a sequential association between thrombus formation and subsequent distal vasoconstriction. Intracoronary injection of nitroglycerin abolished the thrombus-induced vasoconstriction. No significant luminal area changes were observed in 20 patients without angiographic evidence of intracoronary thrombus formation. Intracoronary thrombus formation during PTCA causes focal vasoconstriction of epicardial arteries in patients with CAD. Although caution must be advised in the extrapolation of this phenomenon, which was observed in a manipulated artery during coronary angioplasty, the vasoconstrictor response to intracoronary thrombus formation in vivo may play an important role in the dynamic mechanisms of acute CAD syndromes.

Coronary dissection

Coronary artery dissection is an infrequent but serious complication of PTCA that can lead to periprocedural arterial occlusion, emergency CABG, AMI, or death. Recently a profusion balloon catheter was developed that permits passive perfusion of blood through the central lumen of the catheter. It enables prolonged balloon inflations to be performed and has been used to provide distal blood flow after coronary occlusion. To evaluate the effectiveness of the perfusion balloon catheter in patients with major coronary dissections, Leitschuh and associates[131] from Boston, Massachusetts, compared 36 consecutive patients treated with the perfusion balloon catheter to 46 consecutive patients treated before its availability. The 2 groups were similar in terms of clinical, angiographic and initial procedural characteristics. Use of the perfusion balloon catheter permitted a significantly longer inflation than standard balloon inflation (average 18 ± 5 min). Angiographic success was significantly greater with the perfusion balloon catheter (84 vs 62% for conventional therapy), whereas complications were markedly reduced (48 vs 78%). With the perfusion balloon catheter there were fewer deaths (2 vs 6%), myocardial infarctions (14 vs 40%) and emergency bypass operations (11 vs 25%). The findings of this retrospective comparison demonstrate that the perfusion balloon catheter is effective for the management of major dissections

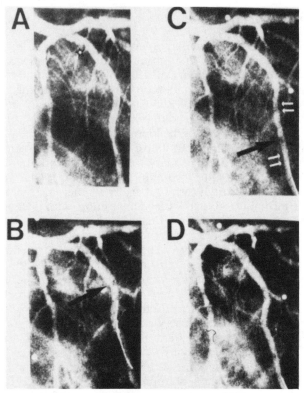

Fig. 2-19. Angiogram of left coronary artery system illustrating vasoconstrictor response to intracoronary thrombus formation (asterisk marks site of balloon dilatation). Panel A: Control angiogram after percutaneous transluminal coronary angioplasty. Panel B: Formation of thrombus adherent to the intracoronary guide wire (black arrow). Panel C: Intense vasoconstriction in response to thrombus formation (white arrows). Advancing guide wire illustrates adherence of thrombus to it (black arrow) and persistence of vasoconstriction, thus excluding passive arterial collapse of vessel segment and development of vasoconstriction at new site (distal white arrows). Panel D: Reduction of vasoconstriction with intracoronary nitroglycerin. Reproduced with permission of Zeiher, et al.[130]

after PTCA. The use of the perfusion balloon catheter should be considered when a major coronary dissection occurs and when emergency bypass surgery is contemplated.

Cripps and associates[132] from Oxford, UK, reviewed findings in 32 patients among 880 undergoing coronary angioplasty during a 9 year period at 1 hospital who had extensive dissection, i.e., involved beyond the limits of the dilated angioplasty balloon, in the coronary artery in which the angioplasty procedure was performed. Two of the 32 patients died as a consequence of the coronary artery dissection. Twelve patients (38%) needed immediate CABG and 11 patients (34%) had an AMI, which in 4 was minor. During follow up, 20 of the 32 patients were successfully managed by medical treatment; only 2 needed further angioplasty procedures. There were no late deaths. Extensive coronary artery dissection is a serious complication of coronary angioplasty, with a high early mortality and a high incidence of infarction and requirement for bypass surgery. None the less, patients with extensive dissection who are free from the manifestations of acute ischemia at the end of the procedure can be managed conservatively and have a good immediate and medium term outlook. Attempts should be made to stabilize extensive dissection during coronary angioplasty so that surgical intervention can be delayed or avoided altogether if possible.

Positive exercise test early

The mechanism responsible for exercise-induced myocardial ischemia early after successful PTCA is poorly understood. El-Tamimi and co-workers[133] in London, UK, studied 12 patients who underwent one-vessel PTCA. Exercise testing was performed before and on day 7 after PTCA, which was repeated after 10 mg sublingual isosorbide dinitrate if the test was positive. Quantitative coronary arteriography was also performed on day 8 after PTCA in the basal state, after intracoronary infusion of 0.9% saline, 1,5,10, and 20 micrograms ergonovine, and after 300 mg nitroglycerin. All patients had a positive exercise test before PTCA but on day 7, 6 patients had a positive exercise test (group 1) and 6 patients (group 2) had a negative exercise test. In group 1, all positive exercise tests on day 7 become negative when repeated after isosorbide dinitrate. Intracoronary ergonovine was associated with a dose-dependent constriction of the PTCA segment, a segment distal to it, and a control segment, with no significant difference in the magnitude of the response between the 2 groups. No angina, ischemic ST segment changes, occlusive, or subocclusive spasm occurred in any patient of either group. The investigators could find no evidence that exercise-induced myocardial ischemia early after PTCA is related to the presence of fixed angiographic restenosis or to dynamic constriction of any epicardial coronary segment. Therefore, inappropriate small coronary vessel constriction responsive to nitrates should be considered as a possible alternative explanation.

Intravascular ultrasonic imaging afterwards

In a study by Werner and associates[134] from Goettingen, Germany, an intravascular ultrasound catheter system was used in patients to assess the effect of PTCA. In 14 out of 16 patients, the intravascular ultrasound catheter could be successfully advanced to the site of a previous dilatation. Qualitative assessment of the cross-sectional images revealed intimal thickening and an increase of ultrasound reflectance and calcification at atherosclerotic coronary arteries. A disruption of the obstructing plaque and evidence for local dissections (11 of 14 cases) were observed after PTCA. The quantitative comparison between angiography and the ultrasound measurement showed a close correlation for vessel sites distant to the dilatation. After PTCA, the quantitative evaluation of the dilated area was possible in 11 cases. The correlation of angiographic and sonographic measurements of these segments was good for the assessment of the vessel diameter, but poor for the determination of the luminal area. This difference reflected the complex morphology of the vessel lumen after PTCA, which would be better assessed by the cross-sectional sonographic technique than by contrast angiography. The intravascular imaging of coronary arteries provides a new and unique method to obtain information on the plaque morphology and composition, and to assess the local effects of interventional procedures and their complications.

Vasomotor changes afterwards

To study the impact of PTCA on coronary vasomotion, El-Tamimi and co-investigators[135] in London, UK, prospectively analyzed spontaneous changes in coronary diameter and the response to the cold pressor test and intracoronary nitroglycerin in 11 patients subjected to successful single-vessel PTCA. All antianginal medications were stopped 48 hours before each study. The minimum diameter of the PTCA segment and the diameter of a distal segment in the angioplastied vessel and of a segment in a control vessel not manipulated by the balloon catheter or guide wire were measured by computerized edge detection immediately before PTCA and 5 minutes after, 4 hours after, and 8 days after PTCA. At 4 hours, PTCA and distal segments were constricted by 38% and 16%, respectively, compared with the values at 5 minutes. Before angioplasty, the cold pressor test caused vasoconstriction of PTCA and distal segments by 23% and 15% respectively, but no constrictor response was elicited at 5 minutes or 4 hours after angioplasty (Figure 2-20). Eight days after PTCA, the basal coronary diameters were similar to those observed 5 minutes after PTCA and the response to the cold pressor test was similar to that ob-

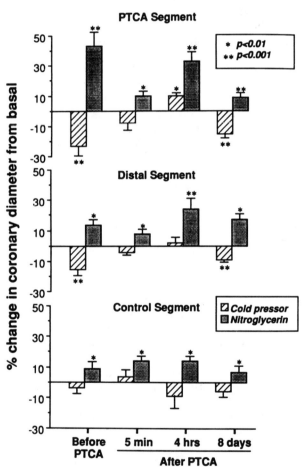

Fig. 2-20. Bar graph of percent changes form basal in coronary diameter (mm) in response to cold pressor test and to nitroglycerin in percutaneous transluminal coronary angioplasty (PTCA) (upper panel), distal (middle panel), and control (lower panel) segments before PTCA, 5 minutes after, 4 hours after, and 8 days after PTCA. PTCA and distal segments constricted significantly in response to cold pressor test before PTCA. This response was lost at 4 hours but had recovered by 8 days. Nitroglycerin induced significant dilatation in all segments. Reproduced with permission of El-Tamimi, et al.[135]

served before PTCA. All segments dilated significantly with nitroglycerin at all times, and no vasoconstriction changes were found in the control segments. Four hours after PTCA, transient spontaneous vasoconstriction of the PTCA and distal segments occurs, which is so intense that the cold pressor test does not cause any further constriction. These abnormalities were solved within 8 days of PTCA.

Risk factors for in-hospital mortality

Simpfendorfer and associates[136] from Cleveland, Ohio, reviewed clinical, angiographic, and procedural findings in 40 in-hospital deaths among 5,000 consecutive PTCA procedures (Table 2-3). Compared to the total group, the mortality group had a higher proportion of women, older age, and more extensive CAD. Angioplasty was performed as an emergency procedure in 21 of the 40 patients who died. Eighteen presented with an evolving AMI and 17 with unstable angina. Most patients presented in critical condition prior to angioplasty: 18 patients were in cardiogenic shock and 5 patients were on cardiopulmonary resuscitation. Among 13 patients who died following elective angioplasty, the salient feature was acute vessel closure or dissection in 7 patients and failed dilatation of a saphenous vein graft in 4 patients.

To better understand the factors predisposing a patient to death after elective PTCA and to gain insight into indications for high-risk PTCA both with and without adjunctive use of support devices, Ellis and associates[137] from 4 USA medical centers reviewed the outcomes of 8,052 consecutive procedures. Death occurred after 32 procedures (0.4%) and was directly related to coronary artery closure in 26 (81%). LV failure due to vessel closure at the dilated site, the most common cause of death, was independently correlated with female sex, "jeopardy score" and PTCA of a proximal right coronary artery site, but not with LVEF or presence of multivessel CAD. RV failure after closure of the proximal right coronary artery, and LM coronary dissection accounted for most of the remaining deaths. Systolic BP immediately after coronary artery closure also correlated closely with jeopardy score and cardiogenic shock was frequent in women with scores ≥3.5 and in men with scores ≥5.0. These data highlight the superiority of the jeopardy score vs EF in the determination of risk, stress the importance of gender in determining outcome and point to the need for better means of RV protection from severe ischemia.

TABLE 2-3. *Comparison of clinical and angiographic characteristics of all PTCA patients and the mortality group. Reproduced with permission from Simpfendorfer, et al.*[136]

	All patients n = 5000 (%)	Mortality group n = 40 (%)
Mean age (years)	58	66
≥70 years old	645 (13)	15 (38)
Women	1280 (26)	20 (50)
Previous myocardial infarction	1737 (35)	13 (33)
Previous coronary artery bypass graft	670 (13)	6 (15)
Extent of disease		
1-vessel	2705 (54)	11 (27)
2-vessel	1579 (32)	13 (33)
3-vessel	641 (13)	16 (40)
Left ventricular dysfunction		
Normal to mild	4438 (89)	13 (48)
Moderate to severe	561 (11)	14 (52)

Therefore, an initial framework for rational use of PTCA and support devices in the high-risk setting is established.

Myocardial ischemia

Titus and Sherman[138] from Los Angeles, California, studied 88 patients undergoing PTCA of 100 coronary stenoses for the presence of factors deemed significant in the etiology of silent myocardial ischemia. Thirty-two patients were asymptomatic during balloon dilations of 36 arteries, and 56 patients had angina during PTCA of 64 arteries. There were no differences in age, sex, prior anginal history, antianginal regimen, extent of CAD and number or duration of inflations between the 2 study groups. Previous infarction (33 vs 12%), Q waves in the target area (31 vs 7%) and diabetes mellitus (36 vs 17%) were present more often in the asymptomatic group (Figure 2-21). Sixty-four percent of all asymptomatic patients had either diabetes or previous infarction in the target territory. Collateral circulation was more frequent in asymptomatic patients, probably reflecting the ability of collateral arteries to ameliorate ischemia. During 2-vessel PTCA, patients without angina during dilation of only 1 of the 2 treated arteries (discordant responders) had previous infarction in that artery's territory (5 of 5, 100%), whereas patients without previous infarction were either symptomatic or asymptomatic (concordant responders) during PTCA of both arteries. This study shows that asymptomatic ischemia occurs frequently during PTCA in patients with symptomatic coronary disease. Prior Q-wave infarction and diabetes mellitus are important, independent factors associated with painless ischemia. It is suggested that infarction produces a localized dysfunction of afferent cardiac pain fibers, whereas diabetes can cause a global cardiac sensory neuropathy.

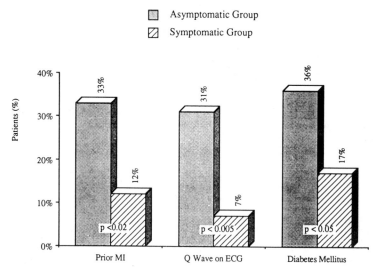

Fig. 2-21. Frequency of major discriminating clinical factors in the 2 groups of patients. ECG = electrocardiogram; MI = myocardial infarction. Reproduced with permission of Titus, et al.[138]

Recovery of ischemic myocardium

Nienaber and associates[139] in Los Angeles, California studied the temporal relations between restorations of coronary blood flow, normalization of tissue metabolism, and recovery of LV segmental function after PTCA in 12 patients. Positron emission tomography and two-dimensional echo were performed before and within 72 hours of revascularization. Ten patients underwent late echos and eight had a late positron emission tomographic study. PTCA significantly increased mean stenosis cross-sectional area from 0.95 ± 0.9 to 2.7 ± 1.4 mm^2 and mean cross-sectional luminal diameter from 0.9 to 1.9. Perfusion defect scores in dependent vascular territories improved after PTCA. The mean perfusion-metabolism mismatch score decreased early after angioplasty and again at late follow-up. However, absolute rates of glucose utilization remained elevated early after revascularization, normalizing only at late follow-up. The average wall motion score did not improve significantly early after PTCA, but a highly significant improvement was observed at late follow-up (Figure 2-22). Perfusion-metabolism mismatch scores before PTCA were linearly related to late improvement in wall motion scores. Thus, restoration of blood flow to ischemic myocardium by PTCA is followed by an early improvement in perfusion and by the initial persistence of an abnormal metabolic and functional state that resolves with time.

Blood flow velocity before and after

Eichhorn and associates[140] in Dallas, Texas, tested the hypothesis that spontaneous coronary blood flow velocity variations occur in some patients with stenosed coronary arteries before or after PTCA. Thirteen patients with severe and limiting angina underwent intracoronary pulsed Doppler velocimetry of their dilated artery immediate before and after PTCA, whereas 9 control patients underwent velocimetry of an angiographically normal coronary artery. A 3F catheter with a 20 MHz Doppler crystal was positioned to achieve a maximal stable signal and the flow velocity signal was recorded continuously for 20 min. Spontaneous flow variations defined as ≥38% change in Doppler frequency shift with wide morphologic changes were present in 3 of the 13 patients tested (Figure 2-23). Spontaneous flow variations occurred before PTCA in one patient, after PTCA in another and both before and after PTCA in a third. In addition, 2 of the 13 patients, 1 with spontaneous coronary artery flow variations before PTCA had frank vasospasm in an adjacent area just distal to the area of coronary dilation immediately after PTCA. These data establish that spontaneous coronary artery blood flow velocity variations occur in some patients with severe and limiting angina before and after PTCA. These variations may be related to platelet aggregation or coronary vasoconstriction, or both, at sites of endothelial injury resulting from plaque fissuring or ulceration and endothelial and medial injury occurring during PTCA.

Effects of esmolol

To assess the effect of the ultrashort-acting beta blocker esmolol on ischemia induced by acute coronary occlusion, Labovitz and associates[141] from St. Louis, Missouri, studied 16 patients undergoing PTCA. Doppler echocardiography and electrocardiographic monitoring were performed

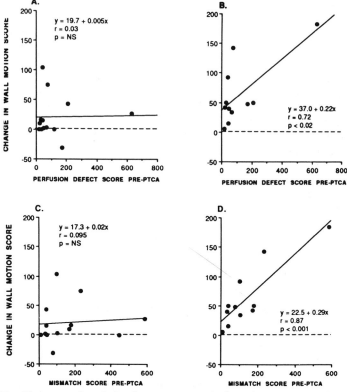

Fig. 2-22. Upper panels, relation between preangioplasty (PRE-PTCA) perfusion defect scores and the improvement in echocardiographic wall motion scores early (A) and late (B) after angioplasty. No relation is noted for the early postangioplasty study, but a weak linear relation is present for the late follow-up study. Lower panels relation between preangioplasty perfusion-metabolism mismatch scores and early (C) and late (D) improvement in wall motion scores after angioplasty. Although no relation is present for the early postangioplasty studies, improvement in wall motion scores at the time of the late follow-up study is linearly related to the preangioplasty perfusion-metabolism mismatch score. The 13 data points in the left panels represent 13 dilated lesions and 13 perfusion territories in 12 patients. The 11 data points in the right panels pertain to 11 perfusion territories in 10 patients; 2 patients (Cases 1 and 6) were excluded from late follow-up wall motion analysis because of early restenosis at the site of angioplasty. Reproduced with permission of Nienaber, et al.[139]

continuously before, during, and after balloon occlusion in the drug-free state and during esmolol infusion. Fourteen of the 16 patients had ST segment elevation during balloon inflation. However, maximal ST segment elevation (2.1 ± 1.5 mm vs 1.7 ± 1.3 mm) and duration of ST segment elevation (68 ± 20 seconds vs 54 ± 19 seconds) were both significantly reduced during esmolol infusion. Furthermore, the decrease in EF seen during drug-free balloon occlusions was significantly blunted during esmolol infusion. In the baseline state EF decreased from 55% to 38% during coronary occlusion compared with no decrease from 52% during esmolol infusion. In addition, esmolol appeared to delay the onset of segmental wall motion abnormalities after coronary occlusion, occurring at a mean of 40 seconds after balloon inflation versus a mean of 31 seconds in the absence of beta blockade. Thus the use of ultrashort-acting beta blockade

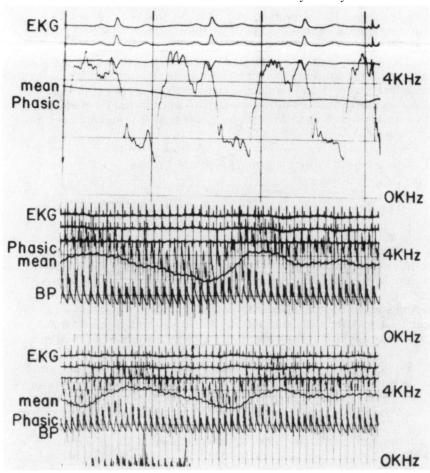

Fig. 2-23. Patient 11A. Representative tracings from a patient with spontaneous coronary artery flow velocity variations. The phasic signal (phasic) was predominantly diastolic (top panel), with wide variations in the mean Doppler (mean) signal morphology (bottom panels) that could not be accounted for by respiratory or pressure (BP) changes. EKG = electrocardiogram. Reproduced with permission of Eichhorn, et al.[140]

appears to diminish the extent and delay the onset of myocardial ischemia during acute coronary occlusion.

Urokinase

In an investigation by Pavlides and associates[142] from Royal Oak, Michigan, 89 of 462 patients were treated with adjunctive urokinase during elective PTCA, 26% for unstable angina, 34% for intracoronary thrombus, 27% for intimal dissection, 10% for abrupt closure, and 3% for saphenous vein graft embolism. The 80 patients treated before abrupt closure (group A) were compared with 167 patients with similar profiles who did not receive urokinase (group B). Procedural success rates were similar. Adverse cardiac events (abrupt closure, AMI, emergency CAB, or death) in group A versus group B occurred in: 1 of 30 (3%) versus 5 of 27 (19%) with intracoronary thrombus, 5 of 45 (9%) versus 18 of 110 (16%) with unstable angina, 1 of 12 (8%) versus 4 of 13 (31%) with unstable angina with intracoronary thrombus, 4 of 33 (12%) versus 14 of 97 (14%) with unstable angina without intracoronary thrombus, and 5 of 24 (21%) versus 6 of 66 (9%) with intimal dissection. Hemorrhage complications occurred in 11% of patients who were treated with urokinase versus 9% of patients who were not. No difference in blood transfusions existed. Thus, urokinase was found to be safe during elective PTCA. In patients with intracoronary thrombus, urokinase appears to decrease the incidence of new adverse cardiac events, whereas in patients with intimal dissection it might have an adverse effect.

Effects of non-ionic vs ionic contrast media on complications

To evaluate the effect of contrast agents on PTCA complications, Lembo and associates[143] from Atlanta, Georgia, randomized 913 patients undergoing 1,058 separate PTCA procedures to receive either nonionic iopamidol (n = 507 PTCA procedures) or ionic contrast media meglumine sodium diatrizoate (n = 551 PTCA procedures). Angioplasty operators, technicians, nurses and patients were blinded to the agent used. All patients were pretreated with 0.6 mg of atropine sulfate intravenously before any contrast injections. Hypotension (mean arterial pressure <65 mm Hg associated with contrast injections) occurred during 8.5% of PTCA procedures in which the patients were receiving iopamidol and during 9.5% of the procedures in which the patients were given diatrizoate (difference not significant). Bradycardia (heart rate of <40 beats/min associated with contrast injections) developed during 5.7% of procedures when patients were given iopamidol and during 5.1% of procedures when patients were given diatrizoate. The need for additional atropine or temporary pacing during the procedure was similar for patients given iopamidol and diatrizoate. The overall incidence of VT or fibrillation, or both, during the procedure occurred less frequently when iopamidol was used compared with diatrizoate (1 vs 2.5%). These serious ventricular arrhythmias were attributable to contrast injections in 0.6% of the PTCA procedures when iopamidol was given and in 2.0% of the cases in which diatrizoate was the contrast agent. Only 1 patient had an allergic reaction to the contrast agent, and this was in a patient who received iopamidol. There were no differences in hospital complications (myocardial infarction, emergency CABG or death) between the 2 groups. It is concluded that in patients undergoing PTCA, iopamidol, compared with meglumine sodium diatrizoate, reduces the overall incidence of serious ventricular arrhythmias but not the frequency of myocardial infarction, the need for surgery, or death.

Restenosis

Cahyadi and associates[144] from Ishikawa, Japan, used serial body surface potential mapping with the departure map technique to evaluate the clinical efficacy of PTCA in various pathophysiologic stages of CAD, and to detect restenosis. The body surface potential mapping was performed prior to, 1 week after, and 1 month after PTCA. A follow-up coronary angiography was performed 3 to 6 months after PTCA, and body surface potential mapping was also performed at the same time. The results of body surface potential mapping were compared with those of thallium-201 single-photon emission computed tomography and radionuclide ventriculography. After PTCA, body surface potential mapping showed a significant reduction in the departure area; the thallium-201 single-photon emission computed tomography also showed a significant reduction in the extent and severity scores, and the LVEF improved significantly. In the cases with restenosis, the departure area, which had decreased in size after PTCA, showed an increase in size. After successful re-PTCA, the size of the departure area again became smaller. It was concluded that body surface potential mapping, which is a simple, non-invasive, and inexpensive method, is useful in the evaluation of the clinical efficacy of PTCA and in the detection of restenosis after successful PTCA.

Restenosis after initial, successful PTCA is due to fibrocellular proliferation. Ueda and co-workers[145] in Amsterdam, The Netherlands studied the nature of fibrocellular tissue in humans by use of immunocytochemical techniques. Four hearts with five coronary arteries were investigated; time lapse between PTCA and death varied between 20 days (2 arteries) and 1 year 7 months. Proliferating cells stained positive with smooth muscle cell-specific monoclonal antibodies. Cells from early proliferative lesions (20 days) have a phenotypic expression different from cells in "old" lesions. Proliferating cells stained positive with vimentin but were negative with desmin, irrespective of the lesions's age. The findings indicated a change in acting insoform expression of smooth muscle cells while adapting to a pathological state.

Johansson and associates[146] from Goteborg, Sweden, analyzed serum levels of total cholesterol, triglycerides, HDL and LDL cholesterol in 157 patients undergoing 161 PTCA procedures (Table 2-4). Follow-up coronary angiograms were performed after 6.0 ± 4.3 months. The restenosis rate was 33%. Treatment with aspirin and a residual stenosis of 25–49% diameter reduction immediately after successful PTCA were the only variables associated with restenosis. Otherwise the clinical and angiographic characteristics were similar in the patients with and without restenosis. There was no relation between restenosis and the levels of total cholesterol, triglycerides, HDL or LDL cholesterol.

Although the association of serum lipid levels with the risk of atherosclerosis is well-recognized, the relation between these levels and

TABLE 2-4. *Serum lipid and lipoprotein levels in patients with and without restenosis on follow-up angiogram after successful PTCA. Reproduced with permission from Johansson, et al.*[146]

	Restenosis (n = 53) Mean ± SD (Range)	No restenosis (n = 108) Mean ± SD (Range)	P value
Total cholesterol (mmol . l⁻¹)	6·50 ± 1·13 (4·01–9·63)	6·76 ± 1·40 (4·44–12·28)	NS
Total triglycerides (mmol . l⁻¹)	2·17 ± 1·07 (0·78–4·04)	2·06 ± 0·98 (0·56–5·83)	NS
HDL (mmol . l⁻¹)	1·07 ± 0·35 (0·48–2·26)	1·14 ± 0·30 (0·48–2·20)	NS
LDL (mmol . l⁻¹)	4·45 ± 1·00 (2·29–6·91)	4·70 ± 1·22 (1·95–9·69)	NS
LDL/HDL	4·47 ± 1·46 (1·67–8·15)	4·36 ± 1·71 (1·69–13·23)	NS

HDL = High density lipoprotein cholesterol, LDL = low density lipoprotein cholesterol, NS = not significant, SD = standard deviation.

restenosis after coronary angioplasty is uncertain. Reis and associates[147] from Boston, Massachusetts, examined 186 patients enrolled in a trial of fish oil for prevention of restenosis. Fasting lipid levels (cholesterol, HDL cholesterol and triglycerides) were measured before angioplasty, and in 90 patients repeated at 6-month follow-up. Fifty-nine patients (32%) developed clinical restenosis confirmed by angiography. Patients who went on to develop restenosis underwent multivessel angioplasty and were more likely to be on lipid-lowering therapy at baseline (27 vs 13%). In addition, they had higher baseline cholesterol/HDL ratios (6.5 ± 2.2 vs 5.9 ± 2.0) and triglyceride levels (233 ± 210 vs 183 ± 112 mg/dl). Multiple logistic regression analysis confirmed cholesterol/HDL ratios at baseline and follow-up to be independent predictors of risk for restenosis. Using these data, regression lines have been developed that predict risk of restenosis based on type of procedure and on lipid values. These results suggest that serum lipid levels may be associated with the risk of clinical restenosis after PTCA.

Prevention of restenosis after successful PTCA remains a major challenge. To determine whether lovastatin could prevent restenosis, between December 1987 and July 1988, a total of 157 patients undergoing successful PTCA were randomly and prospectively assigned to the lovastatin group or a control group in an investigation carried out by Sahni and colleagues[148] from Philadelphia, Pennsylvania. Seventy-nine patients received lovastatin (20 mg daily if the serum cholesterol level was <300 mg/dl and 40 mg daily if the serum cholesterol level was ≥300 mg/dl) in addition to conventional therapy (lovastatin group). Seventy-eight patients received conventional therapy alone (control group). Fifty patients in the lovastatin group and 29 in the control group were evaluated with coronary angiography at an interval of 2 to 10 months (mean 4 months). The restenosis rate was evaluated according to the number of patients showing restenosis, the number of vessels restenosed, and the number of PTCA sites restenosed. Restenosis was defined as the presence of >50% stenosis of the PTCA site. In the lovastatin group 6 of 50 patients (12%) had restenosis compared with 13 of 29 patients (44%) in the control group. When the number of vessels restenosed was considered, only 9 of 72 vessels restenosed in the lovastatin group compared with 13 of 34 vessels (38%) in the control group. Similarly, 10 of 80 (13%) PTCA sites restenosed in the lovastatin group compared with 15 of 36 (42%) in the control group. The serum cholesterol level in the lovastatin group decreased from 212 ± 49 to 175 ± 41 mg/dl, whereas in the control group it only decreased from 207 ± 49 to 196 ± 48 mg/dl. In conclusion, lovastatin significantly reduced the incidence of restenosis after successful PTCA. Possible mechanisms include a decrease in the serum cholesterol level and a decrease in smooth muscle cell proliferation as a result of inhibition of endothelial DNA synthesis by lovastatin.

Bourassa and colleagues[149] in Montreal, Quebec, and Toronto, and Burlington, Canada, conducted a prospective, double-blind placebo-controlled trial with a combination of aspirin and dipyridamole to determine whether these interventions reduced the rate of restenosis within the first 6 months after PTCA. A total of 247 patients and 280 arterial segments had follow-up angiography and quantitative coronary angiographic analysis between 4 and 7 months after PTCA. Two baseline clinical characteristics—angina class and duration of angina in months—were related to the rates of restenosis by univariate analysis. Patient-related stepwise logistic regression analysis identified severity of angina as the only clinical predictor of restenosis. Three univariate baseline anatomic characteristics, including percent diameter stenosis before PTCA, stenosis >10 mm in length, and calcific stenosis and two early post PTCA characteristics, including residual percent diameter stenosis and residual mean pressure gradients as being predictive of restenosis. Of these, only two, including length of stenosis and residual percent diameter stenosis were independently related to restenosis by multivariate analysis. Thus, only a few clinical and anatomic factors appear to be predictive of restenosis after PTCA.

To determine whether angiotensin converting enzyme (ACE) inhibition may reduce the incidence of restenosis after PTCA, Brozovich and associates[150] from Philadelphia, Pennsylvania, retrospectively identified 322 consecutive patients who underwent a successful procedure from June, 1988 to December, 1989. No patients developed chest pain, ST segment elevation, positive cardiac enzymes, or other evidence of abrupt vessel closure following the PTCA. All patients received intravenous heparin after PTCA and aspirin was begun on the day prior to PTCA. Patients were separated into 2 groups: Those at hospital discharge incidentally treated for hypertension or heart failure with ACE inhibitors (n = 36), and those treated with a drug regimen which did not include ACE inhibitors (n = 286). The 2 groups were similar with respect to age (61 ± 13.5 vs 60 ± 12.5) and other demographic characteristics. Restenosis, defined as the presentation to a physician with symptoms of angina within 6 months of the PTCA and the finding on repeat catheterization of a significant restenosis at the site of the PTCA, occurred in 30% of the patients who were discharged on a drug regimen which did not include ACE inhibitors vs. 3% in those treated with an ACE inhibitor. Thus, it appears that the use of ACE inhibitors may significantly reduce the incidence of restenosis after successful PTCA.

Hirshfeld and colleagues[151] in Philadelphia, Pennsylvania, Halifax, Canada, Richmond, Virginia, Miami, Jacksonville, and Orlando and Gainesville, Florida, obtained follow-up angiography in 510 patients with 598 successfully dilated coronary lesions who were enrolled in a controlled trial of the effects of a single dose of 1 g of methylprednisolone on restenosis after PTCA. The overall restenosis rate was 40%. The strongest univariate relations to the restenosis rate were found for lesion location, including saphenous vein graft 68%, LAD 45%, left circumflex artery and right coronary artery 32%; lesion length ≤4.6 mm, 33%; >4.6 mm, 45%; percent stenosis before PTCA ≤73%, 25%; >73%, 43%; percent stenosis after PTCA ≤21%, 33%; >21%, 46%; and arterial diameter <2.9 mm, 44%; ≥2.9 mm, 34% (Figure 2-24). Two multivariate models to predict restenosis probability were developed with use of stepwise logistic regression. The preprocedural model, which included only variables whose values were known before PTCA, entered lesion length, vein graft location, LAD location, percent stenosis before PTCA, and eccentric lesion and arterial diameter. Postprocedural model, which also included variables whose values were known after PTCA, results were similar to those of the preangioplasty model except that it also entered postangioplasty percent stenosis and optimal balloon sizing. These data indicate that the probability of restenosis after PTCA is determined predominantly by the characteristics of the lesion being dilated.

Taylor and associates[152] from Perth, Australia, randomized to treatment with soluble aspirin 100 mg/day or placebo to study the effect of restenosis after angioplasty of a previously untreated native coronary artery and after 2 weeks of aspirin therapy in 216 patients aged <70 years without AMI. Follow-up, defined as angiography at 6 months, earlier

A.

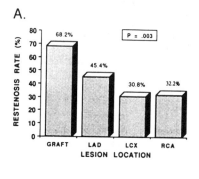

B.

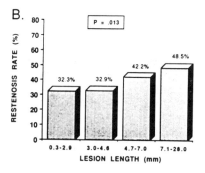

C.

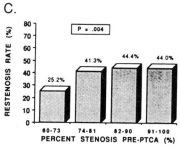

D.

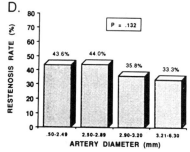

Fig. 2-24. Relation of selected preangioplasty variables to the coronary restenosis rate. In each panel the height of each bar represents the restenosis rate for its group of lesions and the chi-square p value is shown in the box. A, Effect of lesion location with the lesions segregated by location in the coronary system. LAD = left anterior descending coronary artery; LCX = left circumflex coronary artery; RCA = right coronary artery. B, Effect of lesion length (mm) on restenosis with the lesions segregated by quartiles of length. C, Effect of percent stenosis before angioplasty (PTCA) with the lesions segregated by quartile of percent stenosis. D, Effect of the diameter of the arterial segment (mm) immediately adjacent to the dilated lesion with the lesions segregated by arterial diameter. Reproduced with permission of Hirschfeld, et al.[151]

angiographic restenosis or CABG was completed by 108 aspirin- and 104 placebo-treated patients. Restenosis (stenosis ≥50% plus loss of ≥50% of gain, or surgery) occurred in 38 (35%) aspirin- and 45 (43%) placebo-treated subjects. No patient died. Restenosis occurred in 42 of 168 (25%) aspirin- and 51 of 135 (38%) placebo-treated lesions. Aspirin-treated lesions (n = 163) had lost 16 ± 22% (mean ± standard deviation) of lumen and placebo-treated lesions 22 ± 25% of lumen (n = 134) at angiography. There were more left anterior descending lesions in the placebo group and these had a higher recurrence rate than other lesions. The beneficial effect of aspirin was not dependent on this, although significance was reduced in subgroup analysis. Loss of lumen in left anterior descending lesions was 20 ± 24% (n = 57) in the aspirin-treated and 27 ± 25% (n = 70) in the placebo-treated lesions. It is concluded that there is a small beneficial effect of low-dose aspirin on restenosis after PTCA. Alone, this may be of marginal clinical significance but, along with other evidence for benefit from aspirin therapy after coronary events, it suggests that aspirin therapy should be continued after PTCA.

O'Keefe and associates[153] from Kansas City, Missouri, performed a randomized, placebo-controlled, double-blinded trial to evaluate the usefulness of empiric therapy with a calcium antagonist in patients who underwent PTCA. A total of 201 patients were randomized to placebo or to high-dose diltiazem (mean dose, 329 mg/day). Treatment began 24 hours before angioplasty. Restenosis was assessed by percent area stenosis as determined by quantitative angiographic techniques before, immediately and 1 year after angioplasty. All patients also received aspirin and dipyridamole before angioplasty. Heparin and verapamil were administered intravenously during the procedure. The 2 groups were similar with respect to age, extent of CAD, smoking history, and baseline lipid levels. Procedural complications, including death (1 vs 1), Q-wave infarction (0 vs 3), acute occlusion (5 vs 5) and focal spasm (0 vs 0), were not significantly different in the diltiazem and placebo patients, respectively. Freedom from all acute complications was noted in 85% of patients in both groups. One-year angiographic follow-up was obtained in 60% of patients. Restenosis rates were similar: 36% in the diltiazem group and 32% in the placebo group. The incidence of late cardiac events (death, Q-wave AMI, recurrent angina or CABG) was similar in the 2 groups. Thus, diltiazem did not influence the overall restenosis rate or prevent late events after PTCA.

High rates of restenosis after coronary angioplasty have been reported in patients with vasopastic angina. Ardissino and associates[154] from Pavia, Italy, designed a study to determine whether the occurrence of abnormal coronary vasoconstriction, detected by means of hyperventilation testing before angioplasty, influences the risk of restenosis after successful dilatation. Hyperventilation testing was performed 0 to 4 days before coronary angioplasty in 106 consecutive patients with unstable angina and single-vessel CAD. Abnormal coronary vasoconstriction was considered present if hyperventilation-induced myocardial ischemia occurred during the recovery phase of the test. All patients had follow-up angiography 8 to 12 months after angioplasty. Abnormal coronary vasoconstriction was observed in 48 patients (group 1), whereas 58 patients (group 2) had either a negative response throughout the test or a positive response only during the overbreathing phase of the hyperventilation test. Angioplasty was successful in 40 patients in group 1 and 51 in group 2. Restenosis was documented in 29 patients (73%) in group 1 and 13 (25%) in group 2 (relative risk of restenosis, 2.84; 95% confidence interval, 1.69 to 4.28). In a multivariate analysis, the following 3 characteristics were independently related to the risk of restenosis (in descending order of importance): ST-segment elevation during spontaneous ischemic attacks, hyperventilation-induced abnormal coronary vasoconstriction, and the presence of a lesion more than 10 mm long in the left anterior descending coronary artery. In patients with unstable angina and single-vessel CAD who have been selected for PTCA, the presence of hyperventilation-induced abnormal coronary vasoconstriction identifies a subgroup at high risk for restenosis.

To determine the influence of a history of restenosis on subsequent restenosis after PTCA of a new significant narrowing, Bresee and associates[155] from Boston, Massachusetts, retrospectively reviewed the records of 100 patients who underwent successful PTCA at another site ("new narrowing PTCA") ≥2 months after successful initial PTCA. Patients were grouped according to whether initial PTCA resulted in restenosis, which was determined by angiographic follow-up ≥3 months after initial PTCA. Patients in group 1 did not have restenosis after initial PTCA (n = 50), whereas patients in group 2 did (n = 40). All patients were followed for recurrent symptoms, with serial exercise tests, for ≥6 months after new narrowing PTCA. Clinically suspected and angiographically confirmed restenosis occurred in 11 of 50 (22%) patients and 12 of 63 (19%) narrowings in group 1, and in 20 of 40 (50%) patients and 22 of 48 (46%)

narrowings in group 2. Multivariate analysis identified that prior restenosis, left anterior descending artery location of stenosis, and severity of stenosis before PTCA were independently associated with restenosis after new narrowing PTCA. In conclusion, prior restenosis is an independent risk factor for subsequent restenosis after new narrowing PTCA.

CORONARY ATHRECTOMY

Hinohara and associates[156] in Redwood City, California, used directional coronary atherectomy for the treatment of obstructive lesions in coronary arteries by excision and removal of tissue on 447 lesions in 382 procedures. Successful outcome defined as a reduction of the stenosis ≥20% with a <50% residual stenosis was achieved in 90% of lesions and mean stenosis was reduced from 76 ± 13% to 15 ± 22%. Complications included vessel occlusion during the procedure in 2.4%; vessel occlusion after the procedure in 1.3%; new lesion in 0.5%; nonobstructive guiding catheter-induced dissection in 0.3%; perforation in 0.8%; and non-Q wave AMI in 4%. Twelve patients required CABG for these complications. The atherectomy success rate was >80% and the combined atherectomy and angioplasty success rate was >90% for complex morphologic lesions. In the presence of calcific deposits, atherectomy success rate was 52% for primary lesions and 83% for restenosed lesions. Among angiographically complex lesions, calcium was the predictor for failed atherectomy. In summary, directional coronary atherectomy is safe and effective for treatment of obstructive lesions in coronary arteries in selected cases. It achieves a high success rate in lesions with complex morphologic characteristics, but the risk of restenosis following the procedure remains high.

Directional coronary atherectomy has recently become available to treat coronary stenoses. Ellis and co-workers[157] in Ann Arbor, Michigan performed a study to determine the relation of patient characteristics and stenosis morphology to procedural outcome with directional coronary atherectomy to gain insight into which patients might be best treated with this device. Four hundred stenoses from 378 patients consecutively treated at six major referral institutions were analyzed. Angiographic data were assessed at a central angiographic laboratory using standardized morphological criteria and computer-assisted quantitative dimensional analyses. Procedural success was achieved in 88% of stenoses, and major ischemic complications (death, AMI, and emergency CABG) occurred in 6% of patients. Lesion success and complications were closely correlated with recognized modified American College of Cardiology/American Heart Association Task Force lesion morphological criteria. Observed for type A stenoses were 93% success and 3% complication rates; for type B1 stenoses, 88% success and 6% complication rates; and for type B2 stenoses, 75% success and 13% complication rates, respectively. There were too few type C stenoses treated to analyze. Furthermore, multivariate testing demonstrated stenosis angulation, proximal tortuosity, decreased preatherectomy minimum lumen dimension, and calcification to correlate independently with adverse outcome and complex, probably thrombus-associated stenoses to have a favorable outcome. Operator expense and a history of restenosis also favorably influenced outcome. The procedural outcome of directional coronary atherectomy is highly associated with coronary stenosis morphology. Furthermore, after appropriate stratification for morphology and clinical presentation, overall atherectomy procedural outcome may be similar to that achieved with PTCA. However, specific subsets of patients may have relatively better outcome with either atherectomy or balloon angioplasty.

To assess by quantitative analysis the immediate angiographic results of directional coronary atherectomy, Serruys and associates[158] from Rotterdam, The Netherlands, compared the effects of successful atherectomy with those of successful balloon dilatation in 62 patients. Angiographic success on the basis of intention to treat was obtained in 54 patients (87%). In 4 patients the lesion could not be crossed by the atherectomy device; all 4 had an uneventful conventional balloon angioplasty. Four of the 58 patients who underwent atherectomy were subsequently referred for CABG because of failure or complications; 3 of them sustained a transmural infarction. In the successful cases, coronary atherectomy resulted in an increase in the minimal luminal diameter from 1.1 mm to 2.5 mm with a concomitant decrease of the diameter stenosis from 62% to 22%. In the subset of 37 patients in which the changes induced were compared with conventional balloon angioplasty atherectomy increased the minimal luminal diameter more than balloon angioplasty (1.6 vs 0.8 mm). Conventional histology showed media or adventitia in 26% of the atherectomy specimens. In hospital complications occurred in 6 patients who had undergone a successful procedure: 2 transmural infarctions, 2 subendocardial infarctions, 1 transient ischemia attack, and 1 death due to delayed rupture of the atherectomized vessel. All patients were clinically evaluated at 1 and 6 months. One patient had persisting angina (New York Heart Association class II), 1 patient sustained a myocardial infarction, 1 patient underwent a percutaneous transluminal coronary angioplasty for early restenosis, and 1 patient underwent CABG because of a coronary aneurysm formation. At 6 months 80% (36/47) of the patients were symptom free. Coronary atherectomy achieved a better immediate angiographic result than balloon angioplasty; however, in view of the complication rate in this preliminary series, which may be related to a learning curve, a randomized study is needed to show whether this procedure is as safe as a conventional PTCA.

Popma and colleagues[159] in Ann Arbor, Michigan, Rochester, Minnesota, Indianapolis, Indiana, Cleveland and Cincinnati, Ohio, and Atlanta, Georgia, defined the clinical, angiographic and procedural correlates of quantitative coronary dimensions after directional coronary atherectomy in 400 lesions in 378 patients using qualitative morphologic and quantitative angiographic methods. Successful atherectomy, defined by a <75% residual area of stenosis, tissue retrieval and the absence of in-hospital ischemic complications was performed in 351 lesions (88%). After atherectomy, minimal cross-sectional area increased from 1.2 ± 1.1 to 6.6 ± 4.4 mm^2 and percent area of stenosis was reduced from 87 ± 10% to 31 ± 42%. By univariate analysis, device size and left circumflex artery lesion location were associated with a larger final minimal cross-sectional area. Restenosis lesion, lesion length ≥10 mm and lesion calcification were quantitatively associated with a smaller final minimum cross-sectional area. Stepwise multivariate analysis demonstrated that atherectomy device size and left circumflex lesion location were independently associated with a larger final minimal cross-sectional area, whereas restenosis lesion, diffuse proximal disease, lesion length ≥10 mm and lesion calcification were significantly correlated with a smaller final minimal cross-sectional area (Table 2-5). The number of specimens excised, the number of atherectomy passes and atherectomy balloon inflation pressure did not correlate with the final minimal cross-sectional area. There-

TABLE 2-5. *Clinical, angiographic and procedural correlates of final minimal cross-sectional area (mm²) after directional atherectomy. Reproduced with permission from Popma, et al.*[159]

	Univariate		Multivariate	
	Coefficient	p Value	Coefficient	p Value
Constant			3.654	0
Clinical factors				
Restenotic lesion	−1.409	0.002	−1.166	0.010
Male gender	−0.110	NS	—	—
Unstable angina	0.440	NS	—	—
Angiographic factors				
Circumflex artery	2.898	0.004	2.681	0.007
Calcification	−1.499	0.035	−1.615	0.081
ACC/AHA B2/C	−0.105	0.064	−1.531	NS
Diffuse proximal disease	−0.442	NS	−1.374	0.033
Lesion length ≥10 mm	−1.778	0.018	−0.080	0.026
Proximal tortuosity	−0.361	NS	—	—
Bend ≥45°	−0.880	NS	—	—
Irregularity	−0.147	NS	—	—
Bifurcation	−0.618	NS	—	—
Thrombus	−0.266	NS	—	—
Multivessel disease	0.033	NS	—	—
Procedural factors				
Device size	2.139	0.001	1.386	0.003
Number of specimens	0.040	NS	—	—
Number of passes	0.087	NS	—	—
Device/artery ratio	0.264	NS	—	—
Balloon inflation pressure	−0.050	NS	—	—
			Multiple R	0.436
			SEE	3.73
			p	<0.001

fore, directional atherectomy provides marked improvement of coronary lumen dimensions and its effect can be in part predicted by the presence of certain clinical, angiographic and procedural factors at the time of atherectomy.

LASER ANGIOPLASTY

Sanborn and associates[160] in New York, New York, evaluated the initial clinical experience and quantitative angiographic results of percutaneous coronary excimer laser-assisted balloon angioplasty for 55 lesions in 50 patients. With the use of a xenon chloride excimer laser generator and 1.5 to 1.75 mm catheters, excimer laser angioplasty was attempted at 135 ns pulse width, 25 to 40 Hz repetition rate, 2 to 5 s laser delivery time and 30 to 60 mJ/mm² energy fluence. Laser success was achieved in 41 (75%) of 55 lesions, with 100% subsequent balloon angioplasty success. The percent diameter stenosis was reduced from 81 ± 1% to 50 ± 3% after excimer laser angioplasty and to 20 ± 1% after balloon angioplasty. By videodensitometric techniques, the percent area of stenosis decreased from 86 ± 2% to 54 ± 3% after excimer angioplasty and to 26 ± 3% after balloon angioplasty. There were no perforations, need for emergency bypass surgery or deaths. The overall incidence of abrupt closure (3.6%), dissection (1.8%), embolization (1.8%), filling defect (6%), myocardial infarction (5.5%), side branch occlusion (3.6%) or spasm (3.6%) was infrequent and more related to balloon angioplasty than to the laser procedure in the investigators' opinion. During follow-up ranging from 1 to 10 months, mean 7 months, 36 (72%) of the 50 patients remained asymptomatic. Symptoms recurred in 14 patients (28%) in relation to abrupt closure in the first 24 hours in 2 patients (3.6%), late closure in the first week in 2 patients (3.6%) and restenosis in 10 patients (20%). Therefore, percutaneous coronary excimer laser angioplasty appears to be a feasible and safe procedure in selected patients.

An investigation was performed by Geschwind and associates[161] from Créteil, France, to determine the safety and efficacy of coronary pulsed mid-infra-red laser angioplasty. The laser was coupled with a novel 2.0 mm multifiber catheter consisting of 37 optical fibers of 150 μm each arranged concentrically around a 0.018-inch central lumen and a soft leading tapered distal tip to maintain coaxial alignment and position plaque in front of fibers. The laser was operated at 500 millijoules/pulse, 3.5 Hz, and 250 μsec/pulse. Twenty-three patients with stenosis or occlusion of the LAD or right coronary artery were selected for laser treatment. In 3 patients the catheter could not be positioned against the obstruction. In the 20 remaining patients laser angioplasty increased the diameter of the lumen from 0.3 ± 0.3 mm to 1.4 ± 0.3 mm and reduced the stenosis from 91 ± 8% to 57 ± 10%. In 3 patients stand-alone laser treatment was sufficient. In 17 patients PTCA further reduced the stenosis to 20 ± 18%. In 2 patients who had previously undergone unsuccessful PTCA with high inflation pressure, laser angioplasty allowed subsequent successful dilatation with low inflation pressure. There were no deaths, perforations, dissections, or arrhythmias. One patient had abrupt reclosure 24 hours after the procedure. Spasm occurred in 4 patients, and 6 patients had chest sensations during laser emission. Thus mid-infra-red pulsed coronary laser angioplasty is safe and effective for recanalization of stenosed and totally occluded arteries. The efficacy may be sufficient for stand-alone laser treatment. The technique may improve the efficacy of balloon angioplasty in cases of unsuccessful primary dilatation.

CORONARY STENTS

The placement of stents in coronary arteries after coronary angioplasty has been investigated as a way of treating abrupt coronary-artery occlusion related to the angioplasty and of reducing the late intimal hyperplasia responsible for gradual restenosis of the dilated narrowing. From March, 1986 to January, 1988, Serruys and associates[162] from Rotterdam, the Netherlands, and 4 other European medical centers implanted 117 self-expanding stainless steel endovascular stents (Wallstent) in the native coronary arteries (94 stents) or saphenous-vein bypass grafts (23 stents) of 105 patients. Angiograms were obtained immediately before and after placement of the stent and at follow-up at least one month later (unless symptoms required angiography sooner). The mortality after one year was 7.6% (8 patients). Follow-up angiograms (after a mean [± SD] of 5.7 ± 4.4 months) were obtained in 95 patients with 105 stents and were analyzed quantitatively by a computer-assisted system of cardiovascular angiographic analysis. The 10 patients without follow-up angiograms included 4 who died. Complete occlusion occurred in 27 stents in 25 patients (24%); 21 occlusions were documented within the first 14 days after implantation. Overall, immediately after placement of the stent there was a significant increase in the minimal luminal diameter and a significant decrease in the percentage of the diameter with stenosis (changing from a mean [± SD] of 1.88 ± 0.43 to 2.48 ± 0.51 mm and from 37 ± 12 to 21 ± 10%, respectively). Later, however, there was a significant decrease in the minimal luminal diameter and a significant increase in the stenosis of the segment with the stent (1.68 ± 1.78 mm and 48 ± 34% at follow-up). Significant restenosis, as indicated by a reduction of 0.72 mm in the minimal luminal diameter or by an increase in the percentage of stenosis to ≥50%, occurred in 32% and 14% of patent stents, respectively. Early occlusion remains an important limitation of this coronary-artery stent. Even when the early effects are beneficial, there are frequently late occlusions or restenosis. The place of this form of treatment for CAD remains to be determined.

Rab and associates[163] in Atlanta, Georgia, evaluated coronary artery stent sites by follow-up angiography at a medium of 4 months in 29 patients who received the Cook stent for acute coronary closure. Nineteen patients were treated with glucocorticoids administered intravenously or orally, or both, with or without colchicine and results were compared with those in 10 patients who were treated with neither agent. Standard therapy for all patients included routine administration of aspirin and heparin before and warfarin sodium and aspirin after stent placement. Most patients also received dipyridamole and lovastatin during the follow-up period. Six (32%) of the 19 stented arteries showed evidence of coronary artery aneurysm, defined as expansion of the lumen outside the margins of the stent. None of the patients in the control group who did not receive steroids or colchicine developed aneurysms. This pattern of altered vascular healing and stented coronary segments appears to be due to the addition of multiple anti-inflammatory drugs rather than to the stent presence alone. This observation demonstrates the possibility of medical impairment of normal vascular remodeling after acute injury and stent placement.

Fischman and colleagues[164] in Philadelphia, Pennsylvania, Washington, D.C., La Jolla, California, Ann Arbor, Michigan, New Haven, Connecticut, Houma, Louisiana, and San Antonio, Texas, evaluated the effect of the Palmaz-Schatz stent on the angiographic appearance and residual luminal stenosis in 84 consecutive patients (90 lesions) with intimal dissection after PTCA. Coronary angiography was performed before PTCA, after conventional PTCA, and after stent implantation. The degree of intimal disruption was assessed as follows: grade 0, no dissection; grade 1, simple dissection; or grade 2, complex dissection. Quantitative coronary analysis of digitized cineangiograms was performed with the use of a computerized automatic edge detection algorithm. After PTCA, 31 (34%) of 90 lesions demonstrated intimal dissection (18, simple, 13 complex). After stent implantation, intimal dissection improved by ≥1 grade in 29 (94%) of the 31 lesions with 27 (87%) reduced to grade 0. Dissection grade improved after stenting in 16 (89%) of 18 simple dissections and in all 13 complex dissections. Mean diameter stenosis was 77 ± 17% before PTCA, 47 ± 17% after PTCA and 14 ± 10% after stenting. Thus, intracoronary stenting is effective in reducing the residual luminal stenosis and in improving the angiographic appearance of intimal dissections after conventional balloon PTCA.

Haude and associates[165] from Mainz, Germany, described their experience at 1 center with the implantation of balloon-expendable Palmaz-Schatz Stent and focused on device-related complications in the short- and long-term angiographic outcome (Figure 2-25). Stenting was attempted in 50 patients. Restenosis after an initially successful angioplasty procedure, inadequate postangioplasty results, saphenous coronary bypass stenoses, and bail-out situations were regarded as indications. In 49 of 50 attempted patients 61 stents (1–4 per patient) were implanted. Delivery problems occurred in 3 patients and were successfully overcome in 2 patients. Bail-out situations were successfully managed in 16 patients. Complications included acute thrombus formation within the stent immediately after implantation in 1 patient, which was successfully treated by thrombolysis. One patient was sent for CABG the day after implantation; another died 10 days after implantation for unknown reasons. Subacute stent thrombosis occurred in 7 patients 5–9 days after implantation and was successfully treated by thrombolysis or PTCA in 5 patients. Bleeding complications occurred in 9 patients, 5 of whom required blood transfusions. Angiography showed long term vessel patency after 4–6 months in 31 (76%) of the 41 patients who were followed up, restenosis in 6 (14%), and reocclusion in 4 (10%). Late restenosis or reocclusion was found in 5 (15%) of 33 patients with a single stent in contrast to 5 (63%) of 8 patients with multiple stents. Balloon-expandable intracoronary stenting is a feasible method for treating the acute complications of balloon angioplasty. It reduced the rate of restenosis for single stent implantation. Subacute thrombotic events must be regarded as previously unknown and serious complications.

Dissections after coronary balloon angioplasty are risk factors for acute or subacute coronary arterial closure. Intracoronary stenting was devel-

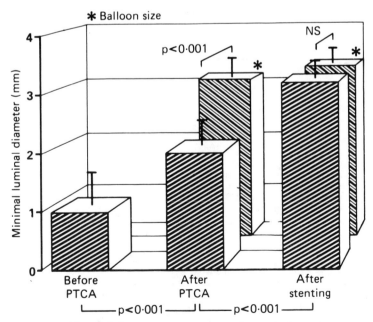

Fig. 2-25. Minimal luminal diameters (mean [1SD]) before and after balloon angioplasty and after implantation of balloon-expandable Palmaz-Schatz stents compared with the maximum balloon diameters used. Reproduced with permission of Haude, et al.[165]

oped to avoid these complications by pressing the intimal and medial flaps against the vessel wall, thus reducing the risk of acute thrombosis formation. Haude and associates[166] from Mainz, Germany, implanted 22 stents into the coronary arteries of 15 patients with dissections after balloon angioplasty which caused angina pectoris or ischemic electrocardiographic changes. Stent delivery was successful in all cases. In 1 patient acute stent thrombosis was documented and treated successfully by thrombolytic therapy. Another patient underwent CABG 24 hours later because of persisting angina. Angiograms after 24 hours documented vessel patency in the remaining 14 patients. Late control angiograms after 4 to 6 months were obtained in 12 of 14 patients. Vessel patency without significant restenosis was observed in 8 patients, restenosis in 3 and reocclusion in 1 patient. All 3 patients with multiple stent implantation had restenosis (n = 2) or reocclusion (n = 1), compared with 1 patient with single stent implantation. Thus, intracoronary stenting appears to be a secure and effective method of handling bailout situations caused by dissection after balloon angioplasty, with good long-term results when only a single stent is implanted.

CORONARY ARTERY BYPASS GRAFTING

Long-term results

Lawrie and associates[167] from Houston, Texas, followed 1,698 patients who underwent CABG using autogenous saphenous veins as conduits. The patients were operated on between 1968 and 1975 and they were followed for up to 20 years (Figures 2-26, 2-27, and 2-28). The age at operation was 54 ± 8 years and 1,485 patients (88%) were men. Angina was present in 1,637 patients (96%). There was single-vessel CAD in 306

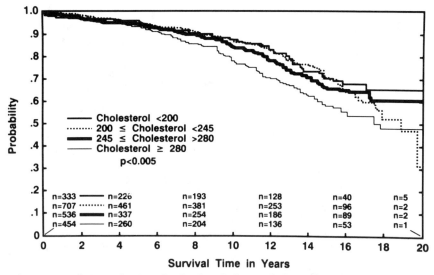

Fig. 2-26. Influence of various levels of total plasma cholesterol on the 20-year patency of saphenous vein grafts analyzed by the Kaplan-Meier technique. The number of patent grafts available for analysis at each interval are shown. Reproduced with permission of Lawrie, et al.[167]

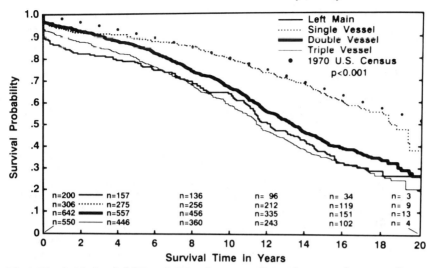

Fig. 2-27. Survival probabilities of 1698 patients according to the extent of coronary disease before operation. Reproduced with permission of Lawrie, et al.[167]

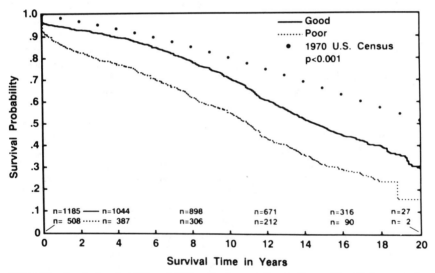

Fig. 2-28. Survival probabilities of 1698 patients according to the quality of left ventricular function before operation. Reproduced with permission of Lawrie, et al.[167]

patients (18%), double-vessel in 642 (38%), triple-vessel in 550 patients (32%) and LM stenosis in 200 (12%). Preoperative LV quality was good in 1,185 (70%), poor in 508 (30%), and unknown in 5 patients. Survival at 20 years was as follows: for single-vessel CAD, 40%; double-vessel, 26%; triple-vessel, 20%; and LM, 25%. At 20 years of follow-up, 67% of surviving patients were asymptomatic and 26% were improved. Antianginal drug therapy consisted of nitrates in 49% of patients and beta-blockers in 26%. Graft patency at 0 to 5 years was 633 or 780 grafts (81%); at 6 to 10 years, 415 of 606 grafts (68%); at 11 to 15 years, 271 of 449 grafts (60%); and at 16 to 20 years, 65 of 140 grafts (46%). Coronary bypass reoperation was performed in 324 patients (19%) and survival of these patients was 62% compared to 37% for non-reoperation patients. Cox analysis demonstrated that the major determinants of survival related to age at operation, extent of CAD, quality of ventricle, history of stroke, and preoperative congestive heart failure. At 20 years of follow-up of this early experience with coronary bypass, 76% of surviving patients had one or more patent grafts and the probability of freedom from reoperation was 0.62.

Changes in patient population and results

Jones and associates[168] from Atlanta, Georgia, attempted to document change in the patient population and results of CABG in recent years compared to earlier years. To document the change, they analyzed 2 groups of patients, 1 in 1981 (n = 1586) and 2 in 1987 (n = 1513), to document preoperative and postoperative variables important in determining immediate mortality and morbidity after isolated CABG. Between 1981 and 1987, patients were found to be older (≥70 years, 8.7% vs 21.8%), more often diabetic (15% vs 24%), have a greater prevalence of triple vessel CAD (14.5% vs 0.54 ± 13) (Table 2-6). To facilitate analysis and because of overlap between subgroups, the authors subdivided patients into 3 subgroups for statistical comparison of the years 1981 and 1987; subgroup I, no prior procedure (n = 1546 in 1981 and 1396 in 1987); subgroup II, optimal group (n = 503 in 1981 and 292 in 1987, and defined as no prior procedure, EF ≥0.50 and age <65 years); subgroup III, patients having reoperations (n = 40 in 1981 and 117 in 1987). Internal mammary artery grafting was infrequently used in 1981 but was used in 72.1% in 1987. Major postoperative morbidity between the 2 years for the total population increased significantly: need for intraaortic balloon pumping, 1.4% versus 4.7%; myocardial infarction, 3.5% versus 5.5%; stroke, 1.4% versus 2.8%; and wound infection, 1.0% versus 3.0%. Wound infection (all types) in 1987 was increased sevenfold in patients having a perioperative myocardial infarction (0.7% vs 5%). For young patients with good LV function (subgroup II), there was no increase in these morbid events between 1981 and 1987. Hospital mortality in the total population increased significantly between 1981 and 1987 from 1.2% to 3.1%, respectively (Figure 2-29). It was lowest for the patients in optimal condition (subgroup II) in both years, 0.8% versus 1.1%, and highest for reoperative patients, 5.3% versus 4.3%. In 1981, 58% of patients (503/870) were in the optimal group compared with 35% (292/828) in 1987. The last 6 years have seen a progressive

TABLE 2-6. *Preoperative characteristics. Reproduced with permission from Jones, et al.[168]*

	1981	1987	p Value
No. of patients	1586	1513	
% Male	81	78	0.031
% Diabetic	15 (135/896)	24 (235/995)	<0.0001
Mean age (yr)	58 ± 9	61 ± 10	<0.0001
% ≥65 yr	22.9	40.1	<0.0001
% ≥70 yr	8.7	21.8	<0.0001
Vessel disease	1.98 ± 0.92 (657)	2.66 ± 0.84 (882)	<0.0001
% Multivessel	65.8	90.8	<0.0001
% 3-vessel	14.5	46.1	<0.0001
% Left main	9.0	14.7	0.0025
EF (No. of patients)	870	828	
Mean	60 ± 14	54 ± 13	<0.0001
% <0.35	4.3	8.2	0.0015
% >0.50	77.6	67.1	0.054
Grafts	3.20 ± 1.14 (1588)	3.37 ± 1.08 (1511)	<0.0001
RI*	1.81 ± 0.91 (657)	1.36 ± 0.62 (880)	<0.0001

EF. Ejection fraction.
*Revascularization index (RI) = number of anastomoses performed/number of diseased arteries.

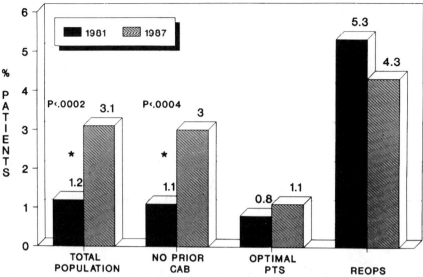

Fig. 2-29. Hospital mortality for all groups of patients. Reproduced with permission of Jones, et al.[168]

TABLE 2-7. *Perioperative complications. Reproduced with permission from Salomon, et al.*[169]

	Group I (n = 6635)	Group II (n = 469)	p Value
Transmural ECG changes*	4.5% (296)	5.1% (24)	NS
Average peak CK-MB	17.47	22.4	p < 0.01
Arrhythmias			
PVC	11.4% (758)	19.8% (93)	p < 0.001
Supraventricular	20.9% (1387)	41.4% (194)	p < 0.001
VT/VF	2.3% (152)	7.5% (35)	p < 0.001
Oliguric renal insufficiency	0.9% (57)	2.3% (11)	p < 0.01
Neurologic complication	1.0% (70)	4.1% (19)	p < 0.001
Prolonged ventilatory support	4.3% (285)	16.2% (76)	p < 0.001
IABP	1.7% (116)	3.4% (16)	p < 0.01
Reoperation for bleeding	4.8% (317)	5.3% (25)	NS
Wound complication	0.6% (40)	0.4% (2)	NS
ICU hours	57.3	68.9	p < 0.05
Days from operation to discharge	8.2	10	p < 0.001
Hospital charges	$19,700	$25,400	p < 0.001

ECG, Electrocardiographic; CK-MB, creatine kinase MB isoenzyme; PVC, premature ventricular contractions; VT/VF, ventricular tachycardia/ventricular fibrillation; IABP, intraaortic balloon pump; ICU, intensive care unit; NS, not significant.
*Or CK-MB > 30 mg/dl.

trend in surgically treating older, sicker patients who have more complex disease, with a significant reduction in the best candidate group. This trend is likely to continue, with a concomitant rise in postoperative complications and hospital mortality.

In older patients

Salomon and associates[169] from Portland, Oregon, reported a consecutive series of 7,104 patients having isolated CABG from 1971 to 1988 and they compared the results of 469 patients >75 years of age at the time of operation to those younger than that age (Table 2-7). Results were analyzed to determine comparative risk factors for morbidity, early and late survival, and functional outcome. Patients younger than 75 years (group I) and patients older than 75 years (group II) were identical for

EF and standard hemodynamic indices. Mean number of grafts and cross-clamp time were greater for group II patients. Mean age of group I was 58.6 years and group II, 77.6 years. Women composed 19.7% (1308/6635) of group I and 36.2% (170/469) of group II patients. Mammary grafts were placed in 57.5% (3830/6635) of group I and 41.6% (195/469) of group II patients. Overall perioperative mortality rate was 2.1% for group I and 6.8% for group II. Perioperative AMI rate was similar for the 2 groups. Ventricular and supraventricular arrhythmias, renal insufficiency, neurologic complications, prolonged ventilatory support, increased hospital cost, and prolonged hospitalization were significantly more prevalent in patients older than 75 years. Five and 10 years postoperatively, there were no significant differences between groups I and II with regard to event-free status including angina, myocardial infarction, and reoperation. The 5-year survival rate was 92% for group I and 80% for group II, similar to that of age-matched control subjects. The significantly increased potential for complications and expense of coronary bypass in patients over 75 years of age mandates judicious patient selection and preoperative counseling. Despite a significantly increased early mortality and an anticipated decreased long-term survival paralleling normal life table survival curves, good intermediate functional improvement can be realized in patients older than 75 years, comparable with that expected in a much younger age group.

Ko and associates[170] from New York, New York, reviewed results of isolated CABG in patients aged 80 years or older and New York Heart Association functional class III (24%) or IV (76%) operated on from 1985 to 1989 at their institution. The operations were elective in 36 patients, urgent in 52, and emergent in 12. Twenty-eight patients had significant disease of the left main coronary artery, with the remainder having an average of 2.8 diseased coronary vessels. Postoperative LVEF was considered good (>50%) in 62 patients, fair (30% to 50%) in 24 patients, and poor (<30%) in 14 patients. An average of 2.8 grafts were performed per patient, and the internal mammary artery was used in 10 patients. Univariate analysis of 36 perioperative factors followed by multivariate logistic regression analysis of the significant variables revealed that the urgency of the operation and LVEF were independent predictors of operative mortality. There were 12 in-hospital deaths, and the mortality was significantly lower in the elective cases (2.8%) than in the urgent (13.5%) and emergent cases (33.3%). Major complications occurred in 14% of the elective cases, in 21% of the urgent cases, and in 67% of the emergent cases. The operative mortality rates for good, fair, and poor LVEF were 4.9%, 12.5%, and 42.9%, respectively. Long-term follow-up averaging 22 months revealed a 77% actuarial probability of survival at 24 months and 51% at 48 months, with only 2 cardiac-related deaths. The authors concluded that CABG can be performed in octogenarians with a favorable outcome when done electively in patients with normal to moderately depressed LV function.

After failed angioplasty

Greene and associates[171] from Louisville, Kentucky, and Chicago, Illinois, described 60 patients who required immediate emergency CABG after PTCA among 1,214 patients having PTCA: 7 of the 60 patients had evidence of AMI before PTCA and they were excluded from the study. Of the remaining 53 patients, 27 (51%) had electrocardiographic and enzyme evidence of post-operative AMI. Two patients died and 10 had postoperative complications (19%). No statistical difference was noted comparing age, sex, incidence of prior AMI or myocardial dysfunction, time for CABG, or average number of grafts completed in those with single-vessel (n = 21) versus multivessel (n = 32) CAD. Postoperatively, those with multi-vessel CAD required intra-aortic balloon pump support and antiarrhythmic medications more frequently than those with single-vessel CAD and had a higher complication rate. The authors concluded that emergency CABG after failed PTCA carries a higher mortality and morbidity than after elective CABG, particularly for patients with multi-vessel CAD.

For stable angina pectoris

Nwasokwa and associates[172] from Bronx, New York, provided a fine review of predictors of survival benefit and strategy for patient selection of coronary artery bypass grafting for stable angina pectoris.

In dialysis patients

To analyze the short- and long-term morbidity and mortality among maintenance dialysis patients who have undergone CABG, Batiuk and associates[173] from Rochester, Minnesota, identified 20 such patients at the Mayo Clinic and 3 recently published large single center studies that provided sufficient detail for meaningful comparison. Two independent observers reviewed the new information with regard to pertinent historical, clinical, and laboratory data. The perioperative mortality was 20%. Among the perioperative survivors, 1- and 2-year survival rates were 95% and 77%, respectively. The 3-year actuarial survival was 70%. Uniformly, the symptoms diminished, and the need for antianginal medication was decreased. In the 3 other large published series, the perioperative mortality ranged from 3 to 20%, and CABG performed earlier after the onset of the symptoms seemed to result in a lower perioperative mortality. The authors concluded that elective CABG in dialysis patients is associated with acceptable short-term morbidity and mortality and effective relief of symptoms. Surgically treated patients may have a survival advantage. Thus, aggressive early investigation and surgical treatment of these patients is advocated.

Atherosclerosis in ascending aorta

Mills and Everson[174] from New Orleans, Louisiana, analyzed 1,735 patients who underwent CABG from January, 1981 to December, 1988 and found that 152 (9%) had mild (4.5%), moderate (2.2%), or severe (2.0%) atherosclerosis of the ascending aorta. Three distinct pathologic patterns were found (Figure 2-30). The prevalence of stroke in patients with the severe type of aortic disease prompted development of a new operative technique that has been used in 16 patients. It involves a "no-touch" technique of the ascending aorta whereupon the proximal saphenous vein anastomoses are performed end to side to internal mammary artery grafts (Figure 2-31). Ages ranged from 49 to 80 years (mean 68.9). The 16 patients had 62 distal artery and vein anastomoses and 26 proximal saphenous vein-internal mammary end-to-side anastomoses. Internal mammary artery free flows ranged from 130 to 420 ml/min. Two hospital deaths were unrelated to the technique. There have been no strokes or recurrences of angina. An inordinately high incidence of LM CAD (50%),

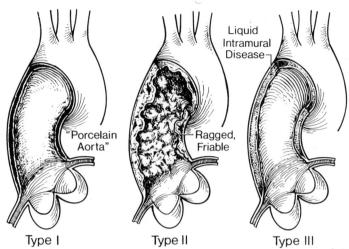

Type I   Type II   Type III

Fig. 2-30. Patterns of ascending aortic atherosclerosis. It is our contention that no clamp is safe on these types of ascending aortic disease. Type I: Circumferential ascending aortic calcification which may be easily diagnosed preoperatively on the angiogram. Palpation of the ascending aorta at operation reveals firm calcification. Embolization or aortic injury that may be difficult to repair may result if the aorta is clamped. Type II: This pattern may be diagnosed preoperatively by noting an irregularity of the normally smooth lining of the ascending aorta on the left ventricular angiogram or aortic root injection. Visualization of the ascending aorta is now considered a mandatory part of workup before CABG. Type III: Intraluminal liquid debris is the most elusive of the three patterns to diagnose before clamping the aorta. A pale appearance of the aorta or adherence of the adventia to the ascending aorta may be the only diagnostic clues. Operative echocardiography will reveal a thickened ascending aorta that will liberate liquid debris if a crossclamp or partial occlusion clamp is applied. Reproduced with permission of Mills, et al.[174]

significant carotid disease (79%), and abdominal aortic occlusive or aneurysm disease (93%) was discovered. Ascending aortic atherosclerosis must be suspected in all coronary bypass patients with associated significant carotid, abdominal aortic, and main left coronary artery disease, aortic wall irregularity on ascending aortic angiography, adhesions between the ascending aorta and its adventitia, pale appearance of the ascending aorta, and minimal bleeding of an aortic cannulation stab wound. A "no-touch" technique that avoids any manipulation of the ascending aorta and that uses the internal mammary arteries as the sole source of blood supply for coronary bypass is an effective method to prevent aortic clamp injury, "trash heart," or stroke from severe ascending aortic disease. Preoperative angiographic visualization of the ascending aorta of all patients undergoing coronary artery bypass is mandatory.

Quality of life afterwards

Caine and associates[175] from Cambridge, UK, measured changes in patients' perceptions of how differing states of health affect their lives and determination of the ability of preoperative variables to predict outcome after CABG. The study was prospective with completion of questionnaires before CABG and at 3 months, 12 months, and 60 months afterwards. One hundred men all aged 60 years at the time of operation were studied. Patients' assessment of their health state in terms of func-

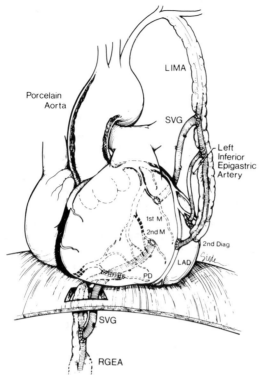

Fig. 2-31. Operation using "no-tough" technique for ascending aortic disease. SV grafts are anastomosed to the IMAs and the right gastroepipoic artery after hypothermic cardiac fibrillation is used with low blood flow or circulatory arrest. The right IMA is not used in diabetic patients because of the significantly increased chance of sternal infection with the use of double IMA grafts. LIMA left internal mammary artery; SVG saphenous vein graft; M, marginal: PD posterior descending; LAD, left anterior descending: RGEA right gastro-epiploic artery. Reproduced with permission of Mills, et al.[174]

tional capacity and aspects of distress, according to the Nottingham health profile and outcome of operation in terms of changes in symptoms, working life, and daily activities determined by self completed study questionnaires before operation and at 3 and 6 months afterwards. In-termediate 1 year results are reported. The differences between the Not-tingham health profile scores before operation and at 3 months afterwards were significantly different indicating an appreciable improvement in general health state, and at 1 year compared favorably with those from a normal male population. Analysis of responses to the study question-naire showed that 65 of 89 patients (73%) were working at 1 year after operation with a further 7 (8%) maintaining that they were fit to work but unable to find employment. The proportion of patients complaining of chest pain fell from 90% (88/98) before grafting to 19% (17/89) at 1 year after CABG, when 91% (81/89) patients maintained that their condition was either completely better or definitely improved. The significant pos-itive factors affecting return to work and home activities were working before operation, short wait for operation, absence of breathlessness, and low physical mobility score in the Nottingham health profile. Improve-ments were evident in general health state, symptoms, and activity at 3 months and 1 year after CABG. Interventions likely to influence outcomes included reduction in waiting times for operation; rehabilitation initiatives; and more attention to the quality of information given to patients, their relatives, and the community.

Differences in mortality

O'Connor and associates[176] from several cities in either Vermont, New Hampshire, or Maine conducted a prospective regional study to determine if the observed differences in in-hospital mortality rates associated with CABG were solely the result of differences in patient case mix. The study presented data for 3,055 CABG patients who underwent operation between 1 July 1987 and 15 April 1989. The data came from 5 regional medical centers. The overall crude in-hospital mortality rate for isolated CABG was 4.3%. The rate varied among centers (range, 3.1% to 6.3%) and among surgeons (range, 1.9% to 9.2%) (Figure 2-32). Predictors of in-hospital mortality included increased age, female gender, small body surface area, greater comorbidity, reoperation, poorer cardiac function as indicated by a lower EF, increased LV end diastolic pressure, and emergent or urgent surgery. After adjusting for the effects of potentially confounding variables, substantial and statistically significant variability was observed among medical centers and among surgeons. The authors concluded that the observed differences in in-hospital mortality rates among institutions and among surgeons in northern New England are not solely the result of differences in case mix as described by these variables and may reflect differences in currently unknown aspects of

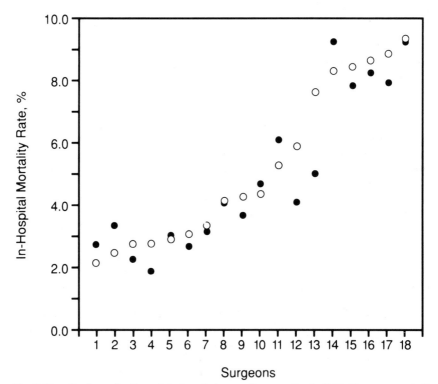

Fig. 2-32. Crude and adjusted in-hospital mortality rates by individual surgeon. Black circles indicate crude rate; and open circles, adjusted rate. Reproduced with permission of O'Connor et al.[176]

patient care. Understanding this variation requires a detailed understanding of the processes of care.

To measure hospital- and surgeon-specific mortality rates for patients having CABG and to examine possible reasons for the differences, Williams and associates[177] from Philadelphia, Pennsylvania, collected 4,613 patients over a 30-month period, operated on at 5 major teaching hospitals in Philadelphia, Pennsylvania. The authors observed differences in in-hospital mortality rates for patients who underwent coronary artery catheterization and CABG during the same admission but not for patients who underwent only CABG surgery during the admission. There were threefold differences in surgeon-specific mortality rates. The hospital mortality rates for coronary artery catheterization and CABG surgery during the same admission changed during the study and coincided with moves of surgeons among study hospitals. Our measures of illness severity did identify patients who were more likely to die, but differences in severity of illness did not explain differences in hospital- or surgeon-specific mortality rates. Patient mortality rates were not associated with the volume of procedures performed by individual surgeons. The authors found inconclusive evidence for an association with surgeons' clinical skills, and, to a lesser extent, with the hospital's volume of procedures and the hospital's organization and staffing. A greater intensity of hospital services was not necessary for a lower mortality rate. The authors concluded that studies of CABG mortality should examine mortality rates by diagnosis related group, collect data from >1 year, examine associations with surgeons' clinical skills, include information on hospital organization and staffing, and cautiously explore more efficient ways of providing care.

Repeat operations

Verheul and associates[178] from Amsterdam, The Netherlands, studied preoperative clinical status in cardiac catheterization data in 200 consecutive patients over a 9-year period to determine clinical outcome and long-term results of a second CABG operation (1979 to 1987) (mean follow up time 34 months, maximum 120). The study group included 169 men and 31 women (mean age 58.4 years [7% >70 years]). Sixty-four percent of patients had severe angina (New York Heart Association class IV), 70% had 3-vessel CAD and 21% had poor LV function. Reoperation was performed after a mean interval of 58 months after the first procedure. A mean of 3.3 distal anastomoses was placed. The operative mortality rate (30 days) was 7.5%, with additional cardiac morbidity (myocardial infarction CHF) in 11.5% of patients. Multivariate analysis showed an increased risk in women (risk ratio 3.6) and in patients with poor LV function (risk ratio 3.1). The cumulative 5-year survival rate was estimated at 84%, with a rate of 77% for patients with poor LV function (difference not significant). The probability of remaining free of a cardiac-related event (myocardial infarction, angioplasty, third operation, cardiac death) was 64% for 5 years. At the end of follow-up, 79% of the surviving patients were in New York Heart Association class I or II and nearly 50% of patients in the fifth year after the reoperation had good functional status. It is concluded that a reoperation is effective but carries an increased, immediate, operative risk. Late survival is good and most patients will be free of cardiac events and be in a good clinical condition in the first 5 years.

Initial reoperative CABG is being performed commonly and an increasing number of patients are being referred for subsequent reoperative CABG. From January, 1980, through June, 1990, 53 patients (52 men) underwent a third or fourth CABG operation and were respectively reviewed by Accola and associates[179] from Atlanta, Georgia. This represented 0.3% (53/17,102) of the CABG procedures done during that time period. The mean age was 59 ± 8 years. The number of grafts placed ranged from 1 to 4 with an average of 2.6 per patient. Internal mammary artery grafts were used in 30 patients (57%). The mean LVEF was 0.52 ± 0.13. Intra-aortic balloon pump support was necessary in 10 patients postoperatively. There were no intraoperative deaths, although 4 patients died in the postoperative hospitalization period. Perioperative myocardial infarctions were diagnosed in 6 patients, 13 patients had perioperative dysrhythmias, and 2 patients sustained a stroke. Superficial wound infections occurred in 5 patients. Late follow-up in 49 patients revealed that 2 other patients have since died, and no further myocardial infarctions have been reported in the survivors. Postoperative 3-year survival is 70%. Although there is increased risk of operative complications and early death after multiple reoperative CABG, both in-hospital and long-term results suggest that it is an appropriate therapeutic strategy.

Bilateral internal mammary arterial grafts

Bilateral internal mammary artery grafting is recognized as the preferred method of myocardial revascularization. Its efficacy in CABG reoperation has not been clearly established. From January 1982 through June 1989 Galbut and associates[180] from Miami, Florida, utilized bilateral internal mammary artery grafts in 88 patients who underwent coronary artery bypass reoperation. Results were compared with those for a subset of 88 patients receiving primary revascularization with bilateral internal mammary artery grafts who were computer-matched for age, sex, LV function, anginal classification, and LM CAD. In each group, 62.5% (55 patients) had unstable angina, 43.2% (38 patients) had reduced EF, and 21.6% (19 patients) in the reoperation group and 20.5% (18 patients) in the reference group had left main CAD. Hospital mortality for the reoperation group was 6.8% (6 patients) and for the reference group, 3.4% (3 patients). No significant difference was found in the incidence of reoperation for bleeding, sternal infection, or stroke in the 2 groups. The incidence of respiratory insufficiency in the reoperation group was 13.6% (12 patients) and in the reference group, 3.4% (3 patients). Recurrent angina occurred in 13.7% (10 patients) of patients in the reoperation group and 13.3% (10 patients) in the reference group. The long-term survival at 5 years for the reoperation group was 85.3% ± 5.6% and for the reference group, 91.6% ± 3.1%. No significant difference was found in the equality of survival distribution for the 2 groups. The results of this comparative study demonstrate that bilateral internal mammary artery grafting can be accomplished with an acceptable operative risk in patients undergoing reoperation. Further, survivors of reoperation experience long-term survival benefits and functional improvement similar to those receiving primary CABG.

Aspirin

Bashein and associates[181] from Seattle, Washington, performed a case-controlled study to estimate the relative risk of reoperation for bleeding after CABG in patients who had taken aspirin within 7 days preceding surgery. Comparison of 90 cases of reoperation with 180 matched control subjects gave an estimated odds ratio for reoperation of 1.82. Although their preoperative coagulation values were similar, cases used significantly more whole blood (cases, 9.5 ± 5.2 units; control subjects, 3.0 ± 2.0 units; median ± interquartile range), packed red blood cells (cases, 2.1 ± 4.0 units; control subjects, 0.9 ± 2.0 units), and platelets (cases, 12.2 ± 12.0 units; control subjects, 2.9 ± 4.0 units) than control subjects. Cases had intensive care unit stays of 4.7 ± 5.7 days (mean ± SD) vs 2.1 ± 1.9 days for control subjects and postoperative hospitalizations of 10.9 ± 1.9 days for control subjects and postoperative hospitalizations of 10.9 ± 8.2 days versus 7.0 ± 3.2 days for control subjects. The authors concluded that aspirin exposure within 7 days before CABG is associated with an increased rate of reoperation for bleeding and that reoperation is associated with large increases in transfusion requirements and intensive care unit and hospital stays.

Although aspirin therapy started before operation improves vein graft patency after CABG, it also causes bleeding. The objective of this prospective, centrally directed, randomized, double-blind, placebo-controlled trial by Goldman and collaborators[182] in Washington, D.C. was to compare the effects of aspirin therapy started before operation with aspirin started 6 hours after operation on early (7–10 day) graft patency. Patients were randomized to receive either aspirin 325 mg or placebo the night before surgery; after operation, all patients received aspirin 325 mg daily, with the first dose administered through the nasogastric tube 6 hours after operation. Angiography was performed in 72% of the analyzed patients an average of 8 days after operation, and the primary end point was saphenous vein graft patency in 351 patients. Internal mammary artery graft patency was also assessed in 246 patients because many individuals received both internal mammary artery and vein grafts. In the patients given preoperative aspirin, the vein graft occlusion rate was 7% compared with 8% in those who received preoperative placebo. In the subgroup of patients receiving Y grafts, 0% of the grafts were occluded in the preoperative aspirin group compared with 7% in the postoperative placebo group. The internal mammary artery occlusion rate was 0% in the aspirin group compared with 2.2% in the placebo group. Patients in the aspirin group received more transfusions than those in the placebo group. The reoperation rate for bleeding in the aspirin group was 6% compared with 2% in the placebo group. Median chest tube drainage within the first 6 hours after operation was 500 ml in the aspirin group compared with 448 ml in the placebo group. Thus preoperative aspirin is associated with increased bleeding complications and offers no additional benefit in early vein graft patency compared with starting aspirin therapy 6 hours after operation. There was a trend, although not significant, toward improved early patency for Y grafts and internal mammary artery grafts with preoperative aspirin.

Transfusion requirements

Goodnough and associates[183] and the Transfusion Medicine Academic Award Group audited 540 patients undergoing elective first-time CABG at 18 institutions to describe the variability in transfusions among institutions and to determine factors that may account for the variability. Mean homologous red blood cell use per patient was 2.9 (± 0.1) U (institutional range, 0.4 to 6.3 U). One hundred seventy-seven patients (32%)

received plasma (institutional range, 0% to 97%), and 119 (22%) received platelets (institutional range, 0% to 80%). After controlling for patient and surgical practice variables, transfusion practice factors still accounted for variation in red blood cell transfusions. Variation in patients receiving plasma and platelet transfusions among institutions was determined in part by prophylactic transfusions. The authors concluded that blood component usage for CABG differs widely among institutions. The variability in use of these components is accounted for in part by unnecessary transfusions in otherwise routine, uncomplicated CABG procedures.

This article was followed by an editorial entitled, "To Treat the Patient or To Treat The Surgeon", by Byron A. Myhre.[184] Myhre made the point that the institutions that use the least blood also use the least platelet concentrates and the least fresh-frozen plasma. Conversely, those that performed the most transfusions also used the most of all the components. Autologous blood, which was underused by all institutions, was employed by those that used fewer blood products. The institutions transfusing the least blood also had a smaller estimated blood loss in their patients.

Sotolol

To investigate the effectiveness and safety of low-dose sotalol in the prevention of SVT and to identify predictors for the occurrence of these arrhythmias shortly after CABG, Suttorp and associates[185] from Amsterdam, The Netherlands, randomized 300 consecutive patients in a double-blind, placebo-controlled study. Patients with severely depressed LV function or other contraindications for B blockers were excluded. Beginning at 4 hours and up to the 6th day after surgery, 150 patients received 40 mg of sotalol every 6 hours and 150 patients received placebo every 6 hours. SVT was observed in 24 (16%) of 150 low-dose sotalol- and in 49 (33%) of 150 placebo-treated patients. In patients receiving sotalol, AF was the only noted tachyarrhythmia, whereas in the placebo group, 42 (28%) patients had AF, 3 (2%) atrial flutter, 1 (0.7%) atrial tachycardia and 3 (2%) sinus tachycardia. Drug-related adverse effects necessitating discontinuation of the drug were noted in only 2 (1%) sotalol-treated patients and 4 (3%) placebo-treated patients. For both groups, univariate analysis indicated that older age, 1- or 2-vessel CAD, long bypass (≥150 minutes) and aorta cross-clamp time (≥120 minutes) were predictive variables for the occurrence of SVTs. Multivariate analysis showed that male sex (odds ratio 2.3), 1- or 2-vessel CAD (odds ratio 2.0) and older age (odds ratio 1.1) were independent risk factors for increased occurrence of postoperative SVT. The prophylactic use of low-dose sotalol [odds ratio 0.3] gave considerable and safe protection against the occurrence of SVTs shortly after CABG.

Supraventricular tachycardia afterwards

Hashimoto and associates[186] from Rochester, Minnesota, evaluated the influence of 45 variables on risk of postoperative SVT by univariate and multivariate analysis from 800 consecutive patients who underwent isolated CABG during a 6-year period. Postoperative supraventricular arrhythmias occurred in 186 patients (23%) but did not contribute to any of the 6 early deaths (30-day mortality rate, 0.8%). Mean length of hospital stay was longer (9.8 ± 5.7 vs 8.3 ± 3.5 days) and mean age was older (65 vs 60 years) in patients with postoperative SVT than in those with regular rhythm. Risk of SVT was increased in patients with a history of atrial arrhythmias (45% versus 22%) or atrial premature complexes on the preoperative electrocardiogram (48% versus 22%). Multiple logistic regression analysis identified age 65 years or more, history of atrial arrhythmia or preoperative atrial premature complexes, and preoperative LV end-diastolic pressure ≥20 mm Hg as independent predictors of postoperative SVT. Six percent of patients converted to sinus rhythm spontaneously; 82% of patients converted within 1.1 ± 1.9 days after onset of SVT on treatment with digoxin or B-adrenergic blocking drugs or both. Only 10% of patients with SVT required electrical cardioversion. The authors concluded that the risk of SVT after CABG is influenced by patient-related variables and is effectively managed by conventional therapy. Prophylactic treatment should be reserved for elderly patients, especially those who have atrial arrhythmias or have preoperative LV end-diastolic pressure ≥20 mm Hg.

Deep venous thrombosis afterwards

The frequency of deep vein thrombosis in patients undergoing CABG has not been established. Therefore to estimate the frequency of clinically silent deep vein thrombosis, Reis and associates[187] from Boston, Massachusetts, performed ultrasound examinations of the leg veins in 29 asymptomatic CABG patients before hospital discharge. They used high-resolution B-mode ultrasonography with color Doppler imaging. Fourteen (48%) had 20 documented leg vein thromboses, and all but 1 patient had deep vein thrombosis limited to the calf veins. Of the 20 thrombi, 10 (50%) were present in the leg ipsilateral and 10 (50%) in the leg contralateral to the saphenous vein harvest site. None of the deep vein thromboses were suspected clinically. Deep vein thrombosis was not associated with any local sign attributed to saphenous vein harvest such as pitting edema, incisional drainage, or local tenderness or with any putative risk factor for deep vein thrombosis such as cigarette use, distant history of malignancy, or varicose veins. Follow-up of these patients 5 to 11 months after CABG showed no clinical evidence of deep vein thrombosis or pulmonary embolism. These findings indicate that asymptomatic deep vein thrombosis of the calf occurs with surprisingly high frequency, 45% after CABG. Future studies in patients undergoing CABG should address the natural history of asymptomatic deep vein thrombosis, determine its clinical importance, and develop optimal strategies for prophylaxis and treatment.

Morphology late afterwards

Atherosclerotic plaque rupture with superimposed thrombosis is recognized as the lesion causing late, acute, thrombotic saphenous vein occlusion. In an investigation by Qiao and associates[188] from Los Angeles, California, to determine the severity of atherosclerosis at the site of plaque rupture, 68 saphenous vein grafts removed at the time of reoperation or at autopsy were studied. The study population consisted of 57 men, 64 ± 9 years old, and 9 women, 70 ± 10 years old. The duration of graft implantation was 7.9 ± 2.7 years. All grafts were dissected from the hearts, fixed, decalcified, cut at 2 to 3 mm intervals, and processed routinely for histologic examination. A planimeter was used to measure total vessel, plaque, thrombus, and luminal cross-sectional areas at the site of plaque rupture with thrombosis in sections projected at 14 power magnification.

At the site of atherosclerotic plaque rupture with superimposed thrombosis, the degree of stenosis due to plaque was: 90 ± 11% for the right coronary artery grafts (n = 19); 94 ± 7% for the LAD grafts (n = 41), and 90 ± 14% for the LC (n = 8) grafts. Thus, in saphenous vein grafts, atherosclerotic plaque rupture with thrombosis usually occurs at sites of severe narrowing (mean 93%) by preexisting atherosclerotic plaque.

KAWASAKI DISEASE

Treatment of the acute Kawasaki syndrome with a 4-day course of intravenous gamma globulin, together with aspirin, has been demonstrated to be safe and effective in preventing coronary-artery lesions and reducing systemic inflammation. Newburger and associates[189] from multiple medical centers in the USA hypothesized that therapy with a single, very high dose of gamma globulin would be at least as effective as the standard regimen. They conducted a multicenter, randomized, controlled trial involving 549 children with acute Kawasaki syndrome. The children were assigned to receive gamma globulin either as a single infusion of 2 g per kilogram of body weight over 10 hours or as daily infusions of 400 mg per kilogram for 4 consecutive days. Both treatment groups received aspirin (100 mg/kg per day through the 14th day of illness, then 3 to 5 mg/kg per day). The relative prevalence of coronary abnormalities, adjusted for age and sex, among patients treated with the 4-day regimen, as compared with those treated with the single-infusion regimen, was 1.94 2 weeks after enrollment and 1.84 7 weeks after enrollment. Children treated with the single-infusion regimen had lower mean temperatures while hospitalized, as well as a shorter mean duration of fever. Furthermore, in the single-infusion group the laboratory indexes of acute inflammation moved more rapidly toward normal, including the adjusted serum albumin level, alpha$_1$-antitrypsin level, and C-reactive protein level. Lower IgG levels on day 4 were associated with a higher prevalence of coronary lesions and with a greater degree of systemic inflammation. The 2 groups had a similar incidence of adverse effects (including new or worsening CAD in 9 children), which occurred in 2.7% of the children overall. All the adverse effects were transient. In children with acute Kawasaki disease, a single large dose of intravenous gamma globulin is more effective than the conventional regimen of 4 smaller daily doses and is equally safe.

TAKAYASU'S ARTERITIS

From 1961 to 1989, Amano and Suzuki[190] from Tokyo, Japan, reviewed 58 patients who had had coronary operations for Takayasu's arteritis and described 5 patients from their own institution who had undergone operations on the coronary arteries for Takayasu's arteritis. Most of the patients were Japanese (86%) and female (86%). The initial clinical manifestation was angina pectoris in 71%. Among 92 lesions, coronary ostia were most frequently involved (73%) followed by nonostial proximal lesions (18%). Forty-two of 62 (67.7%) ostial lesions of the LM coronary artery had >90% or complete, stenosis. Aortic regurgitation was associated in 28 patients (44%). Myocardial revascularization was performed in

49, and transaortic endarterectomy in 12. Concomitant AVR was done in 16 patients. Operative mortality was 5 (7.9%), and late deaths were reported in 3 patients. Postoperative steroid therapy was performed in 22. Operation was repeated in 2 patients because of graft failure. Thus, CAD resulting from Takayasu's arteritis should be suspected in young Asian women with angina pectoris. The timing preferred for surgical intervention is during an inactive phase. Two procedures are commonly chosen for surgical intervention, either transaortic endarterectomy or coronary revascularization with vein grafts. Postoperative steroid therapy is strongly recommended to those patients who are operated on in the clinically or histologically active stage.

References

---

1. MMWR 1991: (July 26);40:493.
2. Mizuno K, Miyamoto A, Satomura K, Kurita A, Arai T, Sakurada M, Yanagida S, Nakamura H: Angioscopic coronary macromorphology in patients with acute coronary disorders. Lancet 1991 (Apr 6);337:809–812.
3. Kragel AH, Gertz SD, Roberts WC: Morphologic comparison of frequency and types of acute lesions in the major epicardial coronary arteries in unstable angina pectoris, sudden coronary death and acute myocardial infarction. J Am Coll Cardiol 1991 (September);18:801–8.
4. Dollar AL, Kragel AH, Fernicola DJ, Waclawiw MA, Roberts WC: Composition of atherosclerotic plaques in coronary arteries in women <40 years of age with fatal coronary artery disease and implications for plaque reversibility. Am J Cardiol 1991 (June 1);67:1223–1227.
5. Gertz SD, Malekzadeh S, Dollar AL, Kragel AH, Roberts WC: Composition of atherosclerotic plaques in the four major epicardial coronary arteries in patients ≥90 years of age. Am J Cardiol 1991 (June 1);67:1228–1233.
6. Graham, SP, Vetrovec GW: Comparison of angiographic findings and demographic variables in patients with coronary artery disease presenting with acute pulmonary edema versus those presenting with chest pain. Am J Cardiol 1991 (Dec 15);68:1614–1618.
7. Valsania P, Zarich SW, Kowalchuk GJ, Kosinski E, Warram JH, Krolewski AS: Severity of coronary artery disease in young patients with insulin-dependent diabetes mellitus. Am Heart J 1991 (September);122:695–700.
8. Maron DJ, Fair JM, Haskell WL and the Stanford Coronary Risk Intervention Project Investigators and Staff: Saturated Fat Intake and Insulin Resistance in Men with Coronary Artery Disease. Circulation 1991 (November);84:2020–2027.
9. Isner JM, Chokshi SK: Cardiovascular complications of cocaine. Current problems in cardiology 1991 (Feb);2:91–123.
10. Kolodgie FD, Virmani R, Cornhill JF, Herderick EE, Smialek J: Increase in atherosclerosis and adventitial mast cells in cocaine abusers: An alternative mechanism of cocaine-associated coronary vasospasm and thrombosis. J Am Coll Cardiol 1991;17:1553–60.
11. Nobuyoshi M, Tanaka M, Nosaka H, Kimura T, Yokoi H, Hamasaki N, Kim K, Shindo T, Kimura K: Progression of coronary atherosclerosis: Is coronary spasm related to progression? J Am Coll Cardiol 1991 (October);18:904–10.
12. Yeung AC, Vekshtein VI, Krantz DS, Vita JA, Ryan TJ Jr, Ganz P, Selwyn AP: The effect of atherosclerosis on the vasomotor response of coronary arteries to mental illness. N Engl J Med 1991 (Nov 28);325:1551–1556.
13. Beitman BD, Kushner MG, Basha I, Lamberti J, Mukerji V, Bartels K: Follow-up status of patients with angiographically normal coronary arteries and panic disorder. JAMA 1991 (Mar 27);265:1545–1549.
14. Ayanian JZ, Epstein AM: Differences in the use of procedures between women and men hospitalized for coronary heart disease. N Engl J Med 1991 (July 25);325:221–225.

15. Steingart RM, Packer M, Hamm P, Coglianese ME, Gersh B, Geltman EM, Sollano J, Katz S, Moye L, Basta LL, Lewis SJ, Gottlieb SS, Bernstein V, McEwan P, Jacobson K, Brown EJ, Jukin ML, Kantrowitz NE, Pfeffer MA: Sex differences in the management of coronary artery disease. N Engl J Med 1991 (July 25);325:226–230.

16. Salem M, Kasinski N, Andrei AM, Brussel T, Gold MR, Conn A, Chernow B: Hypomagnesemia is a frequent finding in the emergency department in patients with chest pain. Arch Intern Med 1991 (Nov);151:2185–2190.

17. Pryor DB, Shaw L, Harrell FE Jr, Lee KL, Hlatky MA, Mark DB, Muhlbaier LH, Califf RM: Estimating the likelihood of severe coronary artery disease. Am J Med 1991 (May);90:553–562.

18. Solomon AJ, Tracy CM: The signal-averaged electrocardiogram in predicting coronary artery disease. Am Heart J 1991 (November);122:1334–1339.

19. Sabia P, Abbott RD, Afrookteh A, Keller MW, Touchstone DA, Sanjiv K: Importance of Two-dimensional Echocardiographic Assessment of Left Ventricular Systolic Function in Patients Presenting to the Emergency Room With Cardiac-Related Symptoms. Circulation 1991 (October);84:1615–1624.

20. Galanti G, Sciagra R, Comeglio M, Taddei T, Bonechi F, Giusti F, Malfanti P, Bisi G: Diagnostic accuracy of peak exercise echocardiography in coronary artery disease: Comparison with thallium-201 myocardial scintigraphy. Am Heart J 1991 (December);122:1609–1616.

21. Sawada SG, Segar DS, Ryan T, Brown SE, Dohan AM, Williams R, Fineberg NS, Armstrong WF, Feigenbaum H: Echocardiographic Detection of Coronary Artery Disease During Dobutamine Infusion. Circulation 1991; (May) 83:1605–1614.

22. Cohen JL, Greene TO, Ottenweller J, Binenbaum SZ, Wilchfort SD, Kim CS, Alston JR: Dobutamin digital echocardiography for detecting coronary artery disease. Am J Cardiol 1991 (June 15);67:1311–1318.

23. Zabalgoitia M, Gandhi DK, Abi-Mansour P, Yarnold PR, Moushmoush B, Rosenblum J: Transesophageal stress echocardiography: Detection of coronary artery disease in patients with normal resting left ventricular contractility. Am Heart J 1991 (November);122:1456–1463.

24. Siegel, RJ, Ariani M, Fishbein MC, Chae J-S, Park JC, Maurer G, Forrester JS: Histopathologic Validation of Angioscopy and Intravascular Ultrasound. Circulation 1991 (July);84:109–117.

25. Nissen SE, Gurley JC, Grines CL, Booth DC, McClure R, Berk M, Fischer C, DeMaria AN: Intravascular Ultrasound Assessment of Lumen Size and Wall Morphology in Normal Subjects and Patients With Coronary Artery Disease. Circulation 1991 (September);84:1087–1099.

26. Scudhir K, Fitzgerald PJ, MacGregor JS, DeMarco T, Ports TA, Chatterjee K, Yock PG: Transvenous Coronary Ultrasound Imaging—A Novel Approach to Visualization of the Coronary Arteries. Circulation 1991 (November);84:1957–1961.

27. Fragasso G, Benti R, Sciammarella M, Rossetti E, Savi A, Gerundini P, Chierchia SL: Symptom-limited exercise testing causes sustained diastolic dysfunction in patients with coronary disease and low effort tolerance. J Am Coll Cardiol 1991 (May);17:1251–5.

28. Akhras F, Jackson G: Raised exercise diastolic blood pressure as indicator of ischemic left ventricular dysfunction. Lancet 1991 (Apr 13);337:899–900.

29. Elder AT, Shaw TRD, Turnbull CM, Starkey IR: Elderly and younger patients selected to undergo coronary angiography. Br Med J 1991 (Oct 19) 303:950–953.

30. Topaz O, Warner M, Lanter P, Soffer A, Burns C, DiSciascio G, Cowley MJ, Vetrovec GW: Isolated significant left main coronary artery stenosis: Angiographic, hemodynamic, and clinical findings in 16 patients. Am Heart J 1991 (November);122:1308–1314.

31. Garber CE, Carleton RA, Camaione DN, Heller GV: The threshold for myocardial ischemia varies in patients with coronary artery disease depending on the exercise protocol. J Am Coll Cardiol 1991 (May);17:1256–62.

32. Dilsizian V, Smeltzer WR, Freedman NMT, Dextras R, Bonow RO: Thallium Reinjection After Stress-Redistribution Imaging-Does 24-Hour Delayed Imaging After Reinjection Enhance Detection of Viable Myocardium? Circulation 1991; (April) 83:1247–1255.

33. Takeishi Y, Tono-oka I, Ikeda K, Komatani A, Tsuiki K. Yasui S: Dilatation of the left ventricular cavity on dipyridamole thallium-201 imaging: A new marker of triple-vessel disease. Am Heart J 1991 (February);121:466–475.

34. Watters TA, Botvinick EH, Dae MW, Cahalan M, Urbanowicz J, Benefiel DJ, Schiller NB, Goldstone G, Reilly L, Stoney RJ: Comparison of the findings on preoperative dipyridamole perfusion scintigraphy and intraoperative transesophageal echocardiography: implications regarding the identification of myocardium at ischemic risk. J Am Coll Cardiol 1991;18:93–100.

35. Pennell DJ, Underwood R, Swanton RH, Walker JM, Ell PJ: Dobutamine thallium myocardial perfusion tomography. J Am Coll Cardiol 1991 (November);18:1471–9.

36. Coyne EP, Belvedere DA, Vande Streek PR, Weiland FL, Evans RB, Spaccavento LJ: Thallium-201 scintigraphy after intravenous infusion of adenosine compared with exercise thallium testing in the diagnosis of coronary artery disease. J Am Coll Cardiol 1991 (May);17:1289–94.

37. Abreu A, Mahmarian JJ, Nishimura S, Boyce TM, Verani MS: Tolerance and safety of pharmacologic coronary vasodilation with adenosine in association with thallium-201 scintigraphy in patients with suspected coronary artery disease. J Am Coll Cardiol 1991 (September);18:730–5.

38. Nishimura S, Mahmarian JJ, Boyce TM, Verani MS: Quantitative thallium-201 single-photon emission computed tomography during maximal pharmacologic coronary vasodilation with adenosine for assessing coronary artery disease. J Am Coll Cardiol 1991 (September);18:736–45.

39. Fleming RM, Kirkeeide RL, Taegtmeyer H, Adyanthaya A, Cassidy DB, Goldstein RA, with the technical assistance of Rodriquez-Bird J, Jones D, Stuart Y, Velasco F: Comparison of technetium-99m teboroxime tomography with automated quantitative coronary arteriography and thallium-201 tomographic imaging. J Am Coll Cardiol 1991 (May);17:1297–302.

40. Kettunen R, Huikuri HV, Heikkila J, Takkunen JT: Usefulness of technetium-99m-MIBI and thallium-201 in tomographic imaging combined with high-dose dipyridamole and handgrip exercise for detecting coronary artery disease. Am J Cardiol 1991 (Sept 1);68:575–579.

41. Stewart RE, Schwaiger M, Molina E, Popma J, Gacioch GM, Kalus M, Squicciarini S, Al-Aouar ZR, Schork A, Kuhl DE: Comparison of rubidium-82 positron emission tomography and thallium-201 SPECT imaging for detection of coronary artery disease. Am J Cardiol 1991 (June 15);67:1303–1310.

42. Kern MJ, Deligonul U, Tatineni S, Serota H, Aguirre F, Hilton TC: Intravenous adenosine: Continuous infusion and low dose bolus administration for determination of coronary vasodilator reserve in patients with and without coronary artery disease. J Am Coll Cardiol 1991 (September);18:718–29.

43. Janowitz WR, Agatston AS, Viamonte M Jr: Comparison of serial quantitative evaluation of calcified coronary artery plaque by ultrafast computed tomography in persons with and without obstructive coronary artery disease. Am J Cardiol 1991 (July 1); 68:1–6.

44. Cohen M, Hawkins L, Greenberg S, Fuster V: Usefulness of ST-segment changes in ≥2 leads on the emergency room electrocardiogram in either unstable angina pectoris or non-Q-wave myocardial infarction in predicting outcome. Am J Cardiol 1991 (June 15);67:1368–1373.

45. Crenshaw JH, Mirvis DM, El-Zeky F, Zwaag RV, Ramanathan KB, Maddock V, Kroetz FH, Sullivan JM: Interactive effects of ST-T wave abnormalities on survival of patients with coronary artery disease. J Am Coll Cardiol 1991 (August);18:413–20.

46. Mark DB, Shaw L, Harrell FE Jr, Hlatky MA, Lee KL, Bengtson JR, McCants CB, Califf RM, Pryor DB: Prognostic value of a treadmill exercise score in outpatients with suspected coronary artery disease. N Engl J Med 1991 (Sept 19);325:849–853.

47. Simari RD, Miller TD, Zinsmeister AR, Gibbons RJ: Capabilities of supine exercise electrocardiography versus exercise radionuclide angiography in predicting coronary events. Am J Cardiol 1991 (Mar 15);67:573–577.

48. Johnson SH, Bigelow C, Lee KL, Pryor DB, Jones RH: Prediction of death and myocardial infarction by radionuclide angiocardiography in patients with suspected coronary artery disease. Am J Cardiol 1991 (May 1);67:919–926.

49. Van Lierde J, Piessens J, Glazier JJ, Vroliz M, De Geest H, Willems JL: Long-term prognosis of male patients with an isolated chronic occlusion of the left anterior descending coronary artery. Am Heart J 1991 (December);122:1542–1547.

50. Cohen M, Merino A, Hawkins L, Greenberg S, Fuster V: Clinical and angiographic characteristics and outcome of patients with rest-unstable angina occurring during regular aspirin use. J Am Coll Cardiol 1991 (November);18:1458–62.

51. Qiu S, Theroux P, Genest J Jr, Solymoss BC, Robitaille D, Marcil M: Lipoprotein (a) blood levels in unstable angina pectoris, acute myocardial infarction, and after thrombolytic therapy. Am J Cardiol 1991 (June 1);67:1175–1179.

52. Eisenberg PR, Kenzora JL, Sobel BE, Ludbrook PA, Jaffe AS: Relation between ST segment shifts during ischemia and thrombin activity in patients with unstable angina. J Am Coll Cardiol 1991 (October);18:898–903.

53. Zalewski A, Shi Y, Nardone D, Bravette B, Weinstock P, Fischman D, Wilson P, Goldberg S, Levin DC, and Bjornsson TD: Evidence for Reduced Fibrinolytic Activity in Unstable Angina at Rest—Clinical, Biochemical, and Angiographic Correlates. Circulation 1991; (May) 83:1685–1691.

54. Wilcox I, Freedman SB, Allman KC, Collins FL, Leitch JW, Kelly DT, Harris PJ: Prognostic significance of a predischarge exercise test in risk stratification after unstable angina pectoris. J Am Coll Cardiol 1991 (September);18:677–83.

55. Brown KA: Prognostic value of thallium-201 myocardial perfusion imaging in patients with unstable angina who respond to medical treatment. J Am Coll Cardiol 1991 (April);17:1053–7.

56. Zhu YY, Chung WS, Botvnick EH, Dae MW, Lim AD, Ports TA, Danforth JW, Wolfe CL, Goldschlager N, Chatterjee K: Dipyridamole perfusion scintigraphy: The experience with its application in one hundred seventy patients with known or suspected unstable angina. Am Heart J 1991 (January);121:33–43.

57. Bilodeau L, Theroux P, Grégoire J, Gagnon D, Arsenault A: Technetium-99m Sestamibi tomography in patients with spontaneous chest pain: correlations with clinical, electrocardiographic and angiographic findings. J Am Coll Cardiol 1991 (December);18:1684–91.

58. Bugiardini R, Pozzati A, Borghi A, Morgagni GL, Ottani F, Muzi A, Puddu P: Angiographic morphology in unstable angina and its relation to transient myocardial ischemia and hospital outcome. Am J Cardiol 1991 (Mar 1);67:460–464.

59. Riemersma RA, Wood DA, MacIntyre CCA, Elton RA, Gey KF, Oliver MF: Risk of angina pectoris and plasma concentrations of vitamins A, C, and E and carotene. Lancet 1991 (Jan 5);337:1–5.

60. Kaski JC, Tousoulis D, Haider AW, Gavrielides S, Crea F, Maseri A: Reactivity of eccentric and concentric coronary stenoses in patients with chronic stable angina. J Am Coll Cardiol 1991 (March);17:627–33.

61. Tousoulis D, Kaski JC, Bogaty P, Crea F, Gavrielides S, Galassi AR, Maseri A: Reactivity of proximal and distal angiographically normal and stenotic coronary segments in chronic stable angina pectoris. Am J Cardiol 1991 (June 1);67:1195–1200.

62. Heller GV, Ahmed I, Tikemeier PL, Barbour MM, Garber CE: Comparison of chest pain, electrocardiographic changes and thallium-201 scintigraphy during varying exercise intensities in men with stable angina pectoris. Am J Cardiol 1991 (Sept 1);68:569–574.

63. Parodi O, Marcassa C, Casucci R, Sambuceti G, Verna E, Galli M, Inglese E, Marzullo P, Pirelli S, Bisi G, Giubbini R, Scopinaro F, for the Italian Group of Nuclear Cardiology: Accuracy and safety of technetium-99m Hexakis 2-methoxy-2-isobutyl isonitrile (Sestamibi) myocardial scintigraphy with high dose dipyridamole test in patients with effort angina pectoris: A multicenter study. J Am Coll Cardiol 1991 (November);18:1439–44.

64. Mangano DT, Hollenberg M, Fegert G, Meyer ML, London MJ, Tubau JF, Krupski WC, and the Study of Perioperative Ischemia (SPI) Research Group: Perioperative myocardial ischemia in patients undergoing noncardiac surgery—I: Incidence and severity during the 4 day perioperative period. J Am Coll Cardiol 1991 (March);17:843–50.

65. McLenachan JM, Weidinger FF, Barry J, Yeung A, Nabel EG, Rocco MB, and Selwyn AP: Relations Between Heart Rate, Ischemia, and Drug Therapy During Daily Life in Patients with Coronary Artery Disease. Circulation 1991; (April) 83:1263–1270.

66. Yeung AC, Barry J, Orav J, Bonassin E, Raby KE, Selwyn AP: Effects of Asymptomatic Ischemia on Long-term Prognosis in Chronic Stable Coronary Disease. Circulation 1991; (May) 83:1598–1604.

67. Barry J, Campbell S, Yeung AC, Raby KE, Selwyn AP: Waking and rising at night as a trigger of myocardial ischemia. Am J Cardiol 1991 (May 15);67:1067–1072.

68. Hinderliter A, Miller P, Bragdon E, Ballenger M, Sheps D: Myocardial ischemia during daily activities: The importance of increased myocardial oxygen demand. J Am Coll Cardiol 1991 (August);18:405–12.

69. Weiner DA, Ryan TJ, Parsons L, Fisher LD, Chaitman BR, Sheffield LT, Tristani FE: Significance of silent myocardial ischemia during exercise testing in patients with diabetes mellitus: A report from the coronary artery surgery study (CASS) registry. Am J Cardiol 1991 (Sept 15);68:729–734.

70. Fleisher LA, Rosenbaum SH, Nelson AH, Barash PG: The predictive value of preoperative silent ischemia for postoperative ischemic cardiac events in vascular and nonvascular surgery patients. Am Heart J 1991 (October);122:980–985.

71. Deedwania PC, Carbajal EV: Usefulness of ambulatory silent myocardial ischemia added to the prognostic value of exercise test parameters in predicting risk of cardiac death in patients with stable angina pectoris and exercise-induced myocardial ischemia. Am J Cardiol 1991 (Nov 15);68:1279–1286.

72. Miranda CP, Lehmann KG, Froelicher VF: Correlation between resting ST segment depression, exercise testing, coronary angiography, and long-term prognosis. Am Heart J 1991 (December);122:1617–1628.

73. Okumura K, Yasue H, Maysuyama K, Matsuyama K, Morikami Y, Ogawa H, Obata K: Effect of H_1 receptor stimulation on coronary artery diameter in patients with variant angina: comparison with effect of acetylcholine. J Am Coll Cardiol 1991 (February);17:338–45.

74. Morikami Y, Yasue H: Efficacy of slow-release nifedipine on myocardial ischemic episodes in variant angina pectoris. Am J Cardiol 1991 (Sept 1);68:580–584.

75. Motz W, Vogt M, Rabenau O, Scheler S, Luckhoff A, Strauer BE: Evidence of endothelial dysfunction in coronary resistance vessels in patients with angina pectoris and normal coronary angiograms. Am J Cardiol 1991 (Oct 15);68:996–1003.

76. Ardissino D, Savonitto S, Mussini A, Zanini P, Rolla A, Barberis P, Sardina M, Specchia G: Felodipine (once daily) versus nifedipine (four times daily) for Prinzmetal's angina pectoris. Am J Cardiol 1991 (Dec 15);68:1587–1592.

77. Dean JD, Jones CJH, Hutchison SJ, Peters JR, Henderson AH: Hyperinsulinemia and microvascular angina ("syndrome X"). Lancet 1991 (Feb 23);337:456–457.

78. Kaski JC, Tousoulis D, Galassi AR, McFadden E, Pereira WI, Crea F, Maseri A: Epicardial coronary artery tone and reactivity in patients with normal coronary arteriograms and reduced coronary flow reserve (syndrome X). J Am Coll Cardiol 1991;18:50–4.

79. Nihoyannopoulos P, Kaski JC, Crake T, Maseri A: Absence of myocardial dysfunction during stress in patients with syndrome X. J Am Coll Cardiol 1991 (November);18:1463–70.

80. Ridker PM, Manson JE, Gaziano JM, Buring JE, Hennekens CH: Low-dose aspirin therapy for chronic stable angina: A randomized placebo-controlled clinical trial. An Intern Med 1991 (May 15);114:835–839.

81. Manson JE, Stampfer MJ, Colditz GA, Willett WC, Rosner B, Speizer FE, Hennekens CH: A prospective study of aspirin use and primary prevention of cardiovascular disease in women. JAMA 1991 (July 24/31);266:521–527.

82. Ridker PM, Manson JE, Buring JE, Goldhaber SZ, Hennekens CH: The effect of chronic platelet inhibition with low-dose aspirin on atherosclerotic progression and acute thrombosis: Clinical evidence from the Physician's Health Study. Am Heart J 1991 (December);122:1588–1592.

83. Wallentin LC, and the Research Group on Instability in Coronary Artery Disease in Southeast Sweden: Aspirin (75 mg/day) after an episode of unstable coronary artery disease: long-term effects on the risk for myocardial infarction, occurrence of severe angina and the need for revascularization. J Am Coll Cardiol 1991 (December);18:1587–93.

84. Force T, Milani R, Hibberd P, Lorenz R, Uedelhoven W, Leaf A, Weber P: Aspirin-Induced Decline in Prostacyclin Production in Patients With Coronary Artery Disease Is Due to Decreased Endoperoxide Shift. Circulation 1991 (December);84:2286–2293.

85. Dubach UC, Rosner B, Sturmer T: An epidemiologic study of abuse of analgesic drugs: Effects of phenacetin and salicylate on mortality and cardiovascular morbidity (1968 to 1987). N Engl J Med 1991 (Jan 17);324:155–160.

86. Cohen MV, Byrne MJ, Levine B, Gutowski T, Adelson R: Low Rate of Treatment of Hypercholesterolemia by Cardiologists in Patients With Suspected and Proven Coronary Artery Disease. Circulation 1991; (April) 83:1294–1304.

87. Hahmann HW, Bunte T, Hellwig N, Hau U, Becker D, Dyckmans J, Keller HE, Schieffer HJ: Progression and regression of minor coronary arterial narrowings by quantitative angiography after fenofibrate therapy. Am J Cardiol 1991 (May 1);67:957–961.

88. Elkayam U: Tolerance to organic nitrates: Evidence, mechanisms, clinical relevance, and strategies for prevention. An Intern Med 1991 (Apr 15);114:667–677.

89. De Milliano PA, Koster RW, Bar FW, Janssen J, De Cock C, Schelling A, Van de Bos A: Long-term efficacy of continuous and intermittent use of transdermal nitroglycerin in stable angina pectoris. Am J Cardiol 1991 (Oct 1);68:857–862.

90. Steering Committee, Transdermal Nitroglycerin Cooperative Study: Acute and chronic antianginal efficacy of continuous twenty-four-hour application of transdermal nitroglycerin. Am J Cardiol 1991 (Nov 15);68:1263–1273.

91. Parker JD, Farrell B, Fenton T, Cohanim M, Parker JO: Counter-Regulatory Responses to Continuous and Intermittent Therapy With Nitroglycerin. Circulation 1991 (December);84:2336–2345.

92. Lehmann G, Reiniger G, Haase HU, Rudolph W: Enhanced effectiveness of combined sustained-release forms of isosorbide dinitrate and diltiazem for stable angina pectoris. Am J Cardiol 1991 (Oct 15);68:983–990.

93. Barth C, Ojile M, Pearson AC, Labovitz AJ: Ultra short-acting intravenous β-adrenergic blockade as add-on therapy in acute unstable angina. Am Heart J 1991 (March);121:782–788.

94. Hohnloser SH, Meinertz T, Klingenheben T, Sydow B, Just H, European Esmolol Study Group: Usefulness of esmolol in unstable angina pectoris. Am J Cardiol 1991 (June 15);67:1319–1323.

95. Frishman WH, Heiman M, Soberman J, Greenberg S, Eff J, Celiprolol International Angina Study Group: Comparison of celiprolol and propranolol in stable angina pectoris. Am J Cardiol 1991 (Apr 1);67:665–670.

96. Hill JA, Gonzalez JI, Kolb R, Pepine CJ: Effects of atenolol alone, nifedipine aline and their combination on ambulant myocardial ischemia. Am J Cardiol 1991 (Apr 1);67:671–675.

97. Ardissino D, Savonitto S, Egstrup K, Marraccini P, Slavich G, Rosenfeld M, Feruglio GA, Roncarolo P, Giordano MP, Wahlqvist I, Rehnqvist N, Barberis P, Specchia G, L'Abbate A: Transient myocardial ischemia during daily life in rest and exertional angina pectoris and comparison of effectiveness of metoprolol versus nifedipine. Am J Cardiol 1991 (May 1);67:946–952.

98. Theroux P, Baird M, Juneau M, Warnica W, Klinke P, Kostuk W, Pflugfelder P, Lavalle E, Chin C, Dempsey E, Grace M, Lalonde Y, Waters D: Effects of Diltiazem on Symptomatic and Asymptomatic Episodes of ST Segment Depression Occurring During Daily Life and During Exercise. Circulation 1991 (July);84:15–22.

99. Di Donato M, Maioli M, Venturi F, Burgisser C, Fantini F, Giamino G, Marchionni N: Acute hemodynamic effects of intravenous diperdipine, a new dihydropyridine derivative, in coronary heart disease. Am Heart J 1991 (March);121:776–781.

100. Singh BN: Comparative efficacy and safety of bepridil and diltiazem in chronic stable angina pectoris refractory to diltiazem. Am J Cardiol 1991 (Aug 1);68:306–312.

101. Santoro G, Savonitto S, Di Bello V, Alberti D, Giusti C: Twenty-four-hour activity of felodipine extended release in chronic stable angina pectoris. Am J Cardiol 1991 (Aug 15);68:457–462.

102. Nesto RW, Phillips RT, Kett KG, McAuliffe LS, Roberts M, Hegarty P: Effect of nifedipine on total ischemic activity and circadian distribution of myocardial ischemia episodes in angina pectoris. Am J Cardiol 1991 (Jan 15);67:128–132.

103. Melandri G, Branzi A, Tartagni F, Esposti DD, Piazzi S, Motta R, Bargossi A, Fallani F, Magnani B: Myocardial metabolic and hemodynamic effects of a sustained intravenous infusion of nifedipine with and without metoprolol in patients with unstable angina. Am Heart J 1991 (January);121:44–51.

104. Egstrup K: Attenuation of circadian variation by combined antianginal therapy with suppression of morning and evening increases in transient myocardial ischemia. Am Heart J 1991 (September);122:648–655.

105. Tzivoni D, Banai S, Botvin S, Ziberman A, Weiss TA, Gavish A, Medina A, Benhorin J, Rogel S, Caspi A, Stern S: Effects of nisoldipine on myocardial ischemia during exercise and during daily activity. Am J Cardiol 1991 (Mar 15);67:559–564.

106. Frishman WH, Heiman M: Usefulness of oral nisolidpine for stable angina pectoris. Am J Cardiol 1991 (Oct 15);68:1004–1009.

107. Katz RJ, Levy WS, Buff L, Wasserman AG: Prevention of Nitrate Tolerance With Angiotension Converting Enzyme Inhibitors. Circulation 1991; (April) 83:1271–1277.

108. Golino P, Piscione F, Willerson JT, Cappelli-Bigazzi M, Focaccio A, Villari B, Indolfi C, Russolillo E, Condorelli M, Chiariello M: Divergent effects of serotonin on coronary-artery dimensions and blood flow in patients with coronary atherosclerosis and control patients. N Engl J Med 1991 (March);324:641–8.

109. McFadden EP, Clarke JG, Davies GJ, Kaski JC, Haider AW, Maseri A: Effect of intracoronary serotonin on coronary vessels in patients with stable angina and patients with variant angina. N Engl J Med 1991 (Mar 7);324:648–654.

110. O'Keefe JH Jr, Gernon C, McCallister BD, Ligon RW, Hartzler GO: Safety and cost effectiveness of combined coronary angiography and angioplasty. Am Heart J 1991 (July);122:49–54.

111. Bentivoglio LG, Holubkov R, Kelsey SF, Holmes DR Jr, Sopko G, Cowley MJ, Myler RK: Short and long term outcome of percutaneous transluminal coronary angioplasty in unstable versus stable angina pectoris: A report of the 1985–1986 NHLBI PTCA Registry. Catheterization and Cardiovascular Diagnosis 1991 (Aug);23:227–238.

112. Bedotto JB, Rutherford BD, McConahay DR, Johnson WL, Giorgi LV, Shimshak TM, O'Keefe JH, Ligon RW, Hartzler GO: Results of multivessel percutaneous transluminal coronary angioplasty in persons aged 65 years and older. Am J Cardiol 1991 (May 15, 1991) 67:1051–1055.

113. Thompson RC, Holmes DR Jr., Gersh BJ, Mock MB, Bailey KR: Percutaneous transluminal coronary angioplasty in the elderly: early and long-term results. J Am Coll Cardiol 1991 (May);17:1245–50.

114. Little T, Milner M, Pichard AB, Mukherjee D, Lindsay J Jr: A comparison of multilesion percutaneous transluminal coronary angioplasty in elderly patients (>70 years) and younger subjects. Am Heart J 1991 (September);122:628–630.

115. Mick MJ, Simpfendorfer C, Arnold AZ, Piedmonte M, Lytle BW: Early and late results of coronary angioplasty and bypass in octogenarians. Am J Cardiol 1991 (Nov 15);68:1316–1320.

116. Jost S, Nolte CWT, Simon R, Amende I, Gulba DC, Wiese B, Lichtlen PR: Angioplasty of subacute and chronic total coronary occlusions: Success, recurrence rate, and clinical follow-up. Am Heart J 1991 (December);122:1509–1514.

117. Plante S, Laarman GJ, de Feyter PJ, Samson M, Rensing BJ, Umans V, Suryapranata H, van den Brand M, Serruys PW: Acute complications of percutaneous transluminal coronary angioplasty for total occlusion. Am Heart J 1991 (February);121:417–426.

118. De Bruyne B, Renkin J, Col J, Wijns W: Percutaneous transluminal coronary angioplasty of the left coronary artery in patients with chronic occlusion of the right coronary artery: Clinical and functional results. Am Heart J 1991 (August);122:415–422.

119. Stevens T, Kahn JK, McCallister BD, Ligon RW, Spaude S, Rutherford BD, McConahay DR, Johnson WL, Giorgi LV, Shimshak TM, Hartzler GO: Safety and efficacy of percutaneous transluminal coronary angioplasty in patients with left ventricular dysfunction. Am J Cardiol 1991 (Aug 1);68:313–319.

120. Savage MP, Goldberg S, Hirshfeld JW, Bass TA, Macdonald RG, Margolis JR, Taussig AS, Vetrovec G, Whitworth HB, Zalewski A, Hill JA, Cowley M, Jugo R, Pepine CJ, for the M-Heart Investigators: Clinical and angiographic determinants of primary coronary angioplasty success. J Am Coll Cardiol 1991 (January) 17:22–8.

121. Vandormael M, Deligonul U, Taussig S, Kern MJ: Predictors of long-term cardiac survival in patients with multivessel coronary artery disease undergoing percutaneous transluminal coronary angioplasty. Am J Cardiol 1991 (Jan 1) 67:1–6.

122. Ellis SG, Cowley MJ, DiSciascio G, Deligonul U, Topol EJ, Bulle TM, Vandormael MG and the Multivessel Angioplasty Prognosis Study Group: Determinants of 2-Year

Outcome After Coronary Angioplasty in Patients with Multivessel Disease on the Basis of Comprehensive Preprocedural Evaluation—Implications for Patient Selection. Circulation 1991; (June) 83:1905–1914.

123. Goudreau E, DiSciascio G, Kelly K, Vetrovec GW, Nath A, Cowley MJ: Coronary angioplasty of diffuse coronary artery disease. Am Heart J 1991 (January);121:12–19.

124. Weintraub WS, Ghazzal ZMB, Cohen CL, Douglas JS, Liberman H, Morris DC, and King SP: Clinical Implications of Late Proven Patency After Successful Coronary Angioplasty. Circulation 1991 (August);84:572–582.

125. Reeves F, Bonan R, Cote G, Crepeau J, deGuise P, Gosselin G, Campeau L, Lesperance J: Long-term angiographic follow-up after angioplasty of venous coronary bypass grafts. Am Heart J 1991 (September);122:620–627.

126. Plokker HWT, Meester BH, Serruys PW: The Dutch experience in percutaneous transluminal angioplasty of narrowed saphenous veins used for aortocoronary arterial bypass. Am J Cardiol 1991 (Feb 15);67:361–366.

127. Jost S, Gulba D, Daniel WG, Amende I, Simon R, Eckert S, Lichtlen: Percutaneous transluminal angioplasty of aortocoronary venous bypass grafts and effect of the caliber of the grafted coronary artery on graft stenosis. Am J Cardiol 1991 (July 1);68:27–30.

128. Dimas AP, Arora RR, Whitlow PL, Hollman JL, Franco I, Raymond RE, Dorosti K, Simpfendorfer CC: Percutaneous transluminal angioplasty involving internal mammary artery grafts. Am Heart J 1991 (August);122:423–429.

129. Bush HS, Ferguson JJ III, Angelini P, Willerson JT: Twelve-lead electrocardiographic evaluation of ischemia during percutaneous transluminal coronary angioplasty and its correlation with acute reocclusion. Am Heart J 1991 (June);121:1591–1599.

130. Zeiher AM, Schächinger V, Weitzel SH, Wollschläger H, Just H: Intracoronary Thrombus Formation Causes Focal Vasoconstriction of Epicardial Arteries in Patients with Coronary Artery Disease. Circulation 1991; (May) 83:1519–1525.

131. Leitschuh ML, Mills RM Jr, Jacobs AK, Ruocco NA Jr, Larosa D, Faxon DP: Outcome after major dissection during coronary angioplasty using the perfusion balloon catheter. Am J Cardiol 1991 (May 15);67:1056–1060.

132. Cripps TR, Morgan JM, Rickards AF: Outcome of extensive coronary artery dissection during coronary angioplasty. Br Heart J 1991 (July);66:3–6.

133. El-Tamimi H, Davies GJ, Sritara P, Hackett D, Crea F, Maseri A: Inappropriate Constriction of Small Coronary Vessels as a Possible Cause of a Positive Exercise Test Early After Successful Coronary Angioplasty. Circulation 1991 (December);84:2307–2312.

134. Werner GS, Sold G, Buchwald A, Kreuzer H, Wiegand V: Intravascular ultrasound imaging of human coronary arteries after percutaneous transluminal angioplasty: Morphologic and quantitative assessment. Am Heart J 1991 (July);122:212–220.

135. El-Tamimi H, Davies GJ, Hackett D, Sritara P, Bertrand O, Crea F, and Maseri A: Abnormal Vasomotor Changes Early After Coronary Angioplasty—A Quantitative Arteriographic Study of Their Time Course. Circulation 1991 (September);84:1198–1202.

136. Simpfendorfer C, Dorosti K, Franco I, Hollman J, Whitlow P: Risk factors for in-hospital mortality associated with coronary angioplasty. Cleve Clin J Med 1991 (Jan–Feb);58:25–27.

137. Ellis SG, Myler RK, King SB III, Douglas JS Jr, Topol EJ, Shaw RE, Stertzer SH, Roubin GS, Murphy MC: Causes and correlates of death after unsupported coronary angioplasty: Implications for use of angioplasty and advanced support techniques in high-risk settings. Am J Cardiol 1991 (Dec 1);68:1147–1451.

138. Titus BG, Sherman CT: Asymptomatic myocardial ischemia during percutaneous transluminal coronary angioplasty and importance of prior Q-wave infarction and diabetes mellitus. Am J Cardiol 1991 (Sept 15) 68:735–739.

139. Nienaber CA, Brunken RC, Sherman CT, Yeatman LA, Gambhir SS, Krivokapich J, Demer LL, Ratib O, Child JS, Phelps ME, Schelbert HR: Metabolic and functional recovery of ischemic human myocardium after coronary angioplasty. J Am Coll Cardiol 1991 (October);18:966–78.

140. Eichhorn EJ, Grayburn PA, Willard JE, Anderson HV, Bedotto JB, Carry M, Kahn JK, Willerson JT: Spontaneous alterations in coronary blood flow velocity before and after coronary angioplasty in patients with severe angina. J Am Coll Cardiol 1991 (January);17:43–52.

141. Labovitz AJ, Barth C, Castello R, Ojile M, Kern MJ: Attenuation of myocardial ischemia during coronary occlusion by ultrashort-acting beta adrenergic blockade. Am Heart J 1991 (May);121:1347–1352.

142. Pavlides GS, Schreiber TL, Gangadharan V, Puchrowicz S, O'Neill WW: Safety and efficacy of urokinase during elective coronary angioplasty. Am Heart J 1991 (March);121:731–745.

143. Lembo NJ, King SB, Roubin GS, Black AJ, Douglas JS Jr: Effects of nonionic versus ionic contrast media on complications of percutaneous transluminal coronary angioplasty. Am J Cardiol 1991 (May 15);67:1046–1050.

144. Cahyadi YH, Takekoshi N, Matsui S: Clinical efficacy of PTCA and identification of restenosis: Evaluation by serial body surface potential mapping. Am Heart J 1991 (April);121:1080–1087.

145. Ueda M, Becker AE, Tsukada T, Numano F, and Fujimoto T: Fibrocellular Tissue Response After Percutaneous Transluminal Coronary Angioplasty—An Immunocytochemical Analysis of the Cellular Composition. Circulation 1991; (April) 83:1327–1332.

146. Johansson SR, Wiklund O, Karlsson T, Hjalmarson A, Emanuelsson H: Serum lipids and lipoproteins in relation to restenosis after coronary angioplasty. Eur Heart J 1991 (Sept);12:1020–1028.

147. Reis GJ, Kuntz RE, Silverman DI, Pasternak RC: Effects of serum lipid levels on restenosis after coronary angioplasty. Am J Cardiol 1991 (Dec 1);68:1431–1435.

148. Sahni R, Maniet AR, Voci G, Banka VS: Prevention of restenosis by lovastatin after successful coronary angioplasty. Am Heart J 1991 (June);121:1600–1608.

149. Bourassa MG, Lesperance J, Eastwood C, Schwartz L, Côté G, Kazim F, Hudon G: Clinical, physiologic, anatomic and procedural factors predictive of restenosis after percutaneous transluminal coronary angioplasty. J Am Coll Cardiol 1991 (August);18:368–76.

150. Brozovich FV, Morganroth J, Gottlieb NB, Gottlieb RS: Effect of angiotensin converting enzyme inhibition on the incidence of restenosis after percutaneous transluminal coronary angioplasty. Catheterization and Cardiovascular Diagnosis 1991 (Aug);23:263–267.

151. Hirshfeld JW Jr., Schwartz JS, Jugo R, Macdonald RG, Goldberg S, Savage MP, Bass TA, Vetrovec G, Cowley M, Taussig AS, Whitworth HB, Margolis JR, Hill JA, Pepine CJ, and the M-Heart Investigators: Restenosis after coronary angioplasty: A multivariate statistical model to relate lesion and procedure variables to restenosis. J Am Coll Cardiol 1991 (September);18:647–56.

152. Taylor RR, Gibbons FA, Cope GD, Cumpston GN, Mews GC, Luke P: Effects of low-dose aspirin on restenosis after coronary angioplasty. Am J Cardiol 1991 (Oct 1);68:874–878.

153. O'Keefe JH, Giorgi LV, Hartzler GO, Good TH, Ligon RW, Webb DL, McCallister BD: Effects of diltiazem on complications and restenosis after coronary angioplasty. Am J Cardiol 1991 (Feb 15);67:373–376.

154. Ardissino D, Barberis P, De Servi S, Merlini PA, Bramucci E, Falcone C, Specchia G: Abnormal coronary vasoconstriction as a predictor of restenosis after successful coronary angioplasty in patients with unstable angina pectoris. N Engl J Med 1991 (Oct 10);325:1053–1057.

155. Bresee SJ, Jacobs AK, Garber GR, Ruocco NA Jr, Mills RM, Bergelson BA, Ryan TJ, Faxon DP: Prior restenosis predicts restenosis after coronary angioplasty of a new significant narrowing. Am J Cardiol 1991 (Nov 1);68:1158–1162.

156. Hinohara T, Rowe MH, Robertson GC, Selmon MR, Braden L, Leggett JH, Vetter JW, Simpson JB: Effect of lesion characteristics on outcome of directional coronary atherectomy. J Am Coll Cardiol 1991 (April);17:1112–20.

157. Ellis SG, De Cesare NB, Pinkerton CA, Whitlow P, King SB, Ghazzal ZMB, Kereiakes DJ, Popma JJ, Menke KK, Topol EJ, Holmes DR: Relation of Stenosis Morphology and Clinical Presentation to the Procedural Results of Directional Coronary Atherectomy. Circulation 1991 (August);84:644–653.

158. Serruys PW, Umans VAWM, Strauss BH, Van Suylen P, Van Den Brand M, Suryapranata H, De Feyter PJ, Roelandt J: Quantitative angiography after directional coronary atherectomy. Br Heart J 1991 (Aug);66:122–129.

159. Popma JJ, De Cesare NB, Ellis SG, Holmes DR Jr., Pinkerton CA, Whitlow P, King SB III, Ghazzal ZMB, Topol EJ, Garratt KN, Kereiakes DJ: Clinical, angiographic and procedural correlates of quantitative coronary dimensions after directional coronary atherectomy. J Am Coll Cardiol 1991 (November);18:1183–9.

160. Sanborn TA, Torre SR, Sharma SK, Hershman RA, Cohen M, Sherman W, Ambrose JA: Percutaneous coronary excimer laser-assisted balloon angioplasty: initial clinical and quantitative angiographic results in 50 patients. J Am Coll Cardiol 1991 (January);17:94–9.

161. Geschwind HJ, Dubois-Rande J-L, Zelinsky R, Morelle JF, Boussignac G: Percutaneous coronary mid-infra-red laser angioplasty. Am Heart J 1991 (August);122:552–558.

162. Serruys PW, Strauss BH, Beatt KJ, Bertrand ME, Puel J, Rickards AF, Meier B, Goy JJ, Vogt P, Kappenberger L, Sigwart U: Angiographic follow-up after placement of a self-expanding coronary-artery stent. N Engl J Med 1991 (Jan 3);324:13–17.

163. Rab ST, King SB III, Roubin GS, Carlin S, Hearn JA, Douglas JS Jr.: Coronary aneurysms after stent placement: A suggestion of altered vessel wall healing in the presence of anti-inflammatory agents. J Am Coll Cardiol 1991 (November);18:1524–8.

164. Fischman DL, Savage MP, Leon MB, Schatz RA, Ellis SG, Cleman MW, Teirstein P, Walker CM, Bailey S, Hirschfeld JW, Goldberg S: Effect of intracoronary stenting on intimal dissection after balloon angioplasty: Results of quantitative and qualitative coronary analysis. J Am Coll Cardiol 1991 (November);18:1445–51.

165. Haude M, Erbel R, Straub U, Dietz U, Meyer J: Short and long term results after intracoronary stenting in human coronary arteries: Monocenter experience with the balloon-expandable Palmaz-Schatz stent. Br Heart J 1991 (Nov);66:337–345.

166. Haude M, Erbel R, Straub U, Dietz U, Schatz R, Meyer J: Results of intracoronary stents for management of coronary dissection after balloon angioplasty. Am J Cardiol 1991 (Apr 1);67:691–696.

167. Lawrie GM, Morris GC Jr, Earle N: Long-term results of coronary bypass surgery: Analysis of 1698 patients followed 15 to 20 years. Ann Surg 1991 (May);213:377–387.

168. Jones EL, Weintraub WS, Craver JM, Guyton RA, Cohen CL: Coronary bypass surgery: Is the operation different today? J Thorac Cardiovasc Surg 1991 (Jan);101:108–115.

169. Salomon NW, Page US, Bigelow JC, Krause AH, Okies JE, Metzdorff MT: Comparative results in a consecutive series of 469 patients older than 75 years. J Thorac Cardiovasc Surg 1991 (Feb);101:209–218.

170. Ko W, Kreiger KH, Lazenby WD, Shin YT, Goldstein M, Lazzaro R, Isom OW: J Thorac Cardiovasc Surg 1991 (Oct);102:532–538.

171. Greene MA, Gray LA Jr, Slater D, Ganzel BL, Mavroudis C: Emergency aortocoronary bypass after failed angioplasty. Ann Thorac Surg 1991 (Feb);51:194–199.

172. Nwasokwa ON, Koss JH, Friedman GH, Grunwald AM, Bodenheimer MM: Bypass surgery for chronic stable angina: Predictors of survival benefit and strategy for patient selection. An Intern Med 1991 (June 15);114:1035–1049.

173. Batiuk TD, Kurtz SB, Oh JK, Orszulak TA: Coronary artery bypass operation in dialysis patients. Mayo Clin Proc 1991 (Jan);66:45–53.

174. Mills NL, Everson CT: Atherosclerosis of the ascending aorta and coronary artery bypass. J Thorac Cardiovasc Surg 1991 (Oct);102:546–553.

175. Caine N, Harrison SCW, Sharples LD, Wallwork J: Prospective study of quality of life before and after coronary artery bypass grafting. Br Med J 1991 (Mar 2);302:511–514.

176. O'Connor GT, Plume SK, Olmstead EM, Coffin LH, Morton JR, Maloney CT, Nowicki ER, Tryzelaar JF, Hernandez F, Adrian L, Casey KJ, Soule DN, Marrin CAS, Nugent WC, Charlesworth DC, Clough R, Katz S, Leavitt BJ, Wennberg JE: A regional prospective study of in-hospital mortality associated with coronary artery bypass grafting. JAMA 1991 (Aug 14);266:803–809.

177. Williams SV, Nash DB, Goldfarb N: Differences in mortality from coronary artery bypass graft surgery at five teaching hospitals. JAMA 1991 (Aug 14);266:810–815.

178. Verheul HA, Moulijn AC, Hondema S, Schouwink M, Dunning AJ: Late results of 200 repeat coronary artery bypass operations. Am J Cardiol 1991 (Jan 1);67:24–30.

179. Accoal KD, Craver JM, Weintraub WS, Guyton RA, Jones EL: Multiple reoperative coronary artery bypass grafting. Ann Thorac Surg 1991 (Oct);52:738–744.

180. Galbut DL, Traad EA, Dorman MJ, Dewitt PL, Larsen PB, Kurlansky PA, Button JH, Ally JM, Gentsch TO: Bilateral internal mammary artery grafts in reoperative and primary coronary bypass surgery. An Thorac Surg 1991 (July);52:20–28.

181. Bashein G, Nessly ML, Rice AL, Counts RB, Misbach GA: Preoperative aspirin therapy and reoperation for bleeding after coronary artery bypass surgery. Arch Intern Med 1991 (Jan);151:89–93.

182. Goldman S, Copeland J, Moritz T, Henderson W, Zadina K, Ovitt T, Kern KB, Sethi G, Sharma GVRK, Khuri S, Richards K, Grover F, Morrison D, Whitman G, Chesler E, Sako Y, Pacold I, Montoya A, DeMots H, Floten S, Doherty J, Read R, Scott S, Spooner T, Masud Z, Haakenson C, Harker LA, and the Department of Veterans Affairs Cooperative Study Group: Starting Aspirin Therapy After Operation—Effects on Early Graft Patency. Circulation 1991 (August);84:520–526.

183. Goodnough LT, Johnston MFM, Toy PTCY, Transfusion Medicine-Academic Award Group: JAMA 1991 (Jan 2);265:86–90.

184. Myhre BA: To treat the patient or to treat the surgeon. JAMA 1991 (Jan 2);265:97–98.

185. Suttorp MJ, Kingma JH, Peels HOJ, Koomen EM, Tijssen JGP, Van Hemel NM, DeFauw JAM, Ernst SMPG: Effectiveness of sotolol in preventing supraventricular tachyarrhythmias shortly after coronary artery bypass grafting. Am J Cardiol 1991 (Nov 1);68:1163–1169.

186. Hashimoto K, Ilstrup DM, Schaff HV: Influence of clinical and hemodynamic variables on risk of supraventricular tachycardia after coronary artery bypass. J Thorac Cardiovasc Surg 1991 (Jan);101:56–65.

187. Reis SE, Polak JF, Hirsch DR, Cohn LH, Creager MA, Donovan BC, Goldhaber SZ: Frequency of deep venous thrombosis in asymptomatic patients with coronary artery bypass grafts. Am Heart J 1991 (August);122:478–482.

188. Qiao J-H, Walts AE, Fishbein MC: The severity of atherosclerosis at sites of plaque rupture with occlusive thrombosis in saphenous vein coronary artery bypass grafts. Am Heart J 1991 (October);122:955–958.

189. Newburger JW, Takahashi M, Beiser AS, Burns JC, Bastian J, Chung KJ, Colan SD, Duffy CE, Fulton DR, Glode MP, Mason WH, Meissner HC, Rowley AH, Shulman ST, Reddy V, Sundel RP, Wiggins JW, Colton T, Melish ME, Rosen FS: A single intravenous infusion of gamma globulin as compared with four infusions in the treatment of acute kawasaki syndrome. N Engl J Med 1991 (June 6);324:1633–1639.

190. Amano J, Suzuki A: Coronary artery involvement in Takayasu's arteritis: Collective review and guideline for surgical treatment. J Thorac Cardiovasc Surg 1991 (Oct);102:554–560.

3

Acute Myocardial Infarction and Its Consequences

Factors delaying hospitalization

Prior studies have had difficulty identifying factors that significantly explain patients' delay in responding to symptoms of AMI. Kenyon and colleagues[1] in Detroit, Michigan therefore examined factors affecting the time between symptom onset and hospital arrival for 103 AMI patients admitted to a Detroit metropolitan hospital between October 1989 and January 1990. Variables evaluated included demographic and medical history factors, psychological characteristics of somatic and emotional awareness, and type A behavior. The mean prehospital delay time was 9 hours. Delay time was not significantly associated with demographic or medical history categories or with type A behavior. Of study variables that can be identified prior to evolution of an AMI, somatic and emotional awareness were the only factors significantly predictive of delay time. Patients who were more capable of identifying inner experiences of emotions and/or bodily sensations sought treatment significantly earlier than patients with low emotional or somatic awareness (low emotional awareness median delay, 13 hours; high emotional awareness median delay, 4 hours; low somatic awareness median delay, 7 hours; high somatic awareness median delay, 4 hours). Variations in sensitivity to bodily sensations and emotions appear to play an important role in treatment seeking and thus potentially in treatment outcome for AMI patients. Assessment of these characteristics in patients with coronary risk factors could allow early identification of persons at risk of excessive delay in responding to symptoms of AMI.

Circadian variation in pain onset

Thompson and associates[2] from Leicester, UK, studied prospectively the time of onset of chest pain in 1154 consecutive patients admitted to a coronary care unit with AMI during a 5-year period (Figure 3-1). Statistical analysis confirmed a previous finding in a retrospective study of a bimodal frequency distribution with peaks in the time of onset of chest pain between 2330 and 0030 hours and between 0630 and 0830 hours.

In black patients

Maynard and associates[3] from Seattle, Washington, reported observations in 641 black and 11,892 white patients with chest pain of presumed cardiac origin admitted to the coronary care unit in 19 hospitals in metropolitan Seattle. Black men and women were younger (58 vs 66), more often admitted to central city hospitals, and developed evidence of AMI less often (19 vs 23%). In the subset of 2,870 AMI patients, blacks (n = 121) were younger (59 vs 67) and had less prior CABG surgery (2 vs 10%) and more prior hypertension (67 vs 46%). During hospitalization, whites (n = 2,749) had higher rates of coronary angioplasty (18 vs 10%) and CABG (10 vs 4%), although thrombolytic therapy and cardiac catheterization were used equally in the 2 groups. Hospital mortality was

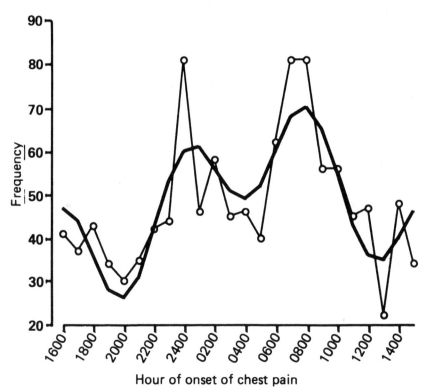

Fig. 3-1. Hourly frequency of onset of chest pain in acute myocardial infarction. Open circles represent the frequencies and the continuous line the fitted values. Reproduced with permission from Thompson, et al.[2]

7.4% for black and 13.1% for white patients. However, after adjustment for key demographic and clinical variables by logistic regression, this difference was not as apparent. Questions about the premature onset of CAD, excess systemic hypertension, and the differential use of interventions in black persons have been raised by other investigators. Despite differences in age, referral patterns and the use of coronary angioplasty and bypass surgery, black and white patients with AMI in metropolitan Seattle had similar outcomes.

First infarct in smokers

Molstad[4] from Hamar, Norway, studied 484 patients with a first AMI and 155 of them were smokers at the time of the AMI. Their unadjusted survival was superior to the non-smokers at 3 months follow-up, with a relative risk of 0.36 (5% confidence interval 0.22–0.59). Major baseline differences existed between the two populations. When these inequalities were taken into account through a multivariate Cox regression the relative risk was increased to 9.55 (95% confidence interval 0.33–0.93), but was still significantly lower than in non-smokers. No difference in rate of reinfarction was observed between the 2 populations. The smokers tended to have a less serious infarction than the non-smokers. However, adding variables that accounted for this into the Cox model did not cancel the impact of smoking. From the results it is suggested that the reduced mortality in smokers is due to a thrombus occurring at an earlier stage of the CAD. Thus, at the time of infarction smokers' LV function tends to be less affected, and this is reflected in the improved survival rate among smokers in the first months after an AMI.

When on aspirin

Ridker and collaborators[5] in Boston, Massachusetts examined the influence of prophylactic low-dose aspirin on the clinical characteristics of subsequent nonfatal AMI in the Physicians' Health Study, a randomized, double-blind placebo-controlled trial of alternate-day aspirin (325 mg) among 22,071 US male physicians. During 60 months of follow-up, 342 incident cases of nonfatal AMI were confirmed: 129 on aspirin and 213 on placebo. Despite this statistically extreme reduction in occurrence of a first nonfatal AMI attributable to aspirin, there were no significant differences in the size, location, electrocardiographic features, or post-AMI, LVEF between the aspirin and placebo groups. Furthermore, among those undergoing angiography, there were no differences in the distribution or number of coronary vessels obstructed. These data indicate that chronic platelet inhibition with alternate-day aspirin therapy reduces the risk of a first AMI but does not appear to have a significant effect on the clinical characteristics of events that are survived. This finding may result from a direct effect of aspirin or from an aspirin-induced shift in infarction severity. Regardless of mechanism, these clinical observations suggest that treatment decisions for AMI patients should be made independently of a history of aspirin use.

Relation to alcohol intake

Kono and associates[6] from Tokorozawa and Fukuoka, Japan, examined the relation between alcohol and nonfatal AMI in a case-control study of 89 men and 271 control subjects in Fukuoka, Japan. Patients admitted for the first AMI at 2 hospitals in Fukuoka City were aged 40 to 69 years, and control subjects were recruited based on the telephone directory of the city. Information on alcohol drinking and potential coronary risk factors was obtained by using a self-administered questionnaire, and past drinkers were separated from lifelong abstainers in the analysis. After adjustment for age, occupation, cigarette smoking, strenuous exercise, body mass index, hypertension, diabetes mellitus and parental heart disease, the risk of AMI was progressively less with increasing levels of alcohol consumption. With those who never drank as a referent, adjusted odds ratios for current drinkers consuming <30, 30 to 59, and ≥60 ml/day of alcohol were 1.11 (95% confidence interval 9.51 to 2.42), 0.31 (0.11 to 0.83), and 0.13 (0.05 to 0.36), respectively. These findings add to the body of data showing that alcohol drinkers are less likely to have AMI.

DIAGNOSIS AND EARLY TESTING

By chest pain in the emergency room

Karlson and associates[7] from Goteborg, Sweden, assessed the possibility of early prediction of AMI in 7,157 consecutive patients coming to their emergency room during a 21 month period with chest pain or other symptoms suggestive of AMI. Of these patients 921 developed an AMI during the first 3 days in the hospital. Of the 4, 690 patients admitted to hospital, 1,576 (34%) had a normal admission electrocardiogram, and 90 of these (6%) developed AMI. Of 1,964 patients with an abnormal electrocardiogram without signs of acute ischemia (42% of those admitted), 268 (14%) developed AMI, and 563 (51%) of 1,109 patients with acute ischemia on the electrocardiogram (24%) developed AMI. All patients were prospectively classified in the emergency room on the basis of history, clinical examination and electrocardiogram into 1 of 4 categories, according to the initial degree of suspicion of AMI. Of 279 admitted patients judged to have an obvious AMI (6% of the 4,690), 245 (88%) actually developed AMI; of 1,426 with a strong suspicion of AMI (30%), 478 (34%) developed one; of 2,519 with a vague suspicion of AMI (54%), 192 (8%) developed one; and of 466 with no suspicion of AMI (10%), 6 (1%) developed one. Thus, only a low percentage of the patients with a normal initial electrocardiogram or a vague initial suspicion of AMI developed a confirmed AMI.

From "rule-out" myocardial infarction cases

Although many investigators have suggested that 24 hours is required to exclude AMI in patients who are admitted to a coronary care unit for the evaluation of acute chest pain, Lee and associates[8] from Boston, Massachusetts, New Haven, Connecticut, and Cincinnati, Ohio, hypothesized that a 12-hour period might be adequate for patients with a low probability of AMI at the time of admission. Using a Bayesian model, the authors developed a strategy to identify candidates for a shorter period of observation from an analysis of a derivation set of 976 patients with acute chest pain who were admitted to 3 teaching and 4 community hospitals. In the derivation set, patients whose clinical characteristics in the emergency room predicted a low (≤7%) probability of myocardial infarction had only a 0.4% risk of infarction if they had neither abnormal levels of cardiac enzymes nor recurrent ischemic pain during the first 12 hours of hospitalization. In an independent testing set of 2,684 patients from the 7 hospitals, 957 admitted patients (36%) were classified as candidates for this 12-hour period of observation according to a previously published multivariate algorithm. Few of these patients were actually transferred from a monitored setting at 12 hours. Of the 771 candidates for a 12-hour period of observation who did not have enzyme abnormalities or recurrent pain during the first 12 hours, 4 (0.5%) were subsequently found to have AMI, and only 3 (0.4%) died after primary cardiac arrests, all of which occurred 3 to 5 days after admission. Rates of other major cardiovascular complications were low in the patients who might have been transferred from the coronary care unit after 12 hours with this strategy. In patients with a higher initial risk of infarction, the standard strategy of 24-hour observation identified all but 11 of 739 AMI (1%). Emergency room clinical data can be used to identify a large subgroup of patients for whom a 12-hour period of observation is normally sufficient to exclude AMI. Patient-specific evaluation and treatment can then proceed without the restrictions imposed by "rule-out" protocols for myocardial infarction.

Gaspoz and associates[9] from Boston, Massachusetts, established for emergency room patients with a low probability of AMI, a new short-stay coronary observation unit, a 2-bed nonintensive care unit with telemetry monitoring adjacent to the emergency room. Of 512 consecutive admissions to the coronary observation unit, these investigators discharged 425 (83%) patients home without evidence of AMI or serious complications (mean length of stay, 1.2 days; median length of stay, 1 day); 87 (17%) were transferred to other hospital beds. The rate of AMI was 3%. No deaths and only 1 serious complication occurred in the coronary observation unit. At 6 month follow-up, the cardiac survival rate was 99% for patients sent home directly from this unit. It is concluded that the coronary observation unit is safe and adequate for ruling out AMI in a defined subset of patients. Short-stay units, however, encourage early discharges which, when premature, may miss patients who are at risk of having complications shortly thereafter. Strategies such as mandatory but expeditious predischarge stress testing to encourage early but not premature discharge may augment the efficiency of coronary observation units.

By echocardiography

To investigate the quantitative relations between the severity of regional wall motion abnormalities and segmental myocardial infarct size and between the severity of overall LV dysfunction and global myocardial infarct size, Shen and associates[10] from Rochester, Minnesota, performed 2-dimensional echocardiograms within 7 days of death in 30 patients who had at least 1 AMI. The severity of regional wall motion abnormalities was graded for each segment with a 2-D echocardiographic 14-segment model. The severity of global LV dysfunction was calculated as the mean of the visualized regional wall motion scores. On pathologic examination of autopsy specimens, segmental infarct size was estimated as a percentage of the segmental cross-sectional area. The global infarct size was expressed as a percentage of the total LV mass. At the segmental level, regional wall motion score was positively correlated with the segmental infarct size. The sensitivity and specificity of detecting infarcted segments by abnormal wall motion scores were 81 and 71%, respectively. All dys-kinetic segments revealed infarct size of ≥10%. The wall motion score index was positively correlated (r = 0.52) with the global infarct size. The mean global infarct size was 7% for the 8 patients with a wall motion score index of <2, which was significantly lower than the mean of 27% for the 22 patients with a wall motion score index of ≥2. A 2-D echo-cardiogram is sensitive and specific in detecting infarcted segments and can be useful in quantitating myocardial damage after AMI.

By electrocardiogram

Pahim and associates[11] from Winston-Salem and Durham, North Car-olina, and Tampa, Florida, applied an automated version of a subset of 3 criteria from the complete Selvester scoring system for electrocardi-ographic screening of healed myocardial infarction to 1,344 electrocar-diograms from normal subjects (473 normal subjects as determined by cardiac catheterization and 871 apparently normal subjects by history and physical examination) to 706 from subjects with single myocardial infarcts and to 131 from subjects with combined anterior and posterior myocardial infarcts. Of the single infarcts, 366 had inferior, 277 anterior and 63 posterolateral locations. Presence and location of infarcts were judged from left ventriculograms and coronary angiograms. Overall spec-ificity was only 86%, whereas overall sensitivity for the infarct population was 77%. Specificity was lower in men than in women; it was also lower in older than in younger subjects. One of the screening criteria (R≥40 ms in V_1) may possibly be eliminated to augment specificity; this can be done with only minor loss of sensitivity. Differences in wave form meas-urements between the manual and computer methods account for a large part of the deterioration of specificity in this study compared with previously published results. Computer application of the screening cri-teria requires altered criteria limits in comparison with those used in manual application. Probably sex- and age-dependent criteria limits should be used.

By late potentials on signal-averaged electrocardiogram

de Chillou and colleagues[12] in Nancy, France determined the natural history of late potentials on signal-averaged electrocardiograms in 167 patients with a first anterior or inferior AMI. Seventy-four patients re-ceived thrombolytic therapy; the remaining 93 patients were treated con-ventionally. All patients underwent coronary angiography, LVEF measurements and signal-averaged electrocardiogram recordings. Eight variables thought to be correlated with the presence of late potentials were studied, including age, infarct location, number of disease vessels, LVEF, infarct-related coronary artery patency, treatment received, delay between admission and signal-averaged recording and delay between admission and coronary angiography. Statistical analyses showed that two independent factors, coronary artery occlusion and impaired LVEF, were highly correlated with the incidence of late potentials. The occur-rence of late potentials was multiplied by 5 in the case of an occluded infarct-related artery and by 1.75 each time the LVEF decreased by 0.10 (Table 3-1). These data suggest that coronary artery patency is the most important factor that decreases the rate of late potentials after a first AMI, and it occurs independently of infarct location and LV function.

TABLE 3-1. *Clinical and angiographic data and incidence of late potentials according to the treatment received in 167 patients. Reproduced with permission from de Chillou, et al.*[12]

	Thrombolytic Therapy (n = 74)	Conventional Therapy (n = 93)	p Value
Clinical data			
Age (yr)	54 ± 10	56.5 ± 9.5	NS
Male/female	13/61	16/77	NS
Anterior infarct location	49% (36/74)	35% (33/93)	NS
Delay A-C (days)	9 ± 5	23 ± 8	<0.000001
Delay A-SA (days)	21 ± 6	23 ± 8	NS
Coronary angiographic data			
No. of diseased vessels			
1	66% (49/74)	54% (50/93)	NS
2	24% (18/74)	29% (27/93)	NS
3	10% (7/74)	17% (16/93)	NS
LVEF (%)	0.53 ± 0.13	0.54 ± 0.13	NS
Open infarct-related artery	74% (55/74)	47% (44/93)	<0.001
Signal-averaged ECG data			
QRS duration (ms)	109 ± 8	108 ± 8	NS
RMS40 (μV)	45 ± 33	42 ± 27	NS
LP incidence			
All patients	22% (16/74)	18% (17/93)	NS
Open artery	16% (9/55)	0% (0/44)	<0.02
Occluded artery	37% (7/19)	35% (17/49)	NS

Heart period variability

Bigger and associates[13] in New York, New York, evaluated four components of the heart period power spectrum, including ultra low frequency, very low frequency, low frequency, and high frequency power for a 24 hour electrocardiogram recording. To determine the time course and magnitude of recovery for these measurements of heart period variability, 68 patients in the Cardiac Arrhythmia Pilot Study (CAPS) placebo group who had 24 hour electrocardiogram recordings at baseline, 3, 6 and 12 months after AMI were studied. The 24 hour power spectral density was computed with the use of fast Fourier transforms and divided into the four components listed previously. The values for the five frequency domain measures of heart period variability in these patients were similar to those found in 715 patients who participated in the Multicenter Post Infarction Program, indicating that this patient sample is generally representative of postinfarction patients with respect to these measurements. The values for the five measurements were one third to one half of those found in 95 normal persons of similar age and gender. There was a substantial increase in the measurements of heart period variability between the baseline 24 hour and the 3 month electrocardiogram recordings. Between 3 and 12 months, the values were quite stable for the group as a whole as well as for individual patients. However, at 12 months after AMI, values for the five measurements of heart period variability were one half to two thirds the values found in the sample of 95 normal individuals (Figure 3-2).

By creatine kinase

Patients with chest pain lasting >6 hours and suggesting AMI are often excluded from thrombolytic therapy because myocardial necrosis is believed to be largely irreversible beyond that time. To evaluate the relation between time of onset of chest pain and enzymatic evidence of myocardial necrosis, Beek and associates[14] from Amsterdan, The Netherlands, analyzed enzymes on admission in 221 consecutive patients with ≥2 mm ST-segment elevation by electrocardiography on admission and no contraindications to thrombolytic therapy. Patients with symptoms within 6 hours (n = 170, early) received thrombolytic therapy, but those with symptoms after 6 hours did not (n = 51, late). Eventually, 219 (168 early, 51 late) patients had enxymatically proven AMI within 24 hours. Creatine kinase levels on admission less than twice the upper normal limit were found in 155 (91%) early patients, but surprisingly, also in 30 (59%) late patients. By electrocardiography on admission, ST-segment elevation per lead was 2.1 ± 1.1 mm in late patients with low initial enzymes versus 1.1 ± 0.3 mm in those with elevated initial enzymes. Concomitantly, Q waves in leads with ST-segment elevation were present

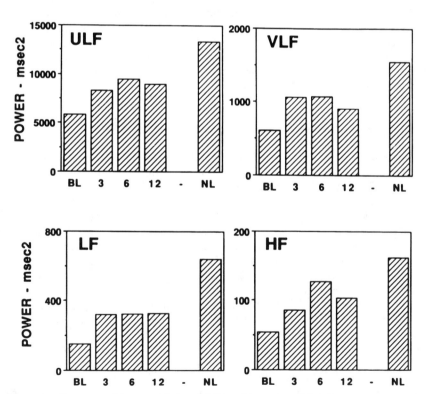

Fig. 3-2. Recovery of heart period variability after myocardial infarction. Because the distributions of the measure of heart period variability are markedly skewed, the median values at baseline (BL) and at 3, 6 and 12 months after myocardial infarction are plotted. For comparison sake, the median values for a group of 95 normal (NL) persons similar in age and gender to the patients in the CAPS placebo group are plotted. Reproduced with permission from Bigger, et al.[13]

in 17 (57%) late patients with low enzymes on admission versus 17 (81%) with elevated enzymes on admission. Eventually, maximal creatine kinase levels were similar in all late patients irrespective of enzyme levels on admission. Therefore, many patients with symptoms of AMI after 6 hours have low enzymes on admission and may still be eligible for thrombolytic therapy. Immediate enzyme testing and the degree of ST-segment elevation by electrocardiography on admission may identify these patients. These data could explain the improved survival reported with "late" thrombolytic therapy for AMI.

Mair and associates[15] from Innsbruck, Austria, examined the diagnostic sensitivity and performance of immunoenzymometric measurements of creatine kinase (CK)-MB mass concentrations in the early diagnosis of AMI and compared them with the sensitivities and performances of CK and CK-MB activity in 36 patients with AMI and 126 patients with chest pain on admission to the emergency room. In the 36 patients with AMI, all of whom were admitted within 4 hours after the onset of chest pain, pathologic increase occurred significantly earlier in CK-MB mass than in both CK and CK-MB activity with a median difference of 1 hour each. In patients coming to the emergency room (51 with AMI, 51 with angina pectoris and 24 with chest pain not related to CAD), CK-MB mass was the best diagnostic measurement for AMI of all markers tested (significantly higher efficiency, Youden index and likelihood ratio than both CK and CK-MB activity). Before initiating thrombolytic therapy, the sensitivity of CK-MB mass is significantly higher than CK-MB activity during the 0- to 6-hour period and significantly higher than CK activity during the 2- to 4-hour period after the onset of chest pain. Consequently, it is often possible to diagnose an AMI on the basis of increased CK-MB mass concentrations even at a time when CK and CK-MB activities are still within the reference interval.

Plasma endothelin-1

Stewart and colleagues[16] in Montreal, Canada, measured plasma endothelin-1 concentration using a radioimmunoassay in serial venous samples from 22 patients over a 72 hour period after AMI (14 patients with uncomplicated infarction, group I) and 8 patients with hemodynamic or ischemic sequelae (group II). Twenty-two normal subjects and 7 patients with stable angina served as the controls. Endothelin-1 levels in patients with stable coronary disease were not different from those of normal subjects. In group I, plasma levels of endothelin-1 rose sharply after AMI reaching a peak of 4.95 ± 0.78 pg/ml at 6 hours after the onset of chest pain and returning rapidly toward normal by 24 hours. Patients with complicated AMI (group II) had a similar rapid increase in plasma endothelin levels to a peak value of 8 ± 1.95 pg/ml; however, plasma endothelin-1 remained elevated in these patients and became different from values in group I at 48 and 72 hours. There was no correlation between peak increases in creatine kinase and peak endothelin-1 in either group. LVEF did not correlate with the increase in endothelin-1 in group I patients, but there was a significant inverse relation between LVEF and plasma endothelin-1 in group II patients. Thus, the rapid increase in plasma endothelin-1 associated with the onset of AMI suggests that this peptide may provide a marker of endothelial perturbation in the early phases of myocardial ischemia or contribute to alterations in myocardial perfusion.

Technetium-99 Sestamibi tomography

Patients who have chest pain without electrocardiographic ST elevation are not candidates for thrombolytic therapy in most clinical trials. Christian and colleagues[17] in Rochester, Minnesota examined the value of technetium-99 Sestamibi tomographic imaging to assess myocardial perfusion in patients during chest pain without ST elevation. Technetium-99m-Sestamibi was injected in 14 patients who had chest pain without ST elevation, who subsequently developed enzymatic evidence of AMI within 24 hours. Tomographic imaging was performed 1–6 hours after injection. Thirteen of 14 patients showed significant perfusion defects indicative of AMI consistent with absent perfusion; one patient had normal images. Because of the absence of definitive electrocardiographic changes, only five patients received reperfusion therapy within 6 hours of the onset of chest pain. Regional wall motion abnormalities were present in nine of nine patients undergoing contrast ventriculography and correlated with the location of the technetium-99m-Sestamibi perfusion defect. At the time of subsequent coronary angiography, total arterial occlusion was present in 11 of the 14 patients. The infarct-related artery could be identified in 13 of the 14 patients. In six of these 13 patients, the LC was the infarct-related artery. Patients who have chest pain without electrocardiographic ST elevation may have arterial occlusion and significant myocardium at risk. Technetium-99m-Sestamibi imaging may be of benefit in identifying these patients early so that they can be considered for acute reperfusion therapy.

Positron emission tomography

Mody and associates[18] in Los Angeles, California, used blood flow imaging using N-13 ammonia and evaluated myocardial metabolism using F-18 2-deoxyglucose with positron emission tomography to determine whether one may distinguish cardiomyopathy of CAD from nonischemic dilated cardiomyopathy in 21 patients with severe LV dysfunction. The origin of left ventricular dysfunction had been determined by coronary angiography to be ischemic in 11 patients or nonischemic in 10. Images were analyzed by three observers on a graded scale in seven LV segments and revealed fewer defects in dilated cardiomyopathy compared with ischemic cardiomyopathy for N-13 ammonia and F-18 deoxyglucose. An index incorporating extent and severity of defects revealed more homogeneity with fewer and less severe defects in subjects with nonischemic than in those with ischemic cardiomyopathy as assessed by imaging of flow and metabolism. Diagnostic accuracy for distinguishing the two subgroups by visual image analysis was 85%. Using previously published circumferential count profile criteria, patients with dilated cardiomyopathy had fewer ischemic segments and infarcted segments than in patients with cardiomyopathy of coronary disease (Figure 3-3). The sensitivity for differentiating the two clinical subgroups was 100% and the specificity 80%. Therefore, noninvasive positron emission tomographic imaging with N-13 ammonia and F-18 deoxyglucose is helpful in distinguishing patients with severe LV dysfunction secondary to CAD from those with nonischemic cardiomyopathy.

To test the hypothesis that simultaneous dual energy single photon emission computed tomography with technetium-99 pyrophosphate and thallium-201 can provide an accurate estimate of the size of myocardial infarction and to assess the correlation between infarct size and peak

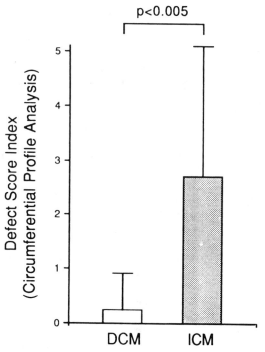

Fig. 3-3. Defect score index (summation of percent activity above normal data in all sectors contributing to segment defect). Open bar demonstrates lower score index and thus more homogeneity with fewer and less severe defects in subjects with dilated cardiomyopathy (DCM) compared with those with ischemic cardiomyopathy (ICM). Reproduced with permission from Mody, et al.[18]

serum creatine kinase activity, 165 patients with AMI underwent single photon emission computed tomography 3.2 ± 1.3 days after the onset of AMI. In the present study by Kawaguchi and colleagues[19] from Nagoya and Ogaki, Japan, the difference in the intensity of technetium-99m-pyrophosphate accumulation was assumed to be attributable to difference in the volume of infarcted myocardium, and the infarct volume was corrected by the ratio of the myocardial activity to the osseous activity to quantify the intensity of technetium-99m-pyrophosphate accumulation. The correlation of measured infarct volume with peak serum creatine kinase activity was significant. There was also a significant linear correlation between the corrected infarct volume and peak serum creatine kinase activity. Subgroup analysis showed a high correlation between corrected volume and peak creatine kinase activity in patients with anterior infarctions, but a poor correlation in patients with inferior or posterior infarctions. In both the early reperfusion and the no reperfusion groups, a good correlation was found between corrected infarct volume and peak serum creatine kinase activity. Thus the infarct volume, as determined by single photon emission computed tomography, correlated well with peak serum creatine kinase activity, and the correlation became closer when infarct volume was corrected by the heart/bone ratio. Simultaneous dual energy single photon emission computed tomography was useful in accurate quantification of AMI, and the quantification improved further when infarct size was corrected by the ratio of myocardial to osseous technetium-99m-pyrophosphate accumulation.

Magnetic resonance imaging

In an investigation by Krauss and associates[20] from Leiden and Utrecht, The Netherlands, spin-echo cardiac magnetic resonance imaging (MRI) studies were performed in 20 patients with a first 7- to 14-day old (mean 10) AMI. The MRI findings were compared with coronary angiography (14 patients), myocardial enzyme release (18 patients), radionuclide angiography (19 patients), and thallium-201 perfusion scintigraphy (19 patients). Regional T2 relaxation times determined from the signal intensities at echo times 30 msec and 90 msec were significantly prolonged in the infarcted areas. Based on abnormal T2 times for every patient, a regional and a total myocardial damage score was determined. The infarct-related artery was correctly identified in 93% of patients by MRI, in 79% of patients by thallium-201 scintigraphy, and in 62% of patients by radionuclide angiography. The total damage score correlated well with enzymatic infarct size. The correlation was close between LV end-systolic volume index determined by MRI and by radionuclide angiography. The LV end-systolic volume index correlated significantly with enzymatic infarct size, total damage score, and radionuclide LVEF. Correlations were also close between the MRI damage score and the thallium-201 perfusion score for the exercise images, and for the redistribution images. This study shows that spin-echo MRI is quite comparable with the established noninvasive imaging modalities currently used in AMI patients.

Coronary angiography

Most patients do not undergo acute reperfusion after AMI, and the selection of these patients for coronary angiography is still debated. Nicod and co-workers[21] in San Diego, California analyzed 1-year clinical outcomes and rates of coronary angiography performed as late as 60 days after AMI in 3,804 patients admitted between 1979 and 1988 and followed in six different centers. Patients less than 75 years old were classified into low-, medium-, and high-risk groups using a multivariate analysis of historical and clinical variables gathered during the first 8 hospital days. Patients who underwent early reperfusion after 1984 were analyzed separately. To analyze time trends, patients were compared before and after mid-1984. Mortalities from day 9 through 1 year were similar for the two time periods in the low- and medium-risk groups, but mortality was lower for the high-risk group after 1984 (32% vs 20%). The proportion of patients undergoing coronary angiography increased dramatically in each group after 1984 (low risk, 18% vs 48%; medium risk, 23% vs 49%; high risk, 10% vs 32%, before and after 1984, respectively). Furthermore, a large percentage of patients in the low-risk group did not have at least one of the indications for coronary angiography recently recommended by a joint task force. Among patients undergoing coronary angiography, the proportion of patients with three vessel CAD decreased after 1984, whereas the proportion undergoing mechanical revascularization in the year after AMI increased in all risk groups. Despite the recent development of non-invasive techniques with high sensitivity for detecting high-risk patients after AMI, coronary angiography is being performed increasingly in all patients, including those determined to be at low risk for complications based on clinical data. The economic consequences of such a trend could be considerable, and its impact requires careful analysis.

PROGNOSTIC INDICES

Combination of factors

In a large population of patients (n = 3666) who were discharged from the hospital after AMI and followed up for 1 year, factors associated with recurrent nonfatal (n = 171) or fatal (n = 74) infarction were identified by Gilpin and associates[22] from San Diego, California, and Vancouver, Canada. Also, the effects of combining various end points (recurrent nonfatal or fatal infarction and other cardiac death) in multivariate analyses, a practice common in many small studies that evaluate the predictive value of various treatments or special tests, was examined. In univariate analyses, patients with nonfatal recurrent infarction did not differ with respect to age or gender from infarct-free survivors, but they more often had a history of previous myocardial infarction, CHF, angina pectoris, and diabetes; more severe pulmonary congestion was present on chest x-ray during the admission, and a non-Q wave index infarction was more frequent. Patients with either a fatal or nonfatal recurrent infarction had more angina pectoris during follow-up (55% to 60%) compared with 27% in event-free survivors and 31% in patients who died of other cardiac causes in whom this factor could be assessed before death. In multivariate analyses, historical and clinical prognostic factors were ranked differently for fatal or nonfatal reinfarction and other cardiac causes of death; angina pectoris at follow-up was highly related to recurrent infarction (fatal or nonfatal), along with a history of diabetes, and a non-Q wave index infarction. These factors were not independently related to other causes of cardiac death. When angina pectoris at follow-up was used in the multivariate analysis of recurrent infarction (fatal plus nonfatal), it was the most important factor. This finding supports the general practice of referring patients with angina pectoris during follow-up (34% of the population) for coronary angiography in an effort to identify those with severe disease who might benefit from revascularization, which is aimed at the prevention of recurrent AMI.

A logical sequence of testing in evaluating prognosis early in AMI would be to use the clinical data first, then add noninvasive data, and finally add invasive data. Griffin and associates[23] from Los Angeles, California, obtained the incremental prognostic information concerning 1-year survival from such a sequence in 107 patients with AMI using logistic regression and receiver-operating characteristic curves. Cardiac mortality was 24% at 1 year. Clinical data obtained soon after admission (prior AMI, heart rate, BP, age) were 78 ± 5% accurate in the prediction of 1-year survival. The addition of radionuclide-estimated LVEF or invasive hemodynamic data in the clinical model at this time improved prognostic accuracy to 84 ± 5% and 87 ± 4%, respectively (Figure 3-4). The further addition of invasive data to the model containing clinical and LVEF data provided a further increment in prognostic accuracy to 89 ± 4%, whereas no significant increase in accuracy was seen on addition of LVEF to the model containing clinical and invasive data. It is concluded that clinical data provide important prognostic information concerning late survival early in the course of AMI. This may be improved by the logical application of noninvasive and invasive studies at this time.

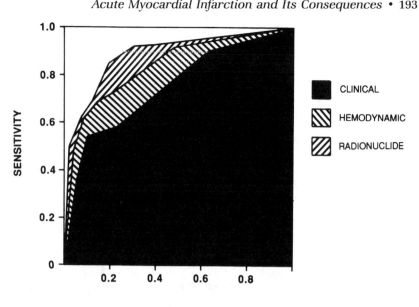

Fig. 3-4. Receiver-operating characteristic curves for the sequence of logistic regression models based on clinical data (step 1) in which invasive hemodynamic data (step 2A) are first added, followed by radionuclide data (step 3). Reproduced with permission from Griffin, et al.[23]

When ineligible for thrombolytic therapy

To determine what proportion of patients with AMI are not eligible for thrombolytic therapy and to assess their natural history, Cragg and associates[24] from Royal Oak, Michigan, retrospectively reviewed all patients with AMI hospitalized during a 27 month period. Of 1,471 patients with AMI, 230 (16%) received thrombolytic therapy according to protocol and an additional 97 (7%) received nonprotocol thrombolytic therapy, primary coronary balloon angioplasty, or both because of contraindications. The other 1,144 patients (78%) did not receive reperfusion therapy. The patients who did not receive thrombolytic therapy were older, more likely to be women, and more likely to have a history of hypertension, previous AMI, or chronic angina (Figure 3-5). An average of 1.9 reasons for exclusion were identified per patient among the ineligible patients. Mortality was 5-fold higher among ineligible patients (19%) than among protocol-treated patients (4%) (Figure 3-6). In-hospital mortality rates for excluded patients were 28% in elderly patients (age, 76 years; n = 396); 29% in patients with stroke or bleeding risk (n = 209); 17% in patients with delayed presentation (>4 hours after the onset of chest pain; [n = 599]); 14% in patients with an ineligible electrocardiogram (n = 673); and 26% in patients with a miscellaneous reason for exclusion (n = 243). Independent predictors of increased mortality were: age greater than 76 years, stroke or other bleeding risk, ineligible electrocardiogram, or the presence of 2 or more exclusion criteria. Thrombolytic therapy is currently used in the USA for only a minority of patients with AMI: those who have low-risk prognostic characteristics.

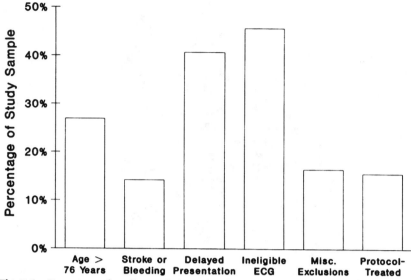

Fig. 3-5. Percentage of study sample in each subgroup. The mean number of exclusions was 1.9 per patient. (ECG = electrocardiogram; Misc. = miscellaneous). Reproduced with permission from Cragg, et al.[24]

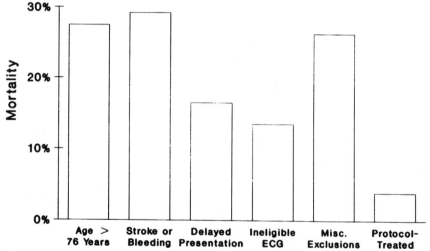

Fig. 3-6. Mortality rates for each exclusion subgroup (including patients with multiple exclusions) and for patients treated according to protocol. (ECG = electrocardiogram; Misc. = miscellaneous). Reproduced with permission from Cragg, et al.[24]

Age

To further evaluate contemporary risk and practice patterns in AMI, Montague and associates[25] from Edmonton, Canada, studied 402 consecutive patients with AMI between July 1988 and June 1989. The clinical investigations, medical therapy and outcome of patients aged ≥70 years (n = 132; group 1) were compared with patients aged <70 years (n = 270; group 2). In group 1, 20% of patients had no typical cardiac pain versus 6% in group 2. History of previous AMI, Q-wave AMI and peak creatine kinase were not different in the 2 groups. In-hospital mortality was markedly higher in group 1 (27%) than in group 2 (8%). Multivariate analysis revealed previous AMI, presentation without typical pain and age ≥70 years to be independently associated with the greatest relative risk. Post-AMI exercise testing, EF calculations and coronary angiography were all performed less often; proven effective medical therapies, including thrombolysis, B blockers, acetylsalicylic acid and nitrates were all used less frequently. The very high mortality and less aggressive management of elderly patients with AMI confirm similar data from the 1987 AMI patient cohort and other recently reported AMI patient outcome analyses. However, it remains uncertain why older patients with AMI are investigated and treated differently from younger patients. Further studies are warranted.

Diastolic blood pressure

To examine the hypothesis that a J curve relation between BP and death from CAD is confined to high risk subjects with AMI, D'Agostino and associates[26] from Boston, Massachusetts, and Manchester, UK, followed up 5,209 subjects in the Framingham study cohort by a person-examination approach. Among subjects without AMI, non-cardiovascular disease deaths were twice to 3 times as common as CAD deaths. Furthermore, there was no significant relation between non-cardiovascular disease death and diastolic or systolic BP. Also CAD deaths were linearly related to diastolic and systolic BP (Figure 3-7). Among high risk patients (that is, people with AMI but free of CAD) death from CAD was more common than non-cardiovascular disease death. There was a significant U shaped relation between CAD death and diastolic BP. Although there was an apparent U shaped relation between CAD death and systolic BP, it did not attain statistical significance when controlling for age and

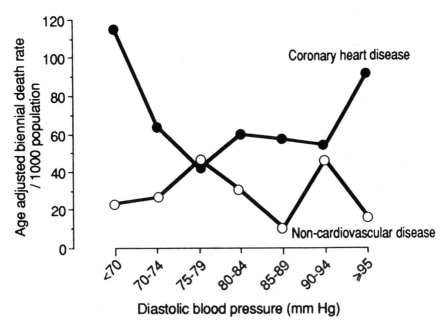

Fig. 3-7. Coronary heart disease deaths and non-cardiovascular disease deaths relative to diastolic blood pressure in men and women with previous myocardial infarction. Reproduced with permission from D'Agostino et al.[26]

change in systolic BP from the pre-myocardial infarction level. None of the above conclusions changed when adjustments were made for risk factors such as serum cholesterol concentration, antihypertensive treatment, and LV function. The U shaped relation between diastolic BP and high risk subjects existed for both those given antihypertensive treatment and those not. These data suggest that an age and sex independent U curve relation exists for diastolic BP and CAD deaths in patients with AMI but not for low risk subjects without AMI. The relation seems to be independent of LV function and antihypertensive treatment.

Serum total cholesterol

To determine the relation between serum cholesterol levels and the long-term risk for reinfarction, death from CAD, and all-cause mortality in persons who recovered from AMI, Wong and associates[27] from Irvine, California, and Framingham, Massachusetts, performed a prospective, long-term study involving 260 men and 114 women aged 33 to 88 years of age (mean 62) who had a history of AMI. A complete physical examination, including electrocardiographic evaluation, BP measurement, height and weight measurements, determination of smoking habits, and casual determinations of blood glucose and serum cholesterol, was done approximately 1 year after recovery from initial AMI. Patients were followed after AMI for the occurrence of reinfarction or death (mean follow-up, 10.5 years; range, 0.8 to 31.6 years). The mean total cholesterol level after infarction was 5.21 mmol/L (243 mg/dL); 20% of patients had levels below 5.17 mmol/L (200 mg/dL), and 22% had levels ≥7.11 mmol/L (275 mg/dL) (Table 3-2). Compared with patients who had cholesterol levels below 5.17 mmol/L, patients with levels ≥7.11 mmol/L were at increased risk for reinfarction (relative risk, 3.8), death from CAD (relative risk, 2.6), and all-cause mortality (relative risk, 1.9) based on multivariate Cox regression analyses adjusted for other coronary risk factors. Intermediate cholesterol levels were generally not associed with increased risk. The association between elevated serum cholesterol and increased risk was strongest in men; however, elevated cholesterol levels were found to be most strongly related to death from CAD and to all-cause mortality in persons who were 65 years of age or more. Patients who have recovered from an AMI and who have high cholesterol levels are at an increased long-term risk for reinfarction, death from CAD, and all-cause mortality. The authors

TABLE 3-2. *Cardiovascular risk factors and follow-up status by cholesterol level in patients with a previous myocardial infarction.* *Reproduced with permission from Wong, et al.*[27]

Risk Factor	Cholesterol Level			
	Men		Women	
	< 6.22 mmol/L (< 240 mm/dL)	≥ 6.22 mmol/L (≥ 240 mm/dL)	< 6.22 mmol/L (< 240 mm/dL)	≥ 6.22 mmol/L (≥ 240 mm/dL)
Age, y	62.2 (142)	57.8† (118)	66.1 (49)	64.7 (65)
Systolic blood pressure, *mm Hg*	137.0 (140)	138.0 (118)	149.1 (46)	149.0 (65)
Relative weight, *% of ideal weight*	117.5 (141)	121.6‡ (117)	116.9 (47)	126.2‡ (65)
Diabetes, %	12.6 (142)	10.2 (118)	22.4 (49)	15.4 (65)
Currently smoking, %	55.0 (129)	59.6 (109)	30.4 (46)	24.2 (62)
Abnormal electrocardiogram, %	82.4 (142)	85.6 (118)	75.0 (48)	83.1 (65)
End points, %§				
Reinfarction	26.8 (142)	34.7 (118)	43.0 (49)	36.9 (65)
Death from coronary heart disease	35.9 (142)	47.5 (118)	30.6 (49)	32.3 (65)
Death from all causes	62.0 (142)	75.4† (118)	53.1 (49)	60.0 (65)

* Numbers in parentheses indicate the sample size under analysis.
† *P* < 0.01 when cholesterol-level categories are compared.
‡ *P* < 0.05 when cholesterol-level categories are compared.
§ Percent of patients experiencing the end point.

results confirm the prognostic value of cholesterol levels measured after AMI and support the role of lipid management in this population.

Platelet size

Although platelet characteristics have an important influence on CAD, the nature of the association of platelet size and platelet count with death and reinfarction after an index AMI is unknown. Martin and associates[28] from London, UK, measured mean platelet volume, a determinant of platelet reactivity, in 1716 men 6 months after AMI. Death and recurrent myocardial ischemic events were then assessed at 2 years. Mean platelet volume was greater in 126 men who had a further fatal or nonfatal ischemic event than in the 1590 men who had no further AMI. In addition, the mean platelet volume was larger in men who died than in those who did not. There was no difference in platelet count between these groups. When analyzed by quartiles, consistent trends of increasing age-adjusted relative odds of death and recurrent ischemic events were noted for mean platelet volume. Mean platelet volume did not correlate with known CAD risk factors such as BP, blood lipids, fibrinogen, white cell count, or plasma viscosity. The authors believe that mean platelet volume is a further independent risk factor for recurrent AMI.

Heart rate variability index

Odemuyiwa and associates[29] from London, UK, compared heart rate variability index and LVEF for the prediction of all-cause mortality, arrhythmic events and sudden death in 385 survivors of AMI. For arrhythmic events, where, for a sensitivity of 75%, heart rate variability index had a specificity of 76%, EF had a specificity of only 45%. An EF of <40% had a sensitivity of 42% and a specificity of 75% for arrhythmic events; for the same sensitivity a heart rate variability index of 20 U had a specificity of 92%. An EF <40% had a sensitivity of 40% and a specificity of 73% for sudden death; heart rate variability index had a specificity of 83% for the same sensitivity. For all cause mortality, where, for a sensitivity of 75%, heart rate variability index had a specificity of 52%, EF had a specificity of 40%. It is concluded that heart rate variability index appears a better predictor of important postinfarction arrhythmic complications than LV EF, but both indexes perform equally well in predicting all-cause mortality.

Farrell and colleagues[30] in London, UK, studied the value of heart rate variability, ambulatory electrocardiogram variables, and the signal-averaged electrocardiogram in the prediction of arrhythmic events, including sudden death or life-threatening ventricular arrhythmias before hospital discharge in 416 consecutive patients with AMI. During the follow-up period, there were 24 arrhythmic events and 47 deaths. The initial relation between several prognostic factors and arrhythmic events was explored with use of the Kaplan-Meier product limit estimates of survival function. Impaired heart rates variability <20 ms, late potentials, ventricular ectopic beat frequency, repetitive ventricular forms, LVEF <40%, and Killip class were identified as significant univariate predictors of arrhythmic events (Figure 3-8). The combination of impaired heart rate variability and late potentials had a sensitivity of 58%, a positive predictive accuracy of 33% and a relative risk of 18.5 for arrhythmic events and was superior to other combinations. These results suggest that a simple method of assessment based on heart rate variability and the signal-averaged electrocardiogram

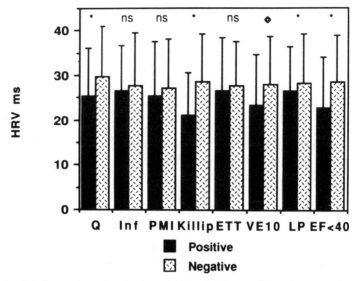

Fig. 3-8. Relations among heart rate variability (HRV) and different prognostic variables such as Q waves (Q), inferior infarction (Inf), history of past myocardial infarction (PMI), Killip class ≥2 on admission, positive exercise text (ETT), ventricular ectopic beat frequency >10 in any hour (VE 10), late potentials (LP) and ejection fraction <40% (EF<40). * = P<0.0001, ♦ = p<0.001. Reproduced with permission from Farrell, et al.[30]

may select a small subgroup of survivors after AMI at high risk of future life-threatening arrhythmias and sudden death.

Exercise testing

The presence or absence of baseline diagnostic Q waves has been believed to compromise the accuracy of standard exercise electrocardiography in identifying severe CAD; therefore, Miranda and coworkers[31] in Long Beach, California, performed a retrospective analysis using a personal computer data base of exercise test responses and cardiac catheterization results to evaluate this premise, and follow-up was performed to observe how Q waves and/or severe CAD impacted on survival. Two hundred fifty-three men who had survived a AMI were studied. Patients on digitalis, those with left BBB or LV hypertrophy on their baseline electrocardiogram, those with previous revascularization procedures, and those with significant valvular or congenital heart disease were excluded. All patients performed either a low-level predischarge or a sign/symptom limited exercise test and underwent diagnostic coronary angiography within 32 days of each test. Long-term follow-up on patients was performed for an average of 45 months. Group with non-Q wave AMI comprised 103 post-myocardial infarction patients lacking Q waves at the time of exercise testing and group Q AMI comprised 150 patients who developed Q waves with their myocardial infarction. The cut points of ≥1 mm and ≥2 mm of exercise-induced ST segment depression were reliable markers of severe CAD. Receiver operating characteristic curve analysis revealed that exercise-induced ST segment depression had discriminating power for the identification of severe CAD in both the Q wave AMI patients and the non-Q wave AMI patients. After 4 years of cumulative follow-up, patients with severe CAD had an infarct-free survival rate of

72%, whereas, those without severe CAD had an 86% infarct-free survival rate. Non-Q wave patients had an infarct-free survival rate of 81%, whereas those with Q waves had an infarct-free survival rate of 85%. The presence or absence of diagnostic Q waves had no significant effect on the ability of the exercise electrocardiogram to identify severe CAD in survivors of AMI. Long-term infarct-free survival of patients with AMI is more related to the presence of severe CAD rather than if they had a non-Q wave or Q wave AMI.

Collateral flow and residual coronary narrowing

Residual high-grade coronary stenosis and collateral flow are frequent findings in the chronic phase after a Q-wave AMI. Gohlke and associates[32] from Bad Krozingen, Germany, analyzed the prognostic importance of a residual stenosis of the infarct artery and of collateral flow to the infarct area in 102 young patients (mean age 35 years, range 22–36) who had survived an anterior wall Q-wave AMI. Patients whose only significant lesion (>50% luminal diameter reduction) was in the proximal portion of the left anterior descending artery were enrolled in the study. A 50 to 74% diameter stenosis was present in 33 of 102 patients (32%), 43 (42%) had a 75 to 99% stenosis and 26% had a total occlusion of the infarct vessel. Collateral vessels, which were evaluated by a scoring system, were present in 52 of 102 patients (51%). Four percent had only faint (score 1), 17 of 102 patients (17%) had moderate and 32 patients (31%) had good collateral flow (score >4). The 8-year cumulative mortality was 15.2%—an 8-fold increase compared with the age-matched general population. No patient with <75% stenosis died during follow-up, whereas the cumulative 8-year mortality was 23 and 17% in patients with a 75 to 99% stenosis or total occlusion, respectively. Patients with at least moderate collateral flow had a mortality rate of 21%, versus 8% for patients without or with faint collateral flow. Thus, a >75% residual stenosis after anterior wall AMI is associated with less favorable survival, compared with a less severe stenosis. Collateral vessels after an anterior wall Q-wave AMI do not protect against adverse events. These results suggest that restoration of anterograde flow could have a favorable influence on long-term prognosis in these patients.

Programmed ventricular stimulation

To determine the influence of timing on the prognostic value of programmed ventricular stimulation after AMI, Nogami and associates[33] from Tokyo and Ibaraki, Japan, studied 32 patients on day 19 (early study) and again on day 36 (late study) after AMI using up to 3 extra stimuli. At the early study, sustained monomorphic VT was induced in 12 patients (38%), sustained polymorphic VT in 8 (25%), nonsustained polymorphic VT in 1 (3%) and no inducible arrhythmia in 10 (31%). At the late study, sustained monomorphic VT, nonsustained monomorphic VT and nonsustained polymorphic VT were induced in 8 patients (25%) each, and no inducible arrhythmia in 8 (25%). Of the 12 patients who had inducible sustained monomorphic VT at the early study, 7 had noninducibility of sustained monomorphic VT at the late study. Of the 20 patients who had noninducibility of sustained monomorphic VT at the early study, 3 had inducible sustained monomorphic VT at the late study. During the follow-up period (mean ± standard deviation 21 ± 8 months), there were 2 sudden cardiac deaths and 3 occurrences of sustained VT. Univariate analysis revealed both inducibilities of sustained monomorphic VT at the early study and at the late study to be predictive of sudden cardiac death or clinical occurrence of sustained VT. However, inducibility of sustained monomorphic VT at the late study had a higher sensitivity (100%), specificity (89%), positive predictive value (63%) and negative predictive value (100%) than at the early study (80, 70, 33 and 95%, respectively). These data suggest that the timing of programmed stimulation study after AMI influences the inducibility of VT and its predictive ability. Programmed ventricular stimulation after AMI may need to be done at least 1 month after AMI for optimal value.

Changes with time

de Vreede and colleagues[34] in Maastricht, The Netherlands, investigated whether survival after AMI has changed between 1960 and 1987. Thirty-six patients were analyzed. They were classified with respect to deaths in the hospital at 1 month and the 5-year mortality rate starting at hospital discharge. Mortality was assessed from all studies by comparing results from different institutions with use of identical inclusion criteria and by analyzing studies reporting on changes in mortality in two or more comparable patient cohorts. The reports on clinical trials in AMI were excluded. Average overall in-hospital mortality decreased from 29% during the 1960s to 21% during the 1970s and 16% during the 1980s. The externally controlled studies also showed a declining trend from1960 to 1969, from 1970 to 1979, and from 1980 to 1987. The overall 1-month mortality rate decreased from 31% during the 1960s to 25% during the 1970s and 18% during the 1980s. Most internally controlled studies also showed significant improvement in in-hospital and 1-month survival. Five year mortality after hospital discharge did not significantly decrease in 33% in 1960 and 33% from 1970 to 1979. Thus, in the pre-thrombolytic era, short-term prognosis after AMI has improved since 1960. Changes in long-term prognosis after hospital discharge could not be demonstrated in this study.

COMPLICATIONS

Ventricular arrhythmias

During a 3-year period, 11 patients developed polymorphous VT 1–13 days after anterior AMI (7 patients) or inferior (4 patients) and the clinical course was followed by Wolfe and colleagues[35] in San Francisco, California. None of the 11 patients had sinus bradycardia but 3 had a sinus pause immediately before the onset of polymorphous VT. In all 11 patients, the QT interval and corrected QT interval were normal or minimally prolonged. None had significant hypokalemia or a grossly abnormal serum magnesium or calcium concentration. Immediately before the onset of polymorphous VT symptoms and/or electrocardiographic changes consistent with recurrent myocardial ischemia occurred in 9 of 11 patients. One patient died before drug therapy could be initiated. Lidocaine was used in 10 patients and proved to be effective in only 1. Intravenous procainamide was used in 6 patients: one improved, and 5 had recurrence of polymorphous VT. Bretylium was used in 5 patients and was ineffective in all cases. Overdrive pacing was used in 4 patients and failed to suppress recurrent arrhythmias in all cases. Four patients with persistent polymorphous VT unresponsive to lidocaine, procainamide, or bretylium responded to intravenous amiodarone. One patient with polymorphous VT that was consistently preceded by ST segment elevation responded to intravenous nitroglycerin. Two patients with persistent polymorphous VT and obvious recurrent ischemia unresponsive to pharmacological intervention responded to emergency CABG. A third patient who experienced recurrent angina and polymorphous VT was initially stabilized with pharmacological therapy but subsequently underwent elective CABG and has remained stable without antiarrhythmic therapy. Post-AMI polymorphous VT is not consistently related to an abnormally long QT interval, sinus bradycardia, preceding sinus pauses, or electrolyte abnormalities. This arrhythmia has a variable response to class I antiarrhythmics but may be suppressed by intravenous amiodarone therapy. It is often associated with signs or symptoms of recurrent myocardial ischemia. Furthermore, CABG appears to be effective in preventing the recurrence of polymorphous VT when associated with recurrent postinfarction angina.

The relation between ventricular late potentials and the occurrence of acute (in-hospital) and hyperacute (before hospital admission) VT or VF was studied by Hong and associates[36] from Los Angeles, California, in 281 consecutive patients with uninterrupted AMI. The prevalence of late potentials was significantly higher in patients with than without VT/VF (65 vs 22%). These relations persisted among patients with left BBB, although a different definition was used for identifying late potentials in these patients. Multivariate analysis showed that presence of late potentials and peak creatine kinase enzyme level were the only 2 independent variables associated with early VT/VF. Total in-hospital mortality, as well as in-hospital cardiac mortality, was significantly higher among patients with than without acute VT/VF. However, at 1 year, mortality rates did not differ between the 2 groups. The following conclusions were drawn from this study: (1) Late potentials are closely related to VT/VF in hyperacute and acute phases of infarction. (2) Presence of left BBB does not mitigate against the finding of late potentials in these patients. (3) Early VT/VF in acute infarction is related to large infarctions and to a high in-hospital mortality rate.

Atrial fibrillation

To elucidate the role of inflammatory and hemodynamic factors in the genesis of AF in AMI, 228 patients with a first Q wave anterior AMI were studied by Sugiura and associates[37] from Osaka, Japan. Forty-nine patients had pericarditis (detection of pericardial rub by careful auscultation), and 36 patients had echocardiographically demonstrated hydropericardium (presence of pericardial effusion without pericardial rub). During the first 3 days after admission, transient episodes of AF were observed in 10 patients (20%) with pericarditis (group 1), 15 patients (42%) with hydropericardium (group 2), and 20 patients (14%) without pericarditis and hydropericardium (group 3). Although there was no significant difference in the incidence of AF between groups 1 and 3, patients in group 2 had a significantly higher incidence of AF than those in groups 1 and 3. PA wedge pressure and the number of advanced asynergic segments were found to be the important factors discriminating the 3 groups by multivariate analysis. Therefore AF after Q wave anterior AMI was not related to the inflammatory infiltration involving the atria but to the increase in atrial pressure resulting from hemodynamic change caused by more extensive myocardial damage.

Sick sinus syndrome

Alboni and associates[38] from Cento, Italy, evaluated a possible role of sinus node (SN) artery disease in the pathogenesis of sick sinus syndrome (SSS) in patients with an inferior wall AMI. Coronary angiography and electrophysiologic studies of the SN, both in the basal state and after pharmacologic autonomic blockade, were performed in 23 study patients (mean age 60 years) with SSS and a previous inferior wall AMI and in another 23 control patients (mean age 57 years) with normal sinus rate and a previous inferior AMI. Stenosis of the SN artery (or that proximal to its origin) >50% was present in 13 study patients (56%) and in 8 control patients (34%). In the study group, the intrinisic heart rate was abnormal in 5 of the 6 patients (83%) with severe SN artery stenosis (≥75% narrowing), in 3 of the 7 (43%) with moderate stenosis (50 to 75% narrowing) and in 3 of the 10 (30%) with insignificant stenosis (<50% narrowing). In the study group, the correlation between the SN measures (heart rate, corrected SN recovery time and sinoatrial conduction time) and the severity of SN artery stenosis was good after autonomic blockade (r between 0.59 and 0.64) and poor in the basal state. These data provide evidence for a role of SN artery disease in the pathogenesis of SSS in patients with an inferior wall AMI.

Right bundle branch block

Ricou and colleagues[39] in San Diego, California and Vancouver, Canada, evaluated 932 patients with Q wave anterior AMI to determine the short- and long-term prognostic significance of the presence of right BBB. Compared with 754 patients without right BBB, 178 patients with this abnormality after AMI showed an increased incidence of LV CHF (72% versus 52%) and increased in-hospital (32% versus 8%) and 1 year after hospital discharge (17% versus 7%) cardiac mortality rates (Figures 3-9 and 3-10). The presence of right bundle branch block was an independent predictor of increased in-hospital and 1-year mortality when entered in a multivariate analysis. However, the absence of LV failure identified a subgroup of patients with right BBB with low in-hospital (4%) and 1 year postdischarge (5%) cardiac mortality rates comparable to those in patients with neither failure nor right BBB (2% and 5% respectively). In the presence of LV failure, patients with associated right BBB had higher in-hospital (43% vs 14%) and 1 year postdischarge (24% vs 9%) cardiac mortality rates than those patients with CHF but no right BBB. Thus, the presence of right BBB after anterior Q wave AMI is an independent marker of poor prognosis but this is found only in patients with evidence of LV failure. These patients may benefit from early evaluation and therapy.

Okabe and associates[40] from Fukuoka, Japan, evaluated whether necrosis of the right bundle branch was responsible for development of right BBB in AMI. Twenty patients with anteroseptal AMI were studied: 10 with right BBB (group A) and 10 without (group B)—to evaluate by serial sectioning the pathological extent of the infarct surrounding the right bundle branch and also that of right bundle branch necrosis. Myocardial infarction reached the right bundle branch more than 8 mm above the moderator band in only 3 patients in Group B. Nine hearts in group

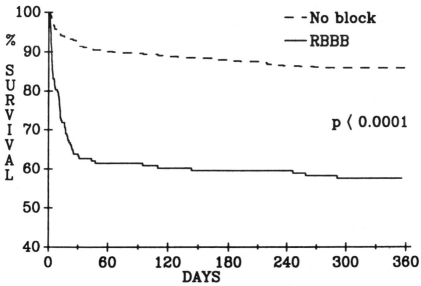

Fig. 3-9. Survival curves for patients without block (dashed line) and those with right bundle branch block (RBBB) (solid line). Survival was significantly better in patients without block than in patients with right bundle branch block. Reproduced with permission from Ricou, et al.[39]

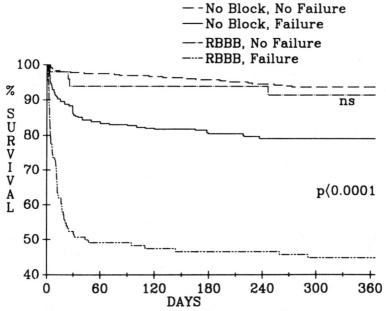

Fig. 3-10. Survival curves for patients without block and those with right bundle branch block grouped according to the absence or presence of signs of left ventricular failure. In the absence of failure, survival was good and not significantly different between the two groups. In the presence of failure, patients with right bundle branch block had a lower survival rate than that of patients without block. Reproduced with permission from Ricou, et al.[39]

A showed significant necrosis of the right bundle branch. In group B and in 1 case with transient right BBB no necrosis was found. The occurrence of right BBB was almost entirely explained by necrosis of the right bundle branch, but transient right BBB did develop without necrosis of the right bundle branch.

Complete heart block

Previous studies report larger myocardial infarcts and increased in-hospital mortality rates in patients with inferior wall AMI and complete AV block, but the clinical implications of these complications in patients treated with reperfusion therapy have not been addressed. Accordingly, Clemmensen and associates[41] from 4 medical centers studied the clinical course of 373 patients—50 (13%) of whom developed complete AV block—admitted with inferior wall AMI and given thrombolytic therapy within 6 hours of symptom onset. Acute patency rates of the infarct artery after thrombolytic therapy were similar in patients with or without AV block. Ventricular function measured at baseline and before discharge in patients with complete AV block showed a decrement in median EF (-3.5 vs -0.4%) and in median regional wall motion (-0.14 vs $+0.24$ standard deviations/chord). The reocclusion rate was higher in patients with complete AV block (29 vs 16%). Patients with complete AV block had more episodes of VF or tachycardia (36 vs 14%), sustained hypotension (36 vs 10%), pulmonary edema (12 vs 4%) and a higher in-hospital mortality rate (20 vs 4%), although the mortality rate after hospital discharge was identical (2%) in the 2 groups. Multivariable logistic regression analysis revealed that complete AV block was a strong independent predictor of in-hospital mortality. Thus, despite initial successful reperfusion, patients with inferior wall AMI and complete AV block have higher rates of in-hospital complications and mortality.

Cardiogenic shock

Cardiogenic shock resulting from AMI is a serious complication with a high mortality rate, but little is known about whether its incidence or outcome has changed over time. As part of an ongoing population-based study of AMI, Goldberg and associates[42] from Worcester, Massachusetts, examined trends over time in the instance and mortality rate of cardiogenic shock after AMI. They studied 4,762 patients with AMI who were admitted to 16 hospitals in the Worcester, Massachusetts, metropolitan area between 1975 and 1988. They determined the incidence of and short-term and long-term mortality due to cardiogenic shock in each of the 6 years during the study (Figure 3-11). The incidence of cardiogenic shock complicating AMI remained relatively constant, averaging 7.5%. Multivariate regression analysis that controlled for variables affecting incidence revealed significant though inconsistent temporal trends in the incidence of cardiogenic shock. As compared with the risk in 1975, the adjusted relative risk was 0.83 in 1978, 0.96 in 1981, 0.68 in 1984, 1.16 in 1986, and 1.65 in 1988. The overall in-hospital mortality rate among patients with cardiogenic shock was significantly higher than that among patients without this complication (77.7% vs 13.5%) (Figure 3-12). The in-hospital mortality among the patients with shock did not improve between 1975 (73.7%) and 1988 (81.7%). Long-term survival during the 14-year follow-up period was significantly worse among patients who survived cardiogenic shock during hospitalization than among patients who did not have shock. The

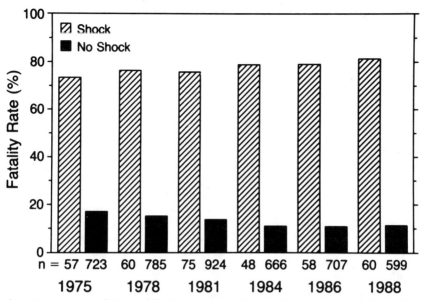

Fig. 3-11. In-Hospital Case Fatality Rates among Patients with Acute Myocardial Infarction, According to the Year Studied and the Occurrence of Cardiogenic Shock. Reproduced with permission from Goldberg, et al.[42]

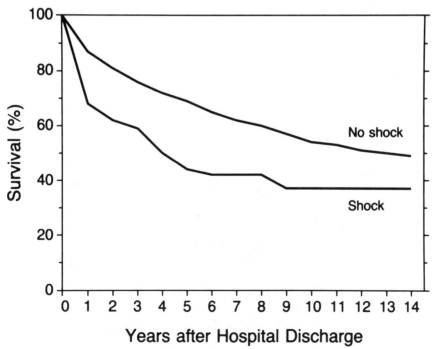

Fig. 3-12. Long-Term Survival after Hospital Discharge among Patients with Acute Myocardial Infarction, According to Occurrence of Cardiogenic Shock during Hospitalization. Reproduced with permission from Goldberg, et al.[42]

results of this observational, community-wide study suggest that neither the incidence nor the prognosis of cardiogenic shock resulting from AMI has improved over time. Both in-hospital and long-term survival remain poor for patients with this complication.

Mitral regurgitation

Intraoperative transesophageal Doppler color flow imaging affords the opportunity to assess mitral valve competency immediately before and after cardiopulmonary bypass. Sheikh and colleagues[43] in Durham, North Carolina assessed the utility of transesophageal flow imaging to assist in the selection and operative treatment of ischemic MR. Two hundred forty-six patients undergoing surgery for ischemic heart disease were prospectively studied. All had preoperative cardiac catheterization. Catheterization and pre-bypass transesophageal flow imaging were discordant in their estimation of MR in 112 patients. Compared with patients in whom both techniques agreed in estimation of MR, patients with discordance in MR were more likely to have had unstable clinical syndromes at the time of catheterization or to have received thrombolytics. Pre-bypass transesophageal flow imaging resulted in a change in the operative plan with respect to the mitral valve in 27 patients. Because less MR was found by transesophageal color flow imaging than catheterization, 22 patients had only CABG when combined CABG and mitral valve surgery had been planned. Because more MR was found by transesophageal flow imaging than catheterization, five patients had combined CABG and mitral valve surgery when CABG alone had been planned. Unsatisfactory results noted by transesophageal flow imaging following mitral valve surgery in 5 patients resulted in immediate corrective surgery. Cox regression analysis identified residual MR at the completion of surgery to be an important predictor of survival after surgery—more important than patient age or LV EF. These results indicate that transesophageal Doppler color flow imaging is useful in guiding patient selection and operative treatment of ischemic MR and that in such patients, intraoperative transesophageal flow imaging should be routinely performed.

Over a 5-year period, Hendren and associates[44] from Cleveland, Ohio, performed operations on native mitral valves in 1,292 patients. Myocardial ischemia was the cause of the MR in 84 patients (6.5%) (Figure 3-13). Sixty-

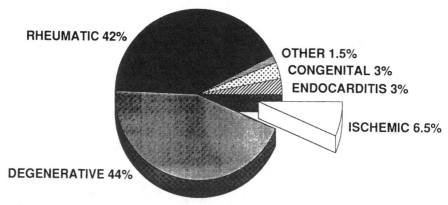

Fig. 3-13. From 1985 through 1989, 1,292 patients underwent surgical procedures on their native mitral valve. Ischemic insufficiency was the cause of the mitral disease in 6.5%. Reproduced with permission from Hendren, et al.[44]

five of the 84 patients had mitral valve repair. Mean age was 66 ± 10 years; 35 patients (53.8%) were women. Mean degree of preoperative MR was 3.2 ± 0.7; mean preoperative New York Heart Association functional class was 3.3 ± 0.7. Eleven patients (16.9%) had acute and 54 (83.1%) had chronic MR. MVP was present in 26 patients (40%). Restrictive leaflet motion secondary to regional or global LV dilatation occurred in 39 patients (60%). All patients had associated myocardial revascularization followed by transatrial valvuloplasty. There were 6 (9.2%) hospital deaths (acute, 9.1%; chronic, 9.3%; prolapse, 11.5%; restrictive, 7.7%). The mean degree of postoperative MR was 0.6 ± 0.8 in 51 patients. At a mean follow-up of 3.1 ± 1.6 years, patient survival was 96% for patients with MVP and 48% for those with restrictive leaflet motion. New York Heart Association functional class was improved in all groups. Ischemic MR is an uncommon cause of mitral valve disease that is amenable to repair in most cases of both acute and chronic onset. The operative mortality is low, and operation is associated with superior survival in patients with MVP.

Left ventricular aneurysm

Although LV aneurysm is associated with increased mortality rates, its independent prognostic significance is controversial. To determine the effect of LV aneurysm on risk, Hassapoyannes and associates[45] from Columbia, South Carolina, and Augusta, Georgia, studied 121 patients with healed myocardial infarction (MI), 55 manifesting akinesia on ventriculography (MI group) and 66 characterized by diastolic deformity (eccentricity) and systolic dyskinesia (LV aneurysm group). At a mean follow-up of 5.7 years, there were 32 cardiac deaths (12 MI vs 20 LV aneurysm), including 9 sudden deaths (1 MI vs 8 LV aneurysm) (Figure 3-14). Multivariate analysis revealed decreasing EF to be the best predictor of total cardiac death, and revascularization to be protective. Nonsudden cardiac death was predicted by EF, absence of revascularization and right CAD, whereas sudden cardiac death was predicted by LV aneurysm and the frequency of ventricular ectopic complexes on Holter monitoring. In the MI group, EF was the only significant predictor of total cardiac death and nonsudden cardiac death. In the LV aneurysm group, total cardiac death, as well as nonsudden cardiac death, were predicted by EF, VT, and right CAD, whereas VT predicted sudden cardiac death. It is concluded that the risk profile for total cardiac death differs between LV aneurysm and MI patients, and that LV aneurysm constitutes an inde-

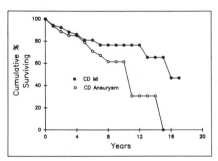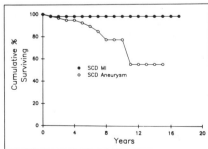

Fig. 3-14. (A) Cumulative percent survival comparing aneurysm and myocardial infarction (MI) groups for total cardiac death (CD). (B) Cumulative percent survival comparing aneurysm and myocardial infarction (MI) groups for sudden cardiac death (SCD). Reproduced with permission from Hassapoyannes, et al.[45]

pendent predictor of late sudden cardiac death after MI. Moreover, on a substrate of LV aneurysm, the risk factors for sudden cardiac death and nonsudden cardiac death differ, with ventricular tachycardia being the sole predictor of sudden cardiac death. Furthermore, Holter monitoring is valuable in identifying patients at persistent risk of sudden cardiac death.

Baciewicz and associates[46] from Atlanta, Georgia, assessed clinical and operative data on a large group of patients in whom LV aneurysm was repaired to determine factors that might predict in-hospital and long-term outcome. Long-term follow-up study was obtained in 296 of 298 patients undergoing LV aneurysm repair with or without CABG between 1974 and 1986 (Figure 3-15). No patient had sustained an AMI within 2 weeks of surgery or was undergoing other concurrent cardiac surgery. The average age of the study patients was 57 ± 9 years and the average EF was 35 ± 13%. Ninety percent of the patients underwent concurrent CABG, with an average of 2.2 ± 1.3 grafts placed. Fourteen (5%) patients died in the hospital, with most deaths attributable to LV dysfunction. Advanced age and less extensive revascularization were correlates of in-hospital mortality. The 10-year survival was 57%, AMI-free survival 43%, and freedom from death, AMI and reoperative CABG 41%. Advanced age, systemic hypertension, significant LM coronary artery narrowing and emergent operative status were multivariate correlates of long-term mor-

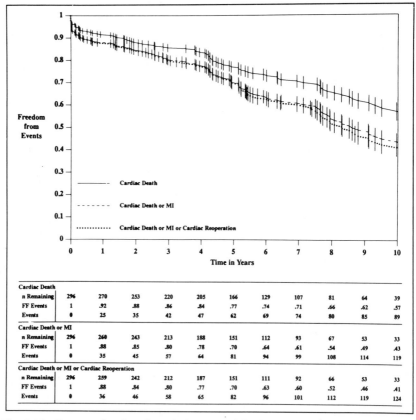

Cardiac Death											
n Remaining	296	270	253	220	205	166	129	107	81	64	39
FF Events	1	.92	.88	.86	.84	.77	.74	.71	.66	.62	.57
Events	0	25	35	42	47	62	69	74	80	85	89
Cardiac Death or MI											
n Remaining	296	260	243	213	188	151	112	93	67	53	33
FF Events	1	.88	.85	.80	.78	.70	.64	.61	.54	.49	.43
Events	0	35	45	57	64	81	94	99	108	114	119
Cardiac Death or MI or Cardiac Reoperation											
n Remaining	296	259	242	212	187	151	111	92	66	53	33
FF Events	1	.88	.84	.80	.77	.70	.63	.60	.52	.46	.41
Events	0	36	46	58	65	82	96	101	112	119	124

Fig. 3-15. Ten-year freedom from (FF) events of death, death or recurrent myocardial infarction (MI), and death, recurrent MI or cardiac reoperation respectively. Vertical bars on lines represent standard error. Reproduced with permission from Baciewicz, et al.[46]

tality. A low-risk population was defined by the absence of these risk factors, and high-risk by the presence of ≥1 risk factors. The 10-year survival was 71% in the low-risk and 41% in the high-risk groups. The 10-year AMI-free survival was 55% in the low-risk and 31% in the high-risk groups. LV aneurysm repair may be performed with acceptable in-hospital mortality, and the long-term risk may be stratified. However, in the absence of controlled studies, uncertainty remains as to the appropriate patients for LV aneurysm repair.

Kulakowski and associates[47] from Warsaw, Poland, performed signal-averaged electrocardiograms and Holter monitors and subsequently followed-up 53 ambulatory patients with LV aneurysms after AMI. Of the 53 patients, 25 (47%) had an abnormal signal-averaged electrocardiogram. The abnormal signal-averaged electrocardiogram correctly identified 9 of 10 cases with a history of sustained VT. Complex ventricular arrhythmias were detected on Holter monitoring in 23 patients: in 5 of 28 (18%) with normal and in 18 of 25 (72%) with abnormal signal-averaged electrocardiograms. During a mean follow-up of 19 months sustained VT and/or cardiac arrest occurred in 8 cases in which 7 had an abnormal signal-averaged electrocardiogram. The authors concluded that an abnormal signal-averaged electrocardiogram identifies those patients after AMI with LV aneurysm who are prone to complex ventricular arrhythmias and that a normal signal-averaged electrocardiogram and an absence of a history of sustained VT strongly indicate that the risk of developing arrhythmic events is low.

Rupture of the ventricular septum

The diagnostic accuracy of Doppler color flow imaging in the diagnosis of postinfarction VSD has not been established. In this study by Fortin and colleagues[48] from Durham, North Carolina, 43 patients with unexplained hypotension or a new murmur in the periinfarct period were evaluated with conventional 2-dimensional echocardiography and Doppler color flow imaging. The presence of a VSD was confirmed by oximetry, ventriculography, operative repair, or autopsy in each case. Both 2-dimensional and Doppler color flow imaging were 100% specific in excluding a VSD. Doppler color flow imaging correctly identified the 12 confirmed VSDs in this study (100% sensitivity), whereas any combination of 2-dimensional criteria only correctly identified 7 (58% sensitive). Doppler color flow imaging is superior to conventional 2-dimensional imaging in the diagnosis of a postinfarction VSD. In addition, Doppler color flow imaging localized the VSD, and thus guided therapy and technique for repair. Carefully performed Doppler color flow examination can exclude or result in the rapid diagnosis of a VSD, which eliminates the need for further time-consuming confirmatory testing.

Cerebrovascular accident

Behar and associates[49] from Tel Hashomer, Israel, reported on the incidence, antecedents, and clinical significance of clinically recognized cerebrovascular accidents (CVA) or transient ischemic attacks (TIA) complicating AMI. During 1981-1983, a secondary prevention study with nifedipine (SPRINT) was conducted in 14 hospitals in Israel among 2,276 survivors of AMI. During the study, demographic, historical, and medical data were collected on special forms for all patients with diagnosed AMI in 13 of these 14 hospitals (the SPRINT registry, n = 5,389). Mortality follow-up was completed for 99% of hospital survivors for a mean follow-up of 5.5 years (range: 4.5 to 7 years). The incidence of CVA-TIA was 0.9% (54 of 5,839). The latter rate increased significantly only with age, from 0.4% among patients up to 59 years old to 1.6% among those aged greater than or equal to 70 years. Multivariate analysis identified age, CAD, and history of stroke as predictors of CVA-TIA during the acute phase of AMI. Patients with CVA-TIA exhibited a complicated hospital course, with a 15-day mortality rate of 41%. Subsequent mortality rates in survivors at 1 and 5 years were 34% and 59%, respectively. Rates at the same time points in patients without CVA-TIA were 16%, 11%, and 29%. In a multivariate analysis that included age, gender, CAD, history of previous AMI, and hypertension, CVA-TIA was independently associated with increased 15-day mortality (covariate-adjusted odds ratio [OR] = 2.62), as well as subsequent 1-year (OR = 3.29) and long-term (mean follow-up = 5.5 years) mortality (OR = 2.46). In this large cohort of consecutive patients with AMI, CVA-TIA was a relatively infrequent complication of AMI. Factors independently favoring the occurrence of CVA-TIA were old age, previous CVA, and CAD. CVA-TIA occurring during AMI independently increased the risk of early death 3-fold as well as the risk of long-term mortality in early-phase survivors.

GENERAL TREATMENT

Beta adrenergic blockade

Curtis and associates[50] from Chapel Hill, North Carolina, studied the effect of propranolol administration on risk assessment based on submaximal exercise testing performed early after AMI. A total of 70 patients with recent AMI underwent modified Bruce treadmill testing with simultaneous measurement of expired gases in the absence of antianginal agents including β-antagonists. Among these, 31 patients who had ≤1 of the following abnormalities—ST depression ≥1 mm (22 patients), chest pain (4 patients), or treadmill time <360 seconds (12 patients)—were studied in a randomized double-blind fashion and received either placebo or 240 mg of propranolol/day. A total of 28 patients completed the randomized phase and were able to undergo repeat exercise testing an average of 3.4 ± 1.8 days later. Randomized groups were equivalent at baseline except for a higher peak oxygen consumption and carbon dioxide production in the propranolol compared with the placebo group; these differences were taken into account in statistical analyses of the study data. Resting heart rate (59 ± 1.2 vs 82 ± 4.2 beats/min) and peak heart rate × systolic BP (14,208 ± 496 vs 20,075 ± 1,062) were both significantly less after propranolol than after placebo. Eight of 9 patients treated with placebo maintained ST depression ≥1 mm from the initial to the randomized exercise test, compared with only 4 of 13 receiving propranolol. In those with continued ST depression, time to positivity was significantly longer in those receiving propranolol compared with those taking placebo (538 ± 73 vs 318 ± 44 seconds). In contrast, the peak ratio between carbon dioxide production and oxygen consumption was higher in those receiving propranolol compared with those receiving placebo (0.93 ± 0.04 vs 0.81 ± 0.03). It was concluded that propranolol therapy reduces evidence of ischemia and changes traditional estimates of potential cardiac risk derived from submaximal postinfarction exercise testing.

Previous studies have shown that long-term survival after AMI is improved by B-adrenergic blockade and anterograde flow in the infarct artery. Glamann and associates[51] from Dallas, Texas, assessed the influence of B blockade on mortality in survivors of AMI without anterograde flow. Over 9.5 years, 113 subjects (87 men and 26 women, aged 26 to 66 years) with AMI and no anterograde flow in the infarct artery and no disease of the other arteries were medically treated for 48 ± 28 (mean ± standard deviation) months. Forty-six patients received long-term B blockade (group I), whereas 67 did not (group II). The groups were similar in age, sex, cardioactive medications, LV performance and infarct artery. Of the 46 group I subjects, 1 (2%) died of cardiac causes; in contrast, 20 (30%) of the group II patients died of cardiac causes. Thus, in survivors of AMI without anterograde flow in the infarct artery, mortality is markedly reduced by long-term B blockade.

Despite extensive investigation, the prognostic significance of the first non-Q wave AMI, when compared with Q wave AMI, remains controversial. The placebo arm of the Beta-Blocker Heart Attack Trial provides a unique opportunity to compare the long-term cardiac events in patients suffering from their first and uncomplicated Q wave or non-Q wave AMI as reported by Gheorghiade and colleagues[52] from Detroit, Michigan. Of a total 3837 patients enrolled in the Beta-Blocker Heart Attack Trial, 3375 were classifiable in terms of appearance or absence of Q waves during the prerandomization period. Of these, 1444 patients with their first AMI were randomized to placebo. Of these, 1186 experienced a Q wave AMI; the remaining 258 suffered a non-Q wave AMI. At 36 months of follow-up, the mortality was 8.4% in the Q wave AMI group and 7.4% in the non-Q wave AMI group. Sudden death was 5.4% in the Q wave AMI group and 4.7% in the non-Q wave AMI group. The reinfarction rate was 5.5% in the Q wave AMI patients and 7.4% in the non-Q wave AMI patients. More patients developed angina (45%) in the non-Q wave AMI group compared with 35% in the Q wave AMI group. Despite similar long-term cardiac event rates within the 2 groups, the 1-year mortality rate for patients with Q wave AMI appeared higher than in the non-Q wave AMI group, 5.2% versus 3.1% respectively. In contrast, the rate of reinfarction appeared higher at the 12-month follow-up period in the non-Q wave AMI group, 4.7% versus 3.4% respectively. Although statistically not different, it appeared that initially the non-Q wave AMI group had a higher reinfarction rate and a lower mortality when compared with the Q wave AMI group. However, over time there was an attenuation of these differences, suggesting a different clinical course for the 2 types of AMI.

Diltiazem

Boden and associates[53] from the Multicenter Diltiazem Post-Infarction Trial Research Group assessed the effect of diltiazem on long-term outcome after AMI in 2,377 patients enrolled in the Multicenter Diltiazem Post-Infarction Trial and subsequently followed for 25 ± 8 months. The study population included 855 patients (36%) with at least 1 prior AMI before the index infarction and 1,522 patients (64%) with a first AMI, of whom 409 (27%) had a first non-Q-wave AMI, 664 (44%) a first inferior Q-wave AMI, and 449 (30%) a first anterior Q-wave AMI. This post hoc analysis revealed that, among patients with first non-Q-wave and first inferior Q-wave AMI, there were fewer cardiac events during follow-up in the diltiazem than in the placebo group, and that the reverse was true for patients with first anterior Q-wave AMI or prior infarction. The diltiazem: placebo Cox hazard ratio (95% confidence limits) for the trial primary end point (cardiac death or nonfatal reinfarction, whichever occurred first) was: first non-Q-wave AMI—0.48 (0.26, 0.89); first inferior Q-wave AMI—0.66 (0.40, 1.09); first anterior Q-wave AMI—0.82 (0.51, 1.21); and prior AMI—1.11 (0.85, 1.44). Use of cardiac death alone as an end point gave an even more sharply focused treatment difference: first non-Q-wave AMI—0.46 (0.18, 1.21); first inferior Q-wave AMI—0.53 (0.27, 1.06); first anterior Q-wave AMI—1.28 (0.68, 2.40); prior infarction—1.26 (0.90, 1.77). Further analysis revealed that these differences in the effect of diltiazem in large part reflected the different status of the 4 electrocardiographically defined subsets in terms of LV function. Mean (± standard deviation) EF for patients with first non-Q-wave AMI (placebo, 0.53 ± 0.13; diltiazem, 0.54 ± 0.12) was comparable to that of patients with a first inferior Q-wave AMI (placebo, 0.52 ± 0.10; diltiazem, 0.52 ± 0.11), and both these first AMI subsets had a lower frequency of radiographic pulmonary congestion range (10 to 16%) during the acute infarction than did patients with first anterior Q-wave or prior AMI. Mean EF for the subset of patients with first anterior Q-wave AMI (placebo, 0.38 ± 0.13; diltiazem, 0.40 ± 0.12) was comparable to that of patients with at least 1 prior AMI (placebo, 0.44 ± 0.15; diltiazem, 0.43 ± 0.14) and the frequency of pulmonary congestion in these 2 infarct subsets ranged from 24 to 26%. The differential effect of diltiazem on postinfarction outcome in these electrocardiographically categorized AMI subsets appears closely linked to the bidirectional effect of diltiazem (beneficial in the majority of patients with well-preserved LV function, harmful in the minority with impaired LV function) that was elucidated in the primary Multicenter Diltiazem Post-Infarction Trial analysis. In patients with multiple infarctions complicated by LV dysfunction, diltiazem appears to be detrimental. Patients with first non-Q-wave or first inferior Q-wave AMI generally have well-preserved LV function and appear to benefit from diltiazem.

Moss and associates[54] of the Multicenter Diltiazem Postinfarction Trial Research Group investigated the effect of diltiazem on long-term outcome in patients with AMI with and without a history of systemic hypertension in 2,466 patients using the Multicenter Diltiazem Postinfarction Trial database. The baseline variables were comparable in the diltiazem and placebo-treated patients within the groups with and without hypertension. The initial 60-mg dose of diltiazem was associated with a significant but modest (3%) reduction in BP and heart rate in both groups with and without hypertension. Univariate and multivariate analyses revealed a meaningful overall reduction in first recurrent cardiac events (cardiac death or nonfatal reinfarction, whichever occurred first) and cardiac death in patients with hypertension treated with diltiazem compared with results in those treated with placebo. Similar effects were not observed in patients without a history of hypertension. When first recurrent cardiac events were used as the end point, the diltiazem: placebo hazard ratio was 0.77 for the total hypertension group, and 0.67 and 1.32 for patients with hypertension with and without pulmonary congestion during the AMI, respectively. Similar results were observed using cardiac death as the end point. Beta blockers had a negligible effect on the hypertension-diltiazem relation. These findings suggest that diltiazem may exert a long-term beneficial effect in most patients with hypertension who do not have pulmonary congestion during an AMI, and a detrimental effect in the minority who have pulmonary congestion.

Digitalis

Mental depression is frequently seen in patients following AMI, many of whom are receiving digitalis glycosides, beta-blockers, or other agents that may exert central nervous system effects. In a prospective study of the clinical significance of post-AMI depression carried out by Schleifer and associates[55] from New York, New York, 335 patients were assessed using a standardized diagnostic interview for depression at 8 to 10 days, and 190 were reinterviewed at 3 to 4 months. Patients prescribed digitalis, beta-blockers, or other cardioactive medications at hospital discharge were identified. Logistic regression analyses were performed to determine the contribution of these agents to depression at 3 to 4 months, controlling for medical and sociodemographic factors as well as for baseline depression. Treatment with digitalis predicted depression at 3 to 4 months; no other medications, including beta-blockers, predicted depression. Digitalis may have central nervous system effects that contribute to depression post-AMI and this finding should be considered in the differential diagnosis of depression in cardiac patients.

Captopril

In a double-blind study, Oldroyd and associates[56] from Glasgow, UK, randomly assigned 99 patients (82 men, age range 40-75 years) with AMI to receive captopril or placebo. Treatment began within 24 hours of admission. Serial echocardiographic measurements of endocardial segment lengths and LV volumes, and EF were obtained. The 2 groups were matched at baseline except for an excess of previous AMI in the placebo group (13 of 50 vs 2 of 49 patients). The increase in anterior segment length, from baseline to 2 months, was significantly less in the captopril than in the placebo group (2.8 ± 1.6 vs 10.4 ± 2.4 mm). The increase in posterior segment length was also less in the captopril group, but the difference was not significant (3.2 ± 1.2 vs 7.0 ± 1.8 mm). Fewer patients in the captopril group demonstrated increases in segment length >2 standard deviations of the measurement error (14 of 70 [20%] vs 29 of 72 [40%] patients). In patients with anterior AMI, the infarct-containing anterior segment length increased by 4.5 ± 2.3 mm in the captopril versus 12.4 ± 3.1 mm in the placebo group, and fewer patients in the captopril group demonstrated infarct expansion (6 of 20 [30%] vs 13 of 21 [62%] patients). In patients with inferoposterior AMI, the infarct-containing posterior segment length increased by 3.1 ± 1.6 mm in the captopril versus 9.8 ± 2.4 mm in the placebo group. No significant treatment effects were seen in LV volumes or maximal exercise performance. This study suggests that early treatment with captopril after AMI can attenuate infarct expansion and favorably influence early LV remodeling.

Heparin

A splendid review of heparin by Hirsch[57] from Hamilton, Canada, appeared in the New England Journal of Medicine May 30, 1991.

Warfarin

Jack Hirsh[58] from Hamilton, Canada, provided a superb summary on oral anticoagulant drugs.

Continuous positive airway pressure

Severe cardiogenic pulmonary edema is a frequent cause of respiratory failure, and many patients with this condition require endotracheal intubation and mechanical ventilation. Bersten and associates[59] from Adelaide, Australia, investigated whether continuous positive airway pressure delivered by means of a face mask had physiologic benefit and would reduce the need for intubation and mechanical ventilation. The authors randomly assigned 39 consecutive patients with respiratory failure due to severe cardiogenic pulmonary edema to receive either oxygen alone or oxygen plus continuous positive airway pressure delivered through a face mask. It was not possible to blind the investigators to the assigned treatment. Physiologic measurements were made over the subsequent 24 hours, and the patients were followed to hospital discharge. After 30 minutes, both respiratory rate and arterial carbon dioxide tension had decreased more in the patients who received oxygen plus continuous positive airway pressure. The mean ($\pm$ SD) respiratory rate at 30 minutes decreased from 32 $\pm$ 6 to 33 $\pm$ 9 breaths per minute in the patients receiving oxygen alone and from 35 $\pm$ 8 to 27 $\pm$ 6 breaths per minute in those receiving oxygen plus continuous positive airway pressure; the arterial carbon dioxide tension decreased from 64 $\pm$ 17 to 62 $\pm$ 14 mm Hg in those receiving oxygen alone and from 58 $\pm$ 8 to 46 $\pm$ 4 mm Hg in those receiving oxygen plus continuous positive airway pressure. The patients receiving continuous positive airway pressure also had a greater increase in the arterial pH (oxygen alone, from 7.15 $\pm$ 0.11 to 7.18 $\pm$ 0.18; oxygen plus continuous positive airway pressure, from 7.18 $\pm$ 0.08 to 7.28 $\pm$ 0.06); and in the ratio of arterial oxygen tension to the fraction of inspired oxygen (oxygen alone, from 136 $\pm$ 44 to 126 $\pm$ 47; oxygen plus continuous positive airway pressure, from 138 $\pm$ 32 to 206 $\pm$ 126). After 24 hours, however, there were no significant differences between the 2 treatment groups in any of these respiratory indexes. Seven (35%) of the patients who received oxygen alone but none who received oxygen plus continuous positive airway pressure required intubation and mechanical ventilation. However, no significant difference was found in in-hospital mortality (oxygen alone, 4 of 20 patients; oxygen plus continuous positive airway pressure, 2 of 19) or the length of the hospital stay. Continuous positive airway pressure delivered by face mask in patients with severe cardiogenic pulmonary edema can result in early physiologic improvement and reduce the need for intubation and mechanical ventilation. This short-term study could not establish whether continuous positive airway pressure has any long-term benefit or whether a larger study would have shown a difference in mortality between the treatment groups.

THROMBOLYSIS

Selection bias

To determine whether clinical selection for thrombolytic therapy for AMI results in a skewed population for subsequent adverse cardiovascular events, Pfeffer and associates[60] from multiple USA medical centers compared clinical features of patients in the survival and ventricular enlargement study who either had or had not received thrombolytic therapy (Figure 3-16). Hospitalized patients with AMI from 112 broadly

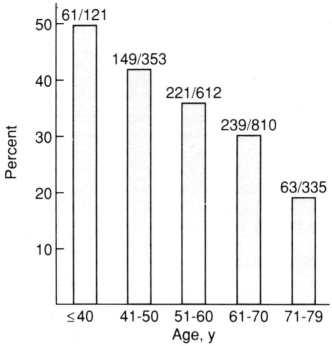

Fig. 3-16. Utilization of thrombolytic therapy during the acute phase of the Survival and Ventricular Enlargement Study qualifying myocardial infarction with respect to age. The influence of age on the use of thrombolytic therapy could not just be attributed to major differences among older patients (≥71 years) since the frequency of thrombolytic use decreased progressively with age, even in the individuals younger than 71 years. Numbers on top of bars indicate actual numbers of patients. Reproduced with permission from Pfeffer, et al.[60]

representative, private, academic, and government hospitals in the USA and Canada were studied. All patients in the survival and ventricular enlargement study had had an AMI less than 16 days earlier and had an LVEF of 40% or less. Thrombolytic therapy was administered to 733 patients and was not given to 1498. The comparisons with respect to use of thrombolytic therapy were formulated after the completion of enrollment and indicated that most patients did not receive thrombolytic therapy. The 1498 (67.1%) patients who did not receive thrombolytic therapy were at higher risk (older age, lower functional capacity, greater likelihood of a history of prior AMI, angina, diabetes, and hypertension) for subsequent cardiovascular events and, as anticipated, were more likely to have concomitant gastrointestinal and neurological diseases. A multiple logistic regression analysis indicated that older age, prior AMI, impaired functional status, employment status, diabetes, and neurological diseases were predictors of use of thrombolytic therapy. Although the Survival and Ventricular Enlargement Study population was selected for LV dysfunction, the majority of patients who currently are judged clinically as unsuitable for thrombolytic therapy have a higher risk for adverse cardiovascular events.

Weaver and associates[61] in Seattle, Washington studied 3,256 consecutive patients hospitalized for AMI to tabulate the history, treatments and outcome of thrombolytic therapy in the elderly. One thousand eight hundred and forty-eight patients (56%) were >65 years of age, including

28% who were ≥75 years of age. The incidence of prior angina, hypertension, and CHF increased with age. Twenty-nine percent of patients <75 years of age were treated with a systemic thrombolytic drug compared with only 5% of patients older than 75 years. Mortality rates increased strikingly with advanced age (Figure 3-17). Both the incidence of complicating illness and nondiagnostic electrocardiogram increased with age. In a multivariate analysis of outcome in older patients ≥65 years, adverse events were related to both prior history of CHF and increasing age (Table 3-2). Outcome was not improved by treatment with thrombolytic drugs, but these agents were prescribed to only 12% of patients >65 years of age. These findings demonstrate that the elderly frequently develop acute AMI in the setting of prior complications from CAD.

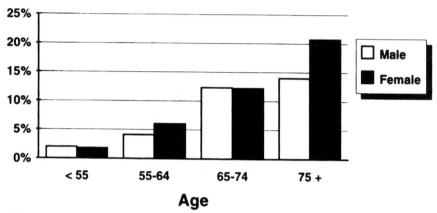

Fig. 3-17. Mortality rates by age for the 3,256 patients with acute myocardial infarction. No patient <47 years of age died during hospitalization, whereas the overall mortality rate in patients ≥75 years was 18%. Gender-specific mortality rates were similar in all but the last stratum. The median age of men and women in the group ≥75 years of age was 80 and 82 years, respectively. Age-adjusted mortality rates for men and women were not significantly different (9.1% and 11.3% respectively). Reproduced with permission from Weaver, et al.[61]

TABLE 3-3. *Clinical event rates (%) by age strata in the subset of patients treated by thrombolytic therapy or emergency angiography, or both, within 12 hours of admission. Reproduced with permission from Weaver, et al.[61]*

	Age (years)				
	<55	55–64	65–74	≥75	All
Mortality					
Treatment	2.5	4.6	11.7	11.5	6.5
No treatment	1.5	4.6	12.5	18.4	11.6
Stroke					
Treatment	1.2	1.3	1.8	5.1	1.7
No treatment	1.5	1.1	2	3.8	2.4
CHF					
Treatment	18	25	31	37	25
No treatment	12	23	31	30	26
Mortality, CHF or stroke					
Treatment	19	23	37	46	29
No treatment	13	26	38	42	34

CHF = congestive heart failure.

Use in Israel

Thrombolysis is now generally accepted as the initial treatment for patients with AMI. The extent to which this therapy is implemented in daily practice and the reasons for exclusion from thrombolytic therapy among 413 consecutive patients with AMI hospitalized in 18 coronary care units in Israel during a 1-month survey were prospectively investigated by Behar and associates[62] from Tel Hashomer, Israel. Thrombolytic therapy administered to 145 patients (35%) was given to 38% of men versus 29% of women, to 38% of patients <75 years old compared with18% of the very elderly, and more often to patients with a first or anterior AMI (40 and 48%) than to counterparts with recurrent or inferior AMI (23 and 31% respectively). The 2 most frequent reasons for excluding patients from thrombolysis were late arrivals to coronary care units (33%) and lack of ST elevation on the admission electrocardiogram (28%). Hospital mortality was 6% in the thrombolytic group versus 20% in patients found ineligible for thrombolysis. The significance of this difference is not clear as treatment was not randomized.

After cardiopulmonary resuscitation

Cardiopulmonary resuscitation (CPR) is often considered a contraindication to thrombolytic therapy for AMI. Tenaglia and associates[63] from 3 USA medical centers analyzed 708 patients involved in the first 3 Thrombolysis and Angioplasty in Myocardial Infarction trials of lytic therapy for AMI and found that 59 patients required <10 minutes of CPR before receiving lytic therapy (CPR >10 minutes was an exclusion of the trials) or required CPR within 6 hours of treatment. The patients receiving CPR were similar to the remainder of the group with respect to baseline demographics. The indication for CPR was usually VF (73%) or VT (24%). The median duration of CPR was 1 minute, with twenty-fifth and seventy-fifth percentiles of 1 and 5 minutes, respectively. The median number of cardioversions/defibrillations performed was 2 (twenty-fifth and seventy-fifth percentiles of 1 and 3 minutes, respectively). Patients receiving CPR were more likely to have anterior infarctions (66 vs 39%), the left anterior descending artery as the infarct-related artery (63 vs 38%) and lower EFs on the initial ventriculogram (46 $\pm$ 11 vs 52 $\pm$ 12%) than those not receiving CPR. In-hospital mortality was 12 vs 6% with most deaths due to pump failure (57%) or arrhythmia (29%) in the CPR group and pump failure (38%) or reinfarction (25%) in the non-CPR group. At 7 day follow-up the CPR group had a significant increase in EF (+5 $\pm$ 9%) compared with no change in non-CPR group. There were no bleeding complications directly attributed to CPR. In particular, the decrease in hematocrit (median 11) and need for transfusion (37 vs 32%) were the same in both groups. In addition, the CPR group did not spend more days in the cardiac care unit or in hospital than the non-CPR group. In conclusion, patients who have received CPR for 10 minutes had no additional complications attributable to thrombolytic therapy. Therefore, CPR, especially of short duration, should not be considered a contraindication to lytic treatment. In addition, the authors' results suggest that patients requiring CPR during AMI constitute a high-risk subgroup which may particularly benefit from receiving thrombolytic therapy.

ST segment early afterwards

To investigate the incidence of early recurrent ST elevation after intravenous thrombolytic therapy for AMI, Kwon and associates[64] from Sydney, Australia, monitored continuously 12-lead electrocardiograms for 571 ± 326 minutes in 31 patients presenting within 4 hours of symptom onset. The study group comprised 9 women and 22 men (mean age $\pm$ standard deviation 53 ± 12 years), with ST elevation (anterior in 15, inferior in 16) on the initial electrocardiogram, who were given either tissue plasminogen activator (22 patients) or streptokinase (9 patients). Angiography was performed in 30 of 31 patients at 7 to 10 days. Early (<3 hours) resolution of ST elevation occurred in 19 patients (62%) at a median of 94 minutes (interquartile range 57 to 113) after thrombolysis, whereas 12 (39%) had no or late (>6 hours) resolution. Eleven of the 19 with early resolution (58%) had either transient (5 patients) or sustained (6 patients) recurrences of ST elevation. Recurrent ST elevation was equal to or more than the initial peak elevation in 9 of 11 patients, and 75% of initial peak in 2. A total of 25 episodes of recurrent ST elevation were observed in the 11 patients (19 transient and 6 sustained episodes), of which 8 (32%) were silent. The proportion of silent episodes was similar for transient (35%) and sustained (33%) recurrences. All patients with sustained recurrent ST elevation had at least 1 preceding transient recurrence. The median duration of transient recurrent ST elevation was 43 minutes (28 to 63). The median time from initiating thrombolysis to the first transient recurrence was 151 minutes (40 to 192), and 328 minutes (120 to 704) to sustained recurrence. Recurrent ST elevation was associated with a delay in time to peak creatine kinase, and sustained recurrent ST elevation was associated with reduced arterial patency and worse residual stenosis at 7- to 10- day angiography. Recurrent ST elevation occurred in 10 of 15 patients with early ST resolution given tissue plasminogen activator despite conventional heparin therapy administered to 9. Transient recurrent ST elevation after ST resolution from thrombolysis is common, may be silent or prolonged, and may presage sustained recurrent ST elevation. This marked lability of ST segments probably represents recurrent coronary occlusion.

Reperfusion therapy has lowered the mortality in patients suffering AMI. Failure to reperfuse is associated with significantly higher risk of short- and long-term mortality. Detection of reperfusion is thus important. In a prospective study, Dellborg and associates[65] from Göteborg, Sweden, and Ann Arbor, Michigan, used continuous on-line computerized vectorcardiography to monitor 21 patients with AMI treated with reperfusion therapy to noninvasively detect coronary patency. By using trend analysis of QRS vector difference, they were able to correctly blindly identify 15 of 16 patients with a perfused infarct-related artery and 4 of 6 patients with a persistently occluded artery at an early angiogram. The present results suggest that QRS complex and ST segment monitoring with continuous on-line vectorcardiography has substantial potential for monitoring patients with AMI treated with reperfusion therapy.

With the increasing use of thrombolytic therapy, the presence and time course of reperfusion-induced ventricular arrhythmias and ST-segment changes have become of interest. Technical improvements in bipolar Holter monitoring offer the opportunity to record both parameters continuously and simultaneously. Zehender and associates[66] from Hamburg, Federal Republic of Germany, investigated time course and interaction of both parameters independence on the onset of thrombolysis and time of reperfusion in 30 patients with AMI. Reperfusion was achieved in 20 patients after 49 ± 23 minutes and in another 2 patients after 120 minutes (73%, group A). Vascular occlusion persisted in 8 patients for 24 hours (group B). Sudden ST-segment changes (>0.2 mV/15 min) in the bipolar leads indicated reperfusion in 7 of 22 patients (32%). Idioventricular rhythms, most frequent in reperfused patients (group A: 18 of 22 patients, mean 121 beats/hour), were unspecific reperfusion markers (group B: 5 of 8 patients, 1 beat/hour) unless frequent or longer lasting, repetitive episodes were considered. VPCs and couplets were also most frequent in group A (peak frequency 3 to 5 hours after thrombolysis). VT observed in 21 of 22 patients (95%) in group A and in 3 of 8 (38%) in group B attained their peak frequency 7 to 9 hours after thrombolysis. They occurred most often in anterior AMI and were often preceded by frequent singular premature beats. In summary, (1) sudden ST-segment changes in the bipolar leads rarely but reliably predict the time of reperfusion (2) VTs are most likely late after thrombolysis and thus make prolonged corresponding supervision advisable, and (3) the frequency rather than the type of ventricular arrhythmia is useful to noninvasively predict coronary reperfusion.

Effects on left ventricular function

White and associates[67] from Auckland, New Zealand, examined the effect of age on LV function, assessed by contrast ventriculography 3 weeks after a first AMI, in 312 patients who received thrombolytic therapy within 4 hours of the onset of AMI and in 83 patients who received placebo. Streptokinase was given to 188 patients and recombinant tissue-type plasminogen activator (rt-PA) to 124. Patients were divided into 2 age groups: <60 years (n = 244) and ≥60 years (n = 151). Thrombolytic therapy improved EF in both age groups: from 54 ± 13 to 59 ± 11% in the younger group and from 50 ± 14 to 57 ± 13% in the older group. EF was identical in streptokinase- and rt-PA-treated patients. Multifactor analysis of variance revealed that younger age and thrombolytic therapy were independently associated with improved EF. Thrombolytic therapy also reduced end-systolic volume by 14 ml in the elderly and 9 ml in the younger group. Minor bleeding complications were more frequent in the elderly and 3 serious hemorrhages occurred in patients ≥60 years. These findings reveal that thrombolysis improves LV function in all age groups studied. Because increasing age is independently associated with a lower EF after AMI, thrombolytic therapy may confer greater benefits in older patients.

Effect on estimating infarct size

To assess the ability of the 12-lead electrocardiogram to estimate infarct size after reperfusion therapy during AMI, Christian and associates[68] from Rochester, Minnesota, compared the presence or absence of Q-waves and the Sylvester QRS score before and after hospital discharge with radionuclide estimates of infarct size and EF at discharge and 6 weeks later. Regional wall motion at discharge and 6 weeks later and myocardial perfusion defect size were quantitated with Tc-99m-sestamibi. A consecutive series of 43 patients with AMI who received reperfusion therapy and were assessed using 12-lead electrocardiography, radionuclide angiography, and Tc-99m-sestamibi tomographic imaging before discharge. All 43 patients received acute reperfusion therapy; 21

patients received intravenous rt-PA, and 22 patients underwent primary PTCA. The correlation of QRS score and Q waves with 3 radionuclide estimated infarction size. A significant correlation was found between myocardial perfusion defect size at discharge and both LVEF and regional wall motion at discharge and 6 weeks later. Little correlation was found between electrocardiographic findings and radionuclide measurements of LV function and perfusion. Presence or absence of Q waves at discharge was not associated with any difference in EF, regional wall motion, or perfusion defect at discharge. No correlation was found between QRS score and EF or myocardial perfusion defect size at discharge. The QRS score at discharge correlated only weakly with regional wall motion at discharge and 6 weeks later. This lack of correlation was unchanged when electrocardiograms obtained after hospital discharge were analyzed. Although inexpensive and readily available, the 12-lead electrocardiogram does not appear to provide a reliable estimate of infarction size after reperfusion therapy for AMI.

Detecting jeopardized myocardium afterwards

Bolognese and co-workers[69] in Novara, Italy assessed whether dipyridamole echocardiography test could detect jeopardized myocardium after thrombolytic therapy. Seventy-six consecutive patients with a first acute AMI were treated with urokinase within 4 hours of the onset of AMI and underwent high-dose dipyridamole echocardiography 8-10 days after AMI. The results were correlated to the anatomy of the infarct-related vessel. In patients with positive echocardiography, the investigators evaluated the wall motion score index. Wall motion score was derived by summation of individual segment scores divided by the number of interpreted segments. In a 13-segment model, each segment was assigned a score ranging from 1 to 4. Fifty-three patients had positive results on echocardiography. Of these, 42 had dipyridamole-induced new wall motion abnormalities confined to the infarct zone or adjacent segments. Coronary angiography showed a patent infarct related vessel in 53 patients and no or minimal reperfusion in 23 patients. A patent infarct related vessel with critical residual stenosis was found in 35 of 42 patients with dipyridamole-induced wall motion abnormalities in the infarct zone and in 18 of 34 patients without wall motion abnormalities. Among the 23 patients with occluded infarct related vessels, 9 had collateral flow to the distal vessel; 6 of these had a positive dipyridamole echocardiography test. Thus, the sensitivity and specificity for identifying a critically stenotic but patent infarct related vessel or the presence of a collateral-dependent zone were 66% and 93%, respectively. In a subset of 9 patients with a positive echocardiography study in the infarct zone or adjacent segments, dipyridamole echocardiography and a control coronary angiography were repeated 1–3 months after an angiographically successful PTCA in the infarct related vessel. The repeat dipyridamole study was negative in 8 patients and again positive in one patient, who showed restenosis at angiography. Thus, dipyridamole echocardiography can identify the anatomy of the infarct related vessel, and dipyridamole-induced wall motion abnormalities within the infarct zone detect regions with jeopardized myocardium that may benefit from intervention.

Interpreting exercise studies afterwards

Numerous studies have assessed the ability of exercise modalities to predict patient outcome after AMI. Implicit in the use of these prior data to assess the prognosis of patients currently undergoing exercise studies is the assumption that patients selected for exercise assessment are similar over time and that the data generated in the past are therefore applicable to the current patient populations. Lavie and associates[70] from Rochester, Minnesota, assessed retrospectively the clinical, exercise, and rest and exercise radionuclide angiographic data in 791 consecutive patients referred for exercise radionuclide angiography within 1-month of an AMI to determine if the clinical and exercise characteristics of patients referred for exercise evaluation after AMI have changed significantly over time. Most parameters examined demonstrated significant increasing trends, including thrombolytic therapy at the time of AMI, revascularization procedure between AMI and exercise assessment, age, B-blocker usage, Q-wave AMI, inferior infarction, exercise double product, exercise capacity, significant ST-segment depression with exercise, peak EF, and change in EF with exercise. These data indicate that the characteristics of patients selected to undergo exercise after AMI in a large referral center have changed significantly over time. If these data are applicable to other referral centers and to other exercise testing modalities, previously published results regarding exercise assessment after AMI will need to be reconfirmed in patients currently selected for testing, since these results may no longer be applicable in this current era of aggressive medical and interventional management.

After thrombolytic therapy for AMI, increasing emphasis is placed on early submaximal exercise testing, with further intervention advocated only for demonstrable ischemia. Although significant residual coronary artery lesions after successful thrombolysis are common, many patients paradoxically have no corresponding provokable ischemia. Sutton and Topol[71] in Ann Arbor, Michigan studied the relation between significant postthrombolytic residual CAD and a negative early, submaximal exercise thallium-201 tomogram among 101 consecutive patients with uncomplicated AMI and at least 70% residual stenosis of the infarct artery. A negative test occurred in 49 patients with a mean 88% residual infarct artery stenosis. Further characteristics of the group were as follows: mean time treatment was 3.1 hours; mean age was 54 years; 80% male, 47% had anterior AMI; 39% had multivessel disease; mean LVEF was 53%; and mean peak creatine kinase level was 3,820 IU/ml. A similar group of 52 patients, treated within 3.3 hours from symptom onset, with a mean postthrombolysis stenosis of 90%, had a positive exercise test. Characteristics of this group were as follows: age was 58 years; 92% were male; 56% had anterior AMI; 40% had multivessel disease; and mean LVEF was 54%. The peak creatine kinase level associated with the infarction, however, was lower: 2,605 IU/ml. There was no difference in performance at exercise testing with respect to peak systolic pressure, peak heart rate, or time tolerated on the treadmill between the two groups. By multivariate logistic regression, only peak creatine kinase level predicted a negative stress result in the presence of a significant residual stenosis (Figure 3-18). The explanation for the relatively frequent finding of a negative early stress thallium tomogram after apparently successful reperfusion appears to be more extensive myocardial necrosis and not delay in therapy or inadequate exercise performance.

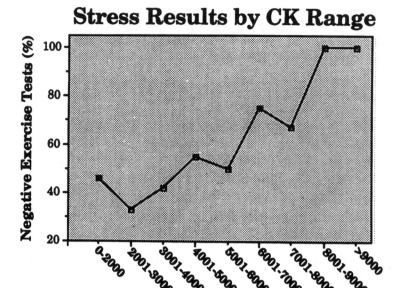

Fig. 3-18. Plot of direct relation between creatine kinase (CK) range and a negative sub-maximal exercise thallium-201 tomogram. Patients were assigned to one of nine categorical ranges for statistical analysis, and only peak CK level (IU/ml) proved to be a significant predictor of a negative exercise test result by logistic regression analysis. Percentages of myocardial infarction patients from each peak CK range who had a negative submaximal stress result are plotted, demonstrating a direct relation. Reproduced with permission from Sutton, et al.[71]

Effect on late potentials on signal-averaged electrocardiogram

Vatterott and colleagues[72] in Rochester, Minnesota evaluated the relation between patency of the infarct-related artery and the presence of late potentials on the signal-averaged ECG in 124 consecutive patients with AMI receiving thrombolytic therapy, PTCA, or standard care. All patients were studied by coronary angiography, measurement of LVEF, and signal-averaged ECG. The infarct-related artery was closed in 51 patients and open in 73. Among patients with no prior AMI undergoing early attempted reperfusion therapy, a patent artery was associated with a decreased incidence of late potentials (20% vs 71% without any difference in LVEF) (Figure 3-19). In the 48 patients receiving thrombolytic agents within 4 hours of symptoms, the incidence of late potentials was 24% and 83% among patients with an open or closed artery, respectively. The best predictors of late potentials were the presence of a closed infarct-related artery, followed by prior AMI and patient age. Among patients receiving thrombolytic agents within 4 hours of symptom onset, the only variable predictive of the presence of late potentials was a closed infarct-related artery. These data demonstrate that reperfusion of an infarct-related artery has a beneficial effect on the electrophysiologic substrate for serious ventricular arrhythmias independent of change in LVEF.

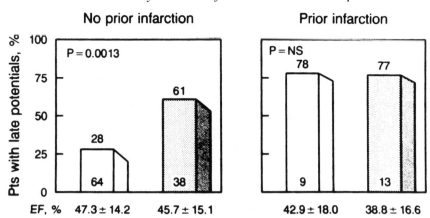

Fig. 3-19. Incidence of late potentials on the signal-averaged electrocardiogram by patency of the infarct-related artery and the presence (right) or absence (left) of prior infarction. Open bar indicates an open infarct-related artery; stippled bar indicates a closed infarct-related artery. Ejection fraction (EF) data are shown as mean values ± standard deviation. Numbers within the bars indicate the number of patients (Pts). Reproduced with permission from Vatterott, et al.[72]

Predicting coronary patency afterwards

Hohnloser and colleagues[73] in Freiburg, Germany, evaluated the predictability of patency of the infarct-related artery assessed by 3 means in 82 patients undergoing thrombolysis for their first AMI. Positive noninvasive markers were defined as follows: 1) early peak creatine kinase activity ≤12 hours after the start of thrombolysis; 2) ≥50% reduction in ST segment elevation; and 3) development of reperfusion arrhythmias within the first 90 minutes of thrombolytic therapy. In 63 (77%) of the 82 patients, Thrombolysis in Myocardial Infarction (TIMI) grade II/III reperfusion was achieved within the first 90 minutes as assessed by coronary angiography. Separate analysis of each marker revealed the following respective values for sensitivity, specificity and positive and negative predictive value regarding prediction of coronary artery patency: creatine kinase ≤12 hours: 84%, 95%, 98% and 64%; reduction of the ST segment elevation ≥50%: 60%, 95%, 97% and 42%; and reperfusion arrhythmias: 63%, 89%, 95%, and 43%. The combined analysis of all three markers utilizing a logistic regression procedure showed that the peak creatine kinase and resolution of the ST segment elevation, but not the development of reperfusion arrhythmias were independent predictors of vessel patency. From this regression procedure, a sensitivity of 100%, specificity of 90%, positive predictive value of 97%, and a negative predictive value of 100% for the prediction of coronary artery patency were obtained. Therefore, the combined analysis of 3 noninvasive markers permits accurate prediction of coronary artery patency in patients with AMI undergoing thrombolytic therapy.

Frequency and significance of minimal coronary narrowing afterwards

Kereiakes and associates[74] in the Thrombolysis and Angioplasty in Myocardial Infarction (TAMI) Study Group evaluated the incidence of minimal residual atherosclerotic coronary obstruction after successful intravenous thrombolytic therapy in 799 patients with AMI. Minimal residual coronary obstruction ($\leq$50%) was observed on selective coronary angiography performed 90 minutes after initiation of therapy in 43 patients (5.5%). In 42 other patients, a >50% but <100% residual stenosis was noted at 90 minutes and demonstrated further resolution of obstruction to <50% at an angiographic follow-up study 7 to 10 days later. Patients with minimal residual coronary obstruction were younger and had less multivessel coronary disease associated with better LVEF's and a lower in-hospital mortality rate than did patients who had a significant residual coronary obstruction after intravenous thrombolysis. Long-term follow-up of patients with a minimal coronary lesion averaging 1.5 $\pm$ 0.6 years and those with significant residual stenoses demonstrated that the incidence of death and recurrent AMI were similar in both groups. Thus, new strategies are needed to prevent coronary rethrombosis in patients with minimal atherosclerosis after thrombolytic therapy for AMI.

Determinants of need for early cardiac catheterization or hospital discharge afterwards

Muller and associates[75] in the TAMI-5 Study Group determined whether clinical variables may be used to identify patients at high risk of recurrent spontaneous myocardial ischemia or hemodynamic compromise during the first four days after intravenous thrombolysis for AMI. Among 288 patients randomly assigned to a conservative postthrombolysis strategy, 54 (19%) required urgent cardiac catheterization within 24 hours. Seventy-five (26%) underwent urgent cardiac catheterization within 4 days of admission. Among the clinical variables examined by multiple logistic regression analysis, only patient age and anterior AMI correlated with the need for urgent cardiac catheterization. Combined with recombinant tissue-type plasminogen activator or urokinase monotherapy, combination therapy with these agents is associated with a lower need for acute intervention during the first 24 hours after admission, but the difference did not reach statistical significance. Among 75 patients undergoing urgent coronary angiography, 39% had an occluded infarct-related artery. Emergent PTCA was performed in 49% of the patients and CABG was performed urgently in 3%. The need for urgent cardiac catheterization was associated with an in-hospital mortality rate of 7%, as compared to 3% in the group not requiring urgent angiography. These data suggest that a large proportion of patients treated conservatively after thrombolytic therapy require early triage to urgent coronary angiography. Baseline clinical characteristics are not good predictors of the need for urgent intervention and despite access to facilities for aggressive intervention, the in-hospital clinical outcome of this group of patients is not as good as that of patients without recurrent ischemia or hemodynamic instability.

Very early day-4 hospital discharge has recently been proposed for selected patients with AMI. Mark and co-workers[76] in Durham, North Carolina proposed a study to determine the most useful factors for identifying AMI patients treated with aggressive interventional therapy who could be safely discharged on day 4. They studied 708 patients enrolled in the Thrombolysis and Angioplasty in Acute Myocardial Infarction trials I-III. Patients dying in the first 3 days and those with early (days 1-3) emergency CABG, late elective CABG ($\geq$day 4), or urgent/emergency CABG resulting from a elective PTCA were excluded. The remaining 580 patients were randomly divided into a training sample (group 1) that was used to build a logistic regression model for predicting the absence of a late major complication and a test sample (group 2) that was used to validate this model. For this study, patients were considered appropriate for day 4 hospital discharge if they did not experience any of the following for 30 days after AMI: death, reinfarction, cardiogenic shock, pulmonary edema, sustained hypotension, sustained VT, high-grade AV block, acute VSD, and recurrent ischemia necessitating urgent CABG. In group 1, 4 variables were independent predictors of freedom from late major complications: absence of early sustained VT or VF, absence of early sustained hypotension or cardiogenic shock, fewer coronary arteries with significant ($\geq$75%) stenosis, and a higher LVEF. In group 2, 23% of patients had a logistic model prediction of a 3% or less chance of a late complication. These patients had no death or reinfarctions by day 30 and 3% late major complication rate. The results of early cardiac catheterization and the absence of selected early major complications do allow identification of a low-risk subgroup of AMI patients that may be suitable for early discharge.

Effect on short-term prognosis

Results of recent studies have suggested that routine cardiac catheterization may be unnecessary after reperfusion therapy for AMI. Therefore to better define the short-term prognostic value of early coronary angiography, and specifically the prognostic significance of multivessel CAD, the angiographic findings of 855 patients consecutively enrolled in 5 phases of the Thrombolysis and Angioplasty in Myocardial Infarction study were correlated with their in-hospital outcome[77]. All patients received intravenous thrombolytic therapy (tissue plasminogen activator, urokinase, or both agents) and underwent cardiac catheterization within 90 minutes of the initiation of therapy. Multivessel disease, defined as the presence of $\geq$75% luminal diameter stenosis in $\geq$2 major epicardial arteries, was documented in 236 patients. When compared with the group of patients without multivessel disease, this group had a higher prevalence of coronary risk factors and more frequently had a history of antecedent ischemic chest pain. Although the severity of the infarct zone dysfunction was similar in the 2 groups, global LVEF was lower in the group with multivessel disease (49 $\pm$ 12% vs 52 $\pm$ 11%). This was associated with a significant difference in the function of the noninfarct zone. Whereas this region was hyperkinetic in the group with minimal or single-vessel disease, it was hypocontractile or dyskinetic in those with multivessel disease. The in-hospital mortality rate, predominantly the result of myocardial failure and cardiogenic shock, was also significantly higher in the multivessel group (11% vs 4%). By means of data from the 708 patients enrolled in the first 3 Thrombolysis and Angioplasty in Myocardial Infarction studies, a statistical model was developed to describe the determinants of in-hospital survival. By logistic regression analysis the strongest independent predictor of in-hospital mortality was the number of diseased arteries. Other parameters that contributed significantly included global LVEF, grade of infarct vessel flow, and patient age. According to this model the prognostic significance of 1 additional year of age was equivalent to a reduction in LV function of 1.1 EF percentage points; 1 additional diseased vessel was equivalent to 15 additional years of age or a reduction in EF of 16 percentage points. These data suggest that more aggressive revascularization procedures should be considered in the early postinfarction period for patients with multivessel disease and noninfarct zone dysfunction. In the absence of reliable noninvasive techniques, coronary angiography remains the procedure of choice for identifying this high-risk subgroup.

Streptokinase

Sheehan and associates[78] from Seattle, Washington, investigated the effect of intravenous streptokinase therapy on the time course of functional recovery in a controlled study of 64 patients randomized within 3 hours after the onset of AMI. Contrast ventriculography was performed 1 to 4 days after AMI and repeated 5 weeks later. Wall motion was analyzed by the centerline method in the central infarct, peripheral infarct and noninfarct regions. In patients with ventriculographic data at the early catheterization, streptokinase-treated patients had less severe hypokinesia in the central infarct region than control patients (-2.9 ± 0.9 [n = 29] vs -3.4 ± 0.7 standard deviations below normal [n = 21]). The benefit of streptokinase was more marked in the peripheral infarct region (-1.5 ± 0.7 vs -2.1 ± 0.6). As a result, the EF was slightly higher in treated versus control groups (46 ± 10 vs $43 \pm 7\%$, respectively). At 5 weeks, function in the streptokinase and control groups had diverged further because of continued improvement in the streptokinase-treated patients. This study shows that streptokinase benefits LV function by 1 to 4 days after AMI, earlier than previously reported. The benefit was not limited to the peripheral infarct region, where ischemia might have been less severe, but was also seen in the central infarct region. The implication is that thrombolytic therapy can improve LV function during the period of myocardial stunning, while myocardial function is still recovering.

Plasmin is capable of degrading extracellular matrix components such as collagen in vitro. To evaluate the significance of this for in vivo conditions, Peuhkurinen and co-investigators[79] in Oulu, Finland set out to study the effect of streptokinase, which acts by converting plasminogen to plasmin, on the serum concentrations of the amino-terminal propeptide of type II procollagen and the carboxy-terminal propeptide of type I procollagen. Twenty-three patients with suspected AMI were included in the study. Seventeen of them received thrombolytic therapy, and six were treated conservatively. Type III and Type I procollagen were assayed with radioimmunoassay. Kinetics of creatine kinase-MB release were determined to differentiate reperfusers from nonreperfusers. Composite curves of creatine kinase-MB release were constructed for different patient subgroups. During streptokinase infusion the serum concentrations of type III procollagen increased rapidly, with a maximum mean increase of 50% in 45 minutes. A similar increase was also observed in two patients who received thrombolytic therapy but did not subsequently develop any AMI determined on the basis of enzyme release. The relative increase in type III procollagen during streptokinase treatment was higher in those AMI patients with probable reperfusion than those with nonprobable reperfusion. Corresponding changes in type III procollagen were not seen in the control group. Two days later there was a second increase in serum type II procollagen for both patients groups. This change coincided with a similar increase in type I procollagen. The investigators concluded that streptokinase, probably by activation of plasminogen to plasmin, stimulates the breakdown of type III collagen during thrombolytic therapy. This phenomenon may decrease the risk of rethrombosis of the affected artery if the exposed collagen is responsible for thrombosis formation, but it could also be involved in the development of hemorrhagic complications during thrombolytic therapy. The second increase in type III procollagen levels probably indicates type III collagen synthesis of the infarcted area.

In a historical follow-up study of 152 hospital patients with AMI, Nielsen and associates[80] from Aalborg, Denmark, compared the frequency of life-threatening arrhythmias (VF, sustained VT, 3rd degree AV-block, 2nd degree AV-block [Mobitz type II], and asystole) and AF in 76 patients treated with streptokinase compared with their frequency in 76 patients who did not receive thrombolytic therapy. Among those treated with streptokinase 2 patients (3%) developed AF, compared with 12 (16%) in the control group. Life-threatening arrhythmias occurred with equal frequency in the 2 groups. Further studies should confirm and clarify the mechanism of the reduced frequency of AF in the streptokinase-treated patients.

In a study carried out by Grip and Ryden[81] from Stockholm, Sweden, of 255 consecutive patients with AMI, 111 were eligible for attempted late thrombolysis. They were randomly assigned to either thrombolytic and antithrombotic treatment (treatment group) or routine treatment (control group). Patients in the treatment group received streptokinase initiated late (mean 32 hours; range 12 to 49) after the onset of symptoms, followed by heparin infusion for at least 5 days and warfarin and dipyridamole for at least 3 months. Patients were examined clinically and by bicycle ergometry on discharge from the hospital and after 3 and 12 months. The 2 groups did not differ with respect to deaths or reinfarctions. There was a trend toward a lower incidence of angina pectoris in the treatment group. Exercise tolerance in this group was significantly higher than in the control group (at 3 months 124 ± 39 W vs 107 ± 41 W). The difference was entirely accounted for by patients with no previous history of infarction or angina pectoris (at 3 months 142 ± 37 W vs 112 ± 45 W). Electrocardiographic signs of myocardial ischemia, silent or symptomatic, occurred at significantly lower levels of exercise among patients in the control group compared with patients in the treatment group. The results support the notion that thrombolytic therapy given as late as 12 to 49 hours after the onset of symptoms may reduce the incidence of residual ischemia during the postinfarction period.

Davies and colleagues[82] in London, UK, analyzed coronary lesion morphology from angiograms in 72 consecutive patients at 1 to 8 days after streptokinase therapy for AMI in relation to subsequent clinical course. All patients were clinically stable at the time of angiography and continued to receive heparin for $\geq$4 days after thrombolysis. The infarct-related artery was patent in 55 patients (76%). In the ten days after angiography, 15 patients developed prolonged episodes of angina at rest; the condition of 4 stabilized with medical therapy, but 11 required urgent medical intervention, including PTCA in 8 and CABG in 3. There were no differences in age, gender, LV function or extent of CAD between those patients who developed unstable angina and those who remained stable. However, the median plaque ulceration index of the infarct-related lesion was 6.7% in the 15 patients with an unstable course versus 3.3% in those with a stable course (Figure 3-20). These data demonstrate that after thrombolysis, the degree of irregularity of the infarct-related artery is a critical determinant of early clinical instability. Among 19 patients with a plaque ulceration index >6, 11 (58%) subsequently demonstrated clinical instability compared with only 4 (8%) of the 53 patients with an ulceration

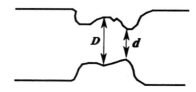

$$U.I. = \frac{\text{maximal intralesional diameter } \; D}{\text{minimal adjacent intralesional diameter } \; d}$$

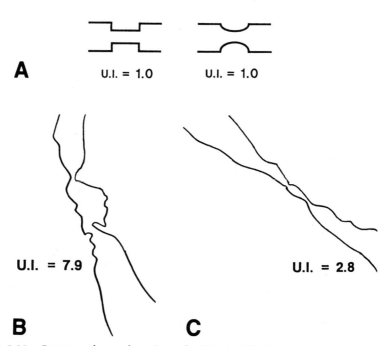

Fig. 3-20. Coronary plaque ulceration index (UI). A, Definition and measurement of the plaque ulceration index. B, Example of a lesion with a high ulceration index. C, Example of a lesion with a low ulceration index. Reproduced with permission from Davies, et al.[82]

index <6. Therefore, quantitative analysis of coronary lesion morphology defines a high risk subset of patients in whom intensive medical therapy or elective intervention may be indicated.

Voth and colleagues[83] in Gottingen, Germany, evaluated LV function up to 3 years after AMI in patients receiving intravenous streptokinase as a thrombolytic intervention. The intravenous streptokinase in Acute Myocardial Infarction trial (I.S.A.M) was a prospective, placebo-controlled, double-blind multicenter trial of high-dose short-term intravenous streptokinase in patients with AMI admitted within 6 hours of symptom onset. Global and regional LVEFs were determined by RNA in a subset of 120 patients 3 days, 4 weeks, 7 months, 18 months, and 3 years after AMI. In patients with anterior AMI, LVEF was higher in the streptokinase than in the placebo treated group 3 days after AMI (49 ± 14% vs 40 ± 11%). This difference of 9 EF units persisted during the 3 year follow-up period.

Among streptokinase-treated patients, regional LVEF was higher within the infarct zone as well as in remote myocardium throughout the follow-up period. Among patients with inferior AMI, no significant differences between the treatment and control groups were demonstrable. Thus, intravenous streptokinase within 6 hours of symptom onset after anterior AMI preserves LV function over a period up to 3 years.

Streptokinase vs recombinant tissue type plasminogen activator

Sherry and Marder[84] from Philadelphia, Pennsylvania, and Rochester, New York, reviewed recent trials in which they concluded that patients with AMI who received either recombinant tissue type plasminogen activator (rt-PA) or streptokinase showed essentially no difference in the amount of myocardial salvage, in mortality reduction, or in the incidence of bleeding complications. These findings thus failed to fulfill the expectation that rt-PA would be twice as effective as streptokinase as a thrombolytic agent. The basis for this mistaken prediction was an unfortunate overemphasis on an inadequate surrogate endpoint, namely, the patency or reperfusion rate at 90 minutes after the start of therapy. Using the 90-minute patency or reperfusion rate as an endpoint has several serious limitations. First, it is an observation made at only 1 point in time during a dynamic process that may change even during the infusion proper. Second, a single view at 90 minutes completely disregards the possibility of subsequent reocclusion which often occurs within 1 hour after treatment. Third, an image at 90 minutes is more a reflection of the speed of thrombolysis than of whether lysis will eventually occur; the pace of clot lysis depends on both the agent used and the age of the thrombus. Fourth, lysis at 90 minutes is of minimal relevance for myocardial salvage unless observed within the time frame when infarction size can be limited significantly, which is generally less than 4 hours between symptom onset and the time that reperfusion is accomplished. Fifth, a stable state of vessel patency is meaningful for mortality reduction even if stabilization occurs after completion of the infarction. Such "late," but lasting, patency is a critical component of the "open vessel" principle and explains, at least in part, the survival benefit that accrues to patients treated even 24 hours after the onset of symptoms. There is currently no evidence that rt-PA has a more beneficial effect on survival or function than does streptokinase or any other plasminogen activator used in treating AMI; nor is there any evidence that patients who receive rt-PA therapy show a decreased incidence of bleeding complications compared with those who receive streptokinase, despite the relative fibrinogen-sparing attribute of rt-PA. Given the poor predictive value of the 90-minute angiogram for ultimate clinical advantage of 1 agent over another, studies that are limited to this endpoint are of marginal use in evaluating treatment regimens used in mortality studies. The best evidence to date indicates that streptokinase and rt-PA are of equivalent value for survival after AMI, a conclusion that can be justifiably challenged only with a valid mortality study.

Cross and associates[85] in Auckland, New Zealand, evaluated regional LV function in 214 patients at 3 weeks after first AMI in a trial in which streptokinase and rt-PA had been compared as thrombolytic interventions. The infarct-related artery was the LAD in 78 patients, the right coronary artery in 122, and a dominant left circumflex artery in 14. Analysis was by the centerline method with a novel correction for the area of myocardium at risk, whereby the search region was determined by the anatomic distribution of the infarct-related artery. Infarct-artery patency at 3 weeks was 73% in the streptokinase group and 71% in the rt-PA group. Global LV function did not differ between the 2 groups. Mean chord motion in the most hypokinetic half of the defined search region was similar in the streptokinase and rt-PA groups. There were no differences in hyperkinesia of the noninfarct zone. Compared with conventional centerline analysis, regional wall motion in the defined area at risk was significantly more abnormal. The 2 methods correlated strongly, however. Patients with a patent infarct-related artery and those with an occluded artery at the time of catheterization had similar global LV function (LVEF 58 ± 12% vs 57 ± 12%). Regional function was also similar in patients with a patent and occluded infarct-related artery on univariate analysis, but multivariate analysis correcting for variation due to infarct site showed that a patent infarct-related artery was associated with improved regional function. Thus, streptokinase and rt-PA in the doses given have similar effects on global and regional LV function measured 3 weeks after a first AMI.

The potential benefits of combination thrombolytic agents in the treatment of AMI remain uncertain. In a small pilot study, Grines and co-investigators[86] in Lexington, Kentucky, demonstrated that combined half-dose rt-PA with streptokinase achieved a high rate of infarct vessel patency and a low rate of reocclusion at half the cost of full dose rt-PA. The investigators designed a prospective trial in which 216 patients were randomized within 6 hours of AMI to receive either the combination of half-dose (50 mg) rt-PA with streptokinase (1.5 MU) during 1 hour or to the conventional dose of rt-PA (100 mg) during 3 hours. Acute patency was determined by angiography at 90 minutes, and angioplasty was reserved for failed thrombolysis. Heparin and aspirin regimens were maintained until follow-up catheterization at day 7. Acute patency was significantly greater after rt-PA/streptokinase (79%) than with rt-PA alone (64%). After angioplasty for failed thrombolysis, acute patency increased to 96% in both groups. Marked depletion of serum fibrinogen levels occurred after rt-PA/streptokinase compared with rt-PA alone at 4 hours and persisted 24 hours after therapy. Reocclusion, reinfarction and need for emergency CABG tended to be less in the rt-PA/streptokinase group. Greater myocardial salvage was apparent in the rt-PA/streptokinase group as assessed by infarct zone function at day 7 (Figure 3-21). In-hospital mortality (6% vs 4%) and serious bleeding (12% vs 11%) were similar between the 2 groups. These results suggest that a less expensive regimen of half-dose rt-PA with streptokinase yields superior 90-minute patency and LV function and a trend toward reduced reocclusion compared with the conventional dose of rt-PA.

Recombinant tissue-type plasminogen activator vs anisoylated plasminogen streptokinase activator complex

Recombinant tissue-type plasminogen activator (rt-PA) and anisoylated plasminogen streptokinase activator complex have been demonstrated to limit infarct size significantly and to preserve LV function when injected soon after AMI. However, as yet, the efficacy and safety of these 2 thrombolytic agents have not been directly compared in 1 trial. Bassand and co-investigators[87] in Clermont-Ferrand, France, randomly allocated 183 patients suffering from a first AMI to either streptokinase complex or rt-PA within 4 hours of the onset of symptoms. Global and regional LV functions were assessed from contract angiography an average of 5

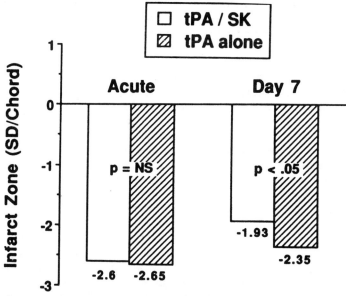

Fig. 3-21. Bar graph showing that despite similarities in acute infarct zone function, patients who received combination therapy had superior function at day 7 follow-up compared with tPA alone. tPA, tissue-type plasminogen activator; SK, streptokinase. Reproduced with permission from Grines, et al.[86]

days after initial therapy. Radionuclide angiography and thallium-201 single-photon emission computerized tomography were performed before hospital discharge. Infarct size was assessed by single-photon emission computerized tomography and expressed in percentage of the total myocardial volume. Ninety patients received streptokinase activator complex and 93 received rt-PA activator within a period of 172 minutes after the onset of symptoms. The 2 groups were similar in age, location of AMI, Killip class, and time of randomization. The patency rate of the infarct-related artery was 72% in the streptokinase activator complex group and 76% in the rt-PA group. Initial and predischarge LV EF as well as infarct size were similar in both therapeutic groups. Bleeding complications requiring blood transfusion occurred in 1 streptokinase activator complex patient and in 2 rt-PA patients. One patient in the plasminogen group died of a massive intracranial hemorrhage. At the end of the 3-week follow-up period, 5 streptokinase activator complex patients and 7 rt-PA patients had died. The early infusion of streptokinase activator complex or rt-PA in AMI produced a similar patency rate, limitation of infarct size, and preservation of LV systolic function with an equivalent rate of bleeding complications.

Recombinant tissue-type plasminogen activator

The effect of thrombolytic therapy on the frequency, time course and sequelae of pericardial effusion after AMI are unknown. Belkin and associates[88] from Valhalla, New York, and Durham, North Carolina, in a prospective, serial, 2-dimensional echocardiographic study of patients with AMI who received recombinant tissue-type plasminogen activator (rt-PA) addressed this issue. The study population comprised 52 of the 112 patients enrolled in the first Thrombolysis and Angioplasty in Myocardial Infarction trial at Duke University Medical Center. Enrollment in the serial echocardiography protocol was determined by equipment and support staff availability. Complete echocardiographic studies were performed within 90 minutes after initiation of thrombolytic therapy (day 0), and on days 1, 3 and 6. Patients undergoing serial echocardiography did not differ in demographic or clinical characteristics from those who did not. Pericardial effusion was present in 3 of 38 patients (8%) at day 0, in 2 of 44 (5%) at day 1, 8 of 43 (19%) at day 3, and in 10 of 42 (24%) at day 6. By day 6, 3 of 10 pericardial effusions were moderate in size, 1 of 10 was large and the remainder were small. No patients developed echocardiographic or hemodynamic signs of cardiac tamponade. The prevalence and time course of pericardial effusion among patients with AMI who received rt-PA in this study are similar to observations reported in earlier studies in which patients did not receive thrombolytic therapy. Adverse sequelae of pericardial effusion after thrombolytic therapy are rare.

Rogers and colleagues[89] for the TIMI II Investigators ascertained whether predischarge coronary arteriography is beneficial in patients with AMI treated with recombinant tissue-type plasminogen activator, heparin and aspirin. One hundred ninety-seven patients in the Thrombolysis in Myocardial Infarction (TIMI) IIA study assigned to conservative management and routine predischarge coronary arteriography were compared with the outcome of 1,461 patients from the TIMI IIB study assigned to conservative management without routine coronary arteriography unless ischemia recurred spontaneously or on predischarge exercise testing. The two groups were similar with regard to baseline variables. During the initial hospital stay, coronary arteriography was performed in 94% of the routine catheterization group and 35% of the selective catheterization group, but the frequency of coronary revascularization (PTCA or CABG) was similar in the two groups (24% and 21%). Coronary arteriograms showed a predominance of zero or one vessel disease (stenosis ≥60%) in both groups. During the first year after infarction, rehospitalization for cardiac reasons and the interim performance of coronary arteriography were more common in the selective catheterization group (38% vs 28% and 29% vs 12%, respectively). However, the interim rates of death, nonfatal reinfarction, and performance of coronary revascularization procedures were similar. At the end of one year, coronary arteriography had been performed one or more times in 99% of the routine catheterization group and 59% of the selective catheterization group, whereas death and nonfatal reinfarction had occurred in 10% vs 7% and 9% vs 9%, respectively. Since the selective coronary arteriography policy exposed approximately 40% fewer patients to the small but finite risks and inconvenience of the procedure without compromising the one year survival or reinfarction rates, it appears appropriate as a management strategy.

Little and associates[90] from Atlanta, Georgia, determined whether reperfusion of AMI by rt-PA or PTCA, or both, would improve LV function when it is measured several months later at rest or maximal bicycle exercise, or both. Radionuclide angiography was performed in 44 patients 5 months (range 6 weeks to 9 months) after AMI to assess function, and tomographic myocardial thallium-201 imaging was performed at maximal exercise and delayed rest to determine whether there was any evidence of myocardial ischemia. As expected, no patient had chest pain or redistribution of a thallium defect during the exercise test, because patients had undergone angioplasty (n = 28) or CABG (n = 5) where clinically indicated for revascularization. The LVEF was plotted as a function of the time elapsed between the onset of chest pain and the time when coronary angiography confirmed patency of the infarct-related artery (achieved in 91% of 44 patients by rt-PA [n = 31] or PTCA [n = 9]). Functional responses differed markedly between patients with anterior (n = 20) versus inferior (n = 24) wall AMI. LVEF during exercise correlated with time to reperfusion in patients with an anterior wall AMI but not in patients with an inferior AMI. LVEF was higher in patients with an anterior AMI reperfused early (≤4.5 hours, n = 8) versus late (>4.5 hours or not at all, n = 12) at rest (44 ± 8 vs 32 ± 9%) and exercise (53 ± 9 vs 33 ± 11%). In contrast, the EF of patients with an inferior wall AMI (n = 24) was not different from that of patients reperfused early (n = 17) versus late or not at all (n = 7), at rest (42 ± 8 vs 46 ± 12%) or exercise (46 ± 12 vs 55 ± 12). It is thus concluded that global LV function and functional reserve during exercise were both improved by reperfusion early (<4.5 hours) in patients with an anterior wall AMI, but not in patients with an inferior wall AMI. Preservation of LV function during exercise was related to how early reperfusion was achieved in patients with anterior but not inferior wall AMI.

This study addressed the need for heparin administration to be continued for more than 24 hours after coronary thrombolysis with rt-PA. Thompson and co-workers[91] in Perth, Australia, treated a total of 241 patients with AMI with a 100 mg rt-PA and a bolus of 5,000 units intravenous heparin followed by 1,000 units/hr intravenous heparin for 24 hours. At 24 hours, 202 patients were randomized to continue intravenous heparin therapy in full dosage or to discontinue heparin therapy and begin an oral antiplatelet regimen of aspirin (300 mg/day) and dipyridamole (300 mg/day). On prospective recording, there were no differences in the pattern of chest pain, reinfarction, or bleeding complications. Coronary angiography on cardiac catheterization at 7-10 days showed no differences in patency of the infarct-related artery. The proportion of patients with total occlusion of the infarct-related artery was 19% in the heparin group and 20% in the aspirin and dipyridamole group. In the patients with an incompletely occluded infarct-related artery, the lumen was reduced by 69% of normal in the heparin group and 67% in the aspirin and dipyridamole group. LV function assessed on cardiac catheterization and radionuclide study at day 2 and at 1 month showed no differences between the 2 groups. LVEF on radionuclide ventriculography at 1 month was 52% in the heparin group and 52% in the aspirin and dipyridamole group. The investigators concluded that heparin therapy can be discontinued 24 hours after rt-PA therapy and replaced with an oral antiplatelet regimen without any adverse effects on chest pain, reinfarction, coronary patency, of LV function.

Morgan and colleagues[92] in Toronto and Hamilton, Canada, evaluated infarct size, LV function, and infarct-related coronary artery patency in 108 patients who were part of a placebo-controlled trial of rt-PA in AMI. Coronary angiography was performed 17 ± 0.8 hours after initiation of therapy in 47 patients (group A) or at 10 days in 61 patients (group B). Both groups had radionuclide ventriculography 3.8 ± 0.8 hours and again on day 9 after treatment and quantitative thallium-201 scintigraphy on day 8. In group A, the infarct-related artery was patent in 53%. These patients had a smaller global and regional fixed thallium-201 defect than did those with an occluded artery. Infarct regional EF improved by 10 ± 2.1% between early and late studies when the infarct-related artery was patent and by 4.8 ± 1.4% if it was occluded. Changes in global and region LVEF were similar irrespective of perfusion status. Infarct regional LVEF and fixed thallium-201 defect were inversely related only when the infarct-related artery was occluded. In group B, 10 day patency of the infarct-related artery was 67%. There was no difference in patency by treatment assignment, in LVEF, or infarct size between patients with and without infarct-related patency. There was no evidence of an effect of rt-PA therapy beyond that expressed through coronary patency alone in either group of patients.

To assess the long-term effect of thrombolytic therapy on LV systolic function, Henzlova and associates[93] from Birmingham, Alabama, assessed LVEF by radionuclide equilibrium angiography at hospital discharge and 1 year later in 222 patients with AMI treated with intravenous rt-PA within 4 hours of symptom onset. Mean EF at hospital discharge (46 ± 12) was similar to that at 1 year (45 ± 13). Stepwise multivariate linear regression analysis identified EF at discharge and patency of the infarct-related artery before discharge as independent predictors of EF change at 1 year. Random assignments to invasive versus conservative treatment strategies or to early versus delayed B-blocker therapy did not affect EF change during follow-up. No significant deterioration of EF was observed in patients with larger infarcts. However, EF decreased from 45 ± 10 at hospital discharge to 39 ± 12 at 1-year follow-up in a subgroup of patients with history of prior AMI. Thus, patients with AMI, treated with intravenous rt-PA early after onset of symptoms, appear to have stable LV function between hospital discharge and 1 year follow-up. The change in EF between hospital discharge and 1 year can be predicted from the EF value at discharge, patency of the infarct related artery before discharge and history of previous AMI.

To evaluate the prevalence of LV thrombi after thrombolytic therapy, 144 consecutive patients with AMI were prospectively studied with two-dimensional echocardiography by Motro and associates[94] from Tel Hashomer and Tel Aviv, Israel, 1 and 8 days after admission. Patients were treated 2.1 ± 0.8 hours after the onset of symptoms. Thrombolytic protocol included 120 mg of recombinant tissue plasminogen activator, 5000 IU of heparin, followed by a continuous infusion of 25,000 IU/24 hours for at least 5 days, and 250 mg of aspirin a day. Seventy-six patients had AMI of the anterior wall; of these 7 (9.2%) developed LV thrombi. The remaining 68 patients had infarcts of the inferior wall; of these, 2 (2.9%) developed LV thrombi. Since anterior wall infarction not treated with thrombolytic therapy is associated with a 25% to 40% rate of LV thrombi, it was concluded that early thrombolytic therapy, heparin, and aspirin reduces the formation of LV thrombus in AMI of the anterior wall. Apical LV thrombi developed more frequently in patients with previous infarctions compared with those without (4 of 17 vs 4 of 127). During the 12-month follow-up period, no patient in the study had manifestations of peripheral emboli.

Munkvad and colleagues[95] in Esbjerg, Denmark and Leiden, The Netherlands studied 20 patients with AMI treated with recombinant rt-PA and measured factor XII-dependent fibrinolytic activity levels throughout the hospital period. The factor XII levels were correlated prospectively with the incidence of recurrent AMI until 8 weeks after hospital discharge. Within the follow-up period, recurrent AMI occurred in 8 patients, whereas the remaining 12 patients showed no clinical evidence of recurrence. The patients in the reinfarction group were characterized by a more pronounced depletion of and sustained lower levels of factor XII-dependent fibrinolytic activity than patients with no reinfarction (Figure 3-22). The

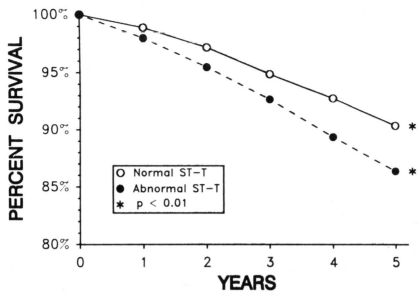

Fig. 3-22. Survival curves depicting the 5-year survival of all patients with and without an ST-T wave abnormality. The two curves are significantly different from each other, indicating a significant effect of ST-T wave changes on survival. Reproduced with permission from Munkvad, et al.[95]

decrease in fibrinolytic activity during rt-PA therapy was associated with a depletion of functional alpha$_2$-antiplasmin, the primary plasmin inhibitor. These results indicate that coronary thrombolysis with rt-PA involved depletion of endogenous factor XII-dependent fibrinolytic activity which also constitutes a risk for early reinfarction.

Bovill and colleagues of the Thrombolysis in Myocardial Infarction (TIMI) Investigators[96] assessed the effects of invasive procedures, hemostatic and clinical variables, the timing of beta-blocker therapy, and the doses of rt-PA on hemorrhagic events. Dose of rt-PA was 150 mg for the first 520 patients and 100 mg for the remaining 2,819 patients. Patients were randomly assigned to an invasive strategy (coronary arteriography with percutaneous angioplasty [if feasible] done routinely 18 to 48 hours after the start of thrombolytic therapy) or to a conservative strategy (coronary arteriography done for recurrent spontaneous or exercise-induced ischemia). Eligible patients were also randomly assigned to either immediate intravenous or deferred beta-blocker therapy. Patients were monitored for hemorrhagic events during hospitalization. In patients on the 100-mg rt-PA regimen, major and minor hemorrhagic events were more common among those assigned to the invasive than among those assigned to the conservative strategy (18.5% vs 12.8%) (Figure 3-23). Major or minor hemorrhagic events were associated with the extent of fibrinogen breakdown, peak rt-PA levels, thrombocytopenia, prolongation of the activated partial thromboplastin time to >90 seconds, weight of ≤70 kg, female gender, and physical signs of cardiac decompensation. Immediate intravenous beta-blocker therapy had no important effect on hemorrhagic events when compared with delayed beta-blocker therapy. Intracranial hemorrhages were more frequent among patients treated with the 150-mg rt-PA dose than with the 100-mg rt-PA dose (2.1% vs 0.5%). The extent of the plasmin-mediated hemostatic defect was also greater

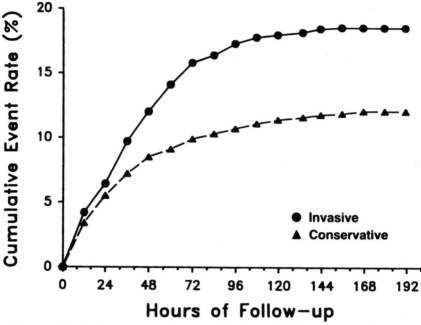

Fig. 3-23. Cumulative event rate of major or minor hemorrhagic events among the patients treated with 100 mg of recombinant tissue-type plasminogen activator and assigned to the conservative (n = 1395) or invasive strategy (n = 1424). Reproduced with permission from Bovill, et al.[96]

in patients receiving the 150 mg dose. Increased morbidity due to hemorrhagic complications is associated with an invasive management strategy in patients with AMI.

In an investigation by Bhatnagar and Al-Yusuf[97] from Kuwait City, Kuwait, and London, United Kingdom, consecutive survivors of a first Q wave anterior AMI were studied to observe the impact of rt-PA therapy on the incidence and associations of LV thrombus. Fifty-four patients received rt-PA <4 hours after the onset of cardiac pain, followed by heparin infusion. Forty-four patients who did not qualify for rt-PA therapy but who were anticoagulated with heparin, served as a control group. Two-dimensional echocardiography was performed in all patients on days 3 and 7 to detect thrombi and analyze wall motion. EF was determined by radionuclide angiography in all patients on day 7. Apical thrombi were detected on day 3 in 3 patients (5.5%) who received rt-PA and in 8 control patients (18%). All patients with a thrombus had apical dyskinesis and 8 of 11 (73%) had an aneurysm. Of the 87 patients without thrombosis, apical dyskinesis and aneurysm were present in 42 (48%) and 11 (13%) patients, respectively. EF and wall motion scores of patients without thrombus were significantly better when compared with data from those with a thrombus. There were fewer patients with apical dyskinesis (17 of 54) in the group receiving rt-PA therapy compared with the control group (36 of 44). EF and wall motion scores were better in patients who received rt-PA compared with control individuals. Thus, rt-PA reduced the incidence of LV thrombosis by 70% in patients with anterior AMI by preserving apical wall motion, and this decrease in relative risk was significant in comparison with the risk in AMI patients receiving heparin therapy.

Sustained infarct artery patency is an important determinant of survival in patients with AMI. Aguirre and associates[98] from St. Louis, Missouri, studied 61 patients with AMI who received intravenous recombinant tissue-type plasminogen activator, aspirin or heparin within 6 hours of symptom onset, to determine if infarct artery patency after intravenous thrombolytic therapy influenced myocardial electrical stability as measured by the prevalence of spontaneous ventricular ectopic activity or late potential activity. Infarct artery patency was determined by angiographic evaluation 2.5 ± 3 days after infarction. Forty-eight patients (79%) had a patent infarct-related artery and 13 (21%) patients had an occluded vessel. The mean number of VPCs per hour and the prevalence of late potentials (54 vs 19%) were significantly higher in patients with an occluded versus patent-infarct related vessel. Although VPC frequency and late potentials were not influenced by the time to thrombolytic treatment, patients with a patent infarct-related artery had a lower prevalence of late potentials regardless of whether treatment was initiated ≤2 hours (25% patent vs 50% occluded) or 2 to 6 hours (16% patent vs 55% occluded) after symptom onset. Thus, successful thrombolysis decreases the frequency of ventricular ectopic activity and late potentials in the early postinfarction phase. The reduction in both markers of electrical instability may help explain why the prognosis after successful thrombolysis is improved after AMI.

McKendall and colleagues[99] in Providence, Rhode Island, New York, New York, and San Francisco, California, studied the safety and efficacy of a new regimen of intravenous rt-PA potentially suitable for either pre- or in-hospital administration in 60 patients with AMI in an open label coronary angiographic study. The regimen consisted of a 20 mg bolus dose followed 30 minutes later by a delayed infusion of 80 mg over 2 hours. This regimen was designed to facilitate prehospital admission of rt-PA. Infarct-related artery patency was observed in 40 of 53 patients at 60 minutes (76%) and in 55 of 60 patients at 90 minutes (92%) after the rt-PA bolus. By 90 minutes, the majority of patients exhibited good coronary blood flow and infarct artery patency at 120 minutes was 85%. During hospitalization, definite recurrent ischemia occurred in nine patients (15%); nonfatal recurrent AMI was noted in one (2%). Four patients (7%) experienced major bleeding, including one with intracranial bleeding. There were seven deaths (12%). Mortality was significantly influenced by the occurrence of cardiogenic shock which was present in five patients at the time of enrollment. Blood fibrinogen levels were obtained before and during rt-PA infusions. At baseline and 30 and 150 minutes after the bolus dose, the mean fibrinogen level was 284 ± 77.4 mg/dl. Compared with the baseline values, there was a significant decrease in fibrinogen at both 30 and 150 minutes. Therefore, a new regimen of intravenous rt-PA has been identified that is well suited for both pre- and in-hospital treatment of patients with AMI. The regimen features an initial 20 mg bolus dose and is capable of achieving infarct artery patency in excess of 90% within 90 minutes after initiation of therapy.

Alteplase

Wilcox and associates[100] from Nottingham, UK, used continuous electrocardiography during the first 24 hours of a stay in a coronary care unit to record ventricular arrhythmias during treatment with rt-PA (alteplase) or placebo. Recordings were made on 378 of the 436 patients admitted to a double blind trial of alteplase or placebo in one participating center of the Anglo-Scandinavian study of early thrombosis (ASSET), patients being selected according to the availability of recorders. Of these, 309 (158 given alteplase and 151 placebo) had >5 hours of analysable data. Most of the arrhythmias were recorded in patients with an in-hospital diagnosis of AMI. Ventricular couplets and VT were significantly more common in the patients treated with alteplase. Further, in patients with myocardial infarction who had VPCs, couplets, or VT type a, the number of hours in which each arrhythmia was recorded was significantly higher in the alteplase group. The various ventricular arrhythmias in the alteplase group tended to cluster in the first 4–12 hours of the recordings. During the first 24 hours admission there were 4 episodes of VF in the alteplase group and 5 in the placebo group of taped patients. By 1 month there had been 18 deaths in these 309 patients (alteplase 4, placebo 14). These bore no relation to any recorded arrhythmia. Clinical records for the patients with no or minimal tape data yielded 6 further episodes of VF during the first 24 hours (3 in the alteplase group and 3 in the placebo group). Of the total 436 patients, 20 of the 218 patients in the alteplase group had died by 1 month compared with 22 of the 218 patients treated with placebo. The use of alteplase increases the incidence of non-life threatening ventricular arrhythmias. These results, however, suggest that arrhythmia after thrombolysis in the pre-hospital phase may be less of a problem than it is perceived to be.

Purvis and associates[101] from Belfast, Northern Ireland, treated 59 consecutive patients presenting within 6 hours of the onset of symptoms of AMI with 150 mg of soluble aspirin orally and either 70 or 100 mg of alteplase divided into 2 intravenous bolus injections separated by 30 minutes. Dosage regimens were either 20 followed by 50 mg (group A), 50 followed by 20 mg (group B), or 50 followed by 50 mg (group C). Coronary angiography 60 minutes after the first bolus showed infarct-related coronary artery patency (Thrombolysis in Myocardial Infarction score 2 or 3) in 13 of 16 (81%) patients in group A, 12 of 17 (71%) in group B, and 10 of 11 (91%) in group C (overall patency rate at 60 minutes: 35 of 44 [80%] patients; 95% confidence interval 68 to 91%). At 90 minutes, patency rates were 15 of 20 (75%) patients in both groups A and B, and 18 of 19 (95%) in group C (overall patency rate 48 of 59 [81%] patients). Residual thrombus was identified with the 90-minute angiogram in 7 patients in group A, 5 in group B, and 3 in group C. Although there was no statistically significant difference in patency between the 3 dosage regimens at either 60 or 90 minutes there was a trend toward increased patency and more complete thrombolysis at 90 minutes in group C. No episodes of bradyarrhythmia, hypotension or cerebrovascular bleeding were observed after double bolus therapy. There were 7 episodes (12%) of reocclusion, and 3 deaths (5%) within 1-month follow-up. Double bolus alteplase therapy is a convenient and highly effective method of promoting early coronary artery patency.

Anistreplase

To see whether early elective angiography with a view to coronary angioplasty or bypass grafting of a narrowed infarct related artery would improve outcome in AMI treated by thrombolysis with anistreplase, the SWIFT (Should We Intervene Following Thrombolysis?) Trial Study Group performed a randomized study of 2 treatment strategies with analysis of results over 12 months[102]. Of 993 patients presenting with clinical and electrocardiographic features of AMI up to 3 hours after the onset of symptoms, 800 patients were included in the study. Intravenous anistreplase 30 units followed by a standard regimen of heparin, warfarin, and timolol and (in patients so randomized) early angiography plus appropriate intervention was the treatment strategy. Three hundred ninety-seven patients were randomized to receive early angiography plus appropriate intervention (PTCA in 169 cases, CABG in 59) and 403 patients to receive conservative care (of these, 12 had angioplasty and 7 bypass grafting during the initial admission). By 12 months mortality (5.8% [23 patients] in the intervention group vs 5.0% [20] in the conservative care group) and rates of reinfarction (15.1% [60 patients] vs 12.9% [52]) were similar in the 2 groups. No significant differences in rates of angina or rest pain were found at 12 months. LVEF at 3 and 12 months was the same in both groups. Median hospital stay was longer in the intervention group (11 days vs 10 days). For most patients given thrombolytic treatment for AMI a strategy of angiography and intervention is appropriate only when required for clinical indications.

In an open multicenter study, Relik-vanWely and associates[103] from multiple European medical centers administered 30 units of anistreplase intravenously over 5 minutes within 4 hours of onset of chest pain in 156 patients with AMI. The patency of the infarct-related artery was determined by coronary angiography 90 minutes after anistreplase treatment, and also 24 hours after treatment, in patients with a patent infarct-related artery at 90 minutes, to assess the reocclusion rate. The investigators categorized the infarct-related vessel as patent or occluded, and 2 independent cardiologists graded the infarct-related vessel according to the Thrombolysis in Myocardial Infarction (TIMI) perfusion criteria. At the 90-minute assessment, 106 of 145 evaluable patients (73%) had patent infarct-related vessels, and 39 of 145 (27%) had occluded infarct-related vessels. Of the 139 independently assessed patients, 98 (71%) had TIMI grades 2 or 3 and 41 (29%) had TIMI grades 0 or 1. At the 24-hour assessment, 98 of 102 patients (96%) had a patent infarct-related vessel, and reocclusion had occurred in 4 of 102 patients (4%). Of the 94 independently assessed patients 90 (96%) had TIMI grades 2 or 3, and 4 (4%) had TIMI grades 0 or 1. The reliability of noninvasive parameters as indicators of achieved patency of the infarct-related vessel was estimated by means of correlation with patency assessed by coronary angiography. A significant correlation of 0.62 was found. The patency rate of 71 to 73% after use of anistreplase in patients with AMI corresponds with findings in earlier studies. The low reocclusion rate of 4% after use of anistreplase probably reflects the prolonged action of anistreplase.

Anistreplase vs streptokinase

Karagounis and associates[104] from Salt Lake City, Utah, examined the effects of thrombolytic therapy on enzymatic and electrocardiographic indexes of AMI in 370 patients who were enrolled within 4 hours of onset of symptoms and were randomized to blinded therapy with intravenous anistreplase (30 U/5 min, n = 188) or streptokinase (1.5 million IU/1 hour, n = 182). Creatine kinase and its MB isoenzyme were initially measured every 4 to 6 hours, and lactic dehydrogenase and its cardiac isoenzyme every 8 to 12 hours. Electrocardiograms were obtained before, and at 90 minutes and 8 hours after starting thrombolysis, and on discharge. Enzymatic and electrocardiographic measures of infarction were compared between drug treatment and patency groups. Early patency was associated with significant reductions in peak values for each of 4 cardiac enzymes (averaging 21 to 25%) even though later rescue procedures were often used in the nonpatent group; times to peaks were also reduced for 3 of the enzymes. Treatment with anistreplase was associated with enzymatics peaks that tended to be lower than with streptokinase (6 to 16%), approaching or reaching significance for lactic dehydrogenase and cardiac isoenzyme; times to peaks were similar. Early patency favorably affected electrocardiographic indexes. Summed ST-segment elevations resolved more rapidly, summed Q-wave amplitude was reduced by 32%, and total QRS infarct score on discharge was 22% less in those achieving early patency. Small differences in electrocardiographic indexes between the 2 drug treatment groups were not significant. These results support use of early reperfusion to reduce infarct size in AMI with administration of streptokinase and anistreplase.

Urokinase

In a randomized trial of the effects on in-hospital mortality of intravenous urokinase plus heparin versus heparin alone, Rossi and Bolognese[105] on behalf of the urokinase in Myocardial Infarction Collaborative Group (USIM) enrolled 2,531 patients with AMI in 89 coronary care units for > 30 months. Patients admitted within 4 hours of the onset of pain were randomized to receive either intravenous urokinase (a bolus dose of 1 million U repeated after 60 minutes) plus heparin (a bolus dose of 10,000 U followed by 1,000 IU/hour for 48 hours) or heparin alone (infused at the same rate). Complete data were obtained in 2,201 patients (1,128 taking urokinase and 1,073 taking heparin). At 16 days, overall hospital mortality was 8% in the urokinase and 8.3% in the heparin group. Among patients with anterior AMI, mortality was 10.3% in the urokinase and 13.9% in the heparin group. The incidence of major bleeding (urokinase 0.44%, heparin 0.37%) as well as the overall incidence of stroke (urokinase 0.35%, heparin 0.20%) was similar in the 2 groups. The rates of major in-hospital cardiac complications (reinfarction, post-infarction angina) were also similar.

Single-chain urokinase-type plasminogen activator ± recombinant tissue-type plasminogen activator

Lipoprotein (a) [Lp(a)] and plasminogen share a high degree of homology as recently evidenced by amino acid and deoxyribonucleic acid analysis. As Lp(a) is enzymatically inactive, it has been suggested that high levels of Lp(a) may suppress the profibrinolytic activity at the cell surface and increase the risk of arteriosclerosis and thrombosis by competitive inhibition of plasminogen. Von Hodenberg and associates[106] from Heidelberg, Germany, evaluated whether high levels of Lp(a) influence thrombolytic therapy in patients with AMI. Forty-one patients with AMI received a combination low-dose thrombolytic therapy with recombinant tissue-type plasminogen activator (rt-PA) and human single-chain urokinase-type plasminogen activator (scu-PA). This regimen did not induce plasminemia or a lytic state as indicated by well-maintained levels of fibrinogen. Coronary patency was assessed angiographically 90 minutes after initiation of treatment. Thrombolysis was successful in 30 and unsuccessful in 11 patients. Patients with high Lp(a) levels (≥25 mg/dl) (n = 9) responded equally well to thrombolytic therapy (8 of 9, patency

89%) as did patients with normal or low levels of Lp(a) (22 of 32, patency 70%, difference >0.1). Lp(a) levels did not differ significantly between patients with successful and unsuccessful thrombolysis. The results demonstrate that high levels of Lp(a) do not affect thrombolysis in patients with AMI when low-dose pharmacologic concentrations of rt-PA and scu-PA are applied in combination.

Kirschenbaum and associates[107] of the Pro-Urokinase for Myocardial Infarction Study Group investigated the effect of simultaneous infusions of low-dose rt-PA and single-chain urokinase-type plasminogen activator (scu-PA, pro-urokinase) on coronary arterial thrombolysis in 23 patients treated within 6 hours (mean 2.6 ± 1.1) of symptoms of an AMI. Infarct artery patency at 90 minutes was achieved in 16 (70%) of 23 patients after a 1-hour intravenous infusion of 20 and 16.3 mg of rt-PA and scu-PA, respectively. At 90 minutes, the fibrinogen concentration decreased from 369 ± 207 to 316 ± 192 mg/dl, while plasminogen decreased to 69 ± 24% and a-2-antiplasmin to 77 ± 24% of pretreatment values. Although no bleeding requiring termination of drug infusion or transfusion occurred, 1 patient with cerebrovascular amyloidosis had a fatal intracerebral hemorrhage. These findings suggest that combination therapy may allow substantial reductions in total thrombolytic doses while still achieving effective fibrin-specific coronary thrombolysis.

PTCA following unsuccessful rt-PA therapy for AMI has been associated with a high incidence of subsequent reocclusion of the infarct-related artery, and a relatively high in-hospital mortality. In contrast, the combination of rt-PA and urokinase, when given intravenously prior to PTCA, appears to be associated with a low incidence of post-rescue PTCA reocclusion. To determine whether intraprocedural urokinase, given at the time of rescue PTCA for failed rt-PA therapy, improves long-term patency of the infarct vessel to the same extent as preangiographic, combination rt-PA/urokinase therapy, 3 thrombolytic treatment strategies were retrospectively compared in a study carried out by Morris and associates[108] from Ann Arbor, Michigan. The first group included 86 patients undergoing rescue PTCA after rt-PA monotherapy (rt-PA alone). The clinical and angiographic outcomes of these patients were compared with those of 24 patients who received intravenous or intracoronary urokinase during rescue PTCA following unsuccessful rt-PA therapy (sequential rt-PA/urokinase therapy) and with those of 34 patients undergoing rescue PTCA following unsuccessful therapy with the combination of intravenous rt-PA and urokinase (simultaneous therapy). There was no difference in postangioplasty patency rate of the infarct-related artery between the 3 groups. However, the sequential rt-PA/urokinase regimen was associated with a subsequent reocclusion rate that was lower than the rate that occurred in the rt-PA monotherapy group but higher than the rate in the simultaneous rt-PA/urokinase group (13 versus 29 versus 2%, respectively). In-hospital mortality in the sequential therapy group was 13% compared with 12% in the rt-PA monotherapy group and 0% in the simultaneous rt-PA/urokinase group. There was no significant difference between the groups in the incidence of bleeding or in the need for emergency CABG. It was concluded that the addition of intracoronary or intravenous urokinase at the time of rescue PTCA may improve the long-term patency of the infarct-related artery following intravenous rt-PA therapy, but that the initial, preangiographic administration of combined rt-PA and urokinase appears to be a preferable treatment regimen for patients in whom rescue PTCA appears likely.

Adjunctive therapy

Popma and Topol[109] from Ann Arbor, Michigan, provided a fine review of adjunctive pharmacologic agents to thrombolytic therapy for AMI. Their data suggest that adjunctive pharmacologic therapy to thrombolytic agents should include aspirin, at least 160 mg administered as soon as possible after the onset of symptoms of myocardial ischemia; intravenous heparin, and, in selected patients without contraindications, intravenous beta-blocking agents.

To assess the risk and possible benefits of use of the percutaneous intraaortic balloon pump in patients given thrombolytic therapy as treatment for AMI, Ohman and associates[110] from Durham, North Carolina, Ann Arbor, Michigan, and Columbus and Cincinnati, Ohio, prospectively evaluated 810 consecutive patients entered into the Thrombolysis and Angioplasty in Myocardial Infarction trials. During hospitalization the 85 patients treated with the intraaortic balloon pump had more cardiac risk factors, were slightly older (58 vs 56 years), and more often had anterior AMI (62% vs 38%). At acute cardiac catheterization, patients treated with the intraaortic balloon pump also had more multivessel CAD (67% vs 43%), more frequent Thrombolysis in Myocardial Infarction grade 0 or 1 flow (44% vs 28%), lower global EF (40% vs 52%), and worse regional infarction and noninfarct zone function. Although mortality rates (32% vs 4%) and in-hospital complications were greater in patients treated with the intraaortic balloon pump, a greater improvement in global and noninfarct zone LV function was observed in patients treated with the intraaortic balloon pump at 1-week follow-up angiography. In addition, no reinfarction or reocclusion of the infarct-related artery occurred while patients were being treated with the intraaortic balloon pump. These results suggest that the intraaortic balloon pump may have a specific role after thrombolytic therapy in treating patients at high risk for reocclusion or at high risk for hemodynamic deterioration because of large infarction or critical stenoses in coronary vessels supplying the noninfarct zone.

Intracerebral hemorrhage afterwards

Maggioni and associates[111] on behalf of the Gruppo Italiano per lo Studio della Streptochinasi nell'Infarto Miocardico (GISSI) analyzed 5,860 patients with AMI treated with 1.5 million units of intravenous streptokinase and 5,852 patients not given fibrinolytic treatment. To determine the frequency of cerebral vascular events, sex, age, BP, history of previous AMI, site of AMI, and Killip class between the 2 groups. Of the 11,712 patients, 99 (0.84%) had a cerebral vascular event. Older age, worse Killip class, and anterior location of infarction seemed to be risk factors for cerebral-vascular events (40/3,201 aged 65 to 75 vs 42/7,295 aged <65, odds ratio 2.18; 9/437 class 3 vs 55/8,277 class I, 1.81; and 57/4,878 anterior vs 24/4,013 posterior, 1.96). No significant difference was found in the rate of cerebral vascular events between patients treated with streptokinase and controls (45/5,852 [0.92%] streptokinase versus 54/5,860 [0.77] control). More patients in the streptokinase group than in the control group had cerebral vascular events (especially hemorrhagic strokes) on day 0-1 after randomization (27 streptokinase vs 7, control), although this was balanced by late events in control patients (54 streptokinase vs 45 control at 1 year). The mortality of patients who had a cerebralvascular event was higher than that of those who did not (47% [47/99] vs 11.6% [1,350/11,613]). Although the incidence of cerebralvascular events complicating AMI was low, they increased morbidity and mortality. Treatment with streptokinase did not significantly alter the incidence, but age and poor hemodynamic state were associated with an increased risk.

Intracerebral hemorrhage is an important concern after thrombolytic therapy for AMI, but risk factors are controversial. Anderson and associates[112] from Salt Lake City, Utah, assessed risk factors in 107 treated patients of whom 4 had intracerebral hemorrhage. Intracerebral hemorrhage occurred at a mean of 25 hours (range 3.5 to 48) after therapy and was fatal in 2 patients. Significant differences were found between patients with and without intracerebral hemorrhage for age (77 ± 7 vs 62 ± 11 years), and initial (161 ± 23 vs 135 ± 23 mm Hg) and maximal (171 ± 30 vs 146 ± 20) systolic BP. Initial and maximal diastolic BP also tended to be higher (101 ± 25 vs 86 ± 16; 104 ± 24 vs 90 ± 13). Differences did not achieve significance for comparisons of gender, height, weight, site of infarction, time to therapy, specific thrombolytic agent used, concomitant therapy, interventions and partial thromboplastin time. It is concluded that age (≥70 years) and elevated BP (≥150/95 mm Hg) are important risk factors for intracerebral hemorrhage. The overall balance of benefit and risk of thrombolysis should continue to be assessed by large mortality trials.

PERCUTANEOUS TRANSLUMINAL CORONARY ANGIOPLASTY

Usefulness

Arnold and colleagues[113] in Rotterdam, The Netherlands, Berlin, West Germany, Leicester, UK, and Leuven, Belgium, analyzed regional ventricular wall motion utilizing three different methods on predischarge left ventriculograms from 291 of 367 patients enrolled in a randomized trial of single chain recombinant tissue-type plasminogen activator, aspirin and heparin with and without immediate PTCA in patients with AMI. With univariate analysis, no differences in regional wall motion variables between the two treatment groups were observed. However, with individual baseline risk assessment by multivariate linear regression analysis using baseline characteristics known to be related to LV function after thrombolytic therapy or outcome of coronary angioplasty, or both, an excess of high risk patients in the invasive treatment group was detected. Multivariate linear analysis regression studies were performed to adjust for the unequal distribution of baseline risk. No benefit of the immediate PTCA was observed after this statistical adjustment. Reocclusion or reinfarction, or both, occurred more frequently in the invasive than in the noninvasive treatment group (18% vs 13%, respectively). Among patients with a patent infarct-related artery on angiography between days 10 and 22 without reinfarction before angiography, there was a trend toward benefit from the invasive strategy, indicating that reocclusion and reinfarction might be responsible for the lack of benefit of the invasive strategy.

Brodie and associates[114] from Greensboro, North Carolina, performed PTCA without prior thrombolytic therapy in 383 patients with AMI. Patients were divided into 2 groups depending on whether they were candidates or non-candidates for thrombolytic therapy. Patients were not considered thrombolytic candidates if they: (1) presented in cardiogenic shock, (2) were ≥75 years of age, (3) had had CABG or, (4) had a reperfusion time of >6 hours. Thrombolytic and nonthrombolytic candidates had similar rates of reperfusion (92 vs 88%), nonfatal reinfarction (6.0 vs 5.9%) and recurrent myocardial ischemia (1.8 vs 0%). Thrombolytic candidates had a lower mortality rate (3.9 vs 24%) and a lower incidence of bleeding (4.6 vs 10.9%). Improvement in LVEF at follow-up angiography was 4.4% in thrombolytic and 10.5% in nonthrombolytic candidates. EF improved most in patients with anterior wall AMI (7.7% in thrombolytic candidates, 15.1% in nonthrombolytic candidates) and in patients with reperfusion times >6 hours (14.2%). These outcomes suggest that direct coronary angioplasty is a viable alternative method of reperfusion in patients with AMI who are candidates for thrombolytic therapy. Nonthrombolytic candidates are a high-risk group of patients. Direct coronary angioplasty may be beneficial in certain subgroups, especially for patients in cardiogenic shock and for patients presenting >6 hours after the onset of chest pain with evidence of ongoing ischemia.

In cardiogenic shock

Lee and colleagues[115] in Ann Arbor, Michigan, performed a retrospective multicenter study to evaluate the role of acute PTCA in the treatment of cardiogenic shock complicating AMI to determine whether early reperfusion altered in-hospital and long-term survival. Sixty-nine patients were treated with emergency PTCA to attempt reperfusion of the infarct-related artery in the time interval 1982 to 1985. PTCA was unsuccessful in 20 patients (group 1) and successful in 49 patients (group 2). Initial clinical and angiographic findings in the groups with unsuccessful and successful PTCA were similar with respect to age, infarct location, and gender. Hemodynamic variables in the two groups, including systolic blood pressures, left ventricular end diastolic pressures, and initial LVEFs were also similar. Twenty-nine patients received thrombolytic therapy with streptokinase and the overall rate of reperfusion was 34%. Group 1 patients had a short-term survival rate of 20% compared with 69% in group 2 patients. Thirty-eight patients survived the hospital period and were followed up for 24 to 54 months (mean 33 months). Five patients died during follow-up; each of these patients was in group 2. Long-term incidence rate of congestive heart failure was 19%, arrhythmias 21%, need for repeat PTCA 17%, and CABG 26%. Twenty-four month survival was significantly better in group 2 patients (54%) versus group 1 patients (11%). Thus, emergency PTCA improved initial and long-term survival in cardiogenic shock complicating AMI with survival contingent on establishing reperfusion.

Emergency PTCA was performed in 62 patients with AMI complicated by hypotension in a study reported by Ghitis and associates[116] from Columbia, Missouri. All patients were treated within 12 hours of the onset of chest pain. PTCA was completely successful (residual lesion ≤50%) in 48 patients, partially successful (patent vessel >50% residual lesion) in 4 patients, and unsuccessful in 10 patients. Patients in whom PTCA was successful had a hospital mortality rate of 19%; those in whom angioplasty was unsuccessful or only partially successful had hospital mortality rates 60% and 50%, respectively. Patients with occlusion of the proximal LAD had the highest failure rate (42%) and the highest mortality rate (67%). Other univariate predictors of hospital mortality were older age and elevated LV end-diastolic pressure. Successful emergency PTCA improves mortality in patients with AMI complicated by hypotension.

Effect on plasma creatine kinase

Klein and associates[117] in Chicago, Illinois, evaluated the incidence and clinical significance of elevated total plasma creatine kinase and MB isoenzyme after apparently successful PTCA in a prospective study of 272 consecutive elective PTCA procedures. Total creatine kinase and creatine kinase MB isoenzymes were measured immediately after successful completion of the procedure and every 6 hours for 24 hours. All non-elective procedures and results not fulfilling all American Heart Association/American College of Cardiology Task Force guideline criteria for a successful result were excluded from analysis. Among the 272 elective procedures, 249 (92%) were successful. Abnormally elevated creatine kinase or creatine kinase MB serum levels, or both, were found in 38 (15%) of the successful outcomes. Three patterns of abnormal enzymes were found: 15 patients with creatine kinase ≥200 IU/liter and creatine kinase MB ≥5% (group 1); 4 patients with creatine kinase ≥200 IU/liter and creatine kinase MB ≤4% (group 2); and 19 patients with creatine kinase <200 IU/liter and creatine kinase MB ≥5% (group 3). The 3 groups were distinguished by the nature of the complications causing the enzyme release. There were significantly more clinically apparent events in group 1 than in the other groups and more events associated with persistent electrocardiogram changes and chest pain. However, there were no clinically important sequelae in any group at hospital discharge. Therefore, abnormal cardiac enzyme release after apparently successful PTCA is 1) relatively common; 2) occurs with apparently minor complications and early reversible impending complications; and 3) does not result in identifiable permanent clinical sequelae.

With fluosol

Forman and colleagues[118] in Nashville, Tennessee, Charlotte, North Carolina, Houston, Texas, and Takoma Park, Maryland, explored whether there is a myocardial reperfusion injury in humans using fluosol as a probe in conjunction with emergency PTCA in 26 patients presenting within 4 hours of a first anterior AMI who were randomized to emergency PTCA or PTCA followed by a 30 minute intracoronary infusion of Fluosol at 40 ml/min. Global and regional ventricular function were assessed immediately and a mean of 12 days after successful PTCA with contrast ventriculography. Infarct size was determined semiquantitatively by thallium-201 single-photon emission computed tomography images before discharge. Twelve patients, including six undergoing PTCA alone, and 6 treated with PTCA and fluosol had emergency cardiac catheterization and were included in the final analysis. At 12 days after successful PTCA, the improvement in regional ventricular function was greater in patients receiving adjunctive therapy with intracoronary Fluosol as compared to those undergoing PTCA alone utilizing both radial shortening and centerline methods of analysis. Tomographic infarct size expressed as a percent of the LV was also reduced. No significant differences in collateral blood flow, extent of CAD or residual stenosis after PTCA were observed. This study suggests that myocardial reperfusion injury may be an important factor in limiting myocardial salvage in patients undergoing reperfusion.

CORONARY ARTERY BYPASS GRAFTING

In a report by Kereiakes and associates[119] from Cincinnati and Columbus, Ohio, Durham, North Carolina, Ann Arbor, Michigan, and Memphis, Tennessee, CABG was performed prior to hospital discharge in 303 (22%) of 1387 consecutive patients enrolled in Thrombolysis and Angioplasty in Myocardial Infarction 1 to 3 and 5 trials of intravenous thrombolytic therapy for AMI. CABG was of emergency nature (<24 hours from treatment with intravenous thrombolytic therapy) in 36 (2.6%) and was deferred (>24 hours) in 267 (19%) patients. The indications for CABG included failed PTCA (12%); LM or equivalent CAD (9%); complex of multivessel CAD (62%); recurrent postinfarction angina (13%); and refractory pump dysfunction, MR, VSD or abnormal predischarge functional test (1% each). Although patients having CABG were older (60 ± 9.8 vs 56 ± 10 years), had more extensive CAD (46% with 3-vessel disease vs 11%), had more frequent diabetes (19% vs 15%), had more prior infarctions, had more severe initial depression in global LVEF (48 ± 12% vs 52 ± 12%) and regional infarct zone and noninfarct zone function than patients not having CABG, no difference in the incidence of death in hospital (7% surgical vs 6% nonsurgical) or death at long-term follow-up of hospital survivors (7% vs 6% nonsurgical) was noted between groups. Surgical patients demonstrated a greater degree of recovery in LVEF (3.4 ± 10% vs 0.16 ± 8.5%) and infarct zone regional function when immediate (90 minutes following initiation of thrombolytic therapy) and predischarge (7 to 14 days after treatment) contrast left ventriculograms were compared than did patients who received only intravenous thrombolytic therapy with or without PTCA. These data suggest a beneficial influence of CABG on LV function and possibly on the clinical outcome of patients initially treated with intravenous thrombolytic therapy for AMI.

References

1. Kenyon LW, Ketterer MW, Gheorghiade M, Goldstein S: Psychological Factors Related to Prehospital Delay During Acute Myocardial Infarction. Circulation 1991 (November);84:1969–1976.

2. Thompson DR, Sutton TW, Jowett NI, Pohl JEF: Circadian variation in the frequency of onset of chest pain in acute myocardial infarction. Br Heart J 1991 (Apr);65:177–178.

3. Maynard C, Litwin PE, Martin JS, Cerqueira M, Kudenchuk PJ, Ho MT, Kennedy JW, Cobb LA, Schaeffer SM, Hallstrom AP, Weaver WD: Characteristics of black patients admitted to coronary care units in metropolitan Seattle: Results from the Myocardial Infarction Triage and Intervention Registry (MITI). Am J Cardiol 1991 (Jan 1);67:18–23.

4. Molstad P: First myocardial infarction in smokers. European Heart Journal 1991 (July);12:753–759.

5. Ridker PM, Manson JE, Buring JE, Goldhaber SZ, Hennekens CH: Clinical Characteristics of Nonfatal Myocardial Infarction Among Individuals on Prophylactic Low-Dose Aspirin Therapy. Circulation 1991 (August);84:708–711.

6. Kono S, Handa K, Kawano T, Hiroki T, Ishihara Y, Arakawa K: Alcohol intake and nonfatal acute myocardial infarction in Japan. Am J Cardiol 1991 (Oct. 15);68:1011–1014.

7. Karlson BW, Herlitz J, Wiklund O, Richter A, Hjalmarson A: Early prediction of acute myocardial infarction from clinical history examination and electrocardiogram in the emergency room. Am J Cardiol 1991 (July 15);68:171–175.

8. Lee TH, Juarez G, Cook EF, Weisberg MC, Rouan GW, Brand DA, Goldman L: Ruling out acute myocardial infarction: A prospective multicenter validation of a 12-hour strategy for patients at low risk. N Engl J Med 1991 (May 2);324:1239–1246.

9. Gaspoz JM, Lee TH, Cook EF, Weisberg MC, Goldman L: Outcome of patients who were admitted to a new short-stay unit to "rule-out" myocardial infarction. Am J Cardiol 1991 (July 15);68:145–149.

10. Shen WK, Khandheria BK, Edwards WD, Oh JK, Miller FA Jr, Naessens JM, Tajik AJ: Value and limitations of two-dimensional echocardiography in predicting myocardial infarct size. Am J Cardiol 1991 (Nov 1);68:1143–1149.

11. Pahlm O, Haisty WK Jr, Wagner NB, Pope JE, Wagner GS: Specificity and sensitivity of QRS criteria for diagnosis of single and multiple myocardial infarcts. Am J Cardiol 1991 (Nov 15);68:1300–1304.

12. de Chillou C, Sadoul N, Briancon S, Aliot E. Factors determining the occurrence of late potentials on the signal-averaged electrocardiogram after a first myocardial infarction: a multivariate analysis. J Am Coll Cardiol 1991 (December);18:1638–42.

13. Bigger JT Jr., Fleiss JL, Rolnitzky LM, Steinman RC, Schneider WJ. Time course of recovery of heart period variability after myocardial infarction. J Am Coll Cardiol 1991 (December);18:1643–9.

14. Beek AM, Verheugt FWA, Meyer A: Usefulness of electrocardiographic findings and creatine kinase levels on admission in predicting the accuracy of the interval between onset of chest pain of acute myocardial infarction and initiation of thrombolytic therapy. Am J Cardiol 1991 (Nov 15);68:1287–1290.

15. Mair J, Artner-Dworzak E, Diensti A, Lechleitner P, Morass B, Smidt J, Wagner I, Wettach C, Puschendorf B: Early detection of acute myocardial infarction by measurement of mass concentration of creatine kinase-MB. Am J Cardiol 1991 (Dec 15);68:1545–1550.

16. Stewart DJ, Kubac G, Costello KB, Cernacek P: Increased plasma endothelin-1 in the early hours of acute myocardial infarction. J Am Coll Cardiol 1991; 18:38–43.

17. Christian TF, Clements IP, and Gibbons RJ: Noninvasive Identification of Myocardium at Risk in Patients With Acute Myocardial Infarction and Nondiagnostic Electrocardiograms with Technetium-99m-Sestamibi. Circulation 1991; (May) 83:1615–1620.

18. Mody FV, Brunken RC, Stevenson LW, Nienaber CA, Phelps ME, Schelbert HR: Differentiating cardiomyopathy of coronary artery disease from nonischemic dilated cardiomyopathy utilizing positron emission tomography. J Am Coll Cardiol 1991 (February);17:373–83.

19. Kawaguchi K, Sone T, Tsuboi H, Sassa H, Okumura K, Hashimoto H, Ito T, Satake T: Quantitative estimation of infarct size by simultaneous dual radionuclide single photon emission computed tomography: Comparison with peak serum creatine kinase activity. Am Heart J 1991 (May);121:1353–1360.

20. Krauss XH, van der Wall EE, van der Laarse A, Doornbos J, Matheijssen NAA, de Roos A, Blokland JAK, van Voorthuisen AE, Bruschke AVG: Magnetic resonance imaging of myocardial infarction: Correlation with enzymatic, angiographic, and radionuclide findings. Am Heart J 1991 (November);122:1274–1283.

21. Nicod P, Gilpin EA, Dittrich H, Henning H, Maisel A, Blacky AR, Smith SC, Ricou F, Ross J: Trends in Use of Coronary Angiography in Subacute Phase of Myocardial Infarction. Circulation 1991 (September);84:1004–1015.

22. Gilpin E, Ricou F, Dittrich H, Nicod P, Henning H, Ross J Jr: Factors associated with recurrent myocardial infarction within one year after acute myocardial infarction. Am Heart J 1991 (February);121:457–465.

23. Griffin BP, Shah PK, Diamond GA, Berman DS, Ferguson JG: Incremental prognostic accuracy of clinical, radionuclide and hemodynamic data in acute myocardial infarction. Am J Cardiol 1991 (Sept 15);68:707–712.

24. Cragg DR, Friedman HZ, Bonema JD, Jaiyesimi IA, Ramos RG, Timmis GC, O'Neill WW, Schreiber TL: Outcome of patients with acute myocardial infarction who are ineligible for thrombolytic therapy. An Intern Med 1991 (Aug 1);115:173–177.

25. Montague TJ, Ikuta RM, Wong RY, Bay KS, Teo KK, Davies NJ: Comparison of risk and patterns of practice in patients older and younger than 70 years with acute myo-

cardial infarction in a two-year period (1987-1989). Am J Cardiol 1991 (Oct 1);68:843–847.

26. D'Agostino RB, Belanger A, Kannel WB, Cruickshank JM: Relation of low diastolic blood pressure to coronary heart disease death in presence of myocardial infarction: The Framingham study. Br Med J 1991 (Aug 17);303:385–389.

27. Wong ND, Wilson PWF, Kannel WB: Serum cholesterol as a prognostic factor after myocardial infarction: The Framingham Study. An Intern Med 1991 (Nov 1);115:687–693.

28. Martin JF, Bath PMW, Burr ML: Influence of platelet size on outcome after myocardial infarction. Lancet 1991 (Dec 7);338:1409–1411.

29. Odemuyiwa O, Malik M, Farrell T, Bashir Y, Poloniecki J, Camm J: Comparison of the predictive characteristics of heart rate variability index and left ventricular ejection fraction for all-cause mortality, arrhythmic events and sudden death after acute myocardial infarction. Am J Cardiol 1991 (Aug. 15);68:434–439.

30. Farrell TG, Bashir Y, Cripps T, Malik M, Poloniecki J, Bennett ED, Ward DE, Camm AJ. Risk stratification for arrhythmic events in postinfarction patients based on heart rate variability, ambulatory electrocardiographic variables and the signal-averaged electrocardiogram. J Am Coll Cardiol 1991 (September);18:687–97.

31. Miranda CP, Herbert WG, Dubach P, Lehmann KG, and Froelicher VF: Post-Myocardial Infarction Exercise Testing Non-Q Wave Versus Q Wave Correlation With Coronary Angiography and Long-term Prognosis. Circulation 1991 (December);84:2357–2365.

32. Gohlke H, Heim E, Roskamm H: Prognostic importance of collateral flow and residual coronary stenosis of the myocardial infarct artery after anterior wall Q-wave acute myocardial infarction. Am J Cardiol 1991 (June 1);67:1165–1169.

33. Nogami A, Aonuma K, Takahashi A, Nitta J, Chun YH, Iesaka Y, Hiroe M, Marumo F: Usefulness of early versus late programmed ventricular stimulation in acute myocardial infarction. Am J Cardiol 1991 (July 1);68:13–20.

34. de Vreede JJM, Gorgels APM, Verstraaten GMP, Vermeer F, Dassen WRM, Wellens HJJ. Did prognosis after acute myocardial infarction change during the past 30 years? A meta-analysis. J Am Coll Cardiol 1991 (September);18:698–706.

35. Wolfe CL, Nibley C, Bhandari A, Chatterjee K, Scheinman M: Polymorphous Ventricular Tachycardia Associated With Acute Myocardial Infarction. Circulation 1991 (October);84:1543–1551.

36. Hong M, Peter T, Peters W, Wang FZ, Xiu Y, Vaughn C, Gang ES: Relation between acute ventricular arrhythmias, ventricular late potentials and mortality in acute myocardial infarction. Am J Cardiol 1991 (Dec 1);68:1403–1409.

37. Sugiura T, Iwasaka T, Takahashi N, Yuasa F, Takeuchi M, Hasegawa T, Matsutani M, Inada M: Factors associated with artrial fibrillation in Q wave anterior myocardial infarction. Am Heart J 1991 (May);121:1409–1412.

38. Alboni P, Baggioni GF, Scarfo S, Cappato R, Percoco GF, Paparella N, Antonioli E: Role of sinus node artery disease in sick sinus syndrome in inferior wall acute myocardial infarction. Am J Cardiol 1991 (June 1);67:1180–1184.

39. Ricou F, Nicod P, Gilpin E, Henning H, Ross Jr., J. Influence of right bundle branch block on short- and long-term survival after acute anterior myocardial infarction. J Am Coll Cardiol 1991 (March);17:858–63.

40. Okabe M, Fukuda K, Nakashima Y, Hiroki T, Arakawa K, Kikuchi M: A quantitative histopathological study of right bundle branch block complicating acute anteroseptal myocardial infarction. Br Heart J (June);65:317–321.

41. Clemmensen P, Bates ER, Califf RM, Hlatky MA, Aronson L, George BS, Lee KL, Kerejakes DJ, Bacioch G, Berrios E, Topol EJ, TAMI Study Group: Complete atrioventricular block complicating inferior wall acute myocardial infarction treated with reperfusion therapy. Am J Cardiol 1991 (Feb 1);67:225–230.

42. Goldberg RJ, Gore JM, Alpert JS, Osganian V, De Groot J, Bade J, Chen Z, Frid D, Dalen JE: Cardiogenic shock after acute myocardial infarction: Incidence and mortality from a community-wide perspective, 1975 to 1988. N Engl J Med 1991 (Oct 17);325:1117–1122.

43. Sheikh KH, Bengtson JR, Rankin JS, deBruijn NP, Kisslo J: Intraoperative Transesophageal Doppler Color Flow Imaging Used to Guide Patient Selection and Operative Treatment of Ischemic Mitral Regurgitation. Circulation 1991 (August);84:594–604.

44. Hendren WG, Nemec JJ, Lytle BW, Loop FD, Taylor PC, Stewart RW, Cosgrove DM III: Mitral valve repair for ischemic mitral insufficiency. Ann Thorac Surg 1991 (Dec);52:1246–1252.

45. Hassapoyannes CA, Stuck LM, Hornung CA, Bergin MC, Flowers NC: Effect of left ventricular aneurysm on risk of sudden and nonsudden cardiac death. Am J Cardiol 1991 (Mar 1);67:454–459.

46. Baciewicz PA, Weintraub WS, Jones EL, Craver JM, Cohen CL, Tao X, Guyton RA: Late follow-up after repair of left ventricular aneurysm and (usually) associated coronary bypass grafting. Am J Cardiol 1991 (July 15);68:193–200.

47. Kulakowski P, Dluzniewski M, Budaj A, Ceremuzynski L: Relationship between signal-averaged electrocardiography and dangerous ventricular arrhythmias in patients with left ventricular aneurysm after myocardial infarction. Eur Heart J 1991 (Nov);12:1170–1175.

48. Fortin DF, Sheikh KH, Kisslo J: The utility of echocardiography in the diagnostic strategy of postinfarction ventricular septal rupture: A comparison of two-dimensional echocardiography versus Doppler color flow imaging. Am Heart J 1991 (January);121:25–32.

49. Behar S, Tanne D, Abinader E, Agmon J, Barzilai J, Friedman Y, Kaplinsky E, Kauli N, Kishon Y, Palant A, Peled B, Reisin L, Schlesinger Z, Zahavi I, Zion M, Goldbourt U, Sprint Study Group: Cerebrovascular accident complicating acute myocardial infarction: Incidence, clinical significance, and short- and long-term mortality rates. Am J Med 1991 (July);91:45–50.

50. Curtis JL, Houghton JL, Patterson JH, Koch G, Bradley DA, Adams KF Jr: Propranolol therapy alters estimation of potential cardiovascular risk derived from submaximal postinfarction exercise testing. Am Heart J 1991 (June); 121:1655–1664.

51. Glamann DB, Lange RA, Hillis LD: Beneficial effect of long-term beta blockade after acute myocardial infarction in patients without anterograde flow in the infarct artery. Am J Cardiol 1991 (July 15);68:150–154.

52. Gheorghiade M, Schultz L, Tilley B, Kao W, Goldstein S: Natural history of the first non-Q wave myocardial infarction in the placebo arm of the Beta-Blocker Heart Attack Trial. Am Heart J 1991 (December);122:1548–1553.

53. Boden WE, Krone RJ, Kleiger RE, Oakes D, Greenberg H, Dwyer EJ, Miller JP, Abrams J, Coromilas J, Goldstein R, Moss AJ, Multicenter Diltiazem Post-Infarction Trial Research Group: Electrocardiographic subset analysis of diltiazem administration on long-term outcome after acute myocardial infarction. Am J Cardiol 1991 (Feb 15);67:335–342.

54. Moss AJ, Oakes D, Rubison M, McDermott M, Carleen E, Eberly S, Brown M, Multicenter Diltiazem Postinfarction Trial Research Group. Am J Cardiol 1991 (Aug. 15);68:429–433.

55. Schleifer SJ, Slater WR, Macari-Hinson MM, Coyle DA, Kahn M, Zucker HD, Gorlin R: Digitalis and ß-blocking agents: Effects on depression following myocardial infarction. Am Heart J 1991 (May);121:1397–1402.

56. Oldroyd KG, Pye MP, Ray SG, Christie J, Ford I, Cobbe SM, Dargie HJ: Effects of early captopril administration on infarct expansion, left ventricular remodeling and exercise capacity after acute myocardial infarction. Am J Cardiol 1991 (Sept 15);68:713–718.

57. Hirsh: Heparin. N Engl J Med 1991 (May 30);324:1565–1574.

58. Hirsh J: Oral anticoagulant drugs. NEJM 1991 (June 27);324:1865–1875.

59. Bersten AD, Holt AW, Vedig AE, Skowronski GA, Baggoley CJ: Treatment of severe cardiogenic pulmonary edema with continuous positive airway pressure delivered by face mask. N Engl J Med 1991 (Dec 26);325:1825–1830.

60. Pfeffer MA, Myoe LA, Braunwald E, Basta L, Brown EJ Jr, Cuddy TE, Dagenais GR, Flaker GC, Geltman EM, Gersh BJ, Goldman S, Lamas GA, Packer M, Rouleau JL, Rutherford JD, Steingart RM, Wertheimer JH: Selection bias in the use of thrombolytic therapy in acute myocardial infarction. JAMA 1991 (July 24/31);266:528–532.

61. Weaver WD, Litwin PE, Martin JS, Kudenchuk PJ, Maynard C, Eisenberg MS, Ho MT, Cobb LA, Kennedy JW, Wirkus MS, The MITI Project Group. Effect of age on use of thrombolytic therapy and mortality in acute myocardial infarction. J Am Coll Cardiol 1991 (September);18:657–62.

62. Behar S, Abinader E, Caspi A, David D, Flich M, Friedman Y, Hod H, Kaplinsky E, Kishon Y, Kristal N, Laniado S, Markiewicz V, Marmor A, Palant A, Pelled B, Reisin L, Rosenfeld T, Roguin N, Sherf L, Rabinowitz B, Schlesinger Z, Sclarovsky S, Zahavi I, Zion M, Goldbourt U: Frequency of use of thrombolytic therapy in acute myocardial infarction in Israel. Am J Cardiol 1991 (Nov 15);68:1291–1294.

63. Tenaglia AN, Califf RM, Candela RJ, Kereiakes DJ, Berrios E, Young SY, Stack RS, Topol EJ: Thrombolytic therapy in patients requiring cardiopulmonary resuscitation. Am J Cardiol 1991 (Oct 15);68:1015–1019.

64. Kwon K, Freedman B, Wilcox I, Allman K, Madden A, Carter GS, Harris PJ: The unstable ST segment early after thrombolysis for acute infarction and its usefulness as a marker of recurrent coronary occlusion. Am J Cardiol 1991 (Jan 15);67:109–115.

65. Dellborg M, Topol EJ, Swedberg K: Dynamic QRS complex and ST segment vector-cardiographic monitoring can identify vessel patency in patients with acute myocardial infarction treated with reperfusion therapy. Am Heart J 1991 (October);122:943–948.

66. Zehender M, Utzolino S, Furtwangler A, Kasper W, Meinertz T, Just H: Time course and inter-relation of reperfusion-induced ST changes and ventricular arrhythmias in acute myocardial infarction. Am J Cardiol 1991 (Nov 1);68:1138–1142.

67. White H, Cross D, Scott M, Norris R: Comparison of effects of thrombolytic therapy on left ventricular function in patients over with those under 60 years of age. Am J Cardiol 1991 (May 1);67:913–918.

68. Christian TF, Clements IP, Behrenbeck T, Huber KC, Chesebro JH, Gersh BJ, Gibbons RJ: Limitations of the electrocardiogram in estimating infarction size after acute reperfusion therapy for myocardial infarction. An Intern Med 1991 (Feb 15);114:264–270.

69. Bolognese L, Sarasso G, Bongo AS, Rossi L, Aralda D, Piccinino C, Rossi P: Dipyridamole Echocardiography Test - A New Tool for Detecting Jeopardized Myocardium After Thrombolytic Therapy. Circulation 1991 (September);84:1100–1106.

70. Lavie CJ, Gibbons RJ, Zinsmeister AR, Gersh BJ: Interpreting results of exercise studies after acute myocardial infarction altered by thrombolytic therapy, coronary angioplasty or bypass. Am J Cardiol 1991 (Jan 15);67:116–120.

71. Sutton, JM and Topol EJ: Significance of a Negative Exercise Thallium Test in the Presence of a Critical Residual Stenosis After Thrombolysis for Acute Myocardial Infarction. Circulation 1991; (April) 83:1278–1286.

72. Vatterott PJ, Hammill SC, Bailey KR, Wiltgen CM, Gersh BJ. Late potentials on signal-averaged electrocardiograms and patency of the infarct-related artery in survivors of acute myocardial infarction. J Am Coll Cardiol 1991 (February);17:330–7.

73. Hohnloser SH, Zabel M, Kasper W, Meinertz T, Just H. Assessment of coronary artery patency after thrombolytic therapy: accurate prediction utilizing the combined analysis of three non-invasive markers. J Am Coll Cardiol 1991;18:44–9.

74. Kereiakes DJ, Topol EJ, George BS, Stack RS, Abbottsmith CW, Ellis S, Candela RJ, Harrelson L, Martin LH, Califf RM, and the Thrombolysis and Angioplasty in Myocardial Infarction (TAMI) Study Group. Myocardial infarction with minimal coronary atherosclerosis in the era of thrombolytic reperfusion. J Am Coll Cardiol 1991 (February);17:304–12.

75. Muller DWM, Topol EJ, Ellis SG, Woodlief LH, Sigmon KN, Kereiakes DJ, George BS, Worley SJ, Samaha JK, Phillips III H, Califf RM, and the TAMI-5 Study Group. Determinants of the need for early acute intervention in patients treated conservatively after thrombolytic therapy for acute myocardial infarction. J Am Coll Cardiol 1991 (December);18:1594–01.

76. Mark DB, Sigmon K, Topol EJ, Kereiakes DJ, Pryor DB, Candela RJ, Califf RM: Identification of Acute Myocardial Infarction Patients Suitable for Early Hospital Discharge After Aggressive Interventional Therapy-Results from the Thrombolysis and Angioplasty in Acute Myocardial Infarction Registry. Circulation 1991; (April) 83:1186–1193.

77. Muller DWM, Topol EJ, Ellis SG, Sigmon KN, Lee K, Califf RM, and the Thrombolysis and Angioplasty in Myocardial Infarction (TAMI) Study Group: Multivessel coronary artery disease: A key predictor of short-term prognosis after reperfusion therapy for acute myocardial infarction. Am Heart J 1991 (April);121:1042–1049.

78. Sheehan FH, Thery C, Durand P, Bertrand ME, Bolson EL: Early beneficial effect of streptokinase on left ventricular function in acute myocardial infarction. Am J Cardiol 1991 (Mar 15);67:555–558.

79. Peuhkurinen KJ, Risteli L, Melkko JT, Linnaluoto M, Jounela A, Risteli J: Thrombolytic Therapy With Streptokinase Stimulates Collagen Breakdown. Circulation 1991; (June) 83:1969–1975.

80. Nielsen FE, Sorennsen HG, Christensen JH, Ravn L, Rasmussen SE: Reduced occurrence of atrial fibrillation in acute myocardial infarction treated with streptokinase. Eur Heart J 1991 (Nov);12:1081–1083.

81. Grip L, Ryden L: Late streptokinase infusion and antithrombotic treatment in myocardial infarction reduce subsequent myocardial ischemia. Am Heart J 1991 (March);121:737–745.

82. Davies SW, Marchant B, Lyons JP, Timmis AD, Rothman MT, Layton CA, Balcon R: Irregular coronary lesion morphology after thrombolysis predicts early clinical instability. J Am Coll Cardiol 1991 (September);18:669–74.

83. Voth E, Tebbe U, Schicha H, Neuhaus K, Schröder R, and the I.S.A.M. Study Group: Intravenous streptokinase in acute myocardial infarction (I.S.A.M.) trial: serial evaluation of left ventricular function up to 3 years after infarction estimated by radionuclide ventriculography. J Am Coll Cardiol 1991 (December);18:1610–6.

84. Sherry S, Marder VJ: Streptokinase and recombinant tissue plasminogen activator (rt-PA) are equally effective in treating acute myocardial infarction. An Intern Med 1991 (Mar 1);114:417–423.

85. Cross DB, Ashton NG, Norris RM, White HD: Comparison of the effects of streptokinase and tissue plasminogen activator on regional wall motion after first myocardial infarction: analysis by the centerline method with correction for area at risk. J Am Coll Cardiol 1991 (April);17:1039–46.

86. Grines CL, Nissen SE, Booth DC, Gurley JC, Chelliah N, Wolf R, Blankenship J, Branco MC, Bennett K, DeMaria AN, and the Kentucky Acute Myocardial Infarction Trial (KAMIT) Group: A Prospective, Randomized Trial Comparing Combination Half-Dose Tissue-Type Plasminogen Activator and Streptokinase With Full-Dose Tissue-Type Plasminogen Activator. Circulation (August);84:540–549.

87. Bassand J-P, Cassagnes J, Machecourt J, Lusson J-R, Anguenot T, Wolf J-E, Maublant J, Bertrand B, Schiele F: Comparative Effects of APSAC and rt-PA on Infarct Size and Left Ventricular Function in Acute Myocardial Infarction - A Multicenter Randomized Study. Circulation 1991 (September);84:1107–1117.

88. Belkin RN, Mark DB, Aronson L, Szwed H, Califf RM, Kisslo J: Pericardial effusion after intravenous recombinant tissue-type plasminogen activator for acute myocardial infarction. Am J Cardiol 1991 (Mar 1);67:496–500.

89. Rogers WJ, Babb JD, Baim DS, Chesebro JH, Gore JM, Roberts R, Williams DO, Frederick M, Passamani ER, Braunwald E, for the TIMI II Investigators. Selective versus routine predischarge coronary arteriography after therapy with recombinant tissue-type plasminogen activator, heparin and aspirin for acute myocardial infarction. J Am Coll Cardiol 1991 (April);17:1007–16.

90. Little T, Crenshaw M, Liberman HA, Battey LL, Warner R, Churchwell AL, Eisner RL, Morris DC, Patterson RE: Effects of time required for reperfusion (thrombolysis or angioplasty, Am J Cardiol 1990 (Apr 15);67:797–805.

91. Thompson PL, Aylward PE, Federman J, Giles RW, Harris PJ, Hodge RL, Nelson GIC, Thomson A, Tonkin AM, and Walsh WF, for the National Heart Foundation of Australia Coronary Thrombolysis Group: A Randomized Comparison of Intravenous Heparin With Oral Aspirin and Dipyridamole 24 Hours After Recombinant Tissue-Type Plasminogen Activator for Acute Myocardial Infarction. Circulation 1991; (May) 83:1534–1542.

92. Morgan CD, Roberts RS, Haq A, Baigrie RS, Daly PA, Gent M, Armstrong PW, for the TPAT Study Group: Coronary patency, infarct size and left ventricular function after thrombolytic therapy for acute myocardial infarction: Results from the tissue plasminogen activator: Toronto (TPAT) Placebo-controlled Trial. J Am Coll Cardiol 1991; 17:1451–7.

93. Henzlova MJ, Bourge RC, Papapietro SE, Maske LE, Morgan TE, Tauxe EL, Rogers WJ: Long-term effect of thrombolytic therapy on left ventricular ejection fraction after acute myocardial infarction. Am J Cardiol 1991 (June 15);67:1354–1359.

94. Motro M, Barbash GI, Hod H, Roth A, Kaplinsky E, Laniado S, Keren G: Incidence of left ventricular thrombi formation after thrombolytic therapy with recombinant tissue plasminogen activator, heparin, and aspirin in patients with acute myocardial infarction. Am Heart J 1991 (July);122:23–26.

95. Munkvad S, Jespersen J, Gram J, Kluft C: Depression of factor XII-dependent fibrinolytic activity characterizes patients with early myocardial reinfarction after recombinant tissue-type plasminogen activator therapy. J Am Coll Cardiol 1991 (August);18: 454–8.

96. Bovill EG, Terrin ML, Stump DC, Berke AD, Frederick M, Collen D, Feit F, Gore JM, Hillis LD, Lambrew CT, Leiboff R, Mann KG, Markis JE, Pratt CM, Sharkey SW, Sopko G, Tracy RP, Chesebro JH: Hemorrhagic events during therapy with recombinant tissue-type plasminogen activator, heparin, and aspirin for acute myocardial infarction: Results of the thrombolysis in myocardial infarction (TIMI), Phase II Trial. An Int Med 1991 (Aug 15);115:256–265.

97. Bhatnagar SK, Al-Yusuf AR: Effects of intravenous recombinant tissue-type plasminogen activator therapy on the incidence and associations of left ventricular thrombus in patients with a first acute Q wave anterior myocardial infarction. Am Heart J 1991 (November);122:1251–1256.

98. Aguirre FV, Kern MJ, Hsia J, Serota H, Janosik D, Greenwalt T, Ross AM, Chaitman BR: Importance of myocardial infarct artery patency on the prevalence of ventricular arrhythmia and late potentials after thrombolysis in acute myocardial infarction. Am J Cardiol 1991 (Dec 1);68:1410–1416.

99. McKendall GR, Attubato MJ, Drew TM, Feit F, Sharaf BL, Thomas ES, Teichman S, McDonald MJ, Williams DO: Safety and efficacy of a new regimen of intravenous recombinant tissue-type plasminogen activator potentially suitable for either pre-hospital or in-hospital administration. J Am Coll Cardiol 1991 (December);18: 1774–8.

100. Wilcox RG, Eastgate J, Harrison E, Skene AM: Ventricular arrhythmias during treatment with alteplase (recombinant tissue plasminogen activator) in suspected acute myocardial infarction. Br Heart J 1991 (Jan);65:4–8.

101. Purvis JA, Trouton TG, Roberts MJD, McKeown P, Mulholland MG, Dalzell GWN, Wilson CM, Patterson GC, Webb SW, Kahn MM, Campbell NPS, Adgey AAJ: Effectiveness of double bolus alteplase in the treatment of acute myocardial infarction. Am J Cardiol 1991 (Dec 15);68:1570–1574.

102. SWIFT: SWIFT trial of delayed elective intervention vs conservative treatment after thrombolysis with anistreplase in acute myocardial infarction. Br Med J 1991 (Mar 9);302:555–560.

103. Relik-Vanwely L, Visser RF, Van Der Pol MJ, Bartholomeus I, Couvee JE, Drost H, Vet AJTM, Klomps HC, Van Ekelen WAAJ, Van Den Berg F, Krauss XH: Angiographically assessed coronary arterial patency and reocclusion in patients with acute myocardial infarction treated with anistreplase: Results of the anistreplase reocclusion multi-center study (ARMS). Am J Cardiol 1991 (Aug 1);68:296–300.

104. Karacounis L, Moreno F, Menlove RL, Ipsen S, Anderson JL, Team-2 Investigators: Effects of early thrombolytic therapy (anistreplase versus streptokinase) on enzymatic and electrocardiographic infarct size in acute myocardial infarction. Am J Cardiol 1991 (Oct 1);68:848–856.

105. Rossi P, Bolognese L: Comparison of intravenous urokinase plus heparin versus heparin alone in acute myocardial infarction. Am J Cardiol 1991 (Sept 1);68:585–592.

106. Von Hodenberg E, Kreuzer J, Hautmann M, Nordt T, Kubler W, Bode C: Effects of lipoprotein (a) on success rate of thrombolytic therapy in acute myocardial infarction. Am J Cardiol 1991 (June 15);67:1349–1353.

107. Kirshenbaum JM, Bahr RD, Flaherty JT, Gurewich V, Levine HJ, Loscalzo J, Schumacher RR, Topol EJ, Wahr DW, Braunwald E, Pro-Urokinase For Myocardial Infarction Study Group: Clot-selective coronary thrombolysis with low-dose synergistic combinations of single-chain urokinase-type plasminogen activator and recombinant tissue-type plasminogen activator. Am J Cardiol 1991 (Dec 15);68:1564–1569.

108. Morris JA, Muller DWM, Topol EJ: Combination thrombolytic therapy: A comparison of simultaneous and sequential regimens of tissue plasminogen activator and uro-kinase. Am Heart J 1991 (August);122:375–380.

109. Popma JJ, Topol EJ: Adjuncts to thrombolysis for myocardial reperfusion. An Intern Med 1991 (July 1);115:34–44.

110. Ohman DM, Califf RM, George BS, Quigley PL, Kereiakes LH, Harrelson-Woodlief L, Candela RJ, Flanagan C, Stack RS, Topol EJ: The use of intraaortic balloon pumping as an adjunct to reperfusion therapy in acute myocardial infarction. Am Heart J 1991 (March);121:895–901.

111. Maggioni AP, Franzosi MG, Farina ML, Santoro E, Celani MG, Ricci S, Tognoni G: Cerebralvascular events after myocardial infarction: Analysis of the GISSI trial. Br Med J 1991 (June 15);302:1428–1431.

112. Anderson JL, Karagounis L, Allen A, Bradford MJ, Menlove RL, Pryor TA: Older age and elevated blood pressure are risk factors for intracerebral hemorrhage after thrombolysis. Am J Cardiol 1991 (July 15);68:166–170.

113. Arnold AER, Serruys PW, Rutsch W, Simoons ML, De Bono DP, Tijssen JGP, Lubsen J, Verstraete M, for the European Cooperative Study Group: Reasons for the lack of benefit of immediate angioplasty during recombinant tissue plasminogen activator therapy for acute myocardial infarction: a regional wall motion analysis. J Am Coll Cardiol 1991 (January);17:11–21.

114. Brodie BR, Weintraub RA, Stuckey TD, Lebauer EJ, Katz JD, Kelly TA, Hansen CJ: Outcomes of direct coronary angioplasty for acute myocardial infarction in candidates and non-candidates for thrombolytic therapy. Am J Cardiol 1991 (Jan 1);67:7–12.

115. Lee L, Erbel R, Brown TM, Laufer N, Meyer J, O'Neill WW: Multicenter registry of angioplasty therapy of cardiogenic shock: initial and long-term survival. J Am Coll Cardiol 1991 (March);17:599–603.

116. Ghitis A, Flaker GC, Meinhardt S, Grouws M, Anderson SK, Webel RR: Early angioplasty in patients with acute myocardial infarction complicated by hypotension. Am Heart J 1991 (August);122:380–384.

117. Klein LW, Kramer BL, Howard E, Lesch M: Incidence and clinical significance of transient creatine kinase elevations and the diagnosis of non-Q wave myocardial infarction associated with coronary angioplasty. J Am Coll Cardiol 1991 (March);17:621–6.

118. Forman MB, Perry JM, Wilson BH, Verani MS, Kaplan PR, Shawl, FA, Friesinger GC: Demonstration of myocardial reperfusion injury in humans: Results of a pilot study utilizing acute coronary angioplasty with perfluorochemical in anterior myocardial infarction. J Am Coll Cardiol 1991 (October);18:911–8.

119. Kereiakes DJ, Califf RM, George BS, Ellis S, Samaha J, Stack R, Martin LH, Young S, Topol EJ and the TAMI Study Group: Coronary bypass surgery improves global and regional left ventricular function following thrombolytic therapy for acute myocardial infarction. Am Heart J 1991 (August);122:390–399.

4

Arrhythmias, Conduction Disturbances, and Cardiac Arrest

THE "SICILIAN GAMBIT"

The Queen's Gambit is an opening move in chess that provides a variety of aggressive options to the player electing it. The Task Force of the Working Group on Arrhythmias of the European Society of Cardiology[1] report represents a similar gambit (the "Sicilian Gambit") on the part of a group of basic and clinical investigators who met in Taormina, Sicily, to consider the classification of antiarrhythmic drugs. Paramount to their considerations were (1) dissatisfaction with the options offered by existing classification systems for inspiring and directing research, development and therapy (Table 4-1), (2) the disarray on the field of antiarrhythmic drug development and testing in this post-CAST era, and (3) the desire to provide an operational framework for consideration of antiarrhythmic drugs that will both encourage advancement and have the plasticity to grow as a result of the advances that occur. The multifaceted approach suggested is a gambit. It is an opening rather than a compendium, and is intended to challenge thought and investigation rather than to resolve issues. The manuscript incorporates first, a discussion of the shortcomings of the present system for drug classification; second, a review of the molecular targets on which drugs act (including channels and receptors) (Figures 4-1, 4-2, and 4-3); third, a consideration of the mechanisms responsible for arrhythmias, including the identification of "vulnerable pa-

254

TABLE 4-1. *Vaughan Williams classification of antiarrhythmic drugs.* Reproduced with permission from European Heart Journal.[1]

	Class I	Class II	Class III	Class IV
	Drugs with direct membrane action (Na channel blockade)	Sympatholytic Drugs	Drugs which prolong repolarization	Calcium channel blocking drugs
IA	Depress phase 0 Slow conduction Prolong repolarization			
IB	Little effect on phase 0 in normal tissue Depress phase 0 in abnormal fibers Shorten repolarization			
IC	Markedly depress phase 0 Markedly slow conduction Slight effect on repolarization			

*This is the classification as modified by Harrison and others.

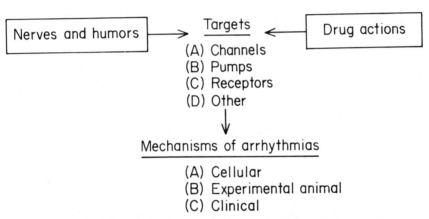

Fig. 4-1. Elements for a classification system. Reprinted with permission from European Heart Journal.[1]

rameters" that might be most accessible to drug effect; and finally, clinical considerations with respect to antiarrhythmic drugs. Information relating to the various levels of information is correlated across categories (i.e., clinical arrhythmias, cellular mechanisms and molecular targets), and a "spread sheet" approach to antiarrhythmic action is presented that considers each drug as a unit, with similarities to and dissimilarities from other drugs being highlighted.

ATRIAL FIBRILLATION/FLUTTER

Stroke prevention

Randomized controlled trials have demonstrated that anticoagulant therapy is very effective at preventing stroke among patients with non-

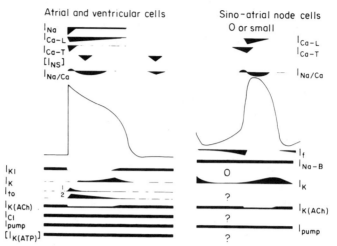

Fig. 4-2. The currents and channels involved in generating the resting and action potential. The time course of a stylized action potential of atrial and ventricular cells is shown on the left, and of sino-atrial node cells on the right. Above and below are the various channels and pumps that contribute the currents underlying the electrical events. See text for identification of the symbols and description of the channels or currents. Where possible, the approximate time courses of the currents associated with the channels or pumps are shown symbolically; their magnitudes relative to each other are not represented. The heavy bars for I c1, I pump, and I K(ATP) only indicate the presence of these channels or pumps, without implying magnitude of currents, since that would vary with physiological and pathophysiological conditions. The channels identified by brackets (Ins and IK[ATP]) imply that they are active only under pathological conditions. For the sino-atrial node cells, I Na and I K1 are small or absent (?) indicates that experimental evidence is not yet available to determine the presence of these channels in sino-atrial cell membranes. Although, it is likely that other ionic current mechanisms exist, they are not shown here because their roles in electrogenesis are not sufficiently well defined. Reprinted with permission of the European Heart Journal.[1]

rheumatic AF. These trials have reported too few strokes for powerful risk factor analysis. Moulton and associates[2] from Providence, Rhode Island, and Boston, Massachusetts, identified all patients discharged from 1 hospital over an 8-year period who met their definition of nonrheumatic AF and ischemic stroke (n = 134), and compared them with contemporaneous control subjects who were discharged with nonrheumatic AF without stroke (n = 131). Cases and controls were similar in terms of duration of AF; proportion with paroxysmal AF; percentage with a past medical history of angina, myocardial infarction, CHF, diabetes, or smoking; and mean left atrial size. In contrast, cases were significantly older than controls (78.5 vs 74.8 years) and more likely to have a history of hypertension (55% vs 38%). The relative odds for stroke was 1.91 for patients with hypertension, 1.73 for patients older than 75 years, and 3.26 for patients with both factors. The authors suggest that age and hypertension should be considered when deciding upon long-term anticoagulant therapy to prevent stroke in patients with nonrheumatic AF.

AF in the absence of rheumatic valvular disease is associated with a 5-fold to 7-fold increased risk of ischemic stroke. In Stroke Prevention in AF Study, a multicenter randomized trial, collaborating investigators[3] in Seattle, Washington, compared 325 mg/day aspirin or warfarin with placebo for prevention of ischemic stroke and systemic embolism and in-

Drug	Channels Na Fast	Na Medium	Na Slow	Ca	K	I$_f$	Receptors α	β	M$_2$	P	Pumps Na K ATPase
Lidocaine	○										
Mexiletine	○										
Tocainide	○										
Moricizine	●										
Procainamide		A			○						
Disopyramide		A			○			○			
Quinidine		A			○		○	○			
Propafenone		A						○			
Flecainide			A		○						
Encainide			A								
Bepridil	○			●	○						
Verapamil	○			●			○				
Diltiazem				○							
Bretylium					●		◐	◐			
Sotalol					●			●			
Amiodarone	○			○	●		○	○			
Alinidine					○	●					
Nadolol								●			
Propranolol	○							●			
Atropine									●		
Adenosine										○	
Digoxin									○		●

Fig. 4-3. This figure summarizes the potentially most important actions of drugs on membrane channels, receptors and ionic pumps in the heart. Included in this table are examples of drugs used to modify cardiac rhythm. Most of these drugs are already marketed as antiarrhythmic agents, but some are not yet approved for this purpose. The drugs (rows) are ordered in a fashion similar to the columns so that, in general, the entries for their predominant action(s) form a diagonal. However, drugs with multiple actions, e.g., amiodarone, depart strikingly from the diagonal trend. The actions of the drugs on the sodium (Na), calcium (Ca) potassium (IK) and i, channels are indicated. Sodium channel blockade is subdivided into three groups of actions characterized by fast (tau <300 ms), medium (tau = 200–1500 ms) and slow (tau >1500 ms) time constants for recovery from block. This parameter is a measure of use dependence and predicts the likelihood that a drug will decrease conduction velocity of normal sodium-dependent tissues in the heart and perhaps the propensity of a drug for causing bundle branch block or proarrhythmia. The rate constant for onset of block might be even more clinically relevant. Blockage in the inactivated (I) or activated (A) state is indicated. Information on the state dependency of the block due to moricizine, propefonone, ecainide and flecainide is especially limited and may be altered with additional research. Drug interaction with receptors alpha (a), beta (B), muscarinic subtype 2 (M) and A purinergic (P) and drug effects on the sodium potassium pump (Na-KATPase) are indicated. Filled circles indicate direct or indirect acting agonists or stimulators. The intensity of the action is indicated by the various shadings as described below. Half-filled circles for bretylium indicate its biphasic action to initially stimulate a and B receptors by release of norepinephrine followed by subsequent block of norepinephrine release and indirect antagonism of these receptors. Relative blocking Potency ◔ = low ● = moderate; ● = high; ○ = agonist; ◑ = agonist, antagonist; A = activated state blockers; I = inactivated state blocker. Reprinted with permission of the European Heart Journal.[1]

cluded 1,330 inpatients and outpatients with constant or intermittent AF. During a mean follow-up of 1.3 years, the rate of primary events in patients assigned to placebo was 6% per year and was reduced by 42% in those assigned to aspirin. In the subgroup of warfarin-eligible patients (most of whom were less than 76 years old), warfarin dose-adjusted to prolong prothrombin time to 1.3-fold to 1.8-fold that of control reduced the risk of primary events by 67%. Primary events or death were reduced 58% by warfarin and 32% by aspirin. The risk of significant bleeding was 1.5%, 1.4%, and 1.6% per year in patients assigned to warfarin, aspirin, and placebo, respectively. Aspirin and warfarin are both effective in reducing ischemic stroke and systemic embolism in patients with AF. Because warfarin-eligible patients composed a subset of all aspirin-eligible patients, the magnitude of reduction in events by warfarin versus aspirin cannot be compared. Too few events occurred in warfarin-eligible patients to directly assess the relative benefit of aspirin compared with warfarin, and the trial is continuing to address this issue. Patients with nonrheumatic AF who can safely take either aspirin or warfarin should receive prophylactic antithrombotic therapy to reduce the risk of stroke.

Connolly and colleagues[4] in Hamilton, Ontario, Canada, randomized 187 patients to warfarin and 191 patients to placebo to determine the potential of warfarin to reduce systemic thromboembolism in patients with AF. The primary outcome of these events were nonlacunar strokes, noncentral nervous systemic embolism and fatal or intracranial hemorrhage. Events were included in the primary analysis of efficacy if they occurred within 28 days of discontinuation of the study medication. Annual rates of the primary outcome event cluster were 3.5% in warfarin-treated and 5.2% in placebo-treated patients with a relative risk reduction of 37% (Figure 4-4). Fatal or major bleeding occurred at annual rates of 2.5% in warfarin-treated and 0.5% in placebo-treated patients. Minor

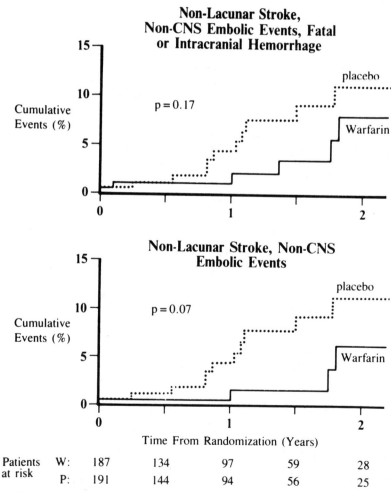

Fig. 4-4. Cumulative rate of events for the two event clusters. CNS = central nervous system; P = placebo; W = warfarin. Reproduced with permission from Connolly, et al.[4]

bleeding occurred in 16% of patients receiving warfarin and 9% of patients receiving placebo. In the warfarin-treated patients, the international normalized ratio was in the target range 44% of the study days, above it 17% of the study days, and below it 40% of the study days. The study was stopped early before completion of its planned recruitment of 630 patients. The data are consistent with a protective effect of warfarin in patients with chronic AF who were without mitral valve or aortic valve prostheses and who had no evidence of MS.

Albers and associates[5] participating in a symposium at Stanford, California, examined 4 large, prospective, randomized trials on the risk and benefits of warfarin therapy for stroke prophylaxis in patients with non-valvular AF (Figure 4-5). All 4 studies showed a substantially reduced risk of stroke and a low incidence of significant bleeding in patients treated with warfarin. One of these studies also showed that aspirin reduced the incidence of stroke. The benefits associated with long-term low-dose warfarin therapy appear to exceed the risks for serious bleeding in most patients with AF. Aspirin may be a viable therapeutic option for patients who are unable to take warfarin or for those in subgroups at a low risk for stroke.

Diltiazem

Ellenbogen and colleagues[6] in Richmond, Virginia; Kansas City, Missouri; Birmingham, Alabama; Loma Linda, California and Memphis, Tennessee, evaluated the safety and efficacy of a 10 to 15 mg/h infusion of intravenous diltiazem in 47 patients with atrial fibrillation or flutter. Forty-four patients responded to the bolus injection and were randomized to double-blind continuous infusion of intravenous diltiazem or placebo for up to 24 hours. A therapeutic response was stated to occur when heart rate decreased to <100 beats/minute, there was a ≥20 beat/minute decrease in heart rate, or conversion to sinus rhythm occurred. Seventeen (74%) of the 23 patients receiving diltiazem infusion and none of the 21 with placebo infusion maintained a therapeutic response for 24 hours.

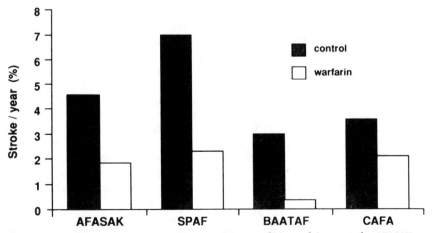

Fig. 4-5. Stroke prevention in patients receiving warfarin and in controls. AFASAK = Copenhagen Atrial Fibrillation, Aspirin, Anticoagulation study; SPAF = Stroke Prevention in Atrial Fibrillation study; BAATAF = Boston Area Anticoagulation Trial for Atrial Fibrillation; CAFA = Canadian Atrial Fibrillation Anticoagulation study. Reprinted with permission of Albers, et al.[5]

Over 24 hours, patients receiving diltiazem infusion lost response significantly more slowly than did those receiving placebo. Nonresponders to the double-blind infusion were given an additional bolus injection of open label intravenous diltiazem and administered an open label 24 hour intravenous diltiazem infusion. The overall proportion of patients maintaining a response to a 24-hour infusion of intravenous diltiazem under double-blind or open label conditions combined was 83%. Efficacy of the 24 hour infusion of intravenous diltiazem was similar in elderly versus young patients, those who did versus those who did not receive digoxin, and those weighing <84 versus ≥84 kg. Intravenous diltiazem appeared to be more effective in patients with atrial fibrillation than those with atrial flutter. No serious side effects were noted. Thus, a bolus dose or doses followed by a 24 hour infusion of diltiazem can be safely administered to patients with atrial fibrillation or flutter and can rapidly and effectively achieve and maintain heart rate control in most patients.

Flecainide

Spontaneous reversion to sinus rhythm is a frequent occurrence in recent-onset AF. In a randomized, double-blind, controlled study, Donovan and associates[7] from Perth, Australia, compared intravenous flecainide (2 mg/kg, maximum dose 150 mg) with placebo in the treatment of recent onset AF (present for ≥30 minutes and ≤72 hours' duration and a ventricular response ≥120 beats/minute). Intravenous digoxin (500 μg) was administered concurrently to all patients in both groups who had not previously taken digoxin. The trial medication was administered over 30 minutes. One hundred two consecutive patients with recent-onset AF were enrolled in the study. All patients underwent continuous electrocardiographic monitoring in the intensive care or coronary care unit. Twenty-nine (57%) patients given flecainide and digoxin, but only 7 (14%) given placebo and digoxin, reverted to sinus rhythm in ≤1 hour after starting the trial mediction infusion and remained in stable sinus rhythm. At the end of the 6-hour monitoring period, 34 patients (67%) in the flecainide-digoxin group were in stable sinus rhythm, whereas only 18 patients (35%) in the placebo-digoxin group had reverted. Severe hypotension, although transient, was more common in the flecainide-digoxin group. Flecainide is effective in reverting recent-onset AF, but should not be given to patients with severe LV dysfunction because the risks may outweigh the potential benefits of reversion to sinus rhythm.

To evaluate the efficacy of flecainide acetate in the prevention of paroxysmal AF and atrial flutter, Pietersen and associates[8] for the Danish-Norwegian Flecainide Multicenter study group randomized blindly 43 patients (23 men) (mean age 53 years) to receive either placebo or 150 mg of flecainide twice per day for consecutive periods of 3 months. Attacks were verified by a minielectrocardiogram event recorder. If intolerable symptoms developed, the protocol allowed patients to cross over between treatments before the end of the first 3-month period. Four patients crossed over prematurely, between 1 week and 1 month, and 15 between 1 month and 3 months. The remaining 24 patients completed both 3-month periods. In all 3 treatment intervals, there was a significant reduction in the number of attacks during flecainide treatment. Complete suppression was seen in 15 of 43 patients (35%) treated with flecainide for 1 week, in 18 of 39 (46%) treated for 1 month and in 12 of 24 (50%) completing all 3 months in each period. Adverse effects were reported in 32 of the 43 patients (74%) treated with flecainide, but only 2 were withdrawals. One patient died suddenly. In comparison, 3 of 43 patients (7%) reported adverse effects in the placebo group. In conclusion, flecainide significantly suppressed the number of attacks of paroxysmal atrial fibrillation and flutter. Adverse effects were frequent but were mostly tolerable.

Cardioversion

Van Gelder and associates[9] from Groningen, the Netherlands, undertook a study to reassess prospectively the immediate and long-term results of direct-current electrical cardioversion in chronic AF or atrial flutter, and to determine factors predicting clinical outcome of the arrhythmia after direct-current cardioversion. Two-hundred forty-six patients underwent direct-current electrical cardioversion and were followed during a mean of 260 days. Multivariate analysis was used to identify factors predicting short- and long-term arrhythmia outcome. Cardioversion was achieved in 70% of patients with AF and in 96% of patients with atrial flutter. Stepwise logistic regression analysis revealed that arrhythmia duration, type of arrhythmia (fibrillation vs flutter) and age independently influenced conversion rate. On an actuarial basis, 42 and 36% of patients remained in sinus rhythm during 1 and 2 years, respectively. Multivariate regression analysis revealed that the type of arrhythmia, low precardioversion functional class and the presence of nonrheumatic mitral valve disease independently increased the length of the arrhythmia-free episode. Rheumatic heart disease shortened this period. In conclusion, patients having a high probability of conversion together with a prolonged post-shock arrhythmia-free episode can be identified.

Surgical treatment

Cox and associates[10] from St. Louis, Missouri, used multipoint computerized electrophysiological mapping systems to map both experimental and human AF (Figure 4-6). On the basis of these studies, a new surgical procedure was developed for AF. Between September 25, 1987, and July 1, 1991, this procedure was applied in 22 patients with paroxysmal atrial flutter (n = 2), paroxysmal AF (n = 11), or chronic AF (n = 9) of 2 to 21 years' duration. All patients were refractory to all antiarrhythmic medications, and each patient failed to receive the desired therapeutic benefits of an average of 5 drugs administered preoperatively. There were no operative deaths and all perioperative morbidity resolved. All 22 patients have been successfully treated for AF with surgery alone. Three patients developed 1 late isolated episode of atrial flutter at 5, 6, and 15 months postoperatively, and each of these patient's symptoms is now controlled by a single antiarrhythmic drug. Preservation of atrial transport function has been documented in all patients postoperatively, and all have experienced marked clinical improvement.

SUPRAVENTRICULAR TACHYCARDIA WITH OR WITHOUT SHORT P-R INTERVAL SYNDROME

Causing syncope

Auricchio and colleagues[11] in Hannover, Federal Republic of Germany, evaluated 36 patients who had reported the occurrence of one or more

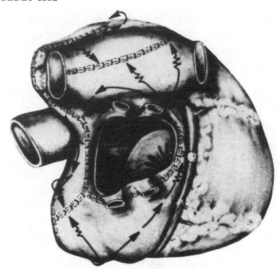

Fig. 4-6. Three-dimensional depiction of the incisions used for performing the maze procedure. Note the presence of the transmural cryolesion (white dot) of the coronary sinus at the site of the posterior left atriotomy. Both atrial appendages have been excised. The only completely solitude portion of the atrium are the orifices of the pulmonary veins. The impulse originates from the region of the SAN and can escape from that region only by passing inferiorly and anteriorly around the base of the right atrium. The impulse continues to propagate around the anterior right atrium onto the top of the interatrial septum. There, it bifurcates into two wave fronts, one passing through the septum in an anterior-to-posterior direction to activate the posteriormedial right and left atria, and the other continuing around the base of the excised left atrial appendage to activate the posterolateral left atrial wall. In this manner, all atrial myocardium, except the pulmonary vein orifices, is activated. The activation of this atrial myocardium is fundamental to the preservation of atrial transport function postoperatively. Reprinted with permission of Cox, et al.[10]

syncopal episodes (group 1) and 65 patients who had no syncope (group 2) with the W-P-W syndrome. These two groups did not differ with regard to age, gender, incidence and characteristics of arrhythmia, clinical history, frequency of arrhythmic events, and presence of associated cardiac disease. There were 10 patients in group 1 and 12 in group 2 who had VF. There were no statistical differences between the 2 groups with respect to the effective refractory period of the right atrium, A-V node, accessory pathway and right ventricle. There were no differences between the 2 groups with respect to cycle length of circus movement tachycardia, mean heart rate during AF, and minimum RR interval during AF. Accessory pathway location was not significantly different between group 1 and 2 patients. The occurrence of syncope could not be predicted from any electrophysiologic finding and this symptom had a low sensitivity and specificity for recognition of dangerous rapid heart rates. Prognostic value of syncope was less accurate and predictive than the shortest RR interval during AF and the anterograde effective refractory period of the accessory pathway for aborted sudden death occurrence. These data indicate that syncope is a relatively common clinical finding in patients with W-P-W syndrome referred for electrophysiologic testing and its occurrence does not identify patients with an increased risk for sudden death.

Flecainide

Allan and associates[12] from London, UK, reported treatment of fetal atrial tachycardia associated with intrauterine cardiac failure in 14 mothers. Conversion to sinus rhythm occurred in 12 of 14 but 1 fetus subsequently died in utero. The remaining fetuses suffered no morbidity and were well 3 months to 2 years after delivery. The 2 fetuses in whom tachycardia did not convert with flecainide were successfully treated with digoxin. Flecainide was stopped after conversion to sinus rhythm in 5 of 12 patients but a second dose or continued flecainide until delivery was required in 4 of 5. Comparison of cord and maternal serum concentrations of flecainide indicated placental transfer of approximately 80% of the drug. These authors report excellent control of fetal atrial tachycardia in the majority of patients in a relatively short period of time. In general, it should be considered a second line drug for use for fetal CHF when digoxin does not result in conversion to sinus rhythm.

Pritchett and colleagues[13] for the Flecainide Supraventricular Tachycardia Study Group evaluated the dose-response relations for efficacy and tolerance of the antiarrhythmic drug, flecainide acetate in 28 patients with paroxysmal SVT (Group 1) and 45 patients with paroxysmal atrial fibrillation of flutter (Group 2). Recurrent symptomatic tachycardia was documented with the use of transtelephonic electrocardiographic recording. Patients received flecainide in doses of 25, 50, 100 and 150 mg twice daily and placebo for 1 month treatment periods. Among 14 patients in Group 1 who qualified for efficacy analysis, 4 (29%) had no tachycardia while taking placebo. The number with no tachycardia increased with progressively larger flecainide doses so that with 150 mg dose twice daily, 12 of 14 patients had no tachycardia. Among 28 patients in Group 2, 2 (7%) had no tachycardia while taking placebo. The number with no tachycardia also increased with progressively larger flecainide doses so that with 150 mg twice daily dose, 17 (61%) of 28 patients had no tachycardia. Noncardiac adverse experiences were the leading cause of premature study discontinuation during flecainide treatment and resulted in five patients in Group 1 and six patients in Group 2 discontinuing the drug.

In a recent clinical trial, the class lc antiarrhythmic drugs encainide and flecainide were found to be associated with an increased mortality risk in patients with new AMI and ventricular arrhythmias. In the present study Pritchett and Wilkinson[14] from Durham, North Carolina, assessed whether an increased mortality risk also accompanied the use of these drugs to treat patients with supraventricular arrhythmias. Data were obtained from the respective pharmaceutical sponsors on the mortality observed with each drug in United States and foreign protocols enrolling patients with supraventricular arrhythmias. Mortality in the encainide population (343 patients) and the flecainide population (236 patients) was compared with that in a research arrhythmic clinic, the Duke population (154 patients). Nine deaths occurred in the combined encainide-flecainide population and 10 deaths occurred in the Duke population; the follow-up periods averaged 488 days and 1,285 days, respectively. The 6-year survival functions of these 2 populations, estimated by the Kaplan-Meier technique, did not differ significantly. The hazard ratio for the combined encainide-flecainide population relative to the Duke population was estimated to be 0.6. These descriptive comparisons did not demonstrate any excess mortality when flecainide and encainide were used in patients with supraventricular arrhythmias.

Adenosine

Several groups have suggested the use of intravenous adenosine or adenosine triphosphate in the diagnosis of regular broad complex tachycardias. The short half-life of these agents has precluded assessment of their effects on refractoriness of accessory connections, and their safety in preexcited arrhythmias has not been demonstrated. Garratt and coworkers[15] in London, UK, examined the effects of intravenous adenosine on accessory AV connections in 30 patients with WPW syndrome. Intravenous adenosine (12 mg, rapid bolus) was administered to 14 patients (group 1) during continuous atrial pacing at a cycle length 20 msec below that required to cause 2:1 conduction block in the accessory connection. After adenosine, transient 1:1 conduction occurred via the accessory connection in 12 of 14 patients, indicating a shortening of antegrade refractoriness. In 3 of 7 patients, this effect was abolished after intravenous propranol. Nineteen patients (group 2) received adenosine during induced, preexcited atrial arrhythmias. The minimum RR interval during preexcited AF transiently decreased after adenosine, but no change in average RR interval was observed. The preexcited ventricular response to atrial flutter was transiently accelerated in 5 of 8 patients due to shortening of flutter cycle length. However, 2:1 accessory connection conduction was maintained in all 8 patients. All effects were short lived, with the decrease in RR intervals during AF occurring for a maximum of 2 RR intervals only. No patient suffered ventricular arrhythmias or hemodynamic deterioration. Adenosine shortens antegrade refractoriness of accessory AV connections, and in some patients this action is mediated by B-adrenergic stimulation. Adenosine may cause acceleration of preexcited atrial arrhythmias, but these effects are transient and should not discourage the use of adenosine as a diagnostic agent in broad complex, regular tachycardias of uncertain origin.

An excellent review of the usefulness of adenosine and supraventricular tachycardia was provided by Camm and Garrett[16] in the December 5, 1991, issue of *The New England Journal of Medicine*.

Propafenone

To test the hypothesis that propafenone orally prevents symptomatic paroxysmal supraventricular arrhythmias, Pritchett and associates[17] from Durham, North Carolina, enrolled 33 patients with either SVT (n = 16) or paroxysmal AF (n = 17). Their arrhythmias were documented by electrocardiogram before enrollment. Twenty-three patients (14 with paroxysmal supraventricular tachycardia and 9 with paroxysmal AF) were randomized and the data obtained from these patients were used in the efficacy analysis. Propafenone (300 mg 3 times daily in 19 patients, 300 mg twice daily in 3 patients, and 150 mg twice daily in 1 patient) and matching placebo tablets were administered in a randomized sequence. Symptomatic arrhythmia was documented by telephone transmission of the electrocardiogram. The time to first recurrence was prolonged for the overall group of 23 patients while they received propafenone. The recurrence rate of arrhythmia during treatment with propafenone was estimated to be approximately one fifth of the recurrence rate during treatment with placebo. Propafenone is effective in reducing symptomatic paroxysmal supraventricular arrhythmias.

Catheter ablation

Van Hare and associates[18] from San Francisco, California, performed 19 catheter ablation procedures in 17 children, aged 10 months to 17 years for the management of malignant or drug-resistant supraventricular tachyarrhythmias. Diagnoses were junctional ectopic tachycardia in 1, atrioventricular node reentry tachycardia in 4 and accessory pathway-mediated tachycardia in 12. Ablation of accessory pathway was performed using 20 to 40 W of energy. The catheter was passed retrograde to the left ventricle in patients with a left-sided pathway and antegrade to the right atrium in patients with a right-sided or posteroseptal pathway. The ablation procedure was successful in 11 of 13 pathways. There were no recurrences of accessory pathway-mediated tachycardia. AV node reentrant tachycardia was treated by AV node modification using 15 W of energy applied until first degree of AV block occurred. After ablation there was a prolonged AH interval, tachycardia was not inducible and tachycardia recurred in only 1 patient. In summary, radiofrequency catheter ablation was initially successful in 17 of 19 procedures and ultimately curative in 14 of 17 with no serious complications. These authors show excellent results for the use of this modality. Hopefully, further follow-up will extend the indications for its use.

Surgical or catheter ablation of accessory pathways by means of high-energy shocks serves as definitive therapy for patients with WPW syndrome but has substantial associated morbidity and mortality. Radiofrequency current, an alternative energy source for ablation, produces smaller lesions without adverse effects remote from the site where current is delivered. Jackman and associates[19] from Oklahoma City, Oklahoma, conducted a study to develop catheter techniques for delivering radiofrequency current to reduce morbidity and mortality associated with accessory pathway ablation. Radiofrequency current (mean power, 30.9 ± 5.3 W) was applied through a catheter electrode positioned against the mitral or tricuspid annulus or a branch of the coronary sinus; when possible, delivery was guided by catheter recordings of accessory-pathway activation. Ablation was attempted in 166 patients with 177 accessory pathways (106 pathways in the left free wall, 13 in the anteroseptal region, 43 in the posteroseptal region, and 15 in the right free wall). Accessory-pathway conduction was eliminated in 164 of 166 patients (99%) by a median of 3 applications of radiofrequency current. During a mean follow-up (± SD) of 8.0 ± 5.4 months, preexcitation or atrioventricular reentrant tachycardia returned in 15 patients (9%). All underwent a second, successful ablation. Electrophysiologic study 3.1 ± 1.9 months after ablation in 75 patients verified the absence of accessory-pathway conduction in all. Complications of radiofrequency-current application occurred in 3 patients (1.8%): atrioventricular block (1 patient), pericarditis (1), and cardiac tamponade (1) after radiofrequency current was applied in a small branch of the coronary sinus. Radiofrequency current is highly effective in ablating accessory pathways, with low morbidity and no mortality.

Calkins and associates[20] from Ann Arbor, Michigan, conducted a study to determine the feasibility of an abbreviated therapeutic approach to the WPW syndrome or paroxysmal SVT in which the diagnosis is established and radiofrequency ablation carried out during a single electrophysiologic test. One hundred six consecutive patients were referred for the management of documented, symptomatic paroxysmal SVT (66 patients) or the WPW syndrome (40 patients). All agreed to undergo a diagnostic electrophysiologic test and catheter ablation with radiofrequency current. No patient had had such a test previously. Among the 66 patients with paroxysmal SVT, the mechanism was found to be AV nodal reentry in 46 (70%) (typical in 44 and atypical in 2), AV reciprocating tachycardia involving a concealed accessory pathway in 16 (24%), atrial tachycardia in 2 (3%), and noninducible paroxysmal SVT in 2 (3%). A successful long-term outcome was achieved in 57 of 62 patients (92%) with paroxysmal SVT in whom ablation was attempted and in 37 of 40 patients (93%) with the WPW syndrome. The only complications were 1 instance of occlusion of the left circumflex coronary artery, leading to AMI, and 1 instance of complete atrioventricular block. The mean (± SD) duration of the electrophysiologic procedures was 114 ± 55 minutes. The diagnosis and cure of paroxysmal SVT or the WPW syndrome during a single electrophysiologic test are feasible and practical and have a favorable risk-benefit ratio. This abbreviated therapeutic approach may eliminate the need for serial electropharmacologic testing, long-term drug therapy, antitachycardia pacemakers, and surgical ablation.

Tachyarrhythmias mediated by an accessory AV pathway and which are refractory to drug therapy have been treated surgically with variable success. Early results of direct-current catheter ablation were encouraging but were associated with complications such as barotrauma and the need for a general anesthetic. Kuck and associates[21] from Hamburg, Germany, investigated the endocardial application of radiofrequency current which is a potentially safer technique. Of 105 patients with an accessory atrioventricular pathway, 79 were located on the left side of the heart and 32 on the right side. Accessory pathway conduction was permanently abolished in 93 (89%) patients. Complications developed in 3 patients: thrombotic occlusion of a femoral artery, arteriovenous fistula formation at the site of groin puncture, and LV rupture with cardiac tamponade after direct-current shocks. There were no deaths from the procedure. The authors concluded that radiofrequency current catheter ablation is both effective and safe for patients with symptomatic tachyarrhythmias mediated by accessory A-V pathways.

Radiofrequency current has been proposed as an alternate energy source. Seventy-three symptomatic patients with WPW syndrome and 19 patients with only retrogradely conducting (concealed) pathways underwent ablative therapy by Shulter and co-workers[22] in Hamburg, Germany, with radiofrequency current. There were 71 accessory pathways located on the left side of the heart and 25 on the right side. In patients with right-sided pathways, ablation was attempted via a catheter positioned at the atrial aspect of the tricuspid annulus. In patients with a left-sided free-wall accessory pathway, a novel approach was used in which the ablation catheter was positioned in the left ventricle directly below the mitral annulus. Accessory pathway conduction was permanently abolished in 79 patients. Growing experience and improved catheter technology resulted in a 100% success rate after the 52nd consecutive patient. Failures were mainly the result of inadequate catheters used initially or an unfavorable approach to left posteroseptal pathways. Catheter ablation of accessory atrioventricular pathways by the use of radiofrequency current is an effective and safe therapeutic modality for patients with symptomatic tachyarrhythmias mediated by these pathways.

Thirty-four patients with W-P-W syndrome and a delta wave pattern indicative of an overt left-sided free-wall accessory pathway underwent attempts by Kuck and Schluter[23] in Hamburg, Germany, at radiofrequency current ablation of the pathway with the use of just one catheter. No patient had a previous electrophysiological study. The catheter was introduced into the left ventricle close to the mitral annulus and was used for pathway localization as well as for ablation. The approach was successful in 30 patients. In one remaining 4 patients, ablation of the pathway was achieved by using the multiple-catheter approach. Overall procedure duration was 2 hours; radiation exposure time was 23 minutes. There were no acute complications. The single-catheter approach to radiofrequency current ablation of overt left-sided free-wall accessory pathways is feasible, safe, and effective in the majority of patients. The approach requires considerable investigator experience but significantly reduces procedure duration and radiation exposure time.

The Catheter Ablation Registry was the first international, multicenter, prospective study of the safety and efficacy of catheter ablation. From August 1987 through March 1990, the study by Evans and co-investigators[24] in San Francisco, California, comprised 136 patients in whom only DC energy was used in attempted production of third-degree atrioventricular block to treat uncontrollable supraventricular tachycardias. Eight patients died during hospitalization for ablation. In 7 (5%), the ablation may have contributed to their deaths. Causes of death included VT (5 patients, 3 with polymorphic VT), progressive heart failure (1 patient), and respiratory failure (2 patients, 1 dying after resuscitation from VF). Compared with survivors, patients who died were more likely to have had prior aborted sudden death (38% vs 2%), congestive heart failure (88% vs 22%), cardiomyopathy (50% vs 16%), lower baseline systolic blood pressure (106 vs 138 mm Hg), prolonged baseline and postablation corrected QT interval, and marked reduced EF (27% vs 52%). Ablation successfully produced third-degree AV block in 88% of the patients who died and in 83% of survivors. Catheter ablation of the AV junction with DC energy carries a significant, previously unrecognized risk of death (5%), particularly from lethal arrhythmias, when applied to patients with severe LV dysfunction. Great care should be taken in these seriously ill patients to guard against postablation ventricular arrhythmias.

VENTRICULAR ARRHYTHMIAS

Association with left ventricular hypertrophy

Ghali and associates[25] in Chicago and Maywood, Illinois evaluated the relationship between ventricular arrhythmias and the presence of LV hypertrophy in 49 hypertensive patients using 24 hour ambulatory electrocardiogram monitoring and echocardiography. These patients had normal coronary arteries by arteriography. Frequency and complexity of ventricular arrhythmias were significantly related to the presence of LV hypertrophy whether it was defined by wall thickness (interventricular septum or posterior wall ≥1.2 cm) or by LV mass indexed to height (LV mass/height ≥163 g/m in men and ≥121 g/m in women). The relationship between LV mass or wall thickness to ventricular arrhythmias was graded and continuous. For every 1 mm increase in the thickness of interventricular septum or posterior wall, there was an associated two- to three-fold increase in the occurrence and complexity of ventricular arrhythmias. Thus, LV hypertrophy is associated with an increase in the frequency and complexity of ventricular arrhythmias in the absence of CAD and the relationship is a continuous one.

Sustained ventricular arrhythmias within 60 days of acute myocardial infarction

Gomes and colleagues[26] in New York, New York, assessed the clinical and electrophysiologic determinants, treatment, and survival of patients with sustained malignant tachyarrhythmias late after AMI in 108 individuals with a mean age of 61 ± 10 years. Thirty-two patients (Group I) had sustained ventricular tachyarrhythmias 8 to 60 days (mean 13 ± 9) after AMI. The remaining 76 patients (Group II) served as a control group and had no sustained ventricular tachyarrhythmias ≤60 days after AMI. The most significant independent determinants of sustained ventricular tachyarrhythmias after AMI were the presence of late potentials defined as an abnormal signal-averaged QRS complex in association with an abnormal root-mean-square voltage in the terminal 40 ms of the QRS complex and an abnormal LVEF of <40%. Sustained VT was induced in 27 (96%) of 28 Group I patients. Among the 32 patients in Group I, antitachycardia therapy included antiarrhythmic drug therapy as the sole preventive measure in 14, map-guided surgery or coronary artery bypass surgery or both in 14, and the automatic cardioverter-defibrillator in 4. The arrhythmias were made noninducible in 83% of patients after map-guided surgery and in 41% after drug therapy. During a follow-up period of 20 ± 14 months, 5 Group I patients (15%) had an arrhythmic event and four (9%) had a cardiac-related death. All five patients who had an arrhythmic event were receiving antiarrhythmic drugs. None of the patients who had successful map-guided surgery had an arrhythmic event. However, the long-term 2-year arrhythmia-free survival and total survival were not significantly different between Group I and II patients. Thus, 1) sustained VT/VF late after AMI is usually due to the presence of well formed substrate rather than the occurrence of acute myocardial ischemia; 2) a marked improvement in survival not significantly different from that of a control group with no sustained ventricular arrhythmias and better LV function was found with aggressive approach consisting of electrophysiologically guided therapy, coronary revascularization, and the automatic implantable defibrillator; and 3) patients with >2 episodes of drug-resistant sustained ventricular tachyarrhythmias do better with early surgery than with antiarrhythmic therapy.

Danger of driving motorized vehicles

Most states have specific laws governing whether patients with seizure disorders can drive motorized vehicles. To learn whether similar laws exist for patients with lethal ventricular arrhythmias, Strickberger and associates[27] from Boston, Massachusetts, surveyed the Departments of Motor Vehicles in all 50 states. In addition, either an arrhythmia specialist (n = 25) or a general cardiologist (n = 25) was chosen randomly from each state and interviewed to study physician awareness of such laws and physician attitudes toward driving by patients with arrhythmias. Forty-two states (84%) have laws restricting driving by patients who have seizures; only 8 states (16%) have specific laws for patients with arrhythmias. No state makes a distinction between driving by patients with arrhythmias who are managed with an implantable cardioverter-defibrillator compared with patients who are managed medically. Seventy-four percent of physicians did not know their own state's laws about driving by patients who have ventricular arrhythmias. Cardiologists were more likely to advise no driving restriction for medically treated patients than for implantable cardio-verter-defibrillator-treated patients. Cardiologists were also more likely to advise permanent restriction for patients with implantable cardio-verter-defibrillators than for patients treated medically. The authors concluded that greater legal and medical consensus is needed to guide physicians in advising patients with lethal ventricular arrhythmias about driving restrictions.

Cardiac sympathetic activity

Although enhanced efferent cardiac sympathetic nervous activity has been proposed as an important factor in the genesis of ventricular arrhythmias and sudden cardiac death, direct clinical evidence has been lacking. Meredith and associates[28] from Melbourne, Australia, measured the rates of total and cardiac norepinephrine spillover into the plasma, which reflect, respectively, overall and cardiac sympathetic nervous activity, in 12 patients who had recovered from a spontaneous, sustained episode of VT or VF outside the hospital 4 to 48 days earlier. The results were compared with those from 3 age-matched reference groups without a history of ventricular arrhythmias: 12 patients with CAD, 6 patients with chest pain but normal coronary arteries, and 12 healthy, normal subjects. The patients who had had ventricular arrhythmias had reduced LVEF, as compared with the patients with CAD or chest pain (mean [± SE], 46 ± 3% vs 58 ± 4% and 69 ± 5%, respectively). The rates of total norepinephrine spillover into the plasma were similar in the 3 reference groups, but 80% higher in the patients with ventricular arrhythmias (Figure 4-7). The rate of cardiac norepinephrine spillover was 450% higher in these patients (176 ± 39 pmol per minute, as compared with 32 ± 8 pmol per minute in the normal subjects), a disproportionate increase relative to the increase in total spillover, which indicated selective activation of the cardiac sympathetic outflow. This increase in cardiac norepinephrine spillover was probably caused by a reduction in LV function. These results suggest that in some patients major ventricular arrhythmias are associated with and perhaps caused by sustained and selective cardiac sympathetic activation. The authors speculate that depressed ventricular function was present before the ventricular arrhythmia occurred, and that this resulted in reflex cardiac sympathetic activation, which in turn contributed to the genesis of the arrhythmia.

More on the Cardiac Arrhythmia Suppression Trial

Pratt and the CAPS investigators[29] from Houston, Texas; Seattle, Washington, Montreal, Quebec, Canada; Richmond, Virginia; and New York, New York analyzed the cardiac arrhythmia pilot study (CAPS) data obtained from a 1 year trial analyzing the safety and efficacy of arrhythmia suppression in 502 patients surviving AMI who had ≥10 VPB's/hour or ≥5 runs of VT on a Holter recording obtained 6 to 60 days after AMI. Since 100 of these patients received placebo in a double-blind fashion for 1 year, a comprehensive objective analysis was performed of spontaneous arrhythmia changes based on real data. In the CAPS placebo group, 19% developed some serious clinical event in 1 year, including death, CHF, or proarrhythmia that might be attributable to antiarrhythmic drug toxicity. A significant reduction in the frequency of VPC's occurred

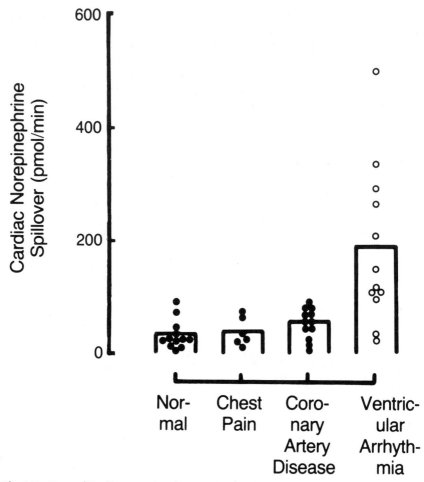

Fig. 4-7. Rates of Cardiac Norepinephrine Spillover into the Plasma in the Three Reference Groups (solid Circles) and the Patients with Ventricular Arrhythmias (open Circles) Bars indicate mean values. Reprinted with permission of Meredith, et al.[28]

in the first few weeks of therapy with a further significant decrease between 3 and 12 months. After initiation of placebo antiarrhythmic therapy, 27% had apparent VPC suppression (≥70% reduction) after one Holter recording evaluation and nearly half (48%) after 6 Holter recordings to assess suppression were performed. Thus, setting a higher percent suppression goal or obtaining multiple baseline Holter recordings decreases the chance of mistaking suppression of VPB's for spontaneous variability.

In the Cardiac Arrhythmia Suppression Trial, designed to test the hypothesis that suppression of ventricular ectopic activity after a myocardial infarct reduced the incidence of sudden death, patients in whom ventricular ectopic activity could be suppressed with encainide, flecainide, or moricizine were randomly assigned to receive either active drug or placebo. The use of encainide and flecainide was discontinued because of excess mortality. Echt and associate CAST investigators[30] examined the mortality and morbidity after randomization to encainide or flecainide or their respective placebo. Of 1,498 patients, 857 were assigned to receive encainide or its placebo (432 to active drug and 425 to placebo) and 641 were assigned to receive flecainide or its placebo (323 to active drug and 318 to placebo). After a mean follow-up of 10 months, 89 patients had died: 59 of arrhythmia (43 receiving drug vs 16 receiving placebo), 22 of nonarrhythmic cardiac causes (17 receiving drug vs 5 receiving placebo), and 8 of noncardiac causes (3 receiving drug vs 5 receiving placebo) (Figure 4-8). Almost all cardiac deaths not due to arrhythmia were attributed to AMI with shock (11 patients receiving drug and 3 receiving placebo) or to chronic CAD (4 receiving drug and 2 receiving placebo). There were no differences between the patients receiving active drug and those receiving placebo in the incidence of nonlethal disqualifying VT, proarrhythmia, syncope, need for a permanent pacemaker, CAD, recurrent myocardial infarction, angina, or need for CABG or angioplasty. There was an excess of deaths due to arrhythmia and deaths due to shock after acute recurrent AMI in patients treated with encainide or flecainide. Nonlethal events, however, were equally distributed between the active-drug and placebo groups. The mechanisms underlying the excess mortality during treatment with encainide or flecainide remain unknown.

Epstein and the CAST Investigators[31] tested the hypothesis that suppression of ventricular arrhythmias by antiarrhythmic drugs after AMI improved survival. This report described the survival experience of all patients enrolled in CAST and compared it with mortality in other studies of patients with ventricular arrhythmias after AMI. As of April 18, 1989, 2,371 patients had enrolled in CAST and entered prerandomization, open label titration: 1,913 (81%) were randomized in double-blind, placebo-controlled therapy (1.775 patients whose arrhythmias were suppressed and 138 patients whose arrhythmias were partially suppressed during open label titration); and 458 patients (19%) were not randomized because they were still in titration, had died during titration or had withdrawn. Including all patients who enrolled in CAST, the actuarial estimate of 1-

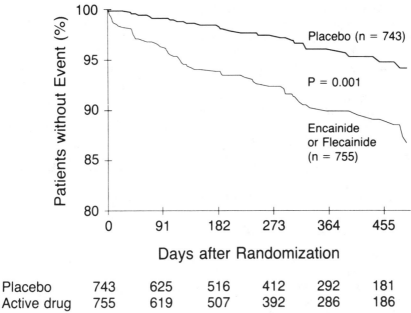

Placebo	743	625	516	412	292	181
Active drug	755	619	507	392	286	186

Fig. 4-8. Actuarial Probabilities of Freedom from Death or Cardiac Arrest Due to Any Cause in 1498 Patients Receiving Encainide or Flecainide or Corresponding Placebo. The number at risk is shown along the bottom. Reprinted with permission of Echt, et al.[30]

year mortality was 10%. To estimate the "natural" mortality rate of patients enrolled in CAST, an analysis was done that adjusted for deaths that might be attributable to the antiarrhythmic agents used, encainide or flecainide treatment during either prerandomization, open label drug titration or after randomization. A minimal 1-year "natural" mortality rate of 6% was estimated by assuming that all deaths during open label titration with encainide or flecainide were due to drug treatment and that after randomization all excess mortality in the group randomized to active treatment was due to drug effect. Maximal 1-year "natural" mortality rate of 8% was estimated by assuming that no deaths upon open label titration with encainide or flecainide were due to drug treatment and that after randomization all excess mortality in the group to active treatment was due to drug effect. Therefore, the "natural" overall mortality rate in CAST of between 6 and 8% is similar to rates observed in other postinfarction natural history studies, suggesting that the low mortality in the group randomized to placebo was largely due to the process of selecting only those enrolled patients for the randomized phase of CAST whose ventricular arrhythmias were suppressed in their prerandomization open label titration phase.

The prevalence, characteristics and significance of ventricular arrhythmias detected by ambulatory electrocardiography were evaluated by Denes and fellow CAST investigators[32] in 1,498 patients who were randomized to encainide, flecainide or placebo in the Cardiac Arrhythmia Suppression Trial (CAST). The mean VPC frequency at baseline was 133 ± 257 VPCs/hour. Nonsustained VT (rate ≥120 beats/min) was present in 22% of patients. Accelerated idioventricular rhythm (rate <120 beats/min) occurred in 22% of subjects. There were 63 deaths/resuscitated cardiac arrests in the active treatment (encainide/flecainide) group and 26 in the placebo group. In the treatment group mortality increased with increasing VPC frequency, whereas in the placebo group such a relation was not present. Mortality/resuscitated cardiac arrest increased in patients with ≥2 VT episodes than in those with ≤1 episode in the active treatment group. There was no significant association between VT and mortality/resuscitated cardiac arrest in the placebo group. The presence of accelerated idioventricular rhythm was not associated with increased mortality/resuscitated cardiac arrest in either the active treatment or placebo groups. However, mortality was lower in patients with accelerated idioventricular rhythm rates <100 beats/min than in those with rates ≥100 beats/min. Thus, in the Cardiac Arrhythmia Suppression Trial the previously described association between mortality/resuscitated cardiac arrest and ventricular arrhythmias (VPC and VT) were only observed in the active treatment group. In addition, based on the results obtained in this highly selected population, it is suggested that the definition of accelerated idioventricular rhythm should be a rate <100 beats/min, and at a rate ≥100 beats/min it should be categorized as VT.

Encainide or flecainide in the young

Fish and colleagues[33] in Chicago, Illinois, and Charleston, South Carolina, evaluated retrospectively collected data from 36 institutions in 579 young patients who were administered encainide or flecainide for treatment of supraventricular arrhythmias or ventricular arrhythmias to assess the frequency of proarrhythmia, cardiac arrest and death during therapy. The two drugs were similar as regards efficacy with flecainide being successful 71% of the time and encainide 60% of the time. The rates of proarrhythmic responses were also similar, including 7% for flecainide and 8% for encainide. However, patients receiving encainide more frequently experienced cardiac arrest or died during treatment. Detailed data were available in 44 patients experiencing one or more adverse events. Patient age, previous drug trials, concomitant therapy and days of inpatient monitoring were similar for patients receiving encainide or flecainide. Echocardiographic LV shortening before treatment was lower among patients receiving encainide than among those receiving flecainide. Plasma drug concentrations were rarely elevated. Cardiac arrest (12 patients) and deaths (13 patients) occurred predominantly among patients with underlying heart disease, especially among patients receiving flecainide for supraventricular tachycardia (8% vs 0.3%). Fifteen patients with apparently normal hearts and ventricular function had proarrhythmia during treatment for supraventricular tachycardia, but only 3 of the 15 had a cardiac arrest or died. Nevertheless, the relatively high incidence of adverse events should be considered when considering therapy with encainide or flecainide, especially among patients with underlying heart disease.

Quinidine

The interim results of the Cardiac Arrhythmia Suppression Trial requires physicians to use a higher threshold for employing antiarrhythmic agents in the treatment of benign or potentially lethal ventricular arrhythmias. Many have managed patients by switching to the traditional class I quinidine despite its known proarrhythmic tendency. To evaluate the relation between quinidine therapy and mortality in patients with benign or potentially lethal ventricular arrhythmias, Morganroth and Goin[34] in Philadelphia, Pennsylvania, performed a meta-analysis on 4 randomized double-blind active controlled parallel trials evaluating 1,009 patients in which quinidine was compared to flecainide, mexiletine, tocainide, and propafenone. All 4 trials had similar patients selection, protocols, and methodology but varying lengths of drug exposure. A total of 12 deaths were reported on quinidine and 4 deaths on the other drugs: 2 on mexiletine, 1 on flecainide, and 1 on tocainide. The statistical analysis of the mortality rates was based on techniques for combining data across separate strata. Based on maximum likelihood estimation, the combined risk of dying on quinidine was statistically significantly higher compared to the other four drugs with a risk difference of 1.6%. The likelihood ratio test for uniformity of the risk difference across strata showed the trials to be homogeneous. There was 1 death recorded for the placebo lead-in period and 7 deaths were reported within 2 weeks on active drug treatment—6 on quinidine and 1 on mexiletine. Furthermore, proarrhythmia was reported in 20 patients on quinidine versus 11 patients on the 4 other drugs. These data suggest that quinidine may have adverse effect on mortality as compared to other class 1 antiarrhythmic agents and that individualized patient selection for the use of this agent be carefully weighted relative to its potential for harm and benefit.

Sotalol

Sotalol is a unique B-blocking drug, possessing significant class III antiarrhythmic activity. Anastasiou-Nana and associates[35] from Salt Lake City, Utah, compared the efficacy and safety of 2 doses of sotalol (320 and 640 mg/day, divided into 2 doses) to placebo in a 6-week randomized, double-blind, multi-center study of 114 patients with chronic VPCs at frequencies of ≥30/hour. Sotalol significantly reduced VPCs in patients receiving both low (n = 38) and high (n = 39) doses, compared with patients (n = 37) receiving placebo (by 75 and 88%, respectively, vs 10%) (Figure 4-9). The individual efficacy criterion (≥75% VPC reduction) was achieved in 34% of low-dose and 71% of high-dose sotalol versus 6% of placebo-treated patients. Repetitive beats were suppressed 25% by placebo (difference not significant), 80% by low-dose and 78% by high-dose sotalol. Sotalol decreased heart rate (by 24 to 25%) and increased PR (by 4 to 6%) and corrected JT intervals (by 12 to 13%), but did not change EF. Proarrhythmia (nonfatal) occurred in 3 sotalol and in 2 placebo patients. Nine discontinued therapy because of adverse effects (1 low dose and 8 high dose). In summary, sotalol is an efficacious antiarrhythmic drug for VPC suppression; in lower doses, it is somewhat less effective but better tolerated.

Amiodarone

Wiersinga and associates[36] from Utrecht, The Netherlands, determined whether long-term amiodarone treatment is associated with a rise in plasma total cholesterol level and if so to analyze its relation to thyroid function. Twenty-three euthyroid patients were studied and they received amiodarone for a mean duration of 17 months (range 6-30). Fasting plasma lipids, thyroid hormones, and peak thyroid stimulating hormone and thyrotropin-releasing hormone were recorded before and every 6 months during amiodarone therapy. Plasma total cholesterol gradually

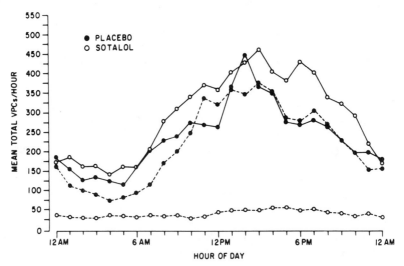

Fig. 4-9. Effect of sotalol (combined treatment groups; open circles) versus placebo (closed circles) on diurnal frequency of total ventricular premature complexes (VPCs). Baseline frequencies for the 2 groups are represented by solid lines and treatment frequencies (6-week end point) by dashed lines. Total VPC frequency is expressed as the logarithmic mean per hour, by the hour of the day. Differences are only significant for the sotalol treatment curve, compared with each of the other 3 curves. Reprinted with permission of Anastasiou, et al.[35]

increased from 5.1 ± 0.2 mmol/L before treatment to 6.9 ± 0.8 mmol/L after 30 months of amiodarone medication. The thyroid hormone levels did not change. When age and sex-specific reference values were applied, 30% of the patients had cholesterol values above the 75th percentile before treatment and this number rose to 69% after 2 years of treatment. The rise in plasma total cholesterol was associated with an equal increase in apoprotein B. Plasma total cholesterol level was not related to the daily dose of amiodarone or to plasma concentrations of amiodarone or to those of the various thyroid hormone levels. There was a positive relation, however, between plasma total cholesterol and cumulative dose of amiodarone. Thus, long-term amiodarone treatment is associated with a dose-dependent increase in plasma total cholesterol that is independent of thyroid function.

Dobs and associates[37] in Baltimore, Maryland determined whether amiodarone causes testicular dysfunction in men treated with this agent chronically. Gonadal function was evaluated in 44 men, including 18 who had been treated with amiodarone for >1 year and 26 survivors of cardiac arrest who had been treated with antiarrhythmic drugs other than amiodarone. Amiodarone-treated men had higher serum follicle-stimulating hormone (42 ± 23 vs 14 ± 10.4) and luteinizing hormone (35 ± 26 vs 10 ± 5) concentrations compared with control individuals. Serum total and free testosterone levels were comparable between the two patient groups, but these levels were inversely correlated with cumulative amiodarone dose. Hyperresponsiveness to the administration of gonadotropin-releasing hormone was noted in the 10 amiodarone-treated men evaluated by this test. Sexual dysfunction was common in both groups (70% of controls and 82% of amiodarone-treated subjects), although atrophic testes were commonly observed in amiodarone-treated men. These data suggest that testicular dysfunction may result from chronic amiodarone treatment.

Atrioventricular node ablation

Yeung-Lai-Wah and colleagues[38] in Vancouver, Canada, used radiofrequency current as an alternative energy source for transcatheter ablation of cardiac arrhythmias to avoid the complications associated with direct current shock. Initial use of radiofrequency current for complete ablation of the AV node yielded only moderate success rates, presumably because of the small size of electrodes and difficulty in localizing the AV node. The use of a larger 4 mm tip electrode for delivery of radiofrequency current and a method to better localize the AV node was studied in 32 patients undergoing catheter ablation procedures. There were 21 men and 11 women with a mean age of 62 ± 12 years. Complete AV block was achieved immediately in 31 patients (97%), and it persisted in 28 patients (88%) during a mean follow-up period of 12 ± 6 months. Three patients who had a return of AV conduction required no drug therapy for control of ventricular rate during AF. The number of radiofrequency pulses used to achieve complete AV block ranged from 1 to 5. In more than 50% of the cases, only one radiofrequency pulse was required. The mean power and duration of radiofrequency pulses were 21 ± 4.5 W and 33 ± 15 seconds, respectively. All patients developed a stable junctional escape rhythm within 45 minutes of successful ablation. The QRS configuration was unchanged in 30 patients. One patient had a new right BBB after ablation. There were no complications related to the ablation procedure. Thus, transcatheter ablation of the AV node is highly efficacious and safe when radiofrequency current is delivered through a large electrode positioned close to the AV node.

Catheter electrical ablation using a relatively low level of energy—40 to 100 joules—was attempted in 12 consecutive patients with drug-refractory sustained VT in a study by Niwano and associates[39] from Niigata, Japan. They had 19 monomorphic VTs, and ischemic heart disease was found as the underlying heart disease in 1, nonischemic heart disease was found in 9, and no structural heart disease was seen in 2 patients. Electrical discharge was delivered at the site of the earliest endocardial activation in 17 VTs and at the slow conduction area in 2 VTs. Among 19 VTs in 12 patients, 12 VTs (63%) in 7 patients (58%) were successfully ablated and became noninducible during electrophysiologic study. There were no major complications, but transient A-V block occurred in 1 patient and transient friction rub occurred in another. Delivered electrical energy and the time interval between the local electrogram and the surface QRS did not correlate with the clinical outcome of the procedure. However, "excellent" pace-mapped QRS morphology was obtained from the site of earliest activation or from the slow conduction area in 9 of 12 VTs in the successful cases but in only 1 of 7 VTs in the unsuccessful cases. Low-energy catheter electrical ablation seems to be a satisfactory therapeutic procedure compared with the conventional method that uses an energy level of 200 joules or higher.

Lawrie and associates[40] from Houston, Texas, described results of direct surgical ablation of arrhythmogenic myocardium in 80 patients with drug-resistant sustained VT. Sixty-nine were men and 11 were women with 1.9 ± 1.1 VT morphologies per patient. The mean number of drugs failed was 3.7 ± 1.6 per patient. The preoperative LVEF was 36.4 ± 14.4%. Complete preoperative endocardial mapping data (>4 endocardial sites in each VT) were available for 60 of the 80 patients (75%) and intraoperative endocardial data in the clinical VT was obtained in 37 (46.3%) of the patients. In 17 patients mapped intraoperatively by computer-assisted techniques, complete epicardial and endocardial data in the clinical VT were obtained in 14 patients (82.4%). Overall, 73 of 80 (91.3%) had some mapping data available. Hospital mortality occurred in 10 patients (12.5%) at a mean interval of 13.5 days, range 0 to 62 days. Postoperatively the clinical VT has not recurred in 65 of 70 surviving patients (93%). Nonclinical ventricular tachycardia occurred in another 4 patients. All 9 patients with postoperative VT responded to drugs. The major factors predictive of hospital mortality were prolonged cardiopulmonary bypass (>150 minutes), preoperative EF <31%, and incomplete preoperative mapping. Hospital mortality in patients with an EF below 31% was significantly associated with a history of amiodarone usage. At 3 years of follow-up, freedom from sudden cardiac death was 96%, and 87% of patients were free of ventricular tachycardia on no antiarrhythmic drugs. These results suggest that direct VT operations are an effective form of therapy for patients with sustained monomorphic VT.

CARDIAC ARREST

In infants sleeping on polystyrene-filled cushions

Infants are at risk for both the sudden infant death syndrome (SIDS) and accidental suffocation. At autopsy it is difficult to distinguish one from the other without information from the scene of the death. Healthy infants are assumed to able to turn their heads and if not otherwise restrained, to obtain fresh air. Kemp and Thach[41] from St. Louis, Missouri, assessed this assumption in an investigation of infant deaths that occurred during sleep on cushions filled with polystyrene beads. The authors obtained data on 24 deaths from the U.S. Consumer Product Safety Commission. They also used mechanical and animal models to study physiologic aspects of ventilation relevant to these results, by simulating the effects on an infant of breathing into a cushion. The authors measured the effects of softness, malleability (molding of the cushion about an infant's head), airflow resistance, and rebreathing of expired gases. All 25 study infants were prone when found dead, and at least 88% were face down with nose and mouth obstructed by the cushion. SIDS was the diagnosis in 19 of the 23 infants who underwent autopsy. The authors findings show, however, that the cushion would have limited movement of the infant's head to obtain fresh air, and the amount of rebreathing estimated to have occurred in the infants was lethal in a rabbit model. Accidental suffocation by rebreathing was the most likely cause of death in most of the 25 infants studied. Consequently, there is a need to reassess the cause of death in the 28 to 52% of the victims of SIDS who are found with their faces straight down. Safety regulations setting standards for softness, malleability, and the potential for rebreathing are needed for infant bedding.

In persons ≤40 years of age

Sports-related sudden cardiac deaths were compared with non-sports-related sudden cardiac death in individuals (14 to 40 years old) who were autopsied from 1981 to 1988 at the Maryland Medical Examiner's Office by Burke and associates[42] from Baltimore, Maryland. Thirty-four of 690 total cases of sudden cardiac death were sports-related which represents 5% of sudden cardiac death in this age group. Causes of death were severe CAD (9 patients), HC (8 patients), coronary artery anomalies (4 patients), idiopathic concentric LV hypertrophy (3 patients), myocarditis (2 patients), arrhythmogenic right ventricle (1 patient), Kawasaki disease (1 patient), and unknown (6 patients). Exercise-related deaths were more likely due to HC compared with 102 age-, sex-, and race-matched controls in the nonexercise group; there was no difference in the frequency of severe CAD. The mean age of individuals with HC was less than that of those with severe CAD (24 vs 32 years).

Drory and associates[43] from 4 Israeli medical centers retrospectively assessed the underlying causes of sudden unexpected death and the occurrence of prodromal symptoms in 162 subjects (aged 9-39 years) over a 10-year period (1976-1985). Underlying cardiac diseases accounted for sudden death in 73% and noncardiac causes in 15% of subjects (Table 4-2). In 12% of subjects, the causes were unidentifiable. Myocarditis (22%), HC (22%), and conduction system abnormalities (13%) were the major causes in 32 subjects aged <20 years. Major causes of 46 deaths in subjects 20 to 29 years were atherosclerotic CAD (24%), myocarditis (22%) and HC (13%). The largest number of deaths in 84 subjects aged ≥30 years was attributed to CAD (58%), followed by myocarditis (11%). Among noncardiac causes of sudden death, intercranial hemorrhage was the most frequent (5%), followed by infectious disease (4%). Prodromal symptoms were reported by 54% of subjects; most frequent were chest pain (25%) in subjects aged ≥20 years, and dizziness (16%) in those aged <20.

TABLE 4-2. *Causes of sudden unexpected death—distribution by age group. Reproduced with permission from Drory, et al.*[43]

Causes of Death	< 20 Years (%)	20–29 Years (%)	≥ 30 Years (%)
Cardiac	21 (66)	35 (76)	62 (74)
Atherosclerotic coronary artery disease	0 (0)	11 (24)	49 (58)*
Myocarditis	7 (22)	10 (22)	9 (11)
Hypertrophic cardiomyopathy	7 (22)	6 (13)	2 (2)
Dilated cardiomyopathy	1 (3)	2 (4)	1 (1)
Endocardial fibroelastosis	2 (6)	0 (0)	0 (0)
Conduction system abnormalities†	4 (13)	2 (4)	0 (0)
Aortic stenosis	0 (0)	1 (2)	0 (0)
Aortic regurgitation	0 (0)	0 (0)	1 (1)
Congenital coronary anomaly‡	0 (0)	1 (2)	0 (0)
Coronary vasculitis	0 (0)	1 (2)	0 (0)
Myocardial fibrosis	0 (0)	1 (2)	0 (0)
Noncardiac	8 (25)	6 (13)	11 (13)
Intracranial hemorrhage	3 (9)	3 (7)	2 (2)
Heat stroke	3 (9)	0 (0)	1 (1)
Respiratory tract infection	1 (3)	1 (2)	2 (2)
Meningococcal meningitis	1 (3)	0 (0)	0 (0)
Pneumococcal sepsis	0 (0)	1 (2)	0 (0)
Hemorrhage due to extrauterine pregnancy	0 (0)	0 (0)	2 (2)
Brain tumor§	0 (0)	0 (0)	2 (2)
Pulmonary embolism	0 (0)	1 (2)	0 (0)
Rupture of aortic aneurysm	0 (0)	0 (0)	1 (1)
Fatty liver	0 (0)	0 (0)	1 (1)
Unidentifiable	3 (9)	5 (11)	11 (13)
Total	32 (100)	46 (100)	84 (100)

*p < 0.001.
†Focal fibrosis in 4 subjects, and presence of inflammatory cells along the His bundle in 2. Mitral valve prolapse was found in 2 of 6 subjects.
‡Anomalous origin of the left coronary artery from the right sinus of Valsalva.
§Meningioma, astrocytoma (1 subject each).

Sudden death, which occurred during routine daily activity in 49% and during sleep in 23% of subjects, was related to physical exercise in 23% and emotional upset in 6% (Table 4-3).

Right ventricular dysplasia as the cause

The frequency of RV dysplasia in an autopsy series of young persons with sudden cardiac death in the USA has not been previously reported. Goodin and associates[44] from Nashville, Tennessee, Washington, D.C., Fairfax, Virginia, and Baltimore, Maryland, reviewed the autopsies from cases of sudden coronary death in young adults in the state of Maryland and found 3 cases of RV dysplasia among 547 cardiac deaths (0.55%). These 3 cases of RV dysplasia in young adults and 3 additional cases from the files of the Armed Forces Institute of Pathology were presented. The 6 patients ranged in age from 19 to 28 years and 5 were men. Five

TABLE 4-3. *Circumstances of sudden unexpected death—distribution by under-lying causes. Reproduced with permission from Drory, et al.*[43]

Circumstances of Death	Cardiac (n = 100) (%)	Noncardiac (n = 21) (%)	Unidentifiable (n = 16) (%)
Routine daily activity	47 (47)	11 (52)	9 (56)
Physical exercise	23 (23)	5 (24)	3 (19)
Sleep	25 (25)	4 (19)	2 (12)
Emotional upset	5 (5)	1 (5)	2 (12)

deaths occurred during strenuous exercise. Three cases had a documented history of arrhythmias and 1 had palpitations. In each case, autopsy disclosed RV dilatation with partial absence of the myocardium and extensive fatty infiltrates with and without fibrosis. In 4 cases, collections of chronic lymphocytic infiltrates were seen and 2 had associated myocyte necrosis. In 1 patient the disease was familial and in the remaining 5 it was sporadic.

Non-fatal arrest

Brooks and associates[45] from Boston, Massachusetts, provided a superb review of current therapy for patients surviving out-of-hospital cardiac arrest.

The CASCADE Investigators[46] from Seattle, Washington, in a randomized study evaluated survivors of out-of-hospital VF not associated with a Q-wave AMI who were deemed to be at a high risk of recurrence of VF. It compares the outcome of treatment with empirically administered amiodarone with the outcome of treatment with other antiarrhythmic agents guided by electrophysiologic testing or Holter recording, or both. The goal of therapy guided by electrophysiologic testing is to suppress inducible VT or VF. Holter recording is used as the primary means of adjusting therapy only if patients are noninducible at the baseline electrophysiologic study. Patients are stratified according to cardiac diagnosis, EF, and whether they had previously received an antiarrhythmic agent that failed to suppress their arrhythmias. The primary end point of the study is total cardiac mortality. The first patient was enrolled in a pilot study on April 26, 1984. By October 1988, 142 patients had been enrolled in the full study and, as of May 1990, 199 patients have been enrolled. Compliance with therapy has been good, with no patients lost to follow-up and 8% of patients, equal in both drug groups, crossing over to alternate therapy. Baseline clinical characteristics remain similar in amiodarone and conventional drug groups. Pulmonary toxicity with amiodarone is 7% of 1 year, with no patients dying of pulmonary toxicity. In the first 142 patients, the overall 1-year cardiac mortality was 19%, with a 17% arrhythmic mortality (either VF or presumed arrhythmic death). Because of this relatively high mortality, even with aggressive evaluation, treatment and follow-up, the investigators concluded that all patients who were participants in the study should also have an automatic defibrillator implanted when possible. Enrollment will continue until March 31, 1991, with follow-up for an additional year thereafter. This study should provide data about the relative efficacy of empirically administered amiodarone compared with other antiarrhythmic agents guided by electrophysiologic study and Holter Monitoring.

In a retrospective survey of 1,195 survivors of out-of-hospital VF, Kudenchuk and associates[47] from Seattle, Washington, identified 43 patients in whom the LVEF was ≥0.50 and in whom no CAD of ≥50% luminal diameter narrowing was present. Thirteen (30%) of these patients had hypokinesia on LV, and 20 patients (47%) had a persistently abnormal electrocardiogram. Seven patients (16%) had recurrent out-of-hospital cardiac arrest during an average follow-up of 86 ± 54 months. The presence of either wall motion or electrocardiographic abnormalities defined patients with a several-fold higher risk of recurrent cardiac arrest than those without such abnormalities. The risk for recurrent cardiac arrest within 5 years was 30% in those with abnormal electrocardiograms versus 5% in the others. Age was an independent predictor of recurrent cardiac arrest in this group; surprisingly, recurrent cardiac arrest was occurring more often among younger patients. Although cardiac arrest is unusual in patients without major structural heart disease, its recurrence in such survivors is common. Patients at relatively high risk for recurrent VF can be identified by their youth and by abnormalities detected on the surface 12-lead electrocardiogram or by contrast LV.

The purpose of this study by Sousa and associates[48] from Ann Arbor, Michigan, was to evaluate the results of electrophysiologic testing and the long-term prognosis of 56 patients with CAD who presented with aborted sudden death unrelated to AMI. The mean age of the patients was 62 ± 8 years and 48 were men. The mean LVEF was 0.34 ± 0.16. During the baseline electrophysiology test, sustained monomorphic VT was inducible in 22 patients who then underwent electropharmacologic testing: 11 patients were treated with antiarrhythmic drugs that suppressed the induction of VT or resulted in the VT becoming hemodynamically stable; 10 patients who failed drug testing received an automatic implantable cardioverter/defibrillator; 1 patient underwent endocardial resection. Among 34 patients who did not have inducible sustained VT, a precipitant of cardiac arrest (severe ischemia, proarrhythmia) was identified and was corrected in 9 of 34. An automatic implantable cardioverter/defibrillator was recommended in the remaining 25 patients; however, 9 patients refused and were treated empirically with antiarrhythmic drugs. The mean follow-up was 22 ± 12 months. The 2-year actuarial incidence of sudden death was 31% in patients who were treated with drugs based on the results of electropharmacologic testing, 26% in patients who were treated with antiarrhythmic drugs on an empiric basis, 0% among patients in whom a correctable etiology for the cardiac arrest was identified, and 9% among patients who underwent implantation of an automatic implantable cardioverter/defibrillator. The 3-year actuarial incidence of sudden death among the 20 patients treated with antiarrhythmic drugs was 53% compared with 9% among the 26 patients who underwent automatic implantable cardioverter/defibrillator implantation. In conclusion, antiarrhythmic therapy, whether guided by electrophysiologic testing or administered on an empiric basis, is associated with a high incidence of recurrent sudden death in patients with CAD and aborted sudden death. Implantation of an automatic implantable cardioverter/defibrillator may be advisable in all patients with CAD and aborted sudden death in whom a correctable precipitant cannot be identified.

Hallstrom and associates[49] from Seattle, Washington, determined survival rates in antiarrhythmic drug use in 941 consecutive patients resuscitated from prehospital cardiac arrest due to VF between March 7, 1970, and March 6, 1985. Of these patients, 18.7% were treated for at least a portion of the period with quinidine, 17.5% with procainamide, and 39.4% received no antiarrhythmic agent. Beta blockers were prescribed for 28.3% of the patients. Unadjusted comparisons of survival estimates showed dramatically lower survival rates for patients who received antiarrhythmic drugs independent of B-blocker therapy and significantly improved survival for patients receiving B-blocker therapy independent of antiarrhythmic use. Patients for whom antiarrhythmic therapy was prescribed also had more adverse baseline risk factors, whereas patients taking B blockers had fewer such risk factors. After adjustment for these baseline risk factors, the use of antiarrhythmics was weakly associated with worsened survival; 2-year survival for procainamide-treated patients was 30% and quinidine-treated patients 55%. Beta-blocker therapy was associated with improved survival. Thus, although neither procainamide nor quinidine appear to have had a benefit on mortality, the effect of procainamide appears to be significantly worse than that of quinidine. The use of antiarrhythmic drug therapy in patients resuscitated from prehospital VF should be regarded as not only unproved, but potentially hazardous, and should probably be restricted to testing in randomized clinical trials.

Supraventricular tachycardia as the cause

Wang and associates[50] in San Francisco, California, studied 290 patients among whom 13 (4.5%) presented with aborted sudden death and had either documented or strong presumptive evidence of supraventricular tachycardia that deteriorated into VF. Six (46%) of the 13 had an accessory conduction pathway and either AF (5 patients) or paroxysmal AV reentrant tachycardia (1 patient) that deteriorated into VF. Three patients with AV node reentrant tachycardia and four with AF and enhanced AV node conduction presented with SVT that deteriorated into VF. Patients were treated with medical, surgical, or catheterization ablative procedure designed to prevent SVT recurrence. Four patients received an implanted automatic defibrillator, but none had an appropriate device discharge. Over a follow-up period of 42 months, 12 patients were alive without symptomatic arrhythmias. One patient died with severe lung disease and CHF. Thus, supraventricular tachycardia was the cause of aborted sudden death in approximately 5% of patients referred for evaluation of sudden cardiac death. Treatment directed at prevention of SVT was associated with an excellent prognosis.

While wearing a Holter monitor

Olshausen and associates[51] from Mainz, Federal Republic of Germany, analyzed the Holter tapes of 61 patients (46 men, mean age 65 ± 11 years) who died suddenly while being monitored. Thirty-eight patients were known to have CAD, 5 had cardiomyopathy, and 7 had aortic valve disease. Etiology remained unknown in 11 patients. Mean New York Heart Association functional class was 2.5 ± 0.7. Thirty patients had received antiarrhythmic drugs and 32 had received digitalis. Sudden death occurred at rest in 73%. In the hours before death, repetitive ventricular arrhythmias were found in 50 patients (82%), with AF in 34%. Patients with bradyarrhythmic death (18%) had less complex ventricular activity compared to patients with tachyarrhythmic death. Lethal arrhythmias—morphic VT, torsades de pointes, primary VF and 1:1 conducting atrial tachycardia—were found in 26 (43%), 15 (25%), 5 (8%), 3 (5%), and 1 patient, respectively. The coupling interval of the final ventricular tachycardia correlated inversely with the initial frequency of ventricular tachycardia. For patients with tachyarrhythmic death, an increase of heart rate within the last 3 hours was noted (83 vs 89 beats/min). VPCs and the proportion of patients with >2 couplets and >2 triplets increased significantly only within the last hour before death. The R-on-T phenomenon was observed in 12 patients (20%), 10 of whom died from tachyarrhythmia. In 6 cases, the arrhythmia was initiated by the R-on-T phenomenon. Thus, monomorphic ventricular tachycardia was the arrhythmia most frequently associated with sudden cardiac death. Increase in heart rate before death was small and clinically insignificant. Increase in complex ectopy was noted only within the last hour. Patients with monomorphic ventricular tachycardia lasting longer than polymorphic tachycardia or torsades de pointes (165 vs 24 or 19 seconds, respectively) have the best chance of successful resuscitation.

Exercise-related arrest

Ciampricotti and associates[52] from Eindhoven, the Netherlands, reported clinical and angiographic findings of 17 resuscitated victims of exercise-related sudden ischemic death in an attempt to elucidate the mechanism(s) of the deaths. Ten survivors developed cardiac arrest during or after sporting activities (group A) and 7 others during or after an exercise stress test (group B). There were 15 men and 2 women. The mean age of group A was 46 years and of group B 55 years. Coronary risk factors, as well as previous angina and myocardial infarction, were more frequent in group B. Only 3 of the 17 survivors had anginal symptoms before sudden death. Sudden death in group A was associated with acute myocardial infarction in 8 and unstable angina in 2 and was associated in group B with acute myocardial infarction in 2, unstable angina in 3 and silent ischemia in 2. Coronary angiography was acutely performed in 15 patients. In most patients the ischemia-related coronary artery was totally or subtotally occluded. Clinical and angiographic findings indicate that exercise-related sudden ischemic death was due to an acute coronary event—in most cases unexpected and unpredictable. It is suggested that exercise-induced intracoronary changes were probably responsible for the development of acute coronary (sub) occlusion and sudden death.

Cardiopulmonary resuscitation

Rapid delivery of defibrillatory shocks increases survival in patients with cardiac arrest. The automated external defibrillator interprets cardiac rhythms and delivers electrical shocks, permitting appropriate defibrillation by persons with minimal training. Haynes and associates[53] from San Diego and Sacramento, California, described a California initiated program for early defibrillation by basic emergency medical technicians using manual or automated external defibrillators and by public safety personnel (fire fighters, peace officers, and public life-guards), using automated external defibrillators. The program includes a system for reporting outcomes statewide. In the first 46 months under this program, 1,487 patients received defibrillatory shocks; 1,009 (68%) of these patients had witnessed VF. Of the latter group, 191 were discharged from the hospital, representing 19% of those with witnessed VF and 13% of all patients who had had shocks applied. California also implemented a framework of training and medical direction for defibrillation by laypersons using automated external defibrillators. Early defibrillation by basic emergency medical technicians and public safety personnel, encouraged by appropriate regulatory changes, results in gratifying survival rates.

Most attempts to resuscitate victims of prehospital cardiopulmonary arrest are unsuccessful, and patients are frequently transported to the emergency department for further resuscitation efforts. Gray and associates[54] from Providence, Rhode Island, evaluated the efficacy and cost of continued hospital resuscitation for patients in whom resuscitation efforts outside the hospital had failed. The authors reviewed the records of 185 patients presenting to their emergency department after an initially unsuccessful, but ongoing, resuscitation for a prehospital arrest (cardiac, respiratory, or both) by an emergency medical team. Prehospital and hospital characteristics of treatment for the arrest were identified, and the patients' outcomes in the emergency room were ascertained. The hospital course and the hospital costs for the patients who were revived were determined. Over a 19-month period, only 16 of the 185 patients (9%) were successfully resuscitated in the emergency department and admitted to the hospital. A shorter duration of prehospital resuscitation was the only characteristic of the resuscitation associated with an improved outcome in the emergency department. No patient survived until hospital discharge, and all but one were comatose throughout hospitalization. The mean stay in the hospital was 12.6 days (range, 1 to 132), with an average of 2.3 days (range, 1 to 11) in an intensive care unit. The total hospital cost for the 16 patients admitted was $180,908 (range per patient, $1,984 to $95,144). In general, continued resuscitation efforts in the emergency department for victims of cardiopulmonary arrest in whom prehospital resuscitation has failed are not worthwhile, and they consume precious institutional and economic resources without gain.

LONG Q-T INTERVAL SYNDROME

In families

The Long QT syndrome is an infrequently occurring familial disorder in which affected individuals have electrocardiographic QT interval prolongation and a propensity to VT syncope and sudden death. Moss and collaborators[55] in Rochester, New York prospectively investigated the clinical characteristics and the long-term course of 3,343 individuals from 328 families in which 1 or more members were identified as affected with Long QT interval. The first member of a family to be identified with Long QT Interval Syndrome, the proband, was usually brought to medical attention because of a syncopal episode during childhood or teenage years. Probands were younger at first contact, more likely to be female, and had higher frequency of preenrollment syncope or cardiac arrest with resuscitation, congenital deafness, a heart rate less than 60 beats/min, a $QTc \geq 0.50$ sec$^{1/2}$ and a history of VT than other affected and unaffected family members. Arrhythmogenic syncope often occurred in association with acute physical, emotional, or auditory arousal. The syncopal episodes were frequently misinterpreted as a seizure disorder. By age 12 years, 50% of the probands had experienced at least one syncopal episode or death. The rates of postenrollment syncope and probable Long QT interval related death for probands were 5% per year and 0.9% per year respectively; these event rates were considerably higher than those observed among affected and unaffected family members. Among 232 probands and 1,264 family members with prospective follow-up, 3 factors made significantly independent contributions to the risk of subsequent syncope or probable long acting QT interval-related death before age 50 years, whichever occurred first: 1) QTc, 2) history of cardiac event, and 3) heart rate.

As a risk factor for cardiac arrest

QTc prolongation has been implicated as a risk factor for sudden death; however a controversy exists over its significance. In the Rotterdam QT Project, Algra and co-workers[56] in Rotterdam, The Netherlands followed 6,693 consecutive patients who underwent 24-hour ambulatory electrocardiography; of these, 245 patients died suddenly. A standard 12-lead electrocardiogram and clinical data at the time of 24-hour ambulatory electrocardiography were collected for all patients who died suddenly and for a random sample of 467 patients from the study cohort. In all patients without an intraventricular conduction defect (176 patients who died suddenly and 390 patients from the sample), QT interval duration was measured in leads, I, II, and III and corrected for heart rate with Bazette's formula (QTc). In patients without evidence of cardiac dysfunction (history of symptoms of pump failure or an EF <40%), QTc of >440 msec was associated with a 2.3 times higher risk for sudden death compared with a QTc of ≤440 msec. In contrast, in patients with evidence of cardiac dysfunction, the relative risk of QTc prolongation was 1.0. Adjustment for age, gender, history of AMI, heart rate, and the use of drugs did not alter these relative risks.

With sinus node dysfunction in children

Although sinus bradycardia and low heart rate with exercise have been found in some patients with long QT syndrome, systematic evaluation, including intracardiac electrophysiologic tests of sinus node function, has not been reported. In an investigation by Kugler[57] from Omaha, Nebraska, records were reviewed of 14 children and adolescents (ages 3 to 16 years) with long QT syndrome (mean QTc 0.51 second) who underwent noninvasive testing and intracardiac electrophysiologic studies because of syncope or cardiac arrest. The resting electrocardiographic sinus heart rate was low for age in only 1 of 13 patients, while the lowest Holter-monitored sinus heart rate was abnormal in 4 of 12. The maximum exercise heart rate was abnormally low in 6 of the 12 who underwent exercise testing. For the electrophysiologic tests, the corrected sinus node recovery time was long in 8 of 14 and the sinoatrial conduction time was long in 6 of the 9 in whom it was calculable. When both noninvasive and electrophysiologic indices are considered, 13 of the 14 patients had some type of sinus node dysfunction.

In Southeast Asian men

Sudden and unexplained deaths of young adults in sleep have been reported among several Southeast Asian populations and Japanese. The victims are predominately men, median age 33 years, in previous good health. Routine toxicological examinations have been negative. The immediate cause of death is VF in the absence of known heart disease. Southeast Asian refugees in Thailand have the highest known rate of sudden death in sleep, but the risk declines greatly after immigration to the United States. Munger and associates[58] from 3 US cities and from several Southeast Asian cities carried out electrocardiographic surveys to find out whether these abnormalities are more common among refugees in Thailand with a high risk of sudden death in sleep than in the same and other groups in the USA who are at lower risk. The mean heart rate corrected QT interval (QTC) was significantly greater among 123 Laotian refugees in Thailand at high risk than in 77 Laotian refugees in the USA at lower risk and 199 non-Asian US residents at negligible risk. Among refugees in Thailand, prolonged QTC interval was associated with poor thiamine status and a history of seizure-like episodes in sleep. Thiamine deficiency, therefore, may be a cause of prolonged QT interval and sudden death in this region.

Treatment with pacemaker

From the international long QT Syndrome Study, Moss and collaborators[59] in Rochester, New York identified 30 patients with corrected QT interval of more than 0.44 second who had permanent pacemakers implanted for management of recurrent syncope or aborted cardiac arrest. Pacemakers were implanted on average 7 years after the onset of the first syncopal episode. Most of the patients were female, the average age at implantation was 19 years, the mean corrected QTc was 0.55 second, and 57% were receiving antiadrenergic treatment for Long QT interval syndrome when the pacemaker was placed. Using birth as the time origin, the median cardiac event rate was significantly reduced by pacing from 0.5 to 0 events per patients per year, with 21 patients experiencing no cardiac events during an average pacemaker follow-up of 49 months per patient. In 10 patients in whom the demand atrial pacing rate was faster than the intrinsic sinus rate, the average heart rate was increased 23 beats/min with pacing with reduction in the QT interval from 0.59 seconds to 0.46 seconds. The beneficial effects of pacing in high-risk long QT syndrome patients probably relate to the prevention of bradycardia, pauses, and the shortening of long QT intervals—factors that are known to be arrhythmogenic in this syndrome. Permanent cardiac pacing reduces the rate of recurrent syncopal events in high-risk Long QT Syndrome patients, but it does not provide complete protection.

BUNDLE BRANCH BLOCK

Matzer and associates[60] in Los Angeles, California, determined whether a new approach to interpretation could improve the accuracy of thallium-201 single photon emission computed tomography for detection of LAD CAD in patients with left BBB. Sixty-nine patients were evaluated. Forty-four had angiographically proven CAD; the remaining 25 were considered to have a low likelihood of disease before thallium-201 scintigraphy. Conventional scintigraphic criteria for detection of LAD disease were compared with a new criterion that required the apex to be abnormal to indicate LAD disease. The normalcy rates in the low likelihood patient group were significantly improved by using the new approach from 16%

to 80% by visual analysis and from 24% to 64% by quantitative single photon emission computed tomography polar map analysis. Sensitivity for LAD disease was similar for the conventional and the new method by visual and quantitative analyses. In contrast, the specificity was significantly improved by using the new approach from 14% to 79% by visual analysis and 14% to 64% by quantitative analysis. Thus, septal and anterior thallium-201 single photon emission computed tomography defects are common in patients with left BBB without CAD resulting in low specificity for the detection of LAD disease. The normalcy rates and accuracy for detection of LAD disease were better when an apical defect was used as the criterion for significant disease.

COMPLETE HEART BLOCK IN FETUSES

Schmidt and associates[61] from Heidelberg, Germany, San Francisco, California, and New Haven, Connecticut, report the clinical course and outcome of 55 fetuses with complete AV block detected perinatally. In 29 fetuses (53%), complete AV block was associated with complex structural heart defects, usually left atrial isomerism in 17 or discordant AV connection in 7. The other 26 fetuses had normal cardiac anatomy; in 19 cases the mother had connective tissue disease or tested positive for antinuclear antibodies. Six fetuses showed progression from sinus rhythm or second degree block to complete AV block. Of the 55 pregnancies, 5 were terminated and 24 fetuses or neonates died; at the end of the neonatal period 26 fetuses were still alive. Fetal or neonatal death correlated significantly with the presence of structural heart defects (4 of 29 surviving), hydrops (0 of 22 surviving), atrial rate ≤120 beats/min (1 of 12 surviving), or a ventricular rate ≤55 beats/min (3 of 21 surviving). Mean atrial and ventricular rates were higher in surviving than in nonsurviving fetuses (142 vs 127 and 64 vs 52 beats/min, respectively). A slow atrial rate, however, was frequently associated with left atrial isomerism. In fetuses without left isomerism, mean atrial rate was not different in surviving and nonsurviving fetuses whereas ventricular rate remained different (64 vs 53 beats/min). In 4 patients transplacental treatment by sympathomimetic drugs to the mother was attempted. Although ventricular rate increased variably, only 1 of these fetuses survived. Postnatal permanent pacemaker implantation was performed in 13 neonates with 9 surviving the neonatal period. These authors emphasize the very poor prognosis in patients with fetal hydrops and complete AV block. Although complete AV block is frequently associated with structural cardiac disease, this is not always the case. The suggestion is made that in a viable fetus with isolated complete block, early delivery and immediate postnatal pacing may be an alternative treatment if fetal hydrops begins to develop.

SYNCOPE

Perry and Garson[62] from Houston, Texas, performed autonomic function testing in 22 patients ages 7 to 18 years with recurrent syncope and a normal heart. Testing consisted of 8 to 9 separate tests and 14 of the 22 patients had reproduction of syncope or symptoms during testing. Patients with a positive test had a lower norepinephrine level while supine and lower norepinephrine level in the upright position than patients with a negative test. The slope of heart rate response versus log isoproterenol dose was greater in patients with a positive test than in those with a negative test. All 5 patients with a positive test who were given intravenous propranolol had elimination of syncope with repeat testing. Atenolol was used in 10 patients with a positive test with 8 having successful treatment, including 2 patients without prior resolution of symptoms after pacemaker implantation for symptoms attributable to bradycardia. These authors show beta-adrenergic hypersensitivity as a cause of recurrent syncope in young patients. Inappropriate heart rate response to standing may elicit the Bezold-Jarisch reflex, resulting in bradycardia or hypotension or both in some patients. Beta-adrenergic blockage may benefit many of these patients. Alternative therapy which has been used include salt loading plus mineralacorticoids in patients who are not treated successfully with beta blockade.

Ninety-one consecutive patients with syncope of unknown origin underwent electrophysiologic studies in a report by Moazez and associates[63] from Los Angeles, California. Univariate analysis identified the following variables: age, positive signal-averaged electrocardiogram, LVEF, history of myocardial infarction, CAD, LV aneurysm, and history of sustained monomorphic VT on Holter; multivariate analysis identified positive signal-averaged electrocardiograms, LVEF, and history of sustained monomorphic VT as risk factors for induction of sustained monomorphic VT at electrophysiologic study. All patients were followed up for 19 ± 8.3 months and 17 had recurrence of syncope. Patients were divided into empiric, electrophysiologic-guided, and no therapy groups. The electrophysiologic-guided therapy group included all patients with sustained monomorphic VT at electrophysiologic study. Recurrence rates among all 3 groups were similar. It was concluded that: (1) Patients who have inducible sustained monomorphic VT at electrophysiologic study can be identified using certain clinical and noninvasive variables. When these patients undergo electrophysiologic-guided therapy, their rate of recurrence of syncope becomes compatible with that of patients who had no arrhythmia induced at electrophysiologic study. (2) Empiric therapy does not offer any benefit over no therapy in reducing the rate of recurrence of syncope.

Muller and associates[64] from Montreal, Canada, performed electrophysiologic studies in 134 patients (87 men, mean age 59 years) with unexplained syncope. Seventy-one patients had organic heart disease (ischemic in 50). Electrophysiologic studies revealed conduction abnormalities and tachyarrhythmias that could account for syncope in 40 patients (30%). Thirty-seven (93%) of these patients received pacing or antiarrhythmic therapy compared with 23 (24%) of the remaining 94 patients who had a negative study and received empiric therapy. Risk of having an abnormal electrophysiologic study was greater in patients with underlying heart disease. During a mean follow-up of 22 ± 17 months, 26 patients (19%) either had recurrent syncope (22 patients) or died (4 patients) suddenly. Men had a higher incidence of recurrent syncope than women (26% versus 6%). Other clinical characteristics, electrophysiologic findings, final diagnosis and therapy at discharge were not predictive of outcome. The authors concluded that (1) 19% of patients investigated for syncope will have a recurrent event, (2) female gender may be an independent predictor of favorable outcome.

Atkins and associates[65] from Pittsburgh, Pennsylvania, determined the postural BP response over time, the prevalence of orthostatic hypotension and the relation of orthostatic hypotension to recurrence of symptoms in patients with syncope. The prospectively evaluated 223 patients with syncope. Orthostatic responses were measured in a standardized fashion at 0, 1, 2, 3, 5, and 10 minutes or until symptoms occurred. Follow-up was obtained at 3-month intervals. Orthostatic hypotension (20 mm Hg or greater systolic BP decline) was found in 69 patients (31%). The median time to reach minimal standing systolic BP was 1 minute for all subjects. In patients with orthostatic hypotension (20 mm Hg or greater), mean time to reach minimum BP was 2.4 minutes. The vast majority of patients with significant orthostatic hypotension had this finding within 2 minutes of standing. Orthostatic hypotension was common in patients for whom other probable causes of syncope were assigned. The recurrence of syncope was not related to the degree of orthostatic hypotension; however, the recurrence of dizziness and syncope as endpoints was lower in patients with 20 mm Hg or greater systolic BP reductions as compared with patients with lesser degrees of orthostatic BP declines. Orthostatic hypotension is common in patients with syncope and is detected in most patients by 2 minutes.

Evaluation of patients with syncope often includes a battery of noninvasive tests. Beauregard and associates[66] from Camden, New Jersey, evaluated 45 patients (26 with suspected neurologic and 19 with suspected cardiac syncope) with simultaneous 24-hour electroencephalographic and 2-channel electrocardiographic recordings. Isolated cardiac rhythm abnormalities were noted in 21 patients, but none of these was symptomatic and no definitive arrhythmias occurred. Isolated electroencephalographic abnormalities were noted in 11 patients, 5 of whom had electroencephalographic abnormalities consistent with seizure disorders. Simultaneous electroencephalographic and electrocardiogram abnormalities were seen in 4 patients. In 2 cases, a previously unsuspected etiology for syncope was found: seizures in 1 patient with heart disease, and sinus pauses in another thought to have a seizure disorder. Thus, combined ambulatory electroencephalographic/electrocardiogram monitoring may prove useful in the evaluation of some patients with syncope.

To verify the role of abnormal neural mechanisms in unexplained syncopes, Brignole and associates[67] from Lavagna and Reggio Emilia, Italy, evaluated the results of carotid sinus massage, eyeball compression, and head-up tilt test in the basal state and during isoproterenol infusion in: 1) 100 consecutive patients affected by syncope which, despite careful cardiovascular and neurologic examination, was of uncertain origin (age 60 ± 18 years; 54 men) and 2) 25 healthy individuals matched 4:1 with the patients of the previous group. All the patients underwent carotid sinus massage and eyeball compression in the supine and standing position for 10 seconds and head-up tilt test at 60 degrees for 60 minutes; if head-up tilt test in the basal state was negative (68 cases), it was repeated during isoproterenol (1 to 5 µg/min) infusion. In the patients with uncertain syncope, spontaneous symptoms were fully reproduced in 49%, 32%, and 16%, of cases respectively by means of carotid sinus massage, eyeball compression, head-up tilt test and head-up tilt test during isoproterenol infusion; overall positivity for ≥1 test was observed in 79% of cases. The results of carotid sinus massage, eyeball compression, or head-up tilt test during isoproterenol infusion were linked to age, sex, and underlying heart disease. In the healthy individuals, syncope was induced by carotid sinus massage, eyeball compression, head-up tilt test, and head-up tilt text during isoproterenol infusion in 1 case each; overall positivity was 16%. In conclusion, neural reflex induction tests reproduced spontaneous symptoms in most patients affected by uncertain syncope, while they evoked normal responses in most healthy individuals. Therefore on the basis of results of induction tests, the diagnosis of neurally mediated syncope can be ascribed to most patients affected by syncope of uncertain origin.

PACING AND PACEMAKERS

Previous studies have shown that single-chamber sensor-driven pacing improves exercise tolerance for patients with chronotropic incompetence. However, long-term single-chamber pacing has a number of inherent problems that limit its usefulness. Although sensor-driven dual-chamber pacing largely obviates the problems inherent with single-chamber sensor-driven pacing, the physiologic benefit of dual-chamber sensor-driven pacing has not yet been demonstrated. Accordingly, the purpose of this study by Proctor and associates[68] from Charleston, South Carolina, was to compare exercise-induced cardiac output for patients with chronotropic incompetence, after programming their pacemakers to either a simulated sensor-driven single or simulated dual-chamber mode. Cardiac output was measured noninvasively at rest and peak exercise using standard Doppler-derived measurements obtained in a blinded fashion. At rest the Doppler-derived resting VVI and DDD cardiac outputs were 4.49 ± 0.3 L/min and 4.68 ± 0.3 L/min, respectively. At peak exercise, the DDD cardiac output was 5.07 ± 0.5 L/min, whereas the simulated activity VVI and DDD cardiac output were 6.33 ± 0.6 L/min and 7.41 ± 0.70 L/min, respectively. Analysis of variance showed that there was an overall significant difference in cardiac output from rest to peak exercise. However, only the simulated activity DDD cardiac output was significantly different from its respective control value. Thus this study shows for the first time that the addition of rate responsiveness to dual-chamber pacing results in a significant improvement in cardiac output for patients with chronotropic incompetence.

CARDIOVERTERS/DEFIBRILLATORS

In a report by Pinski and associates[69] from Cleveland, Ohio, of 125 patients prepared to receive implantable cardioverter-defibrillators with the patch-patch configuration of the defibrillating electrodes, 23 (18%) had high (≥ 25 joules) defibrillation thresholds. These patients had lower LVEF (27 ± 12 vs 34 ± 13) and a higher incidence of previous heart surgery (47% vs 19%) than patients with normal defibrillation thresholds but did not differ in age, type of heart disease, incidence of concomitant heart surgery, or use of antiarrhythmic medication. Defibrillators were implanted in 18 of these 23 patients, 12 during the initial surgery and 6 after repeat defibrillation threshold testing 2 weeks later. After 22 ± 11 months of follow-up, 4 patients with implantable cardioverter-defibrillators died (2 suddenly, and 2 of nonsudden cardiac causes). Two patients without implantable cardioverter-defibrillators died of nonsudden cardiac causes. Appropriate shocks were received by 5 patients (29%) including both who died suddenly later. A high defibrillation threshold may be more common than previously stated. It is associated with poor ventricular function and previous heart surgery. Repeated defibrillation threshold testing may be useful in some patients. A high defibrillation threshold does not preclude successful implantable cardioverter-defibrillator shocks, but other therapies may provide better results.

Levine and co-workers[70] in Baltimore, Maryland, evaluated 218 patients in two-phase approach (time to first appropriate discharge, survival after discharge) to identify factors that may be related to maximal benefit derived from use of an automatic implantable cardioverter-defibrillator. One hundred ninety-seven patients survived implantation of an automatic cardioverter-defibrillator, with or without concomitant cardiac surgery. One hundred five patients had an automatic cardioverter-defibrillator discharge associated with syncope, presyncope, documented sustained VT or VF, or sleep at 9 months after implantation. Patients survived 24 months after automatic cardioverter-defibrillator discharge. LV dysfunction with the EF less than 25% was associated with earlier automatic cardioverter-defibrillator discharge and shortened survival after cardioverter discharge. Beta-Blocker administration and CABG were associated with later automatic cardioverter-defibrillator discharge. CABG but not beta-blockers was associated with more prolonged survival after automatic cardioverter defibrillator discharge. These data suggest that a relatively easy algorithm can be applied to predict which patient will benefit most from automatic cardioverter-defibrillator implantation.

Kim and associates[71] in the Bronx, New York, studied the postoperative course of 68 consecutive patients treated with an implantable defibrillator during the period from 1982 through 1990. In 46 patients (group 1), no concomitant surgery was performed during the implantation. In 22 patients (group 2), concomitant surgery, including coronary artery bypass surgery in 12, valve replacement in 3, or arrhythmia surgery in 7 were performed. All patients in group 1 were clinical stable before surgery receiving an antiarrhythmic agent chosen by serial drug testing. This same regimen was continued postoperatively. Eight of the 46 patients in group 1 whose condition had been stable in the hospital for 19 ± 25 days preoperatively developed multiple episodes of sustained VT 4 ± 9 days after implantation of the defibrillator by receiving the same antiarrhythmic regimen. Although the exacerbation was transient in some patients, six required different antiarrhythmic therapy and one eventually died. Two additional patients had frequent and prolonged episodes of nonsustained VT that could trigger the defibrillator, requiring changes in the antiarrhythmic regimen. Another patient had progressive CHF and died on day 5. A marked increase in asymptomatic ventricular arrhythmias was noted in 42% of the remaining 35 patients. In group 2 patients with combined surgery, one patient developed refractory VT 3 days postoperatively and died, 3 patients developed frequent nonsustained VT postoperatively, requiring changes in the antiarrhythmic regimen. The overall surgical mortality rate was 4% and was due to refractory VT in two patients and CHF in one. Thus, during the postoperative period after defibrillator implantation, exacerbation of ventricular arrhythmias was common and was significant in many patients and included multiple episodes of sustained VT or frequent prolonged nonsustained VT triggering the defibrillator.

Mosteller and associates[72] from Detroit, Michigan, and participating investigators from several medical centers including St Paul, Minnesota, studied operative mortality in 939 consecutive patients undergoing initial implantation of an automatic implantable cardioverter-defibrillator (ÀICD[tm]) at 15 hospitals. Twenty-nine (3.1%) patients died during the first

30 days after surgery. Among patients who survived beyond the first 30 postoperative days, EF data were available in 219; compared with the mortality group, these survivors had a significantly higher EF (34 ± 15 vs 26 ± 10%, respectively), despite similar age, sex, underlying heart disease, type of presenting arrhythmia and prevalence of concomitant surgery. The causes of perioperative death were sudden in 7 (24%), tachyarrhythmic in 9 (31%), and noncardiac in 8 (28%). Twenty-four (83%) of the deaths occurred before hospital discharge, and in all 9 instances of in-hospital sudden and tachyarrhythmic/nonsudden death, the initial recorded rhythm was sustained VT or fibrillation; in 5 (56%) of these 9 patients the AICD had been in a deactivated state since implantation. Other possible contributory factors in the 12 sudden or tachyarrhythmic/nonsudden deaths included acute myocardial ischemia or infarction in 2 (17%), and "device proarrhythmia" in 3 (25%) that were AICD-related in 2 and secondary to an antitachycardia pacemaker in another; defibrillation threshold testing was not performed in 3 patients (1 of whom had terminal VF). Thus, in this multicenter experience with thoracotomy requiring AICD implantation, operative (30-day) mortality was 3.1% and correlated inversely with LVEF. Further studies are needed to explore the potential role of management practices in the occurrence of sudden or tachyarrhythmic/nonsudden death, which accounted for 41% of all postoperative fatalities in this AICD implantation series.

To determine the frequency of loss of consciousness occurring in association with shocks delivered by automatic implantable cardioverter-defibrillators (AICD) in patients who had undergone implantation for VT or VF, Kou and associates[73] from Ann Arbor, Michigan, studied 180 patients who had undergone implantation of an AICD for the ventricular arrhythmia. The AICD used in all patients was one which delivered only high-energy shock. Of the 180 patients who received an AICD, 106 (59%) had AICD shocks during follow-up. Sixteen of the 180 patients (9%) had loss of consciousness; 13 of these 16 patients had syncope and 3 died suddenly, in association with AICD shocks. The absence of syncope during one AICD shock did not always predict the absence of syncope during subsequent shocks. The authors concluded that patients with sustained VT or VF who receive an AICD that delivers only high energy shock therapy are at moderate risk for having loss of consciousness during AICD shock. No clinical variables were found to be predictors of syncope. Therefore, driving and other activities that require patients to be extra vigilant should not be assumed to be safe after implantation of an AICD that delivers only high energy shock.

References

1. The Task Force of the Working Group on Arrhythmias of the European Society of Cardiology: The 'Sicilian gambit': A new approach to the classification of antiarrhythmic drugs based on their actions on arrhythmogenic mechanisms. Eur Heart J 1991 (Nov);12:1112–1131.
2. Moulton AW, Singer DE, Haas JS: Risk factors for stroke in patients with nonrheumatic atrial fibrillation: A case-control study. Am J Med 1991 (Aug);91:156–160.
3. Stroke Prevention in Atrial Fibrillation Investigators: Stroke Prevention in Atrial Fibrillation Study - Final Results. Circulation 1991 (August)84:527–539.
4. Connolly, SJ, Laupacis A, Gent M, Roberts RS, Cairns JA, Joyner C, for the CAFA Study

Coinvestigators. Canadian Atrial Fibrillation Anticoagulation (CAFA) Study. J Am Coll Cardiol 1991 (August);18:349–55.

5. Albers GW, Atwood JE, Hirsh J, Sherman DG, Hughes RA, Connolly SJ: Stroke prevention in nonvalvular atrial fibrillation. An Intern Med 1991 (Nov 1);115:727–736.

6. Ellenbogen KA, Dias VC, Plumb VJ, Heywood JT, Mirvis DM: A placebo-controlled trial of continuous intravenous Diltiazem infusion for 24-hour heart rate control during atrial fibrillation and atrial flutter: A multicenter study. J Am Coll Cardiol 1991 (October);18:891–7.

7. Donovan KD, Dobb GJ, Coombs LJ, Lee KY, Weekes JN, Murdock CJ, Clarke GM: Reversion of recent-onset atrial fibrillation to sinus rhythm by intravenous flecainide. Am J Cardiol 1991 (Jan 15);67:137–141.

8. Pietersen AH, Hellemann H, Danish-Norwegian Flecainide Multicenter Study Group: Usefulness of flecainide for prevention of paroxysmal atrial fibrillation and flutter. Am J Cardiol 1991 (Apr 1);67:713–717.

9. Van Gelder IC, Crijns HJ, Van Gilst WH, Verwer R, Lie KI: Prediction of uneventful cardioversion and maintenance of sinus rhythm from direct-current electrical cardioversion of chronic atrial fibrillation and flutter. Am J Cardiol 1991 (July 1);68:41–46.

10. Cox JL, Boineau JP, Schuessler RB, Ferguson TB Jr, Cain ME, Lindsay BD, Corr PB, Kater KM, Lappas DG: Successful surgical treatment of atrial fibrillation: Review and clinical update. JAMA 1991 (Oct 9);266:1976–1980.

11. Auricchio A, Klein Helmut, Trappe HJ, Wenzlaff P: Lack of prognostic value of syncope in patients with Wolff-Parkinson-White syndrome. J Am Coll Cardiol 1991 (January);17:152–8.

12. Allan LD, Chita SK, Sharland GK, Maxwell D, Priestley K: Flecainide in the Treatment of Fetal Tachycardias. Br Heart J (January) 1991;65:46–48.

13. Pritchett EL, DaTorre SD, Platt ML, McCarville SE, Hougham AJ, for the Flecainide Supraventricular Tachycardia Study Group: Flecainide acetate treatment of paroxysmal supraventricular tachycardia and paroxysmal atrial fibrillation: dose-response studies. J Am Coll Cardiol 1991 (February);17:297–303.

14. Pritchett ELC, Wilkinson WE: Mortality in patients treated with flecainide and encainide for supraventricular arrhythmias. Am J Cardiol 1991 (May 1);67:976–980.

15. Garratt CJ, Griffith MJ, O'Nunain S, Ward DE, Camm AJ: Effects of Intravenous Adenosine on Antegrade Refractoriness of Accessory Atrioventricular Connections. Circulation 1991 (November);84:1962–1968.

16. Camm AJ, Garratt CJ: Adenosine and supraventricular tachycardia. N Engl J Med 1991 (Dec 5);325:1621–1629.

17. Pritchett ELC, McCarthy EA, Wilkinson WE: Propafenone treatment of symptomatic paroxysmal supraventricular arrhythmias: A randomized, placebo-controlled, crossover trial in patients tolerating oral therapy. An Intern Med 1991 (Apr 1);114:539–544.

18. van Hare GF, Lesh MD, Scheinman M, Langberg JJ: Percutaneous radiofrequency catheter ablation for supraventricular arrhythmias in children. J Am Coll Cardiol (June) 1991;17:1613–1620.

19. Jackman WM, Wang X, Friday KJ, Roman CA, Moulton KP, Beckman KJ, McClelland JH, Twidale N, Hazlitt HA, Prior MI, Margolis PD, Calame JD, Overholt ED, Lazzara R: Catheter ablation of accessory atrioventricular pathways (Wolff-Parkinson-White syndrome) by radiofrequency current. N Engl J Med 1991 (June 6);324:1605–1611.

20. Calkins H, Sousa J, El-Atassi R, Roshenheck S, De Buitleir M, Kou WH, Kadish AH, Langberg JJ, Morady F: Diagnosis and cure of the Wolff-Parkinson-White syndrome or paroxysmal supraventricular tachycardias during a single electrophysiologic test. N Engl J Med 1991 (June 6);324:1612–1618.

21. Kuck KH, Schluter M, Geiger M, Siebels J, Duckeck W: Radiofrequency current catheter ablation of accessory atrioventricular pathways. Lancet 1991 (June 29);337:1557–1561.

22. Schluter M, Geiger M, Siebels J, Duckeck W, Kuck K-H: Catheter Ablation Using Radiofrequency Current to Cure Symptomatic Patients With Tachyarrhythmias Related to an Accessory Atrioventricular Pathway. Circulation 1991 (October);84:1644–1661.

23. Kuck K-H, Schluter M: Single-Catheter Approach to Radiofrequency Current Ablation of Left-Sided Accessory Pathways in Patients With Wolff-Parkinson-White Syndrome. Circulation 1991 (December);84:2366–2375.

24. Evans GT, Scheinman MM, Bardy G, Borggrefe M, Brugada P, Fisher J, Fontaine G, Huang

SKS, Huang WH, Josephson M, Kuck K-H, Hlatky MA, Levy S, Lister JW, Marcus F, Morady F, Tchou P, Waldo AL, Wood D: Predictors of In-Hospital Mortality After DC Catheter Ablation of Atrioventricular Junction - Results of a Prospective, International, Multicenter Study. Circulation 1991 (November);84:1924–1936.

25. Ghali JK, Kadakia S, Cooper RS, Liao Y: Impact of left ventricular hypertrophy on ventricular arrhythmias in the absence of coronary artery disease. J Am Coll Cardiol 1991 (May);17:1277–82.

26. Gomes JA, Winters SL, Ergin A, Machac J, Estioko M, Alexopoulous D, Pe E: Clinical and electrophysiologic determinants, treatment and survival of patients with sustained malignant ventricular tachyarrhythmias occurring late after myocardial infarction. J Am Coll Cardiol 1991 (February);17:320–6.

27. Strickberger SA, Cantillon CO, Friedman PL: When should patients with lethal ventricular arrhythmia resume driving? An analysis of state regulations and physician practices. An Intern Med 1991 (Oct 1);115:560–563.

28. Meredith IT, Broughton A, Jennings GL, Esler MD: Evidence of a selective increase in cardiac sympathetic activity in patients with sustained ventricular arrhythmias. N Engl J Med 1991 (Aug 29);325:618–624.

29. Pratt CM, Hallstrom A, Theroux P, Romhilt D, Coromilas J, Myles J, for the CPAS investigators: Avoiding interpretive pitfalls when assessing arrhythmia suppression after myocardial infarction: insights from the long-term observations of the placebo-treated patients in the Cardiac Arrhythmia Pilot Study (CAPS). J Am Coll Cardiol 1991 (January);17:1–8.

30. Echt DS, Liebson PR, Mitchell B, Peters RW, Obias-Manno D, Barker AH, Arensberg D, Baker A, Friedman L, Greene L, Huther ML, Richardson DW, CAST Investigators: Mortality and morbidity in patients receiving encainide, flecainide, or placebo: The Cardiac arrhythmia suppression trial. N Engl J Med 1991 (Mar 21);324:781–788.

31. Epstein AE, Bigger JT Jr., Wyse DG, Romhilt DW, Reynolds-Haertle RA, Hallstrom AP and the CAST Investigators: Events in the cardiac arrhythmia suppression trial (CAST): mortality in the entire population enrolled. J Am Coll Cardiol 1991 (July);18:14–9.

32. Denes P, Gillis AM, Pawitan Y, Kammerlling JM, Wilhelmsen L, Salerno DM, CAST Investigators: Prevalence, characteristics and significance of ventricular premature complexes and ventricular tachycardia detected by 24-hour continuous electrocardiographic recording in the cardiac arrhythmia suppression trial. Am J Cardiol 1991 (Oct 1);68:887–896.

33. Fish FA, Gillette PC, Benson DW Jr., for the Pediatric Electrophysiology Group: Proarrhythmia, cardiac arrest and death in young patients receiving encainide and flecainide. J Am Coll Cardiol 1991 (August);18:356–65.

34. Morganroth J and Goin JE: Quinidine-Related Mortality in the Short-to-Medium-Term Treatment of Ventricular Arrhythmias - A Meta-Analysis. Circulation 1991 (November);84:1977–1983.

35. Anastasiou-Nan MI, Gilbert EM, Miller RH, Singh S, Freedman RA, Keefe DL, Saksena S, MacNeil DJ, Anderson JL: Usefulness of d, 1 sotalol for suppression of chronic ventricular arrhythmias. Am J Cardiol 1991 (Mar 1);67:511–516.

36. Wiersinga WM, Trip MD, Van Beeren MH, Plomp TA, Oosting H: An increase in plasma cholesterol independent of thyroid function during long-term amiodarone therapy: A dose-dependent relationship. An Intern Med 1991 (Jan);114:128–132.

37. Dobs AS, Sarma PS, Guarnieri T, Griffith L: Testicular dysfunction with amiodarone use. J Am Coll Cardiol 1991 (November);18:1328–32.

38. Yeung-Lai-Wah JA, Alison JF, Lonergan L, Mohama R, Leather R, Kerr CR: High success rate of atrioventricular node ablation with radiofrequency energy. J Am Coll Cardiol 1991 (December);18:1753–8.

39. Niwano S, Aizawa Y, Satoh M, Chinushi M, Shibata A: Low-energy catheter electrical ablation for sustained ventricular tachycardia. Am Heart J 1991 (July);122:81–88.

40. Lawrie GM, Pacifico A, Kaushik R, Nahas C, Earle N: Factors predictive of results of direct ablative operations for drug-refractory ventricular tachycardia: Analysis of 80 patients. J Thorac Cardiovasc Surg 1991 (Jan);101:44–55.

41. Kemp JS, Thach BT: Sudden death in infants sleeping on polystyrene-filled cushions. NEJM 1991 (June 27);324:1858–1864.

42. Burke AP, Farb A, Virmani R, Goodin J, Smialek JE: Sports-related and non-sports-related sudden cardiac death in young adults. Am Heart J 1991 (February);121:568–575.

43. Drory Y, Turetz Y, Hiss Y, Lev B, Fisman EZ, Pines A, Kramer MR: Sudden unexpected death in persons <40 years of age. Am J Cardiol 1991 (Nov 15);68:1388–1392.

44. Goodin JC, Farb A, Smialek JE, Field F, Virmani R: Right ventricular dysplasia associated with sudden death in young adults. Modern Pathology 1991:4:702–706.

45. Brooks R, McGovern BA, Garan H, Ruskin JN: Current treatment of patients surviving out-of-hospital cardiac arrest. JAMA 1991 (Feb 13);265:762–768.

46. Cascade Investigators: Cardiac arrest in Seattle: Conventional versus amiodarone drug evaluation (The CASCADE Study). Am J Cardiol 1991 (Mar 15);67:578–584.

47. Kudenchuk PJ, Cobb LA, Greene HL, Fahrenbruch CE, Sheehan FH: Late outcome of survivors of out-of-hospital cardiac arrest with left ventricular ejection fractions ≥50% and without significant coronary arterial narrowing. Am J Cardiol 1991 (Apr 1);67:704–708.

48. Sousa J, Rosenheck S, Calkins H, de Buitleir M, Schmaltz S, Kadish A, Morady F: Results of electrophysiologic testing and long-term prognosis in patients with coronary artery disease and aborted sudden death. Am Heart J 1991 (October);122:1001–1006.

49. Hallstrom AP, Cobb LA, Uy BH, Weaver WD, Fahrenbruch CE: An antiarrhythmic drug experience in 941 patients resuscitated from an initial cardiac arrest between 1970 and 1985. Am J Cardiol 1991 (Oct 15);68:1025–1031.

50. Wang Y, Scheinman MM, Chien WW, Cohen TJ, Lesh MD, Griffin JC: Patients with supraventricular tachycardia presenting with aborted sudden death: incidence, mechanism and long-term follow-up. J Am Coll Cardiol 1991 (December);18:1711–9.

51. Olshausen KV, Witt T, Pop T, Treese N, Bethge KP, Meyer J: Sudden cardiac death while wearing a Holter monitor. Am J Cardiol 1991 (Feb 15);67:381–386.

52. Ciampricotti R, Taverne R, El Gamal M: Clinical and angiographic observations on resuscitated victims of exercise-related sudden ischemic death. Am J Cardiol 1991 (July 1);68:47–50.

53. Haynes BE, Mendoza A, McNeil M, Schroeder J, Smiley DR: A statewide early defibrillation initiative including laypersons and outcome reporting. JAMA 1991 (July 24/31);266:545–547.

54. Gray WA, Capone RJ, Most AS: Unsuccessful emergency medical resuscitation—are continued efforts in the emergency department justified? N Engl J Med 1991 (Nov 14);325:1393–1398.

55. Moss AJ, Schwartz PJ, Crampton RS, Tzivoni D, Locati EH, MacCluer J, Hall WJ, Weithkamp L, Vincent GM, Garson A, Robinson JL, Benhorin J, Choi S: The Long QT Syndrome Prospective Longitudinal Study of 328 Families. Circulation 1991 (September);84:1136–444.

56. Algra A, Tijssen JGP, Roelandt JRTC, Pool J, and Lubsen J: QTc Prolongation Measured by Standard 12-Lead Electrocardiography Is an Independent Risk Factor for Sudden Death Due To Cardiac Arrest. Circulation 1991; (June)83:1888–1894.

57. Kugler JD: Sinus nodal dysfunction in young patients with long QT syndrome. Am Heart J 1991 (April);121:1132–1136.

58. Munger RG, Prineas RJ, Crow RS, Changbumrung S, Keane V, Wangsuphachart V, Jones MP: Prolonged QT interval and risk of sudden death in South-East Asian men. Lancet 1991 (Aug 3);338:280–281.

59. Moss AJ, Liu JE, Gottlieb S, Locati EH, Schwartz PJ, Robinson JL: Efficacy of Permanent Pacing in the Management of High-Risk Patients With Long QT Syndrome. Circulation 1991 (October);84:1524–1529.

60. Matzer L, Kiat H, Friedman JD, Van Train K, Maddahi J, Berman DS: A new approach to the assessment of tomographic thallium-201 scintigraphy in patients with left bundle branch block. J Am Coll Cardiol 1991 (May);17:1309–17.

61. Schmidt KG, Ulmer HE, Silverman NH, Kleinman CS, Copel JA: Perinatal outcome of fetal complete atrioventricular block: A multicenter experience. J Am Coll Cardiol (May) 1991;91:1360–1366.

62. Perry JC and Garson, Jr. A: The Child with Recurrent Syncope: Autonomic Function Testing and Beta-Adrenergic Hypersensitivity. J Am Coll Cardiol (April) 1991;17:1168–1171.

63. Moazez F, Peter T, Simonson J, Mandel WJ, Vaughn C, Gang E: Syncope of unknown origin: Clinical, noninvasive, and electrophysiologic determinants of arrhythmia induction and symptom recurrence during long-term follow-up. Am Heart J 1991 (January);121:81–88.

64. Muller T, Talajic RM, Lemery R, Nattel S, Cassidy D: Electrophysiologic evaluation and outcome of patients with syncope of unknown origin. Br Heart J 1991 (Feb);12:139–143.

65. Atkins D, Hanusa B, Sefcik T, Kapoor W: Syncope and orthostatic hypotension. Am J Med 1991 (Aug);91:179–185.

66. Beauregard LAM, Fabiszewski R, Black CH, Lightfoot B, Schraeder PL, Toly T, Waxman HL: Combined ambulatory electroencephalographic and electrocardiographic recordings for evaluation of syncope. Am J Cardiol 1991 (Oct 15);68:1067–1072.

67. Brignole M, Menozzi C, Gianfranchi L, Oddone D, Lolli G, Bertulla A: Carotid sinus massage, eyeball compression, and head-up tilt test in patients with syncope of uncertain origin and in healthy control subjects. Am Heart J 1991 (December);122:1644–1651.

68. Proctor EE, Leman RB, Mann DL, Kaiser J, Kratz J, Gillette P: Single- versus dual-chamber sensor-driven pacing: Comparison of cardiac outputs. Am Heart J 1991 (September);122:728–732.

69. Pinski SL, Vanerio G, Castle LW, Morant VA, Simmons TW, Trohman RG, Wilocoff BL, Maloney JD: Patients with a high defibrillation threshold: Clinical characteristics, management, and outcome. Am Heart J 1991 (July);122:89–95.

70. Levine, JH, Mellits ED, Baumgardner RA, Veltri EP, Mower M, Grunwald L, Guarnieri T, Aarons D, and Griffith LSC: Predictors of First Discharge and Subsequent Survival in Patients With Automatic Implantable Cardioverter-Defibrillators. Circulation 1991 (August);84:558–566.

71. Kim SG, Fisher JD, Furman S, Gross J, Zilo P, Roth JA, Ferrick KJ, Brodman R: Exacerbation of ventricular arrhythmias during the postoperative period after implantation of an automatic defibrillator. J Am Coll Cardiol 1991 (November);18:1200–6.

72. Mosteller RD, Lehmann MH, Thomas AC, Jackson K: Operative mortality with implantation of the automatic cardioverter-defibrillator. Am J Cardiol 1991 (Nov 15);68:1340–1345.

73. Kou WH, Calkins H, Lewis RR, Bolling SF, Kirsch MM, Langberg JJ, De Buitleir M, Sousa J, El-Atassi R, Morady F: Incidence of loss of consciousness during automatic implantable cardioverter-defibrillator shocks. An Intern Med 1991 (Dec 15);115:942–945.

5

Systemic Hypertension

Ambulatory pressure in normotensive subjects

Ambulatory BP monitoring has become increasingly popular for diagnosing and treating patients with systemic hypertension. Data from normotensive subjects are needed for interpretation of hypertensive readings. Zachariah and associates[1] from Jacksonville, Florida, and Rochester, Minnesota, monitored ambulatory BP in 126 normotensive subjects aged 20 to 84 years. Mean systolic and diastolic BP and BP loads (percentage of systolic readings >140 mm Hg and diastolic readings >90 mm Hg) were obtained and interpreted. Mean awake systolic and diastolic pressures ranged from 125 ± 10 to 137 ± 17 mm Hg and 70 ± 8 to 71 ± 9 mm Hg, respectively. The systolic and diastolic trends of subjects' BP taken during office visits and the 24-hour measurements were similar. Ranged for systolic and diastolic BP loads from youngest to oldest ages were 9% ± 14% to 25% ± 20% and 3% ± 7% to 4% ± 7%, respectively. A comparison of BP means from our sample that were taken during office visits and BP means from a 2122-patient community survey demonstrated that our sample was reflective of an unselected population.

To perform a meta-analysis of published reports in an attempt to determine the mean and range of normal ambulatory BP, Staessen and associates[2] from Leuven, Belgium, reviewed 23 studies including a total of 3,476 normal subjects. Most studies were compatible with a mean 24-hour BP in the range of 115 to 120/70 to 75 mm Hg, a mean daytime BP of 120 to 125/75 to 80 mm Hg, and a mean nighttime BP of 105 to 110/60 to 65 mm Hg. With weighting for the number of subjects included in the individual studies, the 24-hour BP averaged 118/72 mm Hg, the daytime BP 123/76 mm Hg, and the nighttime BP 106/64 mm Hg. The night/day pressure ratio averaged 0.87 for systolic and 0.83 for diastolic BP, with ranges across the individual studies from 0.79 to 0.92 and from 0.75 to

0.90, respectively. If the mean ± 2 standard deviation interval in the various studies was considered normal, the range of normality was on average 97 to 139/57 to 87 mm Hg for the 24-hour BP, 101 to 146/61 to 91 mm Hg for the daytime BP, and 86 to 127/48 to 79 mm Hg for the nighttime BP. Until the results of prospective studies on the relation between the ambulatory BP and the incidence of cardiovascular morbidity and mortality become available, the aforementioned intervals, which summarize the experience of 23 investigators, could serve as a temporary reference for clinical practice.

Ambulatory pressure in hypertensive blacks

Although cigarette smoking raises BP, the office BP measurements of cigarette smokers are the same as, or lower than, those of nonsmokers. Mann and associates[3] from New York, New York, compared office and 24-hour ambulatory BP of 59 untreated hypertensive smokers with 118 non-smoking hypertensive persons matched for age, sex, and race. The office BP of the smoking and non-smoking groups were 141/93 and 142/93 mm Hg, respectively. The awake ambulatory systolic BP was significantly higher in the smokers (145 vs 140 mm Hg). This difference was greater among patients over the age of 50 years (153 vs 142 mm Hg), and absent among patients under 50 years (140 vs 139 mm Hg). BP during sleep did not differ between the 2 groups (121/76 vs 123/77 mm Hg). The authors concluded that among white hypertensives above the age of 50 years smokers maintain a higher daytime ambulatory systolic BP than nonsmokers even though BP measured in the office is similar.

Relation between skin darkness and blood pressure in blacks

To determine the association of skin color, measured by a reflectometer, with BP in U.S. blacks, Klag and associates[4] from 3 USA medical centers studied a community sample of 457 blacks from 3 U.S. cities. Persons taking antihypertensive medications were excluded. Both systolic and diastolic BP were higher in darker persons and increased by 2 mm Hg for every 1-SD increase in skin darkness. However, the association was dependent on socioeconomic status, whether measured by education or an index consisting of education, occupation, and ethnicity, being present only in persons with lower levels of either indicator. Using multiple linear regression, both systolic and diastolic BP remained significantly associated with darker skin color in the lower levels of socioeconomic status, independent of age, body mass index, and concentrations of blood glucose, serum urea nitrogen, serum uric acid, and urinary sodium and potassium. The association of skin color with BP only in low socioeconomic strata may be due to the lesser ability of such groups to deal with the psychosocial stress associated with darker skin color. However, these findings also are consistent with an interaction between an environmental factor associated with low socioeconomic status and a susceptible gene that has a higher prevalence in persons with darker skin color.

This article was followed by an editorial entitled, "Skin Color and Blood Pressure," by Robert F. Murray, Jr.,[5] who concluded that "a combination of disadvantaged socioeconomic status and a behavior pattern of repressed hostility in a dark-skinned individual may be the phenotypic marker of the at-risk person to develop hypertension". The genetic predisposition is important, but environmental factors may still play the pivotal role, even when the genes that are responsible for BP elevation have been identified and their functions elucidated.

Osler's maneuver

In pseudo-hypertension, BP measured indirectly by means of a sphygmomanometer is artifactually high compared with findings when the intra-arterial BP is measured directly. This discrepancy has been attributed either to medical calcification of the arterial wall, known as Monckeberg's calcification, or to advanced atherosclerosis with calcification of the artery. Because the calcified, stiff artery cannot be compressed by the BP cuff, inaccurate high BP readings are recorded. The prevalence of pseudohypertension is unknown because of the inability to diagnose the condition noninvasively with reliability. Messerli et al reintroduced a concept that was originally described in the writings of Sir William Osler. The Osler maneuver is a simple bedside procedure by which patients with true hypertension can be differentiated from patients whose BP readings are elevated because of noncompressible large arteries. Osler's maneuver is performed by assessing the palpability of the pulseless radial or brachial artery distal to the point of occlusion of the artery by direct finger or cuff pressure. Messerli et al found that patients with pseudohypertension had falsely elevated BP readings, with a difference of 10 to 55 mm Hg between cuff and intra-arterial pressures, and that arterial compliance was lower in patients with Osler-positive findings. The prevalence of patients with Osler-positive findings in a general clinic population is unknown. Tsapatsaris and associates[6] from Burlington, Massachusetts, examined the frequency and reproducibility of the findings on Osler's maneuver as performed by general internists and vascular medicine specialists on the hospital population seen at an outpatient clinic. They performed Osler's maneuver on 912 consecutive outpatients aged 60 years or older in a 2-month period by 12 physicians. The incidence of an Osler-positive finding was 7.1% (65/912). The number of positive findings increased with age, ranging from 3.4% in the 60- to 70-year age group to 43.8% in the 86- to 90-year age group. A history of hypertension was present in 58% of patients with Osler-positive findings and in 60% of patients with Osler negative findings. In a group of 48 previously screened patients who were independently examined, concordance was poor when the k test of reliability was used. Positive Osler findings were common in patients older than 70 years, in patients who smoked, and in patients with a high systolic BP. These correlations may be related to a decrease in blood vessel compressibility, which may cause pseudohypertension. The findings on Osler's maneuver, are poorly reproducible, making the procedure an inadequate test.

Obesity-related

Although weight reduction generally lowers BP, it is unclear whether the response is due to concurrent dietary changes or to restricted body mass itself. Weinsier and associates[7] from Birmingham, Alabama, examined independent effects of energy restriction and weight reduction prospectively in 24 obese, hypertensive, normoglycemic women whose dietary intake was tightly controlled. Sodium, potassium, and calcium intake, the polyunsaturated/saturated fat ratio, and the proportional composition of carbohydrate, fat, and protein were constant throughout the 5-month protocol. Hemodynamic and neuroendocrine status was evaluated in four 10-day hospital phases: 2 prior to weight loss (energy balance and then 800-kcal intake), and 2 after an average loss of 13 kg to normal body weight (800 kcal and then return to energy balance). Fasting serum insulin, triiodothyronine: reverse triiodothyronine ratio, resting metabolic rate, and heart rate declined, and sodium and potassium balances were negative during energy restriction. Catecholamines, renin, aldosterone, plasma volume, cardiac output, and BP showed no consistent response to changes in energy intake. By contrast, weight reduction independently lowered BP, plasma volume, cardiac output, and plasma renin activity. Body fat pattern remained unchanged. These results demonstrate that weight loss has a BP-lowering effect that is distinct from energy restriction and that is related to changes in blood volume and cardiac output.

Insulin, glucose, and lipid problems

Essential hypertension is, in some patients, complicated by impairment of insulin-mediated glucose disposal and hyperinsulinemia. Whether this metabolic disturbance is a consequence of the hypertensive process or whether it may precede, and thus possibly promote, the development of hypertension has been unknown. Searching for hereditary or familial defects in hypertension-prone humans, Ferrari and associates[8] from Berne, St. Gallen, and Zurich, Switzerland, prospectively investigated insulin sensitivity, plasma insulin and glucose, and serum lipoproteins in normotensive offspring of essential hypertensive as compared with age- and body habitus-matched offspring of normotensive families. Compared with 78 control subjects 70 offspring of essential hypertensive parents had similar age (mean $\pm$ SEM: 24 $\pm$ 1 vs 24 $\pm$ 1 years, respectively) and body mass index (22.3 $\pm$ 0.2 vs 22.4 $\pm$ 0.2 kg/m^2), a BP of 127/77 $\pm$ 1/1 versus 123/76 $\pm$ 1/1 mm Hg, and significantly elevated fasting plasma insulin levels (9.9 $\pm$ 0.3 vs 8.6 $\pm$ 0.3 $_u$U/mL), serum total triglycerides (1.03 $\pm$ 0.06 vs 0.83 $\pm$ 0.03 mmol/L), total cholesterol (4.37 $\pm$ 0.08 vs 3.93 $\pm$ 0.07 mmol/L), LDL cholesterol (2.45 $\pm$ 0.08 vs 2.14 $\pm$ 0.07 mmol/L), and total/HDL cholesterol ratio (4.3 $\pm$ 0.1 vs 3.7 $\pm$ 0.1). Insulin sensitivity was lower (9.4 $\pm$ 0.7 vs 13.2 $\pm$ 1.1 $\times$ 10^{-4} $\times$ minute^{-1}/$_u$U/mL), while post glucose-load plasma insulin levels were higher in the 41 offspring of essential hypertensive parents than in the 38 offspring of normotensive parents so investigated. These findings demonstrate that young normotensive humans in apparently excellent health but with 1 essential hypertensive parent tend to have an impairment of insulin-mediated glucose disposal, hyperinsulinemia, and dyslipidemia. It follows that a familial trait for essential hypertension seems to coexist commonly with defects in carbohydrate and lipoprotein metabolism that can be detected before or at least at a very early stage of the development of high BP as judged by resting BP measurements.

Various aspects of carbohydrate and lipid metabolism have been studied by Sheu and associates[9] from Palo Alto, California, in 2 groups of patients with mild (diastolic BP between 105 and 95 mm Hg) hypertension before and after 4 months of treatment with either nifedipine (n = 12) or atenolol (n = 12). Mean BP fell to the same degree following treatment with either nifedipine (147 $\pm$ 3/98 $\pm$ 2 to 134 $\pm$ 2/85 + 2 mm Hg) or atenolol (149 $\pm$ 3/99 $\pm$ 2 to 135 $\pm$ 2/86 $\pm$ 3 mm Hg). Circulating plasma glucose, insulin, and triglyceride concentrations were measured at hourly intervals from 8:00 a.m. to 4:00 p.m., before and after breakfast (8:00 a.m.), and at lunch time (noon). The response to treatment was different in the

2 groups. Specifically, plasma glucose concentration were unchanged and insulin concentrations were higher in association with atenolol treatment. In contrast, nifedipine-treated patients had similar plasma insulin, but lower plasma glucose and triglyceride concentrations after 4 months of therapy. The changes in day-long plasma glucose and insulin responses suggested that resistance to insulin-stimulated glucose uptake had increased in association with atenolol treatment and decreased following nifedipine. This conclusion was supported in that measurement of insulin-stimulated glucose disposal showed a decrease in atenolol-treated patients and an increase in nifedipine-treated patients. Finally, plasma lipoprotein cholesterol concentrations did not change following atenolol therapy, whereas plasma HDL cholesterol increased in association with nifedipine administration. These data show that changes in carbohydrate and liquid metabolism observed with treatment of mild hypertension can vary significantly as a function of the drug used, despite similar beneficial effects on BP. As all of the changes noted could modify risk of CAD in patients with hypertension, knowledge of these drug-related differences would seem to be important in planning treatment programs.

To investigate the role of glucose tolerance in the development of systemic hypertension, Salomaa and associates[10] from Helsinki and Espoo, Finland, performed a retrospective analysis of the results of a health checkup in a group of clinically healthy middle-aged men in the late 1960s (median year 1968). The subjects were invited to enter into a primary prevention trial for cardiovascular disease in 1974 when they underwent clinical examination for risk factors. The trial was completed in 1979 when the men were re-examined. Follow-up was in 1986. In all, 3490 men born during 1919–1934 participated in a health checkup in the late 1960s. In 1974, 1815 of these men who were clinically healthy were entered into a primary prevention trial for cardiovascular disease. On clinical examination 1222 of the men were considered at high risk of cardiovascular disease. Of these, 612 received an intervention and were excluded from the study. A total of 593 men were without risk factors. The study comprised all of the men who did not have an intervention. In 1979, 1120 men were re-examined, and in 1986 945 men attended follow-up. There were 2 groups for analysis: 1 comprising all subjects and the other comprising only men who were normotensive in 1968 and for whom complete information was available. By 1979, 103 men were taking antihypertensive drugs, and by 1986, 131 were taking antihypertensive drugs and 12 were taking drugs for hyperglycemia. Blood glucose concentration 1 hour after a glucose load, BP, and body weight were measured in 1968, 1974, and 1979. In 1986 BP and body weight were recorded. Men who were hypertensive in 1986 had significantly higher BP and (after adjustment for body mass index and alcohol intake) significantly higher blood glucose concentrations 1 hour after a glucose load at all examinations than those who were normotensive in 1986. Regression analysis showed that the higher the blood glucose concentration after a glucose load in 1968 the higher the BP during the following years. Those men between the second and third tertiles of blood glucose concentration in 1968 had a significantly higher risk of developing hypertension (odds ratio 1.71) compared with those below the first tertile. In this study men who developed hypertension tended to have shown an increased intolerance to glucose up to 18 years before the clinical manifestation of their disorder. Blood glucose concentration 1 hour after a glucose load was an independent predictor of future hypertension.

Prevalence of resistant hypertension

To determine the prevalence of resistant systemic hypertension in a tertiary care facility, the frequency of its various causes, and the results of treatment, Yakovlevitch and Black[11] from New Haven, Connecticut, reviewed clinical records of all patients seen for the first time in a 3-year period (1986, 1987, and 1988) and found to have met criteria for resistant systemic hypertension. They were examined for appropriateness of their medical regimen, presence of secondary causes of hypertension, non-compliance, interfering substances, drug interactions, office resistance (elevated BP in the office only while receiving treatment), and other potential causes of resistance. Of the 436 charts reviewed, 91 were those of patients who met criteria for resistant hypertension and were seen more than once. The most common cause was a suboptimal medical regimen (39 patients), followed by medication intolerance (13 patients), previously undiagnosed secondary hypertension (10 patients), noncompliance (9 patients), psychiatric causes (7 patients), office resistance (2 patients), an interfering substance (2 patients), and drug interaction (1 patient). BP control, defined as diastolic BP of 90 mm Hg or less and systolic BP of 140 mm Hg or less for patients aged 50 years or less ($\leq$150 mm Hg for those aged 51 to 60 years and >160 mm Hg for those aged >60 years), was achieved in 48 (53%) of those 91 patients. Another 10 had significant improvement in their BP ($\geq$15% decrease in diastolic BP). Of patients whose BP was controlled after they had been on a suboptimal regimen, the 2 most frequently used therapeutic strategies were to add (50%) or modify (24%) diuretic therapy or to add (50%) or increase the dose of (12%) a newer drug, either a calcium entry blocker or angiotensin-converting enzyme inhibitor. The authors concluded that resistant hypertension is common in a tertiary care facility and that a suboptimal regimen is the most common reason. Furthermore, in the majority of these patients, the elevated BP can be controlled or significantly improved.

Effect of potassium depletion

To determine the effects of potassium depletion on BP in patients with hypertension, Krishna and Kapoor[12] from Philadelphia, Pennsylvania, performed a double-blind, randomized, cross-over study involving 12 patients with hypertension with each patient serving as his or her own control. Patients were placed on 10-day isocaloric diets providing a daily potassium intake of either 16 mmol or 96 mmol. The intake of sodium (120 mmol/d) and other minerals was kept constant. On day 11 each patient received a 2-litre isotonic saline infusion over 4 hours. BP, urinary excretion rates for sodium, potassium, calcium, and phosphorous; glomerular filtration rate; renal plasma flow; and plasma levels of vasoactive hormones were measured. With low potassium intake, systolic BP increased by 7 mm Hg and diastolic pressure increased by 6 mm Hg, whereas plasma potassium concentration decreased by 0.8 mmol/L. In response to a 2-litre isotonic saline infusion, the mean arterial pressure increased similarly on both diets but reached higher levels on low potassium intake (115 $\pm$ 2 mm Hg compared with 109 $\pm$ 2 mm Hg). Potassium depletion was associated with a decrease in sodium excretion (83 $\pm$ 6 mmol/d compared with 110 $\pm$ 5 mmol/d). Plasma renin activity and plasma aldosterone concentrations also decreased in patients during low potassium intake, but concentrations of arginine vasopressin and atrial natriuretic peptide, glomerular filtration rate, and renal plasma flow area were unchanged. Further, low potassium intake increased urinary excretion of calcium and phosphorus and of plasma immunoreactive parathyroid hormone levels. Dietary potassium restriction increases BP in patients with essential hypertension. Both sodium retention and calcium depletion may contribute to the increase in BP during potassium depletion.

Associated with mid-ventricular obstruction

Midventricular obstruction is an uncommon finding previously defined by catheterization and angiographic techniques in patients with HC. Harrison and associates[13] from Lexington, Kentucky, described clinical and electrocardiographic findings in 10 patients (mean age 73 years) with severe concentric LV hypertrophy and the unusual finding of a dynamic systolic obstruction located in the midportion of the left ventricle. All patients were known to have chronic hypertension, and none had a history or family history of hypertrophic cardiomyopathy. In each case, a well-defined, high velocity, turbulent jet was identified by Doppler color flow imaging and subsequently confirmed with conventional Doppler techniques. Septal and posterior wall thickness averaged 1.67 and 1.57 cm, respectively. Mean LV mass index was 199 g/m^2 and EF averaged 78%. Peak systolic velocity obtained by continuous-wave Doppler averaged 2.7 m/s and appeared as either a "late-peaking" or a "spike and dome" configuration. Seven of 10 patients gave a history of syncope or severe presyncope at the time of echocardiographic examination. At a mean follow-up of 1 year, syncope or presyncope had resolved in 5 patients in whom medication was adjusted based on the ultrasound study, but persisted in 2 patients in whom diuretic therapy was continued. It is concluded that obstruction to systolic flow can occur at the mid-LV level in some patients with severe concentric LV hypertrophy and avoidance of medication known to lower LV volume may relieve symptoms of transient inadequate cardiac output.

Left ventricular filling and stress

Grossman and associates[14] from New Orleans, Louisiana, evaluated cardiac structure and systolic and diastolic function by 2-dimensional M-mode echocardiography in lean and obese patients who were either hypertensive or normotensive. Diastolic function, as assessed by diminished normalized early peak filling rate and prolonged duration of rapid filling, was decreased in hypertensive patients compared with normotensive patients. When compared with lean patients with similar blood pressure levels, obese patients exhibited a lower normalized peak filling rate but no difference in duration of rapid filling. A significant correlation was observed between the normalized peak filling rate and either body mass index or LV mass. Obese patients had greater LV end-diastolic and systolic dimensions, LV wall thickness and LV mass than lean patients. Impairment of LV filling was most pronounced in obese hypertensive patients. It is concluded that the burden on the LV imposed by obesity causes cardiac enlargement and impairment of LV filling regardless of levels of arterial pressure.

To evaluate whether impaired LV filling determines the hemodynamic responses to isometric and orthostatic stress in patients whose systemic BP is greater than 140/90 mm Hg, Grossman and associates[15] from New Orleans, Louisiana, studied 32 patients with essential hypertension. The patients were divided into those with preserved LV filling (15 patients) and those with impaired LV filling (17 patients). Echocardiograms were obtained before hemodynamic assessment was performed. Isometric stress and head-up tilt tests were done with a recovery period of at least 10 minutes between each to allow for BP and heart rate to return to baseline. Hemodynamic reassessment was performed during the last minute of each test and at the end of the recovery period. Plasma epinephrine, norepinephrine, and dopamine levels were determined by radioenzymatic method. Isometric stress increased mean arterial pressure by 30% by an increase in cardiac output and total peripheral resistance associated with an increase in plasma catecholamine levels. Patients with preserved LV filling had an increase in arterial pressure predominantly through an elevation in cardiac output (17%) associated with a small increase in plasma norepinephrine levels and in peripheral resistance (11%). In contrast, patients with impaired LV filling had an increase in arterial pressure mainly through an increase in peripheral resistance (25%) that was associated with a 45% elevation in plasma norepinephrine levels. Orthostatic stress (passive head-up tilt) caused an exaggerated decrease in stroke volume and cardiac output in patients with impaired LV filling when compared with those with preserved diastolic function. Impaired LV filling blunts the response of the heart to isometric and orthostatic stress.

Use of echocardiographic left ventricular mass and electrolyte intake in predicting hypertension and/or morbidity and mortality

To identify predictors of systemic hypertension, de Simone and associates[16] from New York, New York performed echocardiography, standard blood tests, and 24-hour urine collection at baseline and after an interval of 3 to 6 years (mean 4.7 ± 8) in 132 normotensive adults from a large employed population. At follow-up, 15 subjects (11%; 7 men, 8 women) had a systolic BP >140 mm Hg or a diastolic BP >90 mm Hg or both (mean, 143 ± 7 and 87 ± 6 mm Hg, respectively). At baseline, subjects who developed hypertension had a greater LV mass index than those who did not (92 ± 25 compared with 77 ± 19 g/m² body surface area) and higher 24-hour urinary sodium/potassium excretion ratio (3.6 ± 1.7 compared with 2.6 ± 1.4); there were no differences in race, initial age, systolic or diastolic BP, coronary risk factors, or plasma renin activity. The likelihood of developing hypertension rose from 3% in the lowest quartile of sex-adjusted LV mass index to 24% in the highest quartile; a parallel trend was less regular for quartiles of the sodium/potassium excretion ratio. In multivariate analyses, follow-up systolic pressures in all subjects and in the 117 who remained normotensive were predicted by initial age, systolic BP, black race, and sex-adjusted LV mass index; final diastolic BP was predicted by its initial value, plasma triglyceride levels, urinary sodium/potassium ratio, low renin activity, black race, and plasma glucose level. Echocardiographic LV mass in normotensive adults is directly related to the risk for developing subsequent hypertension. LV mass improves prediction of future systolic pressure, whereas diastolic pressure is more related to initial metabolic status. Black race is also an independent determinant of higher subsequent BP.

Koren and associates[17] from New York, New York, assessed the prognostic significance of LV mass and geometry in 280 patients with essential hypertension evaluated by echocardiogram between 1976 and 1981. Two-hundred and fifty-three subjects or their family members (90%) were contacted for follow-up interview an average of 10.2 years after the initial cardiogram was obtained. The survival status of 27 patients lost to follow-up was ascertained by using National Death Index data. LV mass exceeded 125 g/m² in 69 of 253 patients (27%). Cardiovascular events occurred in a higher proportion of patients with than without LV hypertrophy (26% compared with 12%). Patients with increased ventricular mass were also at higher risk for cardiovascular death (14% compared with 0.5%) and all-cause mortality (16% compared with 2%). Electrocardiographic LV hypertrophy did not predict risk. Patients with normal LV geometry had the fewest adverse outcomes (no cardiac deaths; morbid events in 11%), and those with concentric hypertrophy had the most (death in 21%; morbid events in 31%). In a multivariate analysis, only age and LV mass—but not gender, BP, or serum cholesterol level—independently predicted all 3 outcome measures. Echocardiographically determined LV mass and geometry stratify risk in patients with essential hypertension independently of and more strongly than BP or other potentially reversible risk factors and may help to stratify the need for intensive treatment.

Renal hemodynamics and the renin-angiotensin-aldosterone system in normotensive subjects with hypertensive and normotensive parents

The kidney is important in BP regulation, but its role in the development of essential hypertension is still debated. Van Hooft and associates[18] from Rotterdam, The Netherlands, compared renal hemodynamics, measured in terms of the clearance of para-aminohippuric acid and insulin, and the characteristics of the renin-angiotensin-aldosterone system in 3 groups of normotensive subjects at different degrees of risks of hypertension: 41 subjects with 2 normotensive parents, 52 with 1 normotensive and 1 hypertensive parent, and 61 with 2 hypertensive parents. The subjects ranged in age from 7 to 32 years. The mean renal blood flow was lower in the subjects with 2 hypertensive parents than in those with 2 normotensive parents (mean difference [± SE], 198 ± 61 ml/minute/1.73 m² of body-surface area). Moreover, both the filtration fraction and renal vascular resistance were higher in the subjects with 2 hypertensive parents (filtration fraction: mean difference, 3.0 ± 1.1 percentage points; renal vascular resistance: mean difference, 2.7 ± 0.8 mm Hg/dl/minute/1.73 m²). The subjects with 2 hypertensive parents had lower plasma concentrations of renin (mean difference, 3.3 ± 1.6 mU per liter) and aldosterone (mean difference, 111 ± 36 pmol/L) than those with 2 normotensive parents. The differences could not be explained by the small differences in BP between the groups. The values in the subjects with 1 hypertensive and 1 normotensive parent fell between those for the other 2 groups. Renal vasconstriction is increased and renin and aldosterone secretion is decreased in young persons at risk for hypertension. These findings support the hypothesis that alterations in renal hemodynamics occur at an early stage in the development of familial hypertension.

Relation of renin-sodium profile with risk of myocardial infarction

To test the prognostic value of plasma renin activity prospectively, Alderman and associates[19] from New York, New York, determined the pretreatment renin-sodium profile of 1717 subjects with mild to moderate systemic hypertension (mean age 53 years; 36% white; 67% men) in a systematic work-site treatment program. Renin profiles, obtained by plotting plasma renin activity against the urinary excretion of sodium, were classified as high (12% of the subjects), normal (56%), and low (32%), and there were expected variations according to age, sex, and race. Modified stepped-care treatment for hypertension, prescribed without reference to the renin profile, was similar in the 3 renin groups. Mean (± SD) BP at entry was 151 ± 19/100 ± 10 mm Hg in the subjects with a high renin profile, 151 ± 19/97 ± 10 mm Hg in those with a normal profile, and 151 ± 20/96 ± 11 mm Hg in those with a low profile. During 8.3 years of follow-up, there were 27 myocardial infarctions. As adjusted for age, sex, and race, the incidence of AMI per 1000 person-years was 14.7 among the subjects with a high renin profile, 5.6 among those with a normal profile, and 2.8 among those with a low profile (rate ratio for high vs low, 5.3; 95% confidence interval, 3.4 to 8.3). The rate of mortality from all causes was 9.3 in the high-profile group, 5.3 in the normal-profile group, and 3.9 in the low-profile group. The independent association of a high renin profile with AMI (but not with stroke or noncardiovascular events) was affirmed by Cox analyses (rate ratio for high vs normal plus low, 3.2; 95% confidence interval, 1.2 to 8.4) after adjustment for race, sex, age at entry, serum cholesterol level, smoking status, electrocardiographic evidence of LV hypertrophy, blood glucose level, body-mass index, history of cardiovascular disease or treatment, BP, and use of beta-blockers. In the study population, whose BP before and during treatment was in a narrow range, and after other cardiovascular risk factors had been considered, the renin profile before treatment remained independently associated with the subsequent risk of myocardial infarction.

Effects of caffeine

Caffeine-induced BP elevations are well documented in habitual consumers, occurring through both vasoconstrictive and cardiostimulatory actions. Whether caffeine hinders pressor regulation during exercise has been uncertain, particularly in those at risk for hypertension. Thus effects of caffeine versus placebo were studied during supine bicycle exercise by Pincomb and associates[20] from Oklahoma City, Oklahoma, in healthy men (ages 20 to 35). Hypertension risk was defined during screening: high risk = 135 to 154/85 to 94 mm Hg plus parental hypertension (n = 20); low risk ≤132/84 mm Hg and no parental hypertension. Exaggerated pressor responses (≥230/100 mm Hg) seen during exercise after placebo identified a subgroup of 7 high risk patients indistinguishable at rest from the remaining high risk men. This subgroup shcwed a larger resting diastolic response to caffeine than low risk men and other high risk men. Compared with placebo, caffeine increased the number of low risk (0% to 36%) and high risk (35% to 50%) men reaching abnormal exercise BPs, and blunted normal increments in cardiac index at higher workloads among high risk men. Thus restriction of caffeine before exercise might benefit persons with either risk for hypertension or unusual sensitivity to caffeine.

Coronary angiographic patterns

Patients in this study by De Cesare and associates[21] from Milan, Italy, were assessed by coronary angiography because of classic effort angina and a positive exercise test. Of these patients, 320 had untreated primary hypertension and 320, similar in age and gender distribution, were normotensive. In all patients coronary angiography documented that ≥1 major epicardial branch was restricted by ≥50%. Prevalence of single- and double-vessel disease in the fourth and fifth decades of life was similar in the 2 populations and in both tended to decline with age. Prevalence of triple-vessel disease was also similar in the 2 populations in the fourth and fifth decades; in either population it rose with age and reached a peak at the seventh decade of life. The percentages of hypertensive patients in the sixth and seventh decades with triple-vessel disease was significantly greater (40% and 50%, respectively) than the corresponding values in normotensive individuals (25% and 31%, respectively). The LM was not significantly more involved in the high BP group. Pressure was moderately and similarly raised at any age in hypertension; serum cholesterol and triglyceride levels, blood glucose, and smoking habits were comparable in the 2 populations. These results suggest that hypertension does not accelerate the appearance of significant coronary narrowing or multiple vessel involvement. Starting from the sixth decade, the natural age-related evolution of CAD seems to be aggravated in hypertensive subjects, as reflected by an augmented number of diseased vessels. This process is probably related to high BP itself; whether the severity of hypertension might also exert an influence is not deducible from this study. Although in individuals with high BP coronary disorders other than atherosclerosis have a putative part in coronary events, there is a substantial link between epicardial branch narrowing and classic effort angina.

Accuracy of aneroid sphygmomanometers

Defects of aneroid sphygmomanometers are a source of error in BP measurement. Bailey and associates[22] from Columbia, Missouri, inspected 230 aneroid sphygmomanometers for physical defects and compared their accuracy against a standard mercury manometer at 5 different BP points. An aneroid sphygmomanometer was defined as intolerant if it deviated from the mercury manometer by > ± 3 mm Hg at ≥2 of the test points. The 3 most common physical defects were indicator needles not pointing to the "zero box," cracked face plates, and defective tubing. Eighty (34.8%) of the 230 aneroid sphygmomanometers were determined to be intolerant with the greatest frequency of deviation seen at BP levels ≥150 mm Hg. The authors recommended that aneroid manometers be inspected for physical defects and calibrated for accuracy against a standard mercury manometer at 6-month intervals to prevent inaccurate BP measurements.

The J-curve phenomenon

Farnett and associates[23] from San Antonio, Texas, appraised medical publications to evaluate whether there is a point beyond which BP reduction in hypertensive subjects is no longer beneficial and possibly even deleterious. Twelve studies that stratified cardiovascular outcomes by level of achieved BP in treated hypertensive subjects who had been followed up for at least 1 year were critiqued by 4 independent reviewers (Table 5-1). Data addressing population, protocol, and methodological characteristics were evaluated. Studies did not show a consistent J-shaped relation between treated BP and stroke, but they did demonstrate a consistent J-shaped relation for cardiac events and diastolic BP (Figure 5-1).

TABLE 5-1. *Subject and protocol characteristics of studies that have stratified cardiovascular outcomes by levels of achieved blood pressure. Reproduced with permission from Farnett, et al.[23]*

Study	No. of Subjects	Mean Age, y	% Men	Mean Entry Diastolic BP, mm Hg	Includes Subjects With Cardiovascular Disease	Mean Follow-up Time, y	BP Phase	BP Position	Primary Drugs	Quality Score (0-15)
Cruickshank et al[25]	939	55	61	109	Yes	6.1	V	Sitting	AB, TD, PSD	5
DHCCP[26]	2145	51	50	107	Yes	4	V	Supine	Unclear	4
HDFP[27]	10 053	51	54	90-104	Yes	4	V	Sitting	AB, TD	8
Waller et al[28]	3350	50	50	110	Yes	6.5	V	Unclear	Unclear	5
HEP[29]	884	68	31	98	Yes	4.4	V	Sitting	AB, TD	4
Stewart[30]	169	44	71	124	No	6.25	IV	Unclear	AB, TD	7
NYEC[31]	1765	51	72	102	Yes	4.2	V	Sitting	AB, TD, CCB, ACE	11
EWPHE[32]	840	71	30	90-119	Yes	4.7	V	Sitting	TD, PSD	7
PPT[33]	686	52	100	106	No†	12	V	Sitting	AB, TD	14
IPPPSH[34]	6357	52	50	108	No	3-5	V	Sitting	AB, PSD	5
ANBP[35]	3931	50	55	101	No‡	4	V	Sitting	TD	4
MRC[36]	17 354	52	52	90-109	Yes	5.5	V	Sitting	AB, TD	6

*BP indicates blood pressure; DHCCP, Department of Health and Social Security Hypertension Care Computing Project; HDFP, Hypertension Detection and Follow-up Program; HEP, Hypertension in Elderly Patients; NYEC, the New York Employee Cohort Study; EWPHE, European Working Party on High Blood Pressure in the Elderly; PPT, Primary Prevention Trial; IPPPSH, International Prospective Primary Prevention Study in Hypertension; ANBP, Australian National Blood Pressure Study; MRC, Medical Research Council; AB, adrenergic blocker; TD, thiazide diuretic; CCB, calcium channel blocker; ACE, angiotensin-converting enzyme inhibitor; and PSD, potassium sparing diuretic.

†Excluded subjects with myocardial infarction or stroke within the past 2 years.

‡Excluded subjects with stroke and angina, as well as subjects with myocardial infarction within the past 3 months.

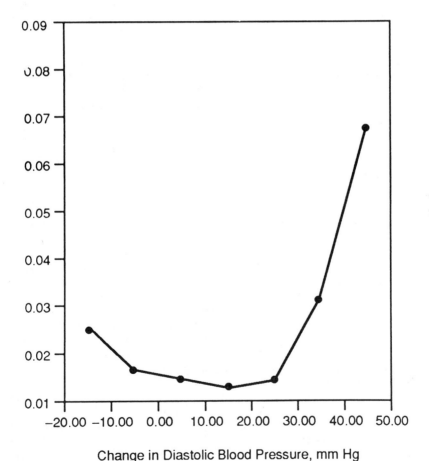

Change in Diastolic Blood Pressure, mm Hg

Fig. 5-1. An increase in mortality is shown in patients with low blood pressure levels (baseline-annuals) enrolled in the Hypertension and Detection Follow-up Program. Adapted from Farnett, et al.[23]

The beneficial therapeutic threshold point was 85 mm Hg. The authors concluded that low treated diastolic BP levels, i.e., <85 mm Hg, are associated with increased risk of cardiac events.

Value of treatment in patients ≥70 years

Although the benefits of antihypertensive treatment in "young" elderly (under 70 years) hypertensive patients are well established, the value of treatment in older patients (70–84 years) is less clear. The Swedish Trial in Old Patients with Hypertension (STOP-Hypertension) was a perspective, randomized, double-blind, intervention study set up to compare the effects of active antihypertensive therapy (3 B-blockers and 1 diuretic) and placebo on the frequency of fatal and non-fatal stroke and AMI and other cardiovascular death in hypertensive Swedish men and women aged 70–84 years[24]. The investigators recruited 1627 patients at 116 health centers throughout Sweden. The enrollees met the entry criteria on 3 separate recordings during a 1-month placebo run-in period of systolic BP between 180 and 230 mm Hg and a diastolic BP of at least 90 mm Hg or a diastolic BP between 105–120 mm Hg irrespective of the systolic pressure. The total duration of the study was 65 months and the average time in the study was 25 months. Eight hundred twelve patients were randomly allocated active treatment and 815 placebo. The mean difference in supine BP between the active treatment and placebo groups at the last follow-up before an endpoint, death, or study termination was 19.5/8.1 mm Hg. Compared with placebo, active treatment significantly reduced the number of primary endpoints (94 vs 58) and stroke morbidity and mortality (53 vs 29) (Figure 5-2). Although the authors did not set out to study an effect on total mortality, they also noted a significantly reduced number of deaths in the active treatment group (63 vs 36). The benefits of treatment were discernible up to age 84 years. The authors concluded that antihypertensive treatment in hypertensive men and women aged 70–84 confers highly significant and clinically relevant reductions in cardiovascular morbidity and mortality as well as in total mortality.

Effect of treatment on renal disease

End-stage renal disease attributed to systemic hypertension has increased annually for the last decade and will probably worsen through the year 2000. Patients with diabetic nephropathy and patients with hypertensive renal disease account for most new cases annually. Evidence reveals that all levels of untreated hypertension are associated with potentially declining renal function. Data from the Hypertension Detection and Follow-up Program and other studies show that antihypertensive treatment can prevent progressive renal failure[25]. An ablation model demonstrates glomerular hyperfiltration as a possible mechanism for progressive renal failure. Human data on the renal effects of antihypertensive agents are limited and inconsistent. Despite the limitations, the Working Group on Hypertension and Chronic Renal Failure concludes that controlled hypertension to <140/90 mm Hg reduces the incidence of end-stage renal disease. Patients with established renal impairment may benefit from individualized treatment to 130/85 mm Hg or less (Table 5-2).

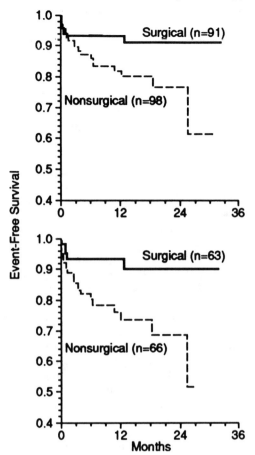

Fig. 5-2. Kaplan-Meier analysis of cumulative event-free survival for ipsilateral stroke or crescendo transient ischemic attacks in surgical vs. nonsurgical patients. The top panel indicates all patients (P = .028); bottom panel, patients with ipsilateral carotid stenosis greater than 70% (P = .010). Reprinted with permission from Dahlof.[24]

TABLE 5-2. *Recommendations for treatment of hypertension to protect the kidney. Reprinted with permission from Archives of Internal Medicine.*[25]

Control blood pressure to <140/90 mm Hg, if practical*
Recognize and evaluate early renal insufficiency
Serum creatinine >124 μmol/L (50% loss of renal function)
Serum creatinine >115 μmol/L (in patients >60 y of age)
Reduce daily dietary sodium to approximately 2 g (5 g of sodium chloride) or <100 mEq of sodium
Use loop diuretics if serum creatinine is >177 μmol/L
Add diuretic to monotherapy if blood pressure is not controlled
Measure serum creatinine and electrolytes frequently
Assess and manage all cardiovascular disease risk factors*

*From the 1988 Report of the Joint National Committee on Detection, Evaluation, and Treatment of High Blood Pressure.

TREATMENT

Salt restriction

To estimate the quantitative relation between BP and sodium intake, Law and associates[26] from London, UK, analyzed data from published reports of BP and sodium intake for 24 different communities (47,000 people) throughout the world. Difference in BP for 100 mmol/24 hour difference in sodium intake was the main outcome measure. Allowance was made for difference in BP between economically developed and undeveloped communities to minimize over-estimation of the association through confounding with other determinants of BP. BP was higher on average in the developed communities, but the association with sodium intake was similar in both types of community. A difference in sodium intake of 100 mmol/24 hours was associated with an average difference in systolic BP that ranged from 5 mm Hg at age 15–19 years to 10 mm Hg at age 60–69. The differences in diastolic BP were about half as great. The standard deviation of BP increased with sodium intake implying that the association of BP with sodium intake in individuals was related to the initial BP—the higher the BP, the greater the expected reduction in BP for the same reduction in sodium intake. For example, at age 60–69 the estimated systolic BP reduction in response to a 100 mmol/24 h reduction in sodium intake was on average 10 mm Hg but varied from 6 mm Hg for those on the fifth BP centile to 15 mm Hg for those on the 95th centile. The association of BP with sodium intake is substantially larger than is generally appreciated and increases with age and initial BP.

Dietary salt restriction is the most common therapeutic recommendation given to patients with systemic hypertension, but past studies have assessed the effect of salt restriction using *resting* BP measurements not the newer technique of 24-hour ambulatory BP monitoring. Moore and associates[27] from Boston, Massachusetts, compared the effect of high (250 mEq of sodium Na/day) and low (10 mEq of sodium Na/day) salt diets on resting versus ambulatory BP in 12 normal and 15 hypertensive subjects. Each diet was given for 7 days. Ambulatory BP was monitored from day 6 to day 7 of each diet; resting supine BP was measured on the morning of day 8. In normal subjects, neither resting nor ambulatory BP changed with sodium restriction. In hypertensives, resting BP fell 14 $\pm$ 3/6 $\pm$ 2 mm Hg (systolic/diastolic) with sodium restriction while ambulatory BP fell only 4 $\pm$ 2/2 $\pm$ 2). The resting BP fall was significantly greater than the ambulatory BP fall for both systolic and diastolic pressure. Ambulatory heart rates were also significantly greater during sodium restriction, suggesting that the low salt diet activated the sympathetic nervous system. This may, in turn, have partially offset the hypotensive effect of sodium restriction. The authors concluded that using resting BP to assess the effect of sodium restriction may overestimate the efficacy of this therapy. Ambulatory BP monitoring should be employed in future studies of sodium restriction.

Dynamic exercise

To quantify the duration of postexercise hypotension at different exercise intensities, Pescatello and co-workers[28] in New Britain, Connecticut studied six unmedicated, mildly hypertensive men matched with 6 normotensive controls. Each subject wore a 24-hour ambulatory BP monitor at the same time of day for 13 consecutive hours on 3 different days. On each of the 3 days, subjects either cycled for 30 minutes at 40% or 70% maximum VO_2 or performed activities of daily living. There was no intensity effect on the postexercise reduction in BP, so BP data were combined for the different exercise intensities. Postexercise diastolic BP and mean arterial pressure were lower by 8 and 7 mm Hg, respectively, than the preexercise values for 13 hours in the hypertensive group. These variables were not different before and after exercise in the normotensive group. Systolic BP was reduced by 5 mm for 9 hours after exercise in the hypertensive group. In contrast, systolic BP was 5 mm higher for 13 hours after exercise in the normotensive group. When the BP response on the exercise days was compared on the nonexercise day, systolic BP and mean arterial pressure were lower on the exercise days in the hypertensive but not in the normotensive group. The investigators found a postexercise reduction in mean arterial pressure for 13 hours independent of the exercise intensity in the hypertensive group. Furthermore, mean arterial pressure was lower on exercise than on nonexercise days in the hypertensive but not in the normotensive group.

N-3 fatty acids

The potential antihypertensive effects after prolonged use of small doses of fish oils remain undefined. Radack and associates[29] from Cincinnati, Ohio, conducted a randomized, double-blind, controlled crossover study comparing low doses of n-3 fatty acid supplementation with n-6 fatty acids on BP in 33 subjects with mild hypertension. After a 6-week stabilization period, subjects ingested either 2.04 g/d of n-3 fatty acids or safflower oil (4.8 g/d of linoleic acid) for 12 weeks, then crossed over to the alternative encapsulated oil for another 12 weeks, after a 4-week washout period. All antihypertensive drug therapy had been discontinued. For the combined data, there were significant reductions from pretreatment values for supine diastolic (-2.4 mm Hg) and sitting systolic (-4.1 mm Hg) BP after fish oil; no significant changes occurred after safflower oil control. Compared with safflower oil, fish oil supplementation was associated with a statistically significant reduction in mean supine diastolic BP of 3.7 mm Hg. Sitting diastolic and mean arterial pressures showed a sequence effect; therefore, only the initial period was used in an analysis of their responses. There were significant decreases from pretreatment values for sitting diastolic (-4.4 mm Hg), mean arterial (-5.1 mm Hg), and systolic (-6.5 mm Hg) BP after fish oil. The differences between groups after the 12-week period remained statistically significant for sitting diastolic and sitting mean arterial BP. No adverse changes were noted in plasma levels of lipids.

Nutritional-hygienic regimen + drugs

There is no consensus for the optimal treatment program for individuals with mild systemic hypertension, including whether treatment should emphasize life-style changes alone, such as weight loss, reduction of sodium and alcohol intake, and increased physical activity, or whether it should also include a pharmacologic component. The dilemma is accentuated by the availability of many drugs from different classes to lower BP. To study the relative efficacy and safety of a combination of pharmacologic and nutritional-hygienic intervention compared with nutrition-hygienic intervention alone, The Treatment of Mild Hypertension Research Group[30] from Minneapolis, Minnesota, initiated a double-blind, controlled clinical trial. Nine hundred two men and women with mild hypertension (average BP, 140/91 mm Hg) were randomized to receive nutritional-hygienic intervention plus 1 of 6 treatments: (1) placebo; (2) diuretic (*chlorthalidone*); (3) B-blocker (acebutolol); (4) a_1-antagonist (*doxazosin mesylate*); (5) calcium antagonist (*amiodipine maleate*); or (6) anglotensin-converting enzyme inhibitor (*enalapril maleate*). After 12 months, weight loss averaged 4.5 kg, urinary sodium excretion was reduced by 23%, and reported leisure-time physical activity was nearly doubled. Systolic and diastolic BP in the group given nutritional-hygienic intervention alone (placebo) were reduced by 10.6 and 8.1 mm Hg, respectively. For participants in the 5 groups receiving antihypertensive medication in addition to nutritional-hygienic treatment, BP reductions were significantly greater than those achieved with nutritional-hygienic treatment alone (range, 16 to 22 mm Hg for systolic and 12 to 14 mm Hg for diastolic BP). Although differences among treatment groups in certain dimensions of quality of life, self-reported side effects, plasma lipid levels, and biochemical measures were observed, no consistent pattern in the differences was noted. Nutritional-hygienic therapy is an effective first-step treatment for persons with mild hypertension, and significant additional BP lowering with minimal short-term side effects can be achieved by adding 1 of 5 different classes of antihypertensive agents.

Potassium

To determine whether an increase of dietary potassium intake from natural foods reduces the need for antihypertensive medication in patients with essential hypertension, Siani and associates[31] from Naples, Italy, randomly assigned 54 patients with well-controlled hypertension into 1 of 2 groups and they were given dietary advice aimed at selectively increasing potassium intake (group 1) or at keeping their customary diet unchanged (group 2). During a 1-year follow-up, drug therapy was reduced in stepwise fashion, according to a fixed protocol, provided that BP remained less than 160/95 mm Hg. Potassium intake was checked monthly by referring to 3-day food records and by measuring 24-hour urinary potassium excretion. Potassium intake increased in group 1 but did not change in group 2. No change was observed in either urinary sodium excretion or in body weight. After 1 year, the average drug consumption (number of pills per day) relative to that at baseline was 24% in group 1 and 60% in group 2. By the end of the study, BP could be controlled using less than 50% of the initial therapy in 81% of the patients in group 1 (confidence interval, 66% to 96%) compared with 29% of the patients in group 2. Patients in group 1 ended the study with a lower number of reported symptoms compared with patients in the control group. Increasing the dietary potassium intake from natural foods is a feasible and effective measure to reduce antihypertensive drug treatment.

Calcium

Calcium supplementation has been reported to reduce BP in pregnant and nonpregnant women. Belizan and associates[32] from Rosario, Argentina, undertook a prospective study to determine the effect of calcium supplementation on the incidence of hypertensive disorders of pregnancy (gestational hypertension and preeclampsia) and to determine the value of urinary calcium levels as a predictor of the response. The authors studied 1194 nulliparous women who were in the 20th week of gestation at the beginning of the study. The women were randomly assigned to receive 2 g per day of elementary calcium in the form of calcium carbonate (593 women) or placebo (601 women). Urinary excretion of calcium and creatinine was measured before calcium supplementation was begun. The women were followed to the end of their pregnancies, and the incidence of hypertensive disorders of pregnancy was determined. The rates of hypertensive disorders of pregnancy were lower in the calcium group than in the placebo group (9.8% vs 14.8%; odds ratio, 0.63) (Figure 5-3). The risk of these disorders was lower at all times during gestation, particularly after the 28th week of gestation, in the calcium group than in the placebo group, and the risk of both gestational hypertension and preeclampsia was also lower in the calcium group. Among the women who had low ratios of urinary calcium to urinary creatinine (≤0.62 mmol per millimole) during the 20th week of gestation, those in the calcium group had a lower risk of hypertensive disorders of pregnancy (odds ratio, 0.56) and less of an increase in diastolic and systolic BP than the

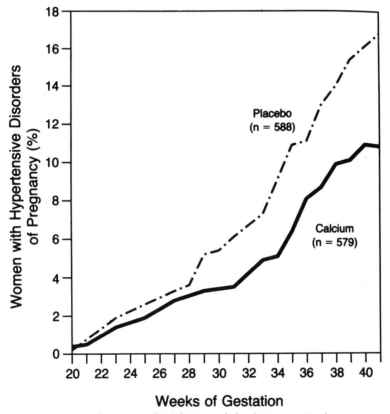

Fig. 5-3. Percentage of Women in the Calcium and Placebo Groups in Whom Hypertensive Disorders of Pregnancy (Gestational Hypertension and Preeclampsia) Developed, According to week of Gestation. The values calculated by life-table analysis. The risk of hypertensive disorders of pregnancy, particularly after the 28th week of gestation, was significantly lower in the calcium group than in the placebo group (P = 0.01 by the log rank test). Reprinted with permission from Belizan, et al.[32]

placebo group. The pattern of response was similar among the women who had a high ratio of urinary calcium to urinary creatinine during the 20th week of gestation, but the differences were smaller. Pregnant women who receive calcium supplementation after the 20th week of pregnancy have a reduced risk of hypertensive disorders of pregnancy.

Diuretics

Thiazide diuretics may preserve bone mass and prevent elderly women's osteopenic fractures, but studies have not distinguished between thiazide preparations or examined former users. Felson and associates[33] from Boston, Massachusetts, and Providence, Rhode Island, performed a case-controlled study looking at thiazide use and subsequent fracture in post-menopausal female members of the Framingham Study cohort. Cases who had experienced a first hip fracture (n = 176) were compared with age-matched controls (n = 672). Results showed a modest protective effect of any recent thiazide use. Recent pure thiazide users experienced significant protection against fracture (odds ratio, 0.31), whereas recent users of combination drugs containing thiazides experienced no protection (odds ratio, 1.16). Combination drugs generally contained only 25 mg of hydrochlorothiazide, suggesting that the small amount of thiazide was insufficient to preserve bone mass. Former thiazide users were not protected against fracture. In sum, recent pure thiazide use in women protects against hip fracture.

To determine whether the high mortality among diabctic patients receiving treatment for systemic hypertension can be explained by associated risk factors or must be attributed to a deleterious effect of antihypertensive therapy, Warram and associates[34] from Boston, Massachusetts, and Milan, Italy, enrolled 759 out-patients with diabetes mellitus and severe retinopathy in a multicenter, randomized clinical trial of laser treatment to prevent blindness and they had an ophthalmological examination every 4 months and annual medical examinations that included measurement of BP and recording of antihypertensive treatment. Only 5.5% of the patients were unavailable for follow-up. When a patient died, the circumstances surrounding the death were reviewed and classified by a mortality review committee. The patients were white and aged 35 to 69 years and all had normal serum creatinine levels at the baseline examination. Patients were classified into 5 groups according to information recorded at the baseline and first annual follow-up examinations: normotensive (diastolic BP <90 mm Hg), untreated hypertensive, hypertensive treated by diuretics alone, hypertensive treated by other agents alone, and hypertensive treated by both agents. Cardiovascular mortality was higher in patients treated for hypertension than in patients with untreated hypertension. The excess was primarily found in patients treated with diuretics alone, although that group had the lowest BP with treatment. After adjusting for differences in risk factors, cardiovascular mortality was 3.8 times higher in patients treated with diuretics alone than in patients with untreated hypertension. In individuals with diabetes, intervention with diuretics to reduce hypertension is associated with excess mortality. Until there is a clinical trial showing a beneficial effect of diuretic treatment in diabetic patients, there is urgent need to reconsider its continued usage in this population.

Hydrochlorothiazide

In a double-blind randomized study, Cushman and associates[35] of a Department of Veterans Affairs Cooperative Study evaluated the effects of 25 mg vs 50 mg of hydrochlorothiazide in 51 elderly patients (aged 69 ± 7 years) with isolated systolic hypertension (BP 160–239 mm Hg systolic and <90 mm Hg diastolic). Dose levels could be increased to twice daily to control BP. The reductions in BP (25.4/6.8 mm Hg and 28.9/7.4 mm Hg) and proportion of patients in whom BP was controlled (78% and 89%) were similar in the lower- and higher-dose groups during the titration phase. However, serum potassium level was reduced more in the higher-dosage (0.57 mmol/L) than the lower-dosage (0.17 mmol/L) group. There were no significant changes in BP during a 24-week maintenance phase. No patient required withdrawal from the study because of adverse effects, and cognitive-behavioral function was well preserved. The authors concluded that hydrochlorothiazide is effective and well tolerated in older patients with isolated systolic hypertension, many of whom may be effectively treated with 25 mg of hydrochlorothiazide once daily.

Chlorthalidone ± atenolol

To assess the ability of antihypertensive drug treatment to reduce the risk of nonfatal and fatal stroke in isolated systolic hypertension, members of the Systolic Hypertension in the Elderly Program (SHEP) performed a multicenter, randomized, double-blind, placebo-controlled study involving community based ambulatory population in tertiary care centers[36]. A total of 4,736 persons (1.06%) from 447,921 screenees aged 60 years and above were randomized (2,365 to active treatment and 2,371 to placebo). Systolic BP ranged from 160–219 mm Hg and diastolic BP was <90 mm Hg. Of the participants, 3,161 were not receiving antihypertensive medication at initial contact and 1,575 were. The average systolic BP was 170 mm Hg; average diastolic BP, 77 mm Hg. The mean age was 72 years, 57% were women, and 14% were black. Participants were stratified by clinical center and by antihypertensive medication status at initial contact. For step 1 of the trial, dose 1 was chlorthalidone, 12.5 mg/d, or matching placebo; dose 2 was 25 mg/d. For step 2, dose 1 was atenolol, 25 mg/d, or matching placebo; dose 2 was 50 mg/d. Average follow-up was 4.5 years. The 5-year average systolic BP was 155 mm Hg for the placebo group and 143 mm Hg for the active treatment group, and the 5-year average diastolic BP was 72 and 68 mm Hg, respectively (Figure 5-4). The 5-year incidence of total stroke was 5.2 per 100 participants for active treatment and 8.2 per 100 for placebo. The relative risk by proportional hazards regression analysis was 0.64. For the secondary end point of clinical nonfatal AMI plus coronary death, the relative risk was 0.73. Major cardiovascular events were reduced (relative risk, 0.68). For deaths from all causes, the relative risk was 0.87. In persons aged 60 years and over with isolated systolic hypertension, antihypertensive stepped-care drug treatment with low-dose chlorthalidone as step 1 medication reduced the incidence of total stroke by 36%, with 5-year absolute benefit of 30 events per 1000 participants. Major cardiovascular events were reduced, with 5-year absolute benefit of 55 events per 1000.

In a multi-center, randomized, placebo controlled trial involving 697 patients aged 21 to 65 years of age with diastolic BP between 90–100 mm Hg and weight between 110% and 160% of ideal weight, Wassertheil-Smoller and associates[37] for the TAIM Research Group randomly assigned

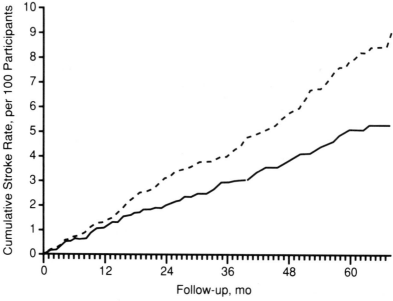

Fig. 5-4. Cumulative fatal plus nonfatal stroke per 100 participants in the active treatment of (solid line) and placebo (broken line) groups during the Systolic Hypertension in the Elderly Program. Reprinted with permission from Shep Cooperative Research Group.[36]

patients to 1 of 3 diets (usual, low-sodium, and high potassium, weight loss) and 1 of 3 agents (placebo, chlorthalidone, and atenolol). Changes in measures of sexual problems, distress, and well-being after 6 months of therapy were analyzed. Low-dose chlorthalidone and atenolol produced few side effects, except in men. Erection-related problems worsened in 28% of men receiving chlorthalidone and usual diet compared with 3% of those receiving placebo and usual diet and 11% of those receiving atenolol and usual diet. The weight loss diet ameliorated this effect. The low-sodium diet with placebo was associated with greater fatigue than was either usual diet or weight reduction. The low-sodium diet with chlorthalidone increased problems with sleep compared with chlorthalidone and usual diet. The weight loss diet benefited quality of life most, reducing total physical complaints and increasing satisfaction with health. Total physical complaints decreased in 57% to 76% of patients depending on drug and diet group, and were markedly decreased by weight loss. In general, low-dose antihypertensive drug therapy (with chlorthalidone or atenolol) improves rather than impairs the quality of life; however, chlorthalidone with usual diet increases sexual problems in men.

Celiprolol

Frohlich and associates[38] from New Orleans, Louisiana, compared the immediate and short-term (2 weeks) hemodynamic and humoral effects of the B-1 antagonist, B-2 antagonist, celiprolol, with those of more prolonged atenolol therapy in 12 patients with essential hypertension. Celiprolol produced an immediate dose-dependent decrease in mean arterial pressure (113 ± 3 to 102 ± 2 mm Hg) and total peripheral resistance (49 ± 3 to 38 ± 1 U/m²) that was associated with an increased heart rate (67 ± 1 to 73 ± 2 beats/min) and cardiac index (2,347 ± 129 to 2,708 ±

111 ml/min/m^2). Both celiprolol and atenolol reduced mean arterial pressure with short-term treatment; this was associated with a reduced total peripheral resistance with celiprolol (from 24 ± 1 to 21 ± 1 U/m^2) and was not observed with atenolol. Moreover, in contrast with atenolol, celiprolol did not change heart rate or stroke and cardiac indexes. Splanchnic and forearm vascular resistances decreased with celiprolol but not with atenolol; neither B-blocking drug altered renal blood flow. These results demonstrate that the hemodynamic effects of celiprolol were strikingly different from atenolol; celiprolol reduced arterial pressure and total peripheral and certain vascular resistances without altering heart rate, cardiac index or regional blood flows. These effects may be explained by celiprolol's cardiac B-1 receptor inhibitory and peripheral B-2 receptor agonistic effects.

Labetalol vs enalapril

Applegate and associates[39] from several medical centers compared the safety and efficacy of labetalol and enalapril as antihypertensive monotherapy for elderly patients. A randomized, open-label, parallel controlled trial was conducted. After completing a 4-week placebo phase, 79 elderly (65 years or older) patients with an average standing diastolic BP 95 mm Hg or above and 114 mm Hg or less were randomized to receive a 12-week course of either labetalol or enalapril in an open-label design. The patients' BP and heart rate were evaluated biweekly by trained observers unaware of the treatment status, and drug dosage was titrated (up to 400 mg twice a day of labetalol or 40 mg daily of enalapril) to achieve a standing diastolic BP of less than 90 mm Hg and a decrease of 10 mm Hg from baseline. Patients underwent 24-hour ambulatory BP monitoring at the end of the placebo phase and again after 8 weeks of active treatment. The treatment groups were comparable in their reduction of supine diastolic BP, with no significant differences between the 2 treatments. Labetalol demonstrated a significantly greater reduction in standing diastolic BP at the end of the titration period compared to enalapril, but this difference was not significant by the end of the study period. Based on 24-hour ambulatory BP monitoring readings, labetalol reduced mean 24-hour diastolic BP and mean heart rate more than enalapril. The labetalol-treated patients were significantly less often above their diastolic BP goal throughout the 24-hour ambulatory BP monitoring period. The 2 treatments were equally well tolerated. The results indicate that labetalol and enalapril are equally effective in lowering supine diastolic BP in the elderly, but labetalol is more effective in lowering ambulatory BP and heart rate throughout the day.

Doxazosin

Doxazosin, a new quinazoline-derivative postsynaptic a$_1$-adrenoceptor antagonist, was studied by Oliveros-Palacios and associates[40] from Maracaibo, Venezuela, in 17 patients over a 12-week period. Its effects on BP, heart rate, metabolic functions and renal hormones were analyzed after administration of a single oral morning dose in a 3-phase fashion when administered to 17 patients (11 women, 6 men, 21 to 59 years) with mild to moderate uncomplicated essential hypertension. After titrating the antihypertensive effective dose biweekly from 1 to 8 mg/day and a mean end titration-point dose of 4.14 ± 0.1 mg at week 8 of treatment, it was adjusted to maintain diastolic BP at levels <90 mm Hg for up to

12 weeks of treatment when, at a final mean dose of 4.35 ± 0.2 mg/day, BP decreased in all patients by a mean 31 ± 3/17 ± 2 (supine) and 39 ± 3/15 ± 3 (standing) mm Hg with no increase in heart rate and no "first-dose phenomenon." Neither the renin-aldosterone system nor electrolyte excretion was significantly affected. Renal function and metabolic parameters also remained unchanged. Urinary kalikrein excretion was augmented 2.47-fold. There was good tolerance; 1 patient discontinued the study because of dry nose. These results suggest that long-term monotherapy with doxazosin is an effective and safe antihypertensive agent for mild to moderate essential hypertension that stimulates urinary kallikrein excretion.

Nifedipine

Frohlich and associates[41] from New Orleans, Louisiana, evaluated in 10 patients with mild to moderate systemic hypertension the hemodynamic and humoral effects and trough-to-peak 24-hour BP responses of 2 nifedipine formulations, capsules and continuous-release once-daily tablets. Both formulations reduced mean arterial pressure similarly from 120 ± 3 (baseline) to 107 ± 2 and 105 ± 2 mm Hg and total peripheral resistance index from 65 ± 9 (baseline) to 47 ± 4 and 45 ± 3 U/m^2, respectively. Renal, splanchnic and total forearm (including skin and skeletal muscle) blood flows were maintained or even increased slightly associated with reductions in regional vascular resistances. Decreases in renal, total forearm and skeletal muscle resistances were significant with the capsules, but the decrease was only significant in renal resistance with the long-acting tablets. Intravascular volume did not expand with reduction in arterial pressure. This antihypertensive effect was not related to baseline plasma renin activity levels or age. Nifedipine tablets provided a better control of mean arterial pressure (66%) than did capsules (44%).

To evaluate the effect of age on the pattern of circadian BP after nifedipine tablets, Kuwajima and associates[42] from Tokyo, Japan, measured ambulatory BP after administration of low and high doses of nifedipine, taken twice daily, over a 24-hour period in 10 elderly and in 8 young hypertensive patients. After a 2-week control period without antihypertensive drug, 10 mg of nifedipine was administered twice daily for 2 weeks (low-dose period), followed by 2 weeks of 20 mg (high-dose period). At the end of each period, ambulatory BP monitoring was conducted every 30 minutes for 24 hours, using an ABPM 630 (Nippon-Colin, Komaki, Japan). In both groups, averages of systolic and diastolic BP for the entire day decreased significantly from the control to the low-dose periods. However, after the high-dose period, only the elderly group had further significant reduction of systolic BP, whereas no further reduction was seen in the young group. Separate analysis of whole-day data into daytime and nighttime values revealed that a further decrease in systolic BP after the high-dose period in the elderly group was a reflection of nighttime decline. It was suggested that circadian BP patterns after administration of nifedipine tablets in the elderly differed from those in young hypertensive patients, especially after administration of the high-dose.

To assess the changes in sodium excretion and sodium balance after initiation of nifedipine treatment and after withdrawal of nifedipine, Cappuccio and associates[43] from London, UK, entered 8 patients with uncomplicated mild to moderate essential hypertension in a single-blind, placebo-controlled study of 39 days duration. Two 7-day periods while on a fixed sodium intake of 150 mmol/day approximately 3 weeks apart was the method used. After 4 days of a placebo and fixed sodium intake, patients were given nifedipine gastrointestinal therapeutic system once a day and carefully studied for the following 4 days. Thereafter, patients continued to receive nifedipine gastrointestinal therapeutic system, and approximately 3 weeks later they were studied again for a week while on a fixed sodium intake. Nifedipine administration was stopped and changes occurring after withdrawal were studied. Nifedipine caused a significant increase in sodium excretion with a cumulative loss of sodium of 38 mmol per subject within the first 4 days of treatment. The withdrawal of nifedipine treatment caused a significant decrease in sodium excretion and a cumulative retention of sodium of 42 mmol per subject within the first 4 days of withdrawal. Nifedipine causes an acute and a sustained reduction in sodium balance in patients with essential hypertension. This prolonged effect may contribute to the mechanism whereby nifedipine lowers BP.

Perindopril vs nifedipine

To compare the efficacy of the angiotensin converting enzyme perindopril with a calcium antagonist, nifedipine, in diabetic patients with microalbuminuria, the Melbourne Diabetic Nephropathy Study Group[44] in a randomized study of diabetic patients with microalbuminuria treated 50 diabetic patients with persistent microalbuminuria with perindopril or nifedipine for 12 months and monitored for 1 or 3 months after stopping treatment, depending on whether they were hypertensive or normotensive. Forty-three patients completed the study: 30 with normotension and 13 with hypertension; 19 had type I and 24 had type II diabetes mellitus. For 12 months 20 patients were given perindopril 2–8 mg daily and 23 were given nifedipine 20–80 mg daily. Albumin excretion rate, BP, and glomerular filtration rate were measured. Both perindopril and nifedipine significantly reduced mean BP. During treatment there was no significant difference between those treated with perindopril and those treated with nifedipine with respect to albuminuria or mean BP. Stopping treatment with both drugs was associated with a sustained increase in albuminuria and mean BP. There was a significant correlation between mean BP and albuminuria and also between the reduction in mean BP and the decrease in albuminuria during treatment with both drugs. In hypertensive patients both drugs caused significant decreases in mean BP and albuminuria. In normotensive patients there was no significant reduction in albuminuria with either regimen. In diabetic patients with microalbuminuria BP seems to be an important determinant of urinary albumin excretion. Perindopril and nifedipine have similar effects on urinary albumin excretion, both preventing increases in albuminuria in normotensive patients and decreasing albuminuria in hypertensive patients.

Felodipine or nifedipine

Bailey and associates[45] from London, Canada, gave 6 men with borderline systemic hypertension 5 mg of felodipine with water, grapefruit juice, or orange juice. The mean felodipine bioavailability with grapefruit juice was 284% (range 164–469%) of that with water. The dehydrofelodipine/felodipine AUC ratio was lower, diastolic BP lower, and heart rate higher with grapefruit juice than with water. Vasodilatation-related side-effects were more frequent. Orange juice had no such effects. Six healthy men took nifedipine 10 mg with water or grapefruit juice; the bioavailability with grapefruit juice was 134 (108–169%) of that with water. This study is the first example of a pharmacokinetic interaction between a citrus fruit and a drug.

Captopril vs nifedipine

Angeli and associates[46] from Padua, Italy, compared sublingual captopril (25 mg) with sublingual nifedipine (10 mg) to determine their effectiveness and safety in the treatment of hypertensive emergencies. In 9 of 10 patients who received sublingual captopril mean (± SD) systolic BP and diastolic BP dropped from 245 ± 39 to 190 ± 25 mm Hg and from 144 ± 8 to 115 ± 8 mm Hg at 50 minutes, respectively. The hypotensive effect of the drug was maintained for a mean of 4 hours. In 6 of 9 responders to sublingual captopril, BP—lowering effect was associated with a clear improvement of end-organ failure within 60 minutes. There were no side effects, including a dangerous fall in BP or reflex tachycardia. Sublingual nifedipine lowered diastolic BP and systolic BP in 8 of 10 patients. The hypotensive effect of nifedipine was more rapid than that of captopril (10 vs 20 minutes for diastolic BP and 20 vs 30 minutes for systolic BP, respectively), but no difference was observed in the time or in the magnitude of peak hypotensive effect between the 2 treatments, nor was a difference observed in the duration of hypotensive effect. In 6 of 8 responders to nifedipine therapy, a clear improvement of symptoms and signs of end-organ failure was observed within 60 minutes. In 3 patients, minor side effects were observed. The authors concluded that sublingual captopril effectively and safely lowers arterial BP in patients with hypertensive emergencies.

Enalapril vs atenolol

To compare the antihypertensive, renal hemodynamic and antiproteinuric effect of enalapril and atenolol in patients with proteinuria of non-diabetic origin, Apperloo and associates[47] from Groningen, The Netherlands, performed a prospective, double-blind, randomized 16-week study after a pre-treatment period of at least 3 weeks in 27 patients with proteinuria (>300 mg protein/day) of nondiabetic origin, moderately impaired renal function (creatinine clearance 30–90 ml/min), and a pretreatment diastolic BP of >80 mm Hg. Treatment with enalapril (10 mg/day, adjusted between 5 and 40 mg, if necessary) or atenolol (50 mg/day, adjusted between 25 and 100 mg if necessary) titrated against a target fall in diastolic BP to <95 mm Hg or of >10 mm Hg, or both. BP, renal hemodynamics, and urinary protein excretion were the main outcome measures. No differences were detected between the 2 groups before treatment. The falls in systolic and diastolic BP during treatment were not significantly different between both groups. Proteinuria fell slightly with atenolol but significantly more with enalapril (mean change −0.38 v −1.2 g/day, respectively) as did filtration fraction (mean change −1.8 v −3.8, respectively). Serum potassium concentration increased with enalapril (mean change 0.63 v 0.19 mmol/l). Enalapril lowers proteinuria more than atenolol in patients with non-diabetic renal disease despite a similar BP lowering effect of both drugs, and its antiproteinuric effect seems to be associated with the characteristic renal hemodynamic effect of angiotensin converting enzyme inhibitors.

7. Weinsier RL, James LD, Darnell BE, Dustan HP, Birch R, Hunter GR: Obesity-related hypertension: Evaluation of the separate effects of energy restriction and weight reduction on hemodynamic and neuroendocrine status. Am J Med 1991 (Apr);90:460–468.

8. Ferrari P, Weidmann P, Shaw S, Giachino D, Riesen W, Allemann Y, Heynen G: Altered insulin sensitivity, hyperinsulinemia, and dyslipidemia in individuals with a hypertensive parent. Am J Med 1991 (Dec);91:589–596.

9. Sheu WHH, Swislocki ALM, Hoffman B, Chen YDI, Reaven GM: Comparison of the effects of atenolol and nifedipine on glucose, insulin, and lipid metabolism in patients with hypertension. Am J Hypertens 1991 (Mar);4:199–205.

10. Salomaa VV, Strandberg TE, Vanhanen H, Naukkarinen V, Sarna S, Miettinen TA: Glucose tolerance and blood pressure: Long term followup in middle aged men. Br Med J 1991 (Mar 2);302:493–496.

11. Yakovlevitch M, Black HR: Resistant hypertension in a tertiary care clinic. Arch Intern Med 1991 (Sept);151:1786–1792.

12. Krishna GG, Kapoor SC: Potassium depletion exacerbates essential hypertension. An Intern Med 1991 (July 15);115:77–83.

13. Harrison MR, Grigsby CG, Souther SK, Smith MD, Demaria AN: Midventricular obstruction associated with chronic systemic hypertension and severe left ventricular hypertrophy. Am J Cardiol 1991 (Sept. 15);68:761–765.

14. Grossman E, Oren S, Messerli FH: Left ventricular filling in the systemic hypertension of obesity. Am J Cardiol 1991 (July 1);68:57–60.

15. Grossman E, Oren S, Messerli FH: Left ventricular filling and stress response pattern in essential hypertension. Am J Med 1991 (Nov);91:502–506.

16. Desimone G, Devereux RB, Roman MJ, Schlussel Y, Alderman MH, Laragh JH: Echocardiographic left ventricular mass and electrolyte intake predict arterial hypertension. An Intern Med 1991 (Feb 1);114:202–209.

17. Koren MJ, Devereux RB, Casale PN, Savage DD, Laragh JH: Relation of left ventricular mass and geometry to morbidity and mortality in uncomplicated essential hypertension. An Intern Med 1991 (Mar 1);114:345–352.

18. Van Hooft IMS, Grobbee DE, Derkx FHM, De Leeuw PW, Schalekamp ADH, Hofman A: Renal hemodynamics and the renin-angiotensin-aldosterone system in normotensive subjects with hypertensive and normotensive parents. N Engl J Med 1991 (May 9);324:1305–1311.

19. Alderman MH, Madhavan S, Ooi WL, Cohen H, Sealey JE, Laragh GH: Association of the renin-sodium profile with the risk of myocardial infarction in patients with hypertension. N Engl J Med 1991 (Apr 18);324:1098–1104.

20. Pincomb GA, Wilson MF, Sung BH, Passey RB, Lovallo WR: Effects of caffeine on pressure regulation during rest and exercise in men at risk for hypertension. Am Heart J 1991 (October);122:1102–1115.

21. De Cesare N, Polese A, Cozzi S, Apostolo A, Fabbiocchi F, Loaldi A, Montorsi P, Guazzi MD: Coronary angiographic patterns in hypertensive compared with normotensive patients. Am Heart J 1991 (April);121:1101–1106.

22. Bailey RH, Knaus VL, Bauer JH: Aneroid sphygmomanometers: An assessment of accuracy at a university hospital and clinics. Arch Intern Med 1991 (July);151:1409–1412.

23. Farnett L, Mulrow CD, Linn WD, Lucey CR, Tuley MR: The J-curve phenomenon and the treatment of hypertension: Is there a point beyond which pressure reduction is dangerous? JAMA 1991 (Jan 23/30);265:489–495.

24. Dahlof B, Lindholm LH, Hansson L, Schersten B, Ekbom T, Wester P-O: Morbidity and mortality in the Swedish trial in old patients with hypertension (STOP-hypertension). Lancet 1991 (Nov 23);338:1281–1285.

25. National High Blood Pressure Education Program: National high blood pressure education program working group report on hypertension and chronic renal failure. Arch Intern Med 1991 (July);151:1280–1287.

26. Law MR, Frost CD, Wald NJ: By how much does dietary salt reduction lower blood pressure? Br Med J 1991 (Apr 6);302:811–815.

27. Moore TJ, Malarick C, Olmedo A, Klein RC: Salt restriction lowers resting blood pressure but not 24-H ambulatory blood pressure. Am J Hypertens 1991 (May);4:410–415.

28. Pescatello LS, Fargo AE, Leach CN and Scherzer HH: Short-term Effect of Dynamic Exercise on Arterial Blood Pressure. Circulation 1991; (May)83:1557–1561.

29. Radack K, Deck C, Huster G: The effects of low doses of n-3 fatty acid supplementation on blood pressure in hypertensive subjects: A randomized controlled trial. Arch Intern Med 1991 (June):151:1173–1180.

30. The Treatment of Mild Hypertension Research Group: The treatment of mild hypertension study: A randomized, placebo-controlled trial of a nutritional-hygienic regimen along with various drug monotherapies. Arch Intern Med 1991 (July):151:1413–1423.

31. Siani A, Strazzullo P, Giacco A, Pacioni D, Celentano E, Mancini M: Increasing the dietary potassium intake reduces the need for antihypertensive medication. An Intern Med 1991 (Nov 15):115:753–759.

32. Belizan JM, Villar J, Gonzalez L, Campodonico L, Bergel E: Calcium supplementation to prevent hypertensive disorders of pregnancy. N Engl J Med 1991 (Nov 14):325:1399–1405.

33. Felson DT, Sloutskis D, Anderson JJ, Anthony JM, Kiel DP: Thiazide diuretics and the risk of hip fracture: Results from the Framingham Study. JAMA 1991 (Jan 16):265:370–373.

34. Warram JH, Laffel LMB, Valsania P, Christlieb AR, Krolewski AS: Excess mortality associated with diuretic therapy in diabetes mellitus. Arch Intern Med 1991 (July):151:1350–1356.

35. Cushman WC, Khatri I, Materson BJ, Reda DJ, Freis ED, Goldstein G, Ramirez EA, Talmers FN, White TJ, Nunn S, Schnaper H, Thomas JR, Henderson WG, Fye C: Treatment of hypertension in the elderly: III. Response of isolated systolic hypertension to various doses of hydrochlorothiazide: Results of a Department of Veterans Affairs cooperative study. Arch Intern Med 1991 (Oct):151:1954–1960.

36. SHEP Cooperative Research Group: Prevention of stroke by antihypertensive drug treatment in older persons with isolated systolic hypertension: Final results of the systolic hypertension in the elderly program. JAMA 1991 (June 26):265:3255–3264.

37. Wassertheil-Smoller S, Blaufox MD, Oberman A, Davis BR, Swencionis C, Knerr MO, Hawkins CM, Langford HG, TAIM Research Group: Effect of antihypertensives on sexual function and quality of life: The TAIM Study. An Intern Med 1991 (Apr 15):114:613–620.

38. Frohlich ED, Ketelhut R, Kaesser UR, Losem CJ, Messerli FH: Hemodynamic effects of celiprolol in essential hypertension. Am J Cardiol 1991 (Aug 15):68:509–514.

39. Applegate WB, Borhani N, DeQuattro V, Kaihlanen PM, Oishi S, Due DL, Sirgo MA: Comparison of labetalol versus enalapril as monotherapy in elderly patients with hypertension: Results of 24-hour ambulatory blood pressure monitoring. Am J Med 1991 (Feb):90:198–205.

40. Oliveros-Palacios MC, Godoy-Godoy N, Colinachourio JA: Effects of Doxazosin on blood pressure, renin-angiotensin-aldosterone and urinary kallikrein. Am J Cardiol 1991 (Jan 15):67:157–161.

41. Frohlich ED, McLoughlin MJ, Losem CJ, Ketelhut R, Messerli FH: Hemodynamic comparison of two nifedipine formulations in patients with essential hypertension. Am J Cardiol 1991 (Nov 15):68:1346–1350.

42. Kuwajima I, Suzuki Y, Shimosawa T, Otsuka K, Kawamura H, Kuramoto K: Effect of nifedipine tablets on ambulatory blood pressure in patients aged >60 and <65 years with systemic hypertension. Am J Cardiol 1991 (Nov 15):68:1351–1356.

43. Cappuccio FP, Markandu ND, Sagnella GA, Singer DRJ, Miller MA, Buckley MG, MacGregor GA: Acute and sustained changes in sodium balance during nifedipine treatment in essential hypertension. Am J Med 1991 (Sept):91:233–238.

44. Melbourne Diabetic Nephropathy Study Group: Comparison between perindopril and nifedipine in hypertensive and normotensive diabetic patients with microalbuminuria. Br Med J 1991 (Jan 26):302:210–216.

45. Bailey DG, Spence JD, Munoz C, Arnold JMO: Interaction of citrus juices with felodipine and nifedipine. Lancet 1991 (Feb 2):337:268–269.

46. Angeli P, Chiesa M, Caregaro L, Merkel C, Sacerdoti D, Rondana M, Gatta A: Comparison of sublingual captopril and nifedipine in immediate treatment of hypertensive emergencies: A randomized, single-blind clinical trial. Arch Intern Med 1991 (Apr):151:678–682.

47. Apperloo AJ, De Zeeuw D, Sluiter HE, De Jong PE: Differential effects of enalapril and atenolol on proteinuria and renal hemodynamics in non-diabetic renal disease. Br Med J 1991 (Oct 5);303:821–824.

48. Applegate WB, Phillips HL, Schnaper H, Shepherd AMM, Schocken D, Luhr JC, Koch GG, Park GD: A randomized controlled trial of the effects of three antihypertensive agents on blood pressure control and quality of life in older women. Arch Intern Med 1991 (Sept);151:1817–1823.

49. Beevers DG, Blackwood RA, Garnham S, Watson M, Mehrzad AA, Admani K, Angell-James JE, Feely M, Kumar S, Husaini MH, Mannering D, Connett C, Long C: Comparison of lisinopril versus atenolol for mild to moderate essential hypertension. Am J Cardiol 1991 (Jan 1);67:59–62.

50. Grossman E, Messerli FH, Oren S, Nunez B, Garavaglia GE: Cardiovascular effects of isradipine in essential hypertension. Am J Cardiol 1991 (July 1);68:65–70.

51. Zing W, Ferguson RK, Vlasses PH: Calcium antagonists in elderly and black hypertensive patients: Therapeutic controversies. Arch Intern Med 1991 (Nov);151:2154–2162.

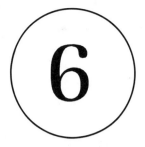

Valvular Heart Disease

Timing valve surgery

Slater and associates[1] in New York, New York, performed a prospective evaluation on 189 consecutive patients with a mean age of 67 years with valvular heart disease considered for surgical treatment on the basis of clinical information to determine whether Doppler echocardiographic or cardiac catheterization data are most valuable in the decision of whether to operate. Three sets of 2 cardiologist decision makers who did not know patient identity were given clinical information in combination with either Doppler echocardiographic or cardiac catheterization data. The combination of Doppler echocardiographic and clinical data were considered inadequate for clinical decision making in 21% of patients with aortic and 5% of patients with mitral valve disease. The combination of cardiac catheterization and clinical data were considered inadequate in 2% of patients with aortic and 2% of patients with mitral valve disease. Among the remaining patients, the cardiologists using echocardiographic or angiographic data were in agreement on the decision to operate or not operate in 113 or 76% of patients overall. When the data were analyzed by specific valve lesion, decisions based on Doppler echocardiographic or cardiac catheterization data were in agreement in 92%, 90%, 83%, and 69%, respectively, of patients with AR, MS, AS, and MR. Differences in cardiac output determination, estimation of valvular regurgitation and information concerning coronary anatomy were the main reasons for different clinical management decisions. These results suggest that for most adult patients with aortic or mitral valve disease, alone or in combination, Doppler echocardiographic data enabled the clinician to make the same decision reached with catheterization data.

Phosphorus-31 magnetic resonance spectroscopy can be used to study intracellular biochemistry non-invasively by measuring the relative proportions of high energy phosphates. Study of deteriorating cardiac metabolism might be useful in the management of hypertrophy and CHF. Conway and associates[2] from Oxford, UK, carried out ^{31}P magnetic resonance spectroscopy in 6 patients with AS and 8 patients with AR. Six patients were receiving treatment for CHF. The phosphocreatine to ATP ratio in these patients was significantly lower than that in 13 controls or in the 8 patients who did not have symptoms of CHF. These findings indicate that CHF in aortic valve disease is associated with low phosphocreatine, which could be due to loss of intracellular creatine. The measurement could eventually have a role in helping to determine the optimum timing for aortic valve replacement.

Percutaneous fiberoptic angioscopy of cardiac valves

The feasibility of percutaneous transluminal angioscopy of the cardiac valves was examined in 8 patients with and in 11 patients without valvular disease in an investigation by Uchida and associates[3] from Tokyo, Funabashi, Gifu, and Hachioji, Japan. In 8 of these patients, a guiding balloon catheter (9F) was introduced into the aortic root, a guide wire (0.014 or 0.025 inch) was introduced through the catheter into the left ventricle to prevent dislocation of the catheter, and a fiberscope (1.6 or 4.6F) was advanced to the distal tip of the catheter. The balloon was then inflated with carbon dioxide and was manipulated against the aortic valve; a body temperature heparinized saline was infused through the catheter for observation. Similarly, the balloon catheter was advanced transseptally into the left atrium for observation of the mitral valve in 4 patients. Also, the balloon catheter was advanced through the right femoral vein into the right atrium for observation of the tricuspid valve in 3 patients. In patients with a normal aortic valve, the aortic cusp surface was smooth and white and the edges were sharp. They opened briskly during systole and coapted each other completely during diastole. In rheumatic AR, the cuspus were thick and blunt and their coaptation insufficiency was observed during diastole. In a patient with rheumatic AS, globular and yellow cusps were observed. Mitral valve leaflets were smooth and white in patients without mitral valvular disease, while the leaflets were yellow, thick, and irregular, and blood regurgitation from the left ventricle into the left atrium could be observed in 2 patients with rheumatic MR. The process of opening and closure of a tricuspid valve was also observed in 3 patients without tricuspid valvular disease. No complications were noted. It was concluded that percutaneous fiberoptic imaging with a balloon-tipped catheter is feasible, safe, and yields highly detailed images of the cardiac valves.

Human leukocyte class II antigens in rheumatic disease

The incidence of rheumatic heart disease is great in Brazil. Guilherme and colleagues[4] in Sao Paulo, Brazil, analyzed the distribution of human leukocyte antigens in a Brazilian population sample with rheumatic fever or rheumatic heart disease, with the aim of better understanding the mechanisms involved. Human leukocyte antigens class I (A, B, and C) and class II (DR and DQ) antigen distribution was studied in 40 patients with diagnosis of rheumatic fever or rheumatic disease and compared with a control group of 617 healthy individuals for class I typing, from which 118 were drawn for class II typing. A strong correlation between rheumatic fever and rheumatic heart disease and human leukocyte antigens-DRw53 (73% in disease group versus 39% in the control group) was found. The investigators also found an increase in the frequency of human leukocyte antigens-DR57, but human leukocyte antigens class I and human leukocyte antigens-DQ typing did not point to any association with these diseases. Thus, human leukocyte antigens-DR57 and DRw53 are markers for susceptibility to rheumatic fever and rheumatic heart disease in Brazil. These results could be explained by genetic differences resulting from racial or geographical diversity.

MITRAL VALVE PROLAPSE

An excellent review of MVP appeared in the May 1991 issue of *Current Problems in Cardiology.* The article was written by Fontana and associates[5] from Columbus, Ohio.

Another review of MVP in virtually all of its various aspects was provided by Wooley and associates[6] from Columbus, Ohio.

Sochowski and associates[7] from Ottawa, Canada, compared the accuracy of transesophageal echocardiography with that of transthoracic echocardiography in the detection of ruptured chordae tendineae (flail mitral leaflet) in 27 patients with MVP who underwent valve repair or replacement for MR. Confirmation of the presence of ruptured chordae resulting in a flail leaflet was available at surgery in all cases. The echocardiographic studies were read blindly by 2 independent observers with any differences resolved by a third. Mean age was 63 ± 13 years. Men (n = 20) outnumbered women (n = 7), and tended to be younger. Flail leaflets were identified in 20 of 27 patients. In 1 patient, both leaflets were involved and in the remaining 19 patients posterior leaflets (15 patients) were more frequently affected than anterior leaflets (4 patients). Transesophageal echocardiography correctly identified all 20 patients with flail leaflets, but 1 false positive study occurred among the 7 patients without a flail leaflet. In contrast, transthoracic echocardiography identified only 12 of 20 patients with flail leaflets, with no false positive studies. Transesophageal echocardiography was more accurate, correctly classifying 26 of 27 (96%) cases versus 19 of 27 (70%) by the transthoracic approach. This study suggests a higher incidence of chordal rupture of the posterior leaflet in patients with MVP and demonstrates improved accuracy of transesophageal over transthoracic echocardiography in the detection of flail leaflets.

To determine the incidence and significance of late potentials in patients with MVP, Jabi and associates[8] from Huntington, West Virginia, performed surface signal-averaged electrocardiography and 24-hour ambulatory electrocardiographic monitoring in 41 patients with moderate to severe MVP on 2-dimensional echocardiograms. Late potentials were defined as the presence of either a root mean square voltage of the last 40 msec of the QRS of <20 μv or a low-amplitude signal duration >39 msec. Despite the absence of clinically significant VT by history and on ambulatory electrocardiographic monitoring, 12 patients had late potentials on their signal-averaged electrocardiograms. Clinical characteristics could not differentiate patients with from patients without late potentials, and all patients were doing well at a mean follow-up of 34 months except for 1 noncardiac death. It was concluded that late potentials on the surface signal-averaged electrocardiogram are a common and benign finding in patients with MVP and their clinical significance should be determined only in the presence of other findings.

MITRAL REGURGITATION

Vasodilator therapy with captopril

Few data exist regarding the effects of angiotensin converting enzyme inhibitors in patients with regurgitant valvular lesions. Wisenbaugh and colleagues[9] in Johannesburg, South Africa, postulated an immediate improvement in cardiac performance with captopril in MR, which, in a hemodynamically compensated group of patients, might be mediated through parasympathetic vasodilation rather than through blockade of angiotensin converting enzyme. Hemodynamics were examined before and 90 minutes after oral captopril (25–50 mg) in 18 patients with chronic, severe MR in New York Heart Association functional class II and III. One group of patients was given captopril alone and a second group was given captopril plus atropine. Captopril alone (group 1) produced decreases in heart rate, mean arterial pressure, systemic resistance, and PA wedge pressure. There was no improvement in either arteriorvenous oxygen difference or thermodilution cardiac output; in fact, the latter slightly declined. Pretreatment with atropine (group 2) diminished the effects of captopril on heart rate, mean arterial pressure, and systemic resistance. In patients with chronic, severe MR, captopril reduced systemic arterial and LV filling pressures but did not immediately augment cardiac output as expected. Furthermore, the modest systemic vasodilator effect of captopril was parasympathetically mediated.

Predicting results of valve replacement

The ability to predict outcome after MVR remains limited in patients with symptomatic chronic MR. The aims of this study were to determine the preoperative predictors of postoperative cardiac-related mortality and to assess the additive prognostic value of tests performed in such patients. Reed and colleagues[10] in Charlottesville, Virginia, followed 176 patients who underwent MVR at least 4 years earlier. Four categories of variables were analyzed to predict postoperative cardiac-related mortality: clinical, laboratory, 2-dimensional echocardiographic and cardiac catheterization. There were 39 cardiac-related deaths (29 due to CHF and 10 sudden). When the 4 categories were analyzed separately, 2 clinical, 1 laboratory, 2-dimensional echocardiographic, and one catheterization variable best predicted postoperative death. When these 6 variables were examined simultaneously, only 3 remained significant predictors of cardiac-related mortality: presence of pulmonary rales, LV size, and the ratio of LV wall thickness to LV cavity dimension in end systole. A model based on these 3 variables may predict cardiac-related death with considerable accuracy. Laboratory data did not add to clinical information for predicting death. Two-dimensional echocardiographic variables provided significant additional information in this regard. Further addition of catheterization variables was not useful. Prognostic value did not change significantly when 50 patients with prior mitral surgery or 49 patients undergoing concomitant AVR or CABG were excluded from analysis.

Anatomic features

Among patients with chronic mitral valve dysfunction severe enough to warrant MVR, associated tricuspid valve dysfunction is relatively common. Most patients having tricuspid valve replacement have simultaneous MVR because of MS (with or without associated MR). Roberts and Eways[11] from Bethesda, Maryland, described certain clinical and morphologic findings in 17 patients having MVR for severe, chronic, pure MR, and simultaneous tricuspid valve replacement for severe tricuspid valve dysfunction. The 17 patients were derived from examination of 113 patients >20 years of age who underwent simultaneous replacement of dysfunctioning native tricuspid and mitral valves at the National Heart, Lung, and Blood Institute between 1963 and 1989. Of the 113 patients, the mitral valve was stenotic before valve replacement in 96 (85%) and purely regurgitant in 17 (15%). The present report focused exclusively on the latter 17 patients. Eight (47%) were women and 9 (53%) were men and their ages ranged from 27 to 73 years (mean 54). None of the 17 patients had evidence of aortic valve dysfunction. Sixteen patients (94%) had pulmonary hypertension, including 8 (47%) with peak pulmonary arterial systolic pressures ≥70 mm Hg. All had clinical evidence of severe TR and none had a pressure gradient between right ventricle and right atrium during ventricular diastole. Five patients had isolated MVP, 2 had MVP associated with HC, and 2 had MVP associated with secundum ASD. Infective endocarditis that healed was the cause of the MR in 4 patients, one of whom also had HC. Two patients had involvement of both the tricuspid and mitral valves by the hypereosinophilic syndrome. In 1 patient the cause of MR was rheumatic heart disease. The etiology of the MR was unclear in 1 patient who had a heavily calcified papillary muscle but angiographically normal coronary arteries. Except for the 2 patients with hypereosinophilic syndrome, the operatively excised tricuspid valve leaflets and chordae tendineae were anatomically normal. The tricuspid valve anuli were described as being dilated at operation in all 17 patients. Five patients died within 2 months of the double valve replacement and 4 others died from 34 to 95 months afterwards. In summary, the type of tricuspid valve dysfunction occurring in association with pure chronic MR is virtually always pure TR and the cause of the TR is usually dilatation of the tricuspid valve anulus.

MITRAL STENOSIS

Use of atrial systole

The importance of the contribution of atrial systole to ventricular filling in MS is controversial. The cause of reduced cardiac output following the onset of AF may be due to an increased heart rate, a loss of booster pump function, or both. Meisner and co-workers[12] in Tel Aviv, Israel, studied the atrial contribution to filling under a variety of conditions by combing noninvasive studies of patients with computer modeling. Thirty patients in sinus rhythm with mild-to-severe stenosis were studied with two-dimensional and Doppler echocardiography for measurement of mitral flow velocity and mitral valve area. The mean standard deviation atrial contribution to LV filling volume was 18% and varied inversely with mitral resistance. Patients with mild MS (mitral valve area, at 1.8 cm²) and severe MS (mitral valve area, of 0.9 cm²) had atrial contributions of 29% and 9%, respectively. The pathophysiological mechanisms responsible for these trends were further investigated by the computer model. In modeled severe MS increasing heart rate from 75 to 150 beats/min caused an increase of 5.2 mm Hg in mean LA pressure, whereas loss of atrial contraction at a heart rate of 150 beats/min caused only a 1.3 mm Hg increase. The atrial booster pump contributes less to ventricular filling in MS than in the normal heart, and the loss of atrial pump function is less important than the effect of increasing heart rate as the cause of decompensation during AF.

Valve area from doppler color flow imaging

Kawahara and colleagues[13] in Osaka, Japan used Doppler color flow imaging to evaluate valve areas in 30 patients with mitral stenosis undergoing cardiac catheterization. Color jet width correlated well with actual orifice diameter (Figure 6-1). In the clinical Doppler study, the mitral valve orifice was assumed to be elliptic and the mitral valve area was calculated from the following equation: $(\pi/4)(a \times b)$, where a = color jet width at the mitral valve orifice in the apical long-axis view (short diameter) and b = the width in the 90° rotated view (long diameter). Mitral valve area was determined by two-dimensional echocardiography and the pressure half-time method, and the results for all three noninvasive methods were compared with those obtained at cardiac catheterization. Mitral valve area was determined in all patients by Doppler color flow imaging, and there was a significant correlation between the Doppler jet and catheterization estimates of mitral valve area (Figure 6-1). Valve area determined by two-dimensional echocardiography corre-

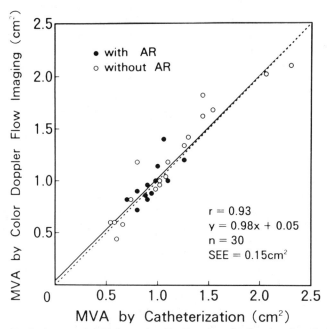

Fig. 6-1. Mitral valve areas (MVA) determined by Doppler color flow imaging plotted against the cardiac catheterization data. Closed circles represent patients with and open circles patients without aortic regurgitation (AR). The correlation coefficient for this relation was 0.93 in 30 patients. Reprinted with permission from Kawahara, et al.[13]

lated well with catheterization measurements in 26 patients, but the area could not be determined in 4 of the 30 because of technical problems. The pressure half-time method tended to overestimate valve area in patients with AR. These data suggest that Doppler color flow imaging provides an accurate estimate of mitral valve area and appears applicable to the assessment of the severity of MS.

Percutaneous balloon valvuloplasty

Percutaneous double balloon mitral valvotomy was performed by Casale and associates[14] in 25 patients with severe MS who were followed for at least 6 months after the procedure. There were 22 women and 3 men, with a mean age of 51 ± 14 years (range 27 to 74). Hemodynamic and angiographic findings were evaluated before and after percutaneous double balloon mitral valvotomy and clinical status was assessed at follow-up. There was a significant decrease in mitral gradient following percutaneous double balloon mitral valvotomy, from 15 ± 5.1 to 5.0 ± 2.6 mm Hg; an increase in cardiac output from 4.6 ± 1.1 to 5.2 ± 1.1 L/min; and an increase in calculated mitral valve area from 0.9 ± 0.2 to 2.2 ± 0.6 cm². MR developed or increased in severity in 6 patients (24%). At the time of follow-up (mean 12 ± 5 months), 3 patients required elective MVR for symptomatic MR and 91% (20 of 22) of the remaining patients had continued improvement in functional class. Percutaneous double balloon mitral valvotomy can safely be performed in properly selected patients with symptomatic MS with good immediate and follow-up results.

Lefèvre and associates[15] in Montreal, Canada, used percutaneous mitral valvuloplasty in 34 of 126 consecutive patients judged to be at high risk for surgery on the basis of age >70 years, New York Heart Association functional class IV, LVEF ≤35%, severe pulmonary hypertension, and need for associated bypass surgery, additional valve surgery or severe pulmonary disease. Clinical features of the high risk group were worse than those of the other patients. Three high risk patients had technical failures and 3 others had major complications. Among the remaining 28 patients, 18 (65%) had a hemodynamic success, 4 (14%) an incomplete success, and 6 (21%) hemodynamic failure. MR did not change after the procedure in 15 (56%) of 27 patients and increased by one grade in the remaining 12 patients. Atrial shunting was detected by dye-dilution curves in 71% of the patients, but only 4 (14%) had a pulmonary to systemic flow ratio >1.5. Three patients (9%) died within 48 hours of the procedure and by 6 months, three additional patients had died. Twenty (80%) of survivors had improved by at least one functional class. Therefore, in patients at high surgical risk, the risk of percutaneous mitral valvuloplasty is also increased, but is acceptable compared with that of surgery.

Turi and co-investigators[16] in Detroit, Michigan, performed a prospective, randomized trial comparing percutaneous balloon commissurotomy with surgical closed commissurotomy in 40 patients with severe rheumatic MS. The data were analyzed by investigators who were masked to treatment assignment or phase of study. Patients randomized to balloon (20) or surgical (20) commissurotomy had severe MS without significant baseline differences (LA pressure, 26 versus 28 mm Hg; mitral valve gradient, 18 versus 20 mm Hg; mitral valve area 1.0 versus 1.0 cm², respectively). At 1-week follow-up after balloon commissurotomy PA wedge pressure was 14 mm Hg; mitral valve gradient 10 mm Hg; and mitral valve area was 1.6 cm². At 1-week follow-up after surgical closed commissurotomy, PA wedge pressure was 14 mm Hg; mitral valve gradient was 9 mm Hg; and mitral valve area was 1.6 cm²). At 8-month follow-up, improvement occurred in both groups: mitral valve area was 1.6 cm² in the balloon commissurotomy group and was 1.0 cm² in the surgical closed commissurotomy group. There was no difference between the groups at 1-week or 8-month follow-up. One case of severe MR occurred in each group; complications were otherwise related to transseptal catheterization. There was no death, stroke, or AMI. Cost analysis revealed that balloon commissurotomy may substantially exceed the cost of surgical commissurotomy in developing countries, whereas it may represent a significant savings in industrialized nations.

Percutaneous transvenous mitral commissurotomy was performed in 219 patients with symptomatic, severe rheumatic MS by Hung and associates[17] from Taiwan, Republic of China. There were 59 men and 160 women, aged 19 to 76 years (mean 43). Pliable, noncalcified valves were present in 139 (group 1), and calcified valves or severe mitral subvalvular lesions, or both, in 80 patients (group 2). AF was present in 133 patients (61%) and 1+ or 2+ MR in 59 (27%). Technical failure occurred with 3 patients in our early experience. There was no cardiac tamponade or emergency surgery. The only in-hospital death occurred 3 days after the procedure in a group 2 premoribund patient in whom last-resort PTMC created 3+ MR. MR appeared or increased in 72 patients (33%); 3+ MR resulted in 12 patients (6%). There were 3 systemic embolisms. Atrial left-to-right shunts measured by oximetry developed in 33 patients (15%). Immediately after commissurotomy, there were significantly reduced LA pressure (24 ± 6 to 15 ± 5 mm Hg), mean PA pressure (40 ± 13 to 31 ± 11 mm Hg) and mitral valve gradient (13 ± 5 to 6 ± 3 mm Hg). Mitral valve area increased from 1.0 ± 0.3 to 2.0 ± 0.7 cm² and cardiac output from 4.4 ± 1.4 to 4.7 ± 1.2 L/min. The results mirrored clinical improvements in 209 patients (97%). Multivariate analysis showed an echo score >8, and valvular calcium and severe subvalvular lesions as independent predictors for suboptimal hemodynamic results. The cardiovascular event-free survival rate for group 1 was 100% up to 42 months; that for group 2 was 91% at 12 months, and held at 76% from 24 to 31 months.

Shrivastava and associates[18] from New Delhi, India, reported results of percutaneous balloon mitral valvuloplasty in 34 patients <20 years of age with rheumatic MS. Of the 34 patients, 26 had successful valvuloplasty: a single balloon technique was used in 20 patients and a double balloon technique in 6 patients. Balloon valvuloplasty resulted in a significant decrease in the transmitral end diastolic pressure gradient from 23 ± 6 to 8 ± 6 mm HG and in a significant increase in mitral valve area, from .65 ± .25 to 1.8 ± 0.9 cm². Mean PA pressure decreased from 44 ± 15 to 34 ± 16 mm HG. The complications encountered were severe MR in 1 patient and cardiac tamponade in another. Angiographic left-to-right shunt was demonstrated immediately after mitral valve dilatation in 15 of 26 patients and oximetry evidence of shunt was seen in 6 of 26 patients (23%). Repeat hemodynamic measurements in 10 patients at 3 to 6 months revealed no change in the transmitral end diastolic gradients compared to those immediately after valvuloplasty.

Anatomic features

Eways and Roberts[19] from Bethesda, Maryland, described certain clinical and morphologic findings in 67 patients (aged 23–76 years [mean 52]; 55 women [82%]) who had MVR for MS (with or without associated MR), and simultaneous tricuspid valve replacement for pure TR (58 patients) or tricuspid stenosis (all with associated regurgitation; 9 patients). Of the 58 patients with pure TR, 21 had anatomically normal and 37 had anatomically abnormal (diffusely fibrotic leaflets) tricuspid valves (Table 6-1). Among these 58 patients, no clinical or hemodynamic variable was useful before surgery in distinguishing the group without from that with anatomically abnormal tricuspid valves. All 9 patients with stenotic tricuspid valves had anatomically abnormal tricuspid valves. The latter group had a lower average RV systolic pressure (tricuspid valve closing pressure) than those with pure TR, and none had severe PA hypertension (present in 20 [30%] of the 58 patients with pure TR).

AORTIC-VALVE STENOSIS

Natural history

Kennedy and associates[20] in Rochester, Minnesota, evaluated the natural history of moderate AS in 66 patients who at the time of cardiac catheterization had an aortic valve between 0.7 and 1.2 cm^2 and who did not have surgical therapy during the first 180 days after cardiac catheterization. During a mean follow-up period of 35 months, 14 patients died of causes attributed to AS and 21 underwent AVR. Estimated probability for remaining free of any complication of AS at the end of the first 4 years was 59%. Symptomatic patients with decreased LVEF or hemodynamic evidence of LV decompensation were at greater risk for these complications. These data suggest that patients with moderate AS are at significant risk for the development of complications, especially those who are symptomatic and have hemodynamic evidence of LV decompensation.

Rapidity of progression

Progression from mild to severe AS is well recognized, but there are few data as to the likely rate of progression. Davies and associates[21] from Leicester, UK, reviewed clinical outcome and cardiac catheterization data in 65 patients with AS. Each patient had been investigated by cardiac catheterization on at least 2 occasions, the interval between studies ranging from 1–17 years (mean 7). In 60 cases the aortic valve gradient had increased from a median of 10 mm Hg (range 0–60) to a median of 52 mm Hg (range 15–120). The mean rate of increase of gradient was 6.5 mm per year and was significantly faster in patients in whom there was aortic valve calcium or AR present at the first catheterization study. This study shows that progression of AS may be very rapid and correlates with valvular calcium and AR.

TABLE 6-1. *Clinical, hemodynamic and anatomic observations in 67 patients having combined mitral and tricuspid valve replacement for mitral and tricuspid valve stenoses or regurgitation, or both. Reproduced with permission from Eways.*[19]

								Pressures (mm Hg)													
								Right Atrium		PAW or LA							Dead After VR				
Group	Type of Valve Dysfunction	Valve Anatomically Abnormal	No. of Pts. (%)	Age (yrs) at VR Range (mean)	Women (%)	Men (%)		Mean	V Wave	Mean	V Wave	RV (s/d) Average	LV (s/d) Average	RVSP ≤40 (%)	RVSP >70 (%)	LVSP >140 (%)	≤60 Days (%)	12 Mos	60 Mos	10 Yrs
1	MS,TR	MV	21 (31)	23–75 (54)	17 (81)	4 (19)	12	21	22	29	61/11	117/12	5 (24)	4 (19)	2 (10)	2/21 (10)	4/19	8/17	11/16
2	MS,TR	MV & TV	37 (55)	25–76 (54)	29 (78)	8 (22)	14	22	26	35	68/13	117/14	7 (19)	16 (43)	3 (8)	8/37 (22)	8/34	10/29	15/23
3	MS,TS	MV & TV	9 (14)	29–55 (40)	9 (100)	0 (0)	13	20	19	32	47/10	121/13	2 (22)	0 (0)	2 (22)	2/9 (22)	3/9	3/9	3/6
Totals or means			67 (100)	23–76 (52)	55 (82)	12 (18)	13	21	23	33	63/12	118/13	14 (21)	20 (30)	7 (10)	12/67 (18)	5/62 (24%)	21/55 (38%)	29/45 (64%)

LA = left atrium; LV = left ventricle; LVSP = left ventricular peak systolic pressure; MS = mitral stenosis (with or without mitral regurgitation); MV = mitral valve; PAW = pulmonary artery wedge; RV = right ventricle; RVSP = right ventricular peak systolic pressure; s/d = peak systole/end-diastole; TR = tricuspid regurgitation; TS = tricuspid stenosis; TV = tricuspid valve; VR = valve replacement.

With bicuspid valve and aortic aneurysm

Pachulski and associates[22] from Ottawa, Canada, identified by 2 dimensional echocardiogram 144 patients with bicuspid aortic valve (BAV) in a 41-month period. Seventeen of the 144 patients were excluded because of greater than trivial AR, 14 because of associated aortic coarctation, 11 because of a mean resting LV outflow gradient <25 mm Hg as determined by continuous wave Doppler, and 1 because of combined AS and AR. The resulting study group, therefore, consisted of 101 patients with a functionally normal or minimally stenotic BAV and they were compared to an age and sex-matched control group of 50 patients with normal echocardiograms during the same interval. The echocardiographic measurements were taken at the sinus level at end diastole. The mean aortic root diameter in patients with a functionally normal or minimally stenotic BAV was 35 ± 6 mm (range 20 to 54 mm), whereas the mean aortic root diameter in the control group was 30 ± 4 mm (range 23 − 40 mm). Fifty-eight percent of the study group and only 20% of the control subjects had an aortic route diameter >34 mm, a conventionally accepted upper limit of normal for the aortic root at the sinus level in adults.

Responses to exercise stress

Patients with heart disease may have myocardial ischemia or LV dysfunction without symptoms. The exercise responses of 14 asymptomatic patients with AS were studied by Clyne and colleagues[23] from Bethesda, Maryland, using treadmill testing, thallium-201 scintigraphy and radionuclide angiography. Compared with age- and gender-matched control subjects, patients with AS demonstrated reduced exercise tolerance (10.7 ± 2.5 vs 13.3 ± 4.2 min) and maximal oxygen consumption (26.7 ± 6.3 vs 36.3 ± 9.5 ml O_2/min/kg) associated with decreased peak systolic BP response to exercise (177 ± 18 vs 214 ± 42 mm Hg). Ten of 14 patients developed ST-segment depression during exercise, only 3 of whom had reversible thallium defects. Patients with AS tended to have greater LVEF at rest (65 ± 11 vs 58 ± 7) and significantly decreased early peak filling rates (4.8 ± 1.3 vs 6.1 ± 0.6 stroke volume/s) compared with those of control subjects. During maximal supine exercise, patients with AS had less of an increase in EF (2 ± 9 vs 15 ± 7%) associated with a decrease in end-diastolic (−7 ± 15 vs + 5 ± 16%) and stroke (−6 ± 17 vs +30 ± 13%) volumes from baseline measurements. The limitation in stroke volume and heart rate to exercise stress in patients with AS was associated with attenuation of the cardiac output response during exercise compared with that of control subjects (73 ± 48 vs 284 ± 48%), which correlated directly with effort limitation (4 = 0.717). Thus, despite the absence of symptoms patients with AS demonstrate limited effort tolerance with abnormal systemic and LV hemodynamics, which is most likely a consequence of the inability to augment end-diastolic volume during exercise.

Doppler echocardiography findings

To determine the relation of Doppler findings to clinical outcome and the agreement between Doppler and cardiac catheterization in the assessment of AS severity, Galan and associates[24] from Houston, Texas, studied 510 consecutive patients with suspected AS. Adequate echocardiographic and Doppler examinations were obtained in 498 patients or

98% of the population. Clinical data were available for analysis in 497 patients. In 160 patients, Doppler demonstrated an aortic valve area <0.75 cm² or a peak jet velocity >4.5 m/s consistent with critical AS. In the subgroup with cardiac catheterization (n = 105), Doppler was 97% accurate. AVR or balloon valvuloplasty was performed in 109 patients, 106 of whom were symptomatic. Noncritical AS was detected by Doppler in 327 patients, with 95% accuracy in the subgroup with cardiac catheterization (n = 133). AVR was performed in 15 patients with symptoms of AS and with valve areas assessed by Doppler to be between 0.76 and 0.80 cm² or with peak jet velocities >3.5 m/s. In 20 patients, AVR was performed because of moderate to severe AR, and in 11 elderly (>70 years old) patients with valve areas between 0.80 and 1.0 cm², AVR was performed at the time of CABG in an attempt to prevent the need for a repeat surgical procedure in the future. These observations allow the following conclusions. In the symptomatic patient with critical or near critical AS by Doppler, cardiac catheterization does not provide additional information beyond that provided by Doppler. In these patients, the procedure could be limited to coronary arteriography when indicated. Likewise, the asymptomatic patient with noncritical AS by Doppler can be followed noninvasively without catheterization to monitor the progression of AS. In a subgroup of patients with noncritical AS by Doppler in whom symptoms and physical findings suggest significant AS, cardiac catheterization may still be indicated to confirm or exclude the presence of significant AS. Overall, Doppler echocardiography is highly accurate in the assessment of AS severity and its use should allow for a more conservative application of cardiac catheterization in these patients.

Otto and associates[25] of the Balloon Valvuloplasty Registry Echocardiographers analyzed baseline echocardiographic data in 680 adults (mean age 78 years) undergoing balloon aortic valvuloplasty at 24 medical centers to describe the degree of outflow obstruction in patients with symptomatic AS. Maximal aortic jet velocity ranged from 2.3 to 6.6 m/s (mean 4.4 ± 0.8) and continuity equation valve area ranged from 0.1 to 1.4 cm² (mean 0.6 ± 0.2). Of note, 36% had a jet velocity >4.0 m/s but only 3% had a valve area <1.0 cm² due to a high prevalence of impaired systolic function (54%). Outflow tract diameter was poorly correlated with body surface area, although the group mean diameter was smaller in women than in men (1.9 ± 0.2 vs 2.1 ± 0.3 cm). Mean pressure gradient was related closely to maximal gradient (r = 0.92) and to maximal jet velocity (mean $\Delta P = 2.4 V^2 + 0.75$ mm Hg). Simpler measures of AS severity were correlated with Doppler and invasive valve area. This study demonstrates marked variability in AS severity in symptomatic adults referred for balloon aortic valvuloplasty. The absence of a predictable relation between outflow tract diameter and body size emphasizes the importance of this measurement in each patient if definition of valve area is needed. The correlations between mean pressure gradient and maximal jet velocity, and between valve area and the velocity ratio support the potential use of these simpler measures of stenosis severity.

Valve area by transesophageal echocardiography

In an investigation by Stoddard and associates[26] from Louisville, Kentucky, to determine if AS severity could be accurately measured by 2-dimensional transesophageal echocardiography, 62 adults (mean age 66 ± 12 years) with AS had their aortic valve area determined by direct planimetry using transesophageal echocardiography, and with the continuity equation using combined transthoracic Doppler and 2-dimensional echocardiography. Eighteen individuals had aortic valve area calculated by the Gorlin method during catheterization. An excellent correlation was found between aortic valve area determined by transesophageal echocardiography (mean 1.24 ± 0.49 cm²; range 0.40 to 2.26 cm²) and transthoracic Doppler/2-dimensional echocardiography (mean 1.23 ± 0.46 cm²; range 0.40 to 2.23 cm²). The absolute (0.13 ± 0.12 cm²) and percent (10.8 ± 8.9%) differences between aortic valve area determined by transesophageal echocardiography versus transthoracic Doppler/2-dimensional echocardiography were small. Excellent correlations between aortic valve area by transesophageal echocardiography and transthoracic Doppler/2-dimensional echocardiography were also found in subjects with normal systolic function (n = 38) and impaired function (n = 24). Aortic valve area determined by catheterization correlated better with aortic valve area measured by transesophageal echocardiography than aortic valve area measured with transthoracic Doppler/2-dimensional echocardiography. These data demonstrate that aortic valve area can be accurately measured by direct planimetry using transesophageal echocardiography in individuals with AS. Transesophageal echocardiography may become an important adjunct to transthoracic echocardiography in the assessment of AS severity.

Balloon valvuloplasty

Balloon aortic valvuloplasty has been a therapeutic alternative treatment for severe symptomatic aortic stenosis. Previous studies have been unable to predict 1-year outcome because of limited acute and follow-up clinical, invasive and echocardiographic data. Davidson and associates[27] from Durham, North Carolina, performed a study to predict long-term outcome based on comprehensive data obtained at the time of valvuloplasty and at 3 and 6 months after the procedure. Of 170 consecutive patients undergoing valvuloplasty, 108 (mean age 78 years) were at least 1 year from their procedure. Prospective clinical, micromanometer hemodynamic, digital ventriculographic and echocardiographic/Doppler data were collected at baseline and immediately after the procedure. Echocardiographic data were also obtained at 3 and 6 months. With use of Cox model analysis, major events (defined as cardiac death [n = 30], AVR [n = 21] or repeat valvuloplasty [n = 13]) were predicted by advanced age, baseline CHF class, and baseline echocardiographic-determined diastolic LV diameter. Only baseline LVEF proved to be a significant predictor of cardiac death in a multivariate model (Figure 6-2). Absolute values after valvuloplasty (stroke work, first derivative of LV pressure, valve area, end-systolic volume, Fick cardiac output, transvalvular gradient) and acute changes measured by catheterization or echocardiography did not provide additional predictive information over that of postprocedure EF. Similarly, echocardiographic valve area and transvalvular gradient at 3 months added no further prognostic data. With an EF ≥45% (n = 63), cardiac survival at 1 year was 80%, irrespective of age, sex, CHF class or severity of CAD. Thus, prognosis after valvuloplasty can be determined by noninvasive clinical and echocardiographic data obtained before cardiac catheterization. Despite advanced age and concomitant medical problems, patients undergoing valvuloplasty with baseline EF ≥45% have an excellent cardiac survival to 1 year.

Between December 1985 and April 1989, valvuloplasty was performed by Kuntz and associates[28] from Boston, Massachusetts, in 205 patients.

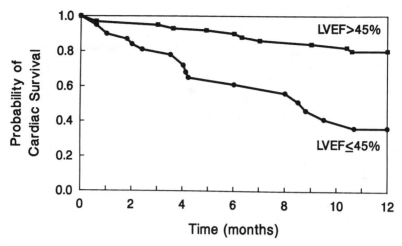

Fig. 6-2. Probability of cardiovascular death based on baseline left ventricular ejection fraction (LVEF). Reprinted with permission of Davidson, et al.[27]

The authors evaluated 40 demographic and hemodynamic variables as univariate predictors of event-free survival by Cox regression analysis and identified independent predictors of event-free survival by stepwise multivariate analysis. Early hemodynamic results indicated a decrease in the peak transaortic-valve pressure gradient from 67 ± 28 to 33 ± 15 mm Hg after valvuloplasty and an increase in aortic-valve area from 0.6 ± 0.2 to 0.9 ± 0.3 cm². The rate of event-free survival (defined as survival without recurrent symptoms, repeated valvuloplasty, or AVR) was 18% over the mean (± SD) follow-up period of 24 ± 12 months (range, 1 to 47) (Figure 6-3). Significant predictors of event-free survival included the LVEF and the LV and aortic systolic pressure before valvuloplasty, and the percent reduction in the aortic-valve pressure gradient; the PA wedge pressure was inversely associated with event-free survival. Although the predicted event-free survival rate for the entire patient group was 50% at 1 year and 25% at 2 years, the probability of event-free survival at 1 year varied between 23 and 65% when patients were stratified according to 3 independent predictors: the aortic systolic pressure, the PA wedge pressure, and the percent reduction in the peak aortic-valve gradient. The most important predictors of event-free survival after balloon aortic valvuloplasty were related to base-line LV performance. The best long-term results after valvuloplasty were observed among patients who would also have been expected to have excellent long-term results after AVR.

In a study by Letac and associates[29] from Rouen, France, to evaluate the restenosis rate after successful balloon aortic valvuloplasty, clinical evaluation and repeat catheterization were performed in 96 patients who had undergone balloon dilatation 7 ± 5 months earlier. Restenosis, defined as a loss of >50% of the benefit in aortic valve area obtained after balloon valvuloplasty, was observed in 48% of the patients. Actuarial analysis showed that the restenosis rate was time dependent and was 80% at 15 months. Functional improvement was observed in most of the patients with or without restenosis. The restenosis rate was not correlated with the degree of enlargement of the aortic orifice produced by the

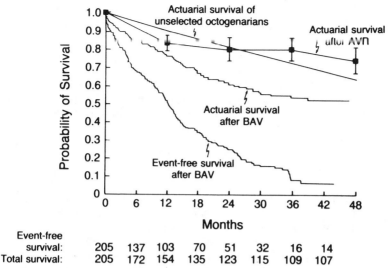

Fig. 6-3. Actuarial total and event-free survival among 205 patients treated by balloon aortic valvuloplasty (BAV). Shown for comparison are the actuarial survival rates among unselected octogenarians in the United States and among octogenarians who undergo aortic-valve replacement (AVR) (reproduced from Levinson et al. with permission of the American Heart Association). The numbers below the figure show how many patients were alive or alive without an event at each follow-up. Reprinted with permission from Kuntz, et al.[28]

valvuloplasty procedure. Because of the high incidence of restenosis, balloon aortic valvuloplasty should be limited to patients who have a contraindication to surgery or are at high risk for surgery, or as a bridge to surgery.

A study by the National Heart, Lung, and Blood Institute Valvuloplasty Registry participants described patients undergoing initial percutaneous aortic balloon valvuloplasty[30]. Extensive baseline procedural and post-procedural data were tabulated in 674 patients during a 24-month period. Complications were defined and divided into procedural, acute (within 24 hours), in-hospital, and within 30 days of the procedure. The patient population was elderly and symptomatic, with 83% >70 years of age. New York Heart Association functional class III or IV CHF was present in 76%, syncope or presyncope was present in 34% and Canadian Heart Association class III or IV angina was present in 23%. Using an overall functional scoring system (0–100), 54% had scores > than 50. Comorbid disease was common. Forty-five percent possessed at least one serious noncardiac disability as a reason for valvuloplasty. Eight percent of those seen by a cardiothoracic surgeon were believed inappropriate for AVR. Hemodynamically, the aortic valve area increased from 0.5 to 0.8 cm², accompanied by a fall in mean and peak aortic valve gradient from 55 and 65 to 29 and 31 mm Hg respectively. Small but significant increases were observed in cardiac output, heart rate, and mean aortic pressure with minor declines in the PA systolic and LV end-diastolic pressure. One hundred sixty-seven (25%) experienced at least one significant complication within 24 hours, and 211 (31%) experienced a significant complication before discharge. Complications before hospital discharge included the need for transfusion (23%), vascular surgery (7%), cerebrovascular accident (3%), other systemic embolus (2%), AMI (2%), acute tubular necrosis (15), or cardiac surgery (1%). Seventeen patients died during the procedure; 16 of these were due to cardiac causes. By hospital discharge, there was an additional 52 total deaths; 37 were due to cardiovascular disease. Between hospital discharge and 30 days 23 additional deaths occurred; 18 were due to cardiac disease. At 30 days, therefore, there was a grand total of 92 (14%) deaths; 71 (11%) were due to cardiovascular-related causes. Of the survivors at 30 days, symptomatic improvement was generally present. These data reveal that percutaneous aortic balloon valvuloplasty in an elderly and debilitated population can be done with low mortality but substantial morbidity. Mortality is greatest in patients with multiorgan failure resulting from poor cardiac output.

Valve replacement age ≥80 years

Culliford and associates[31] from New York, New York, described the results of AVR alone (n = 35) or in combination with CABG without any other valve procedure (n = 36, group 2) in 71 patients aged ≥80 years (mean 82 ± 2 years) with AS or mixed AS and AR. Preoperatively, 91% had severe cardiac limitations (New York Heart Association class III or IV). Hospital mortality was 13% overall (9 of 71), 6% (2 of 35) for group 1 and 19% (7 of 36) for group 2. Perioperatively, 1 patient (1.4%) had a stroke. Survival from late cardiac death at 1 and 3 years was 98.2 and 95.5%, respectively, for all patients, 100% for patients who underwent isolated AVR, and 96 and 91%, respectively, for patients who underwent AVR plus CABG. Eighty-three percent of surviving patients had marked symptomatic improvement. Freedom from all valve-related complications (thromboembolism, anticoagulant, infective endocarditis, reoperation or prosthetic failure) was 93 and 80% at 1 and 3 years, respectively. Thus, short- and long-term morbidity and mortality after AVR for AS in patients aged >80 years are encouragingly low, although the addition of CABG increases short- and long-term mortality.

AORTIC REGURGITATION

Natural history

Many asymptomatic patients with AR and normal LV systolic function remain clinically stable for many years, but others ultimately develop symptoms or LV dysfunction and require operation. To identify indexes of LV function predictive of symptomatic and functional deterioration during the long-term course of asymptomatic patients, Bonow and coworkers[32] in Bethesda, Maryland, studied 104 asymptomatic patients with chronic severe AR and normal LV EF at rest. Serial echocardiographic and radionuclide angiographic studies were obtained over a mean follow-up period of 8 years. By Kaplan-Meier life table analysis, 58% of patients remained asymptomatic with normal EF at 11 years, an average attrition rate of less than 5% per year; 2 patients died suddenly, 4 developed asymptomatic LV dysfunction, and 19 underwent operation because symptoms developed. By univariate Cox regression analysis, many variables on initial study were associated with death, LV dysfunction, or symptoms, including age, LV end-systolic dimension and end-diastolic dimension, fractional shortening, and both rest and exercise EF. The average rates of change of rest EF, fractional shortening, and end-systolic dimension were also associated with death or symptoms by univariate

Cox analysis. When all variables were included in a multivariate Cox analysis, only age, initial end-systolic dimension, and rate of change in end systolic dimension and rest EF during serial studies predicted outcome (Table 6-2). Thus, in addition to indexes of LV function determined on initial evaluation, serial long-term changes in systolic function identify patients likely to develop symptoms and require operation. Patients have a higher risk of symptomatic deterioration if there is progressive change in end-systolic dimension or resting EF during the course of serial studies.

Echocardiography of the Austin-Flint murmur

Rahko[33] in Madison, Wisconsin, investigated the genesis of the Austin-Flint murmur using Doppler and echocardiographic imaging. A total of 51 patients having significant AR and an anatomically normal mitral valve were evaluated. They were divided into two groups; 30 patients had an audible Austin Flint murmur and 21 did not. All patients had a complete M-mode, two-dimensional, and Doppler echocardiographic examination to characterize LV size and function, motion of the mitral valve, transmittal flow velocities, direction of the AR jet, and severity of the AR. There was no significant difference in the severity of AR between groups. There was, however, a significant difference in the direction of the insufficiency jet. In the Austin Flint group compared with the group without the Austin Flint Murmur, for the parasternal long-axis view 24 versus 8 had their AR jet directed at the mitral valve, for the apical 5-chamber view the values were 25 versus 5, and for the apical long-axis view the values were 27 versus 5. There was also a greater frequency of localized anterior mitral leaflet distortion by 2-dimensional echocardiography in patients with Austin-Flint murmur and a greater frequency of Doppler striations overlying the AR jet versus patients without the Austin-Flint Murmur. Regarding transmittal flow velocities, there was no significant difference in filling patterns or absolute velocities during early or late diastole between groups. There was no gradient by Doppler analysis or by hemodynamics

TABLE 6-2. *Multivariate Cox regression analysis of variables on serial studies associated with death or symptoms. Reproduced with permission from Bonow.[32]*

Variable	Initial value	Rate of change
Age	$p<0.05$	. . .
Echocardiogram		
LV end-diastolic dimension	NS	NS
LV end-systolic dimension	$p<0.001$	$p<0.05$
LV fractional shortening	NS	NS
Radionuclide angiogram		
LV EF at rest	NS	$p<0.05$
LV EF during exercise	NS	NS
LV EF response to exercise	NS	NS

LV, left ventricular; EF, ejection fraction; NS, not significant.

across the mitral valve in their group. There also was no difference in the frequency of preclosure of the mitral valve. Systolic function was similar in both groups, but the LV end-diastolic dimension was significantly greater in the Austin Flint Murmur group. This study suggests that the primary factor responsible for the Austin-Flint murmur is the presence of an AR jet directed at the anterior mitral leaflet. This, combined with the biphasic pattern of transmittal flow, distorts the shape of the anterior mitral leaflet as it opens and closes during diastole, making it shudder. The leaflet's shuddering sets up vibrations and shock waves that distort the AR jet, causing the observed Doppler striations and probably the sound of the murmur. There is no evidence from this study to support prior theories that have proposed functional MS or diastolic MR as the source of the murmur.

Mechanisms of left ventricular systolic dysfunction

Starling and colleagues[34] in Ann Arbor, Michigan, tested the hypothesis that the combined use of the time-varying elastance concept and conventional circumferential stress-shortening relations would elucidate differential mechanisms for LV systolic dysfunction with severe, chronic AR and thereby predict the functional response to aortic valve replacement. Thirty-one control patients and 37 patients with aortic regurgitation were studied. The studies included micromanometer LV pressure determinations, biplane contrast cineangiograms under control conditions and radionuclide angiograms under control conditions and during methoxamine or nitroprusside infusions with RA pacing. The patients with AR were classified into three groups: Group I had normal E_{max} and stress-shortening relations; Group II had abnormal E_{max} but normal stress-shortening relations; and Group III had abnormal E_{max} and stress-shortening relations. The LV end-diastolic and end-systolic volumes showed a progressive increase and the EF a progressive decrease from Groups I to III. These values differed from those in control subjects. In Group I, there was a decrease in the LV volumes, but no significant change in LVEF after aortic valve replacement. In contrast, in Group II, reduction in LV volumes was associated with an increase in EF from $50 \pm 8\%$ to $64 \pm 11\%$. Finally, in Group III, reduction in LV volumes was associated with a further decrement in ejection fraction from $35 \pm 13\%$ to $30 \pm 13\%$. Group I patients had compensated adequately for chronic volume overload. However, Group II had LV dysfunction that associated with an increase in LV volume/mass ratio compared with that in control patients and Group I suggesting inadequate hypertrophy and assumption of a spherical geometry. Finally, irreversible myocardial dysfunction had occurred in patients in Group III. Thus, combined analysis of LV chamber performance using the time-varying elastance concept and myocardial performance using conventional circumferential stress-shortening relations provides complementary information that elucidates different mechanisms for LV systolic dysfunction and thereby predicts the functional response to AVR.

Effects of vasodilator therapy

Electrocardiographic abnormalities develop in patients with chronic AR. Although vasodilator drugs may reduce LV volume overload, the effects of such therapy on electrocardiographic abnormalities have not been previously evaluated. Wilson and associates[35] from Portland, Oregon, and San Francisco, California, analyzed electrocardiograms before and after double-blind, randomized administration of either hydralazine or placebo in 54 patients with chronic AR. These patients were without limiting symptoms and had preserved EF on entry in the study. The magnitude of ST-segment depression and Romhilt-Estes point score for LV hypertrophy were assessed. Baseline ST depression and LV hypertrophy scores in the placebo and hydralazine groups were not significantly different. At follow-up, after a mean of 19 ± 6 months, there was a significant reduction in ST depression in patients taking hydralazine (n = 28) compared with patients given placebo (n = 26): −0.023 ± 0.044 vs 0.029 ± 0.055 mV, respectively; and in the LV hypertrophy score (−1.1 ± 2.2 vs 0.9 ± 2.3 points, respectively). Hydralazine-treated patients also had significant decreases in LV end-diastolic and end-systolic volume indexes, and a significant increase in EF. These results suggest that such vasodilator therapy may be beneficial in patients with chronic AR.

INFECTIVE ENDOCARDITIS

Two-dimensional echocardiography

Sanfilippo and associates[36] in Boston, Massachusetts, studied the echo identification of high risk lesions in patients with infectious endocarditis, the medical records and two-dimensional echocardiograms of 204 patients in an attempt to use this information to predict subsequent complications. Specific clinical complications were recorded and vegetations were assessed with respect to predetermined morphologic characteristics. The overall complication rates were roughly equivalent for patients with mitral (53%), aortic (62%), tricuspid (77%) and prosthetic valve (61%) vegetations and for those with nonspecific valvular changes but no discrete vegetations (57%), although the distribution of specific complications varied among these groups. There were fewer complications in patients without discernible valvular abnormalities (27%). In native left-sided valvular endocarditis, vegetation size, extent, mobility and consistency were found to be significant univariate predictors of complications. In multivariate analysis, vegetation size, extent and mobility were the greatest predictors and an echo score based on these factors predicted the occurrence of complications with 70% sensitivity and 92% specificity in mitral valve endocarditis and with 76% sensitivity and 62% specificity in aortic valve endocarditis (Figure 6-4).

Transesophageal echocardiography

Echocardiography is recognized as a method of choice for the noninvasive detection of valvular vegetations in patients with active, infective endocarditis, with transesophageal echocardiography being more accurate than transthoracic echocardiography. The diagnosis of associated abscesses by transthoracic echocardiography is difficult or even impossible in many cases, and it is not known whether transesophageal echocardiography is any better. To determine the value of transesophageal echocardiography in the detection of abscesses associated with active, infective endocarditis, Daniels and associates[37] from Hannover, Germany, and Atlanta, Georgia, studied prospectively by 2-dimensional transthoracic and transesophageal echocardiography 118 consecutive patients with

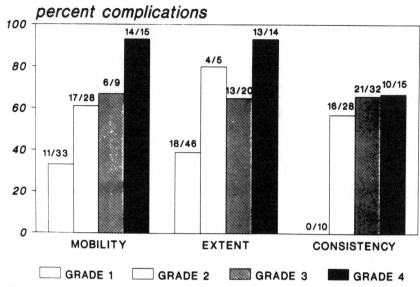

Fig. 6-4. Incidence of complications relative to the degree of morphologic abnormality is illustrated here by vegetation mobility, extent and consistency. The numbers above the bar refer to the absolute number of patients with complications relative to the total in the subgroup. Reprinted with permission from Sanfilippo, et al.[36]

active, infective endocarditis of 137 native or prosthetic valves that was documented during surgery or at autopsy. During surgery or at autopsy, 44 patients (37%) had a total of 46 definite regions of abscess. Abscesses were more frequent in aortic-valve endocarditis than in infections of other valves, and the infecting organism was more often staphyloccoccus (52% of cases) in patients with abscesses than in those without abscesses (16%). The hospital mortality rate was 23% in patients with abscesses, as compared with 13.5% in patients without abscesses. Whereas transthoracic echocardiography identified only 13 of the 46 areas of abscess, the transesophageal approach allowed the detection of 40 regions. Sensitivity and specificity for the detection of abscesses associated with endocarditis were 28 and 99%, respectively, for transthoracic echocardiography and 87 and 95% for transesophageal echocardiography; positive and negative predictive values were 93% and 69%, respectively, for the transthoracic approach and 91% and 92% for the transesophageal approach. Variation between observers was 3.4% for transthoracic and 4.2% for transesophageal echocardiography. The data indicate that transesophageal echocardiography leads to a significant improvement in the diagnosis of abscesses associated with endocarditis. This article was followed by an editorial by Alan S. Pearlman[38] who emphasized that although transesophageal echocardiography is a sound diagnostic technique with important clinical applications that it does not replace transthoracic echocardiography which, in contrast, has no risk.

Shively and colleagues[39] in Albuquerque, New Mexico and San Francisco, California, compared transesophageal and transthoracic echocardiograms in 62 patients and 66 episodes of suspected endocarditis. Echocardiographic results were compared with the presence or absence of endocarditis determined by pathologic or nonechocardiographic data from the subsequent clinical course. All echocardiograms were reviewed blindly. Diagnosis of endocarditis was eventually made in 16 of the 66 episodes of endocarditis. In 7 of the 16 transthoracic and 15 of 16 transesophageal echocardiograms, endocarditis was diagnosed at a probability level of "almost certain" providing sensitivities of 11% and 91%, respectively. In the remaining episodes, 49 of 50 transthoracic and all transesophageal studies provided normal results giving a specificity of 98% and 100%, respectively. Thus, transesophageal echocardiography is highly sensitive and specific for the diagnosis of infective endocarditis and more sensitive than transthoracic echocardiography. The high diagnostic sensitivity of transesophageal echocardiography provides a low probability of the disease when the study yields negative results in a patient with an intermediate likelihood of the disease process.

Prognosis with systemic emboli

To determine whether valvular vegetations visualized on 2-dimensional echocardiography are an independent risk factor for the development of subsequent emboli in patients with active infective endocarditis and to assess the timing of emboli relative to the initiation of antimicrobial therapy, Steckelberg and associates[40] from Rochester, Minnesota, in an investigative blinded, retrospective incidence cohort study studied 207 patients with left-sided native valve infective endocarditis who had 2-dimensional echocardiograms within 72 hours of the beginning of microbial therapy. The crude incidence rate of first embolic events in patients receiving antimicrobial therapy was 6.2 per 1,000 patient-days. The rates in patients with and without vegetations were 7.1 and 4.9 per 1000 patient-days, respectively. The relation between vegetations and risk for emboli was microorganism-dependent: Stratified incidence rate ratios were 6.9 and 1.0 for Viridans streptococcal and Staphylococcus aureus endocarditis, respectively. The rate of first embolic events diminished over time, falling from 13 per 1000 patient-days during the first week of therapy to <1.2/1000 patient-days after completion of the second week of therapy. Overall, the presence of vegetations on echocardiographically visualized vegetations may be microorganism-dependent, with a significantly increased risk seen only in patients with viridans streptococcal infection. The rate of embolic events declines with time after initiation of antimicrobial treatment.

Surgery with septic cerebral emboli

Ting and associates[41] from Chicago, Illinois, and New Brunswick, New Jersey, found cerebral septic emboli in 45 (42%) of 106 patients with active infective endocarditis who underwent valve replacement at their hospital. Of the 45 patients with clinical features typical of cerebral septic emboli, 31 (69%) had symptomatic cerebral septic infarcts and 14 (31%) were asymptomatic. Cerebral tomographic scans preoperatively disclosed ischemic infarcts in 36 patients (80%), hemorrhagic infarcts in 5 (11%), normal studies in 2 patients (4%) and unknown in 2 patients (4%). Neurological complications after valve replacement included strokes in 6 patients, cerebral abscesses in 2 and seizure in 1. The presence of a hemorrhagic infarct preoperatively predisposed to a perioperative stroke. The authors concluded that cerebral septic infarcts, both symptomatic and asymptomatic, are not contraindications to valvular replacement in active infective endocarditis in the absence of a hemorrhagic cerebral infarct.

Surgery with associated heart failure

Middlemost and colleagues[42] in Johannesburg, South Africa, studied 203 consecutive patients selected for early valve replacement at mean of 10 days from time of admission if they had clinical evidence of native valve endocarditis with 1) vegetations on echo, 2) severe valvular lesions, and 3) CHF. Surgery was performed within 7 days of admission in 56% of patients and was done urgently because of hemodynamic deterioration in 108 (53%). All vegetations were identified by echo and confirmed macroscopically at surgery. One hundred ten patients had isolated aortic valve infection, 50 had isolated mitral valve infection, and 43 had double-valve infection. Mean aortic cross-clamp times were 57, 38 and 67 minutes, respectively. Sixty-four patients (32%) had extensive infections involving the anulus or adjacent tissues, or both. Such infections more frequently involved the aortic than the mitral valves. Thirty-eight patients with aortic valve infections had abscess formation compared with one with mitral valve infection. Only eight patients (4%) died in the hospital. There were seven patients (3%) with periprosthetic leaks and five patients (3%) with early prosthetic valve endocarditis. Long-term follow-up data available in 174 hospital survivors (89%) revealed 10 deaths and two new ring leaks at 38 ± 22 months. Therefore, among patients with endocarditis who need surgery for CHF, aortic valve infections are more prevalent than mitral valve infections and are more often associated with extensive infections, including abscess formation. Even the presence of CHF and extensive infection, however, is not necessarily associated with a high risk when surgery is performed early.

Tricuspid valvulectomy

Arbulu and associates[43] from Detroit, Michigan, reviewed their experience since September 1970 in 55 patients who had total excision of the tricuspid valve because of intractable right-sided infective endocarditis. All patients were addicted to heroin. Fifty-three underwent tricuspid valvulectomy without replacement and in addition 2 had pulmonic valve excision (Figure 6-5). Twenty-four patients (49%) returned to their drug addiction. Six patients (11%) required prosthetic heart valve insertion 2 days to 13 years later for medically refractory right-sided heart failure, and 4 of these died. Overall, 16 patients (29%) died, six (11%) within 45 days after the tricuspid valvulectomy. One (2%) of these deaths was related to the operation and 5 were due to uncontrollable infection. Ten (18%) deaths occurred 9 months to 13 years after the tricuspid valvulectomy. Nine were due to drug addiction and 1 to progressive RV failure 2 months after prosthetic heart valve insertion and 10 years after the initial valve removal. Of the 39 patients who are alive, 37 (67%) have not required prosthetic heart valve insertion. From these observations, the authors reached the following conclusions: (1) Drug addiction is a recurrent and lethal disease. Among these patients, tricuspid valvulectomy without replacement is the operation of choice for the management of intractable right-sided endocarditis; (2) after tricuspid valvulectomy without replacement, only 6 of 55 patients (11%) had required prosthetic heart valve insertion to control medically refractory right-sided heart failure; (3) in a small percentage of patients the absence of the tricuspid valve may lead to severe and permanent impairment of RV function.

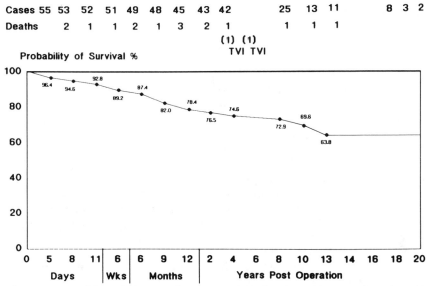

Fig. 6-5. Actuarial survival curve showing survival of patients 20 years after tricuspid valvulectomy without prosthetic replacement. TVI, Tricuspid valve replacement. Reprinted with permission from Arbulu, et al.[43]

VALVE REPAIR OPERATION

Surgical valve repair for MR has significant advantages over MVR, but little is known about the mechanisms of its failure. This echocardiographic study by Marwick and associates[44] from Cleveland, Ohio, examined abnormalities leading to failed mitral valve repair in 2 populations: "immediate failure" of the valve repair in the operating room requiring a second run of cardiopulmonary bypass and "late failure" of valve repair necessitating reoperation on another occasion. Intraoperative echocardiography after cardiopulmonary bypass was performed in 309 patients undergoing valve repair for MR over a 3-year period. Twenty-six (8%) of these patients had immediate failure of the repair demonstrated by intraoperative echocardiography, requiring further repair of MVR during the same thoracotomy. The causes of immediate failure were LV outflow tract obstruction (10 patients), incomplete correction (10 patients), and suture dehiscence (6 patients). Echocardiography was performed on 17 patients requiring reoperation for recurrent MR who had undergone previous primary valve repair. These late failures resulted from progressive degenerative leaflet or chordal disease (n = 9) or suture dehiscence of the annular ring or the leaflet resection site (n = 6). In only 2 patients early in the series did the problem originate from inadequate initial surgery. Intraoperative echocardiography is an effective marker for unsuccessful mitral valve repair, and affords an understanding of the mechanism of the persistent dysfunction. Immediate failure of mitral repair may be reduced by greater attention to the mechanism of valve dysfunction and by changes in valvuloplasty technique to avoid outflow tract obstruction. Late failure after mitral repair occurs predominantly due to progression of disease, particularly in patients with severe myxomatous or annular abnormalities that are prone to progress.

VALVE REPLACEMENT

In the United Kingdom

Taylor[45] from London, UK, reviewed heart valve surgery in UK. Presently about 5,000 artificial valves are implanted each year in the UK in just over 4,500 patients. These totals remained stable in the period 1986–1989, and they were similar to those reported in UK from 1977–1980. These figures contrast considerably to that of CABG in the UK. In the late 1970s, fewer than 4,000 CABG operations were carried out each year, but by 1985 the annual figure had risen to >12,000. Single-valve replacement procedures account for about 90% of all valve operations in the UK, 10% of double-valve replacements, and triple valve replacement operations account for <0.2% of all valve procedures. AVR is the most common procedure, accounting for 60% of procedures with MVR about 40% and only about 1% of valve replacements are tricuspid valve replacements. In 1986 about 54% of artificial valves implanted in the UK were mechanical valves compared to 46% of bioprostheses. Homograph valves accounted for <1% of total implants. In 1987–1988 an increased preference for mechanical valves resulted in a 70% to 30% split between mechanical and bioprosthetic valves. Over the past 4 years single disk valves were the most commonly used mechanical valves. The use of ball valves declined and there was a significant corresponding increase in the use of bileaflet valves. For the year 1989, the figures were 48% single leaflet, 37% bi-leaflet, and 15% ball valves. In the bioprosthetic valve group, the preference for porcine over bovine pericardial valves increased since 1986 when 75% of bioprosthetic valves implanted were porcine. By 1989 the proportion of pericardial valves had fallen to 15%. These data indicate a clear shift in preference in the period 1986–1989 toward the mechanical valve. The average age of patients requiring heart valve surgery continues to increase. It is estimated that 40% of valve surgery patients in the 1990s will be >65 years of age. Conservative valve surgery, particularly in the mitral position, is likely to increase during this decade. Currently, conservative procedures account for about 10% of all mitral valve operations and 0.5% of all aortic procedures. Homograph aortic valve replacements made up around 2% of all aortic valve replacements.

Mechanical prostheses available in the USA

Akins[46] from Boston, Massachusetts, provided a nice review of the various mechanical cardiac valve prostheses available for use in the USA. Only the Starr-Edwards caged silicone rubber ball, Medtronic-Hall, St. Jude Medical, and Omniscience valves remain available in the USA (Figure 6-6). Late follow-up of valve-related complications favors the St. Jude Medical and Medtronic-Hall valves over the other 2 mechanical prostheses (Figure 6-7).

In children

Solymar and colleagues[47] from Riyadh, Saudi Arabia, Gothenburg, Sweden, and Madison, Wisconsin, presented short- and long-term results of prosthetic valve replacement in children. During a 7-year period that

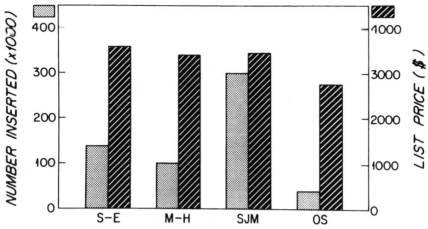

Fig. 6-6. Number of Starr-Edwards (S-E), Medtronic-Hall (M-H), St. Jude Medical (SJM), and Omniscience (OS) valves inserted and their current list prices. Reprinted with permission from Akins, et al.[46]

MECHANICAL VALVE ADVANTAGE

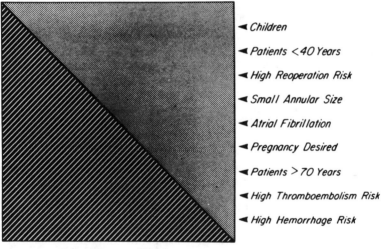

◄ *Children*

◄ *Patients <40 Years*

◄ *High Reoperation Risk*

◄ *Small Annular Size*

◄ *Atrial Fibrillation*

◄ *Pregnancy Desired*

◄ *Patients >70 Years*

◄ *High Thromboembolism Risk*

◄ *High Hemorrhage Risk*

TISSUE VALVE ADVANTAGE

Fig. 6-7. Relative advantage of mechanical valves or tissue valves according to patient-related variables. Reprinted with permission from Akins, et al.[46]

ended in April 1985, 186 children, ages 1 to 20 years, underwent valve replacement; there were 55 (30%) AVRs, 95 (51%) MVRs, and 36 (19%) multiple valve replacements. Ninety-four percent of the lesions were rheumatic in origin, 4% were congenital, and 2% were infectious. Of 223 valves replaced, 175 (78%) were mechanical valves and 48 (22%) were heterografts; the latter were in the mitral position in all but 3 patients. Surgical mortality rates were 3.6%, 4.2%, and 19%, respectively, for AVR, MVR, and multiple valve replacements. Five-year actuarial survival was 91% for AVR, 82% for MVR and 60% for multiple valve replacement. Major events included reoperation in 34 (with 3 deaths), progressive CHF led to death in 10, sudden unexpected death in 2, thromboembolic complications in 19 (death in 5), subacute bacterial endocarditis in 5 (2 deaths), and bleeding that required transfusion in 2 patients. Five-year complication-free actuarial survival rates were 83% for AVR, 63% for MVR, and 57% for multiple valve replacement. The respective 5-year complication-free survival rates were 83%, 48%, and 43%. Significant morbidity and mortality rates are associated with valve replacement. Therefore every effort should be made to preserve the native valve by plastic reparative procedures. When prosthetic replacement of mitral valve is contemplated, these data would suggest that heterografts should not be inserted in children ≤15 years of age with the expectation of valve survival comparable to that of mechanical valves. When complications that are associated with anticoagulant therapy were reviewed, platelet inhibiting drugs seem quite satisfactory in patients with AVR; patients with MVR seem to require warfarin therapy, and warfarin must be used in patients with multiple valve replacement to reduce the risk of thromboembolic complications.

Echocardiography

To compare the hemodynamic results of different anuloplasty techniques of primary valve repair for MR, Unger-Graever and associates[48] from Boston, Massachusetts, prospectively studied 122 patients with Doppler echocardiograms 5 to 10 days after operation. Seventy-seven patients had mitral valve prolapse, 27 had CAD, 13 patients had rheumatic mitral valve lesions and 5 patients had infective endocarditis. Forty-eight patients received the flexible Duran ring, 46 received the more rigid Carpentier ring and 28 patients received no ring. Doppler echocardiography demonstrated a significant decrease in mitral valve area estimated by the pressure half-time method in patients who received either a Carpentier (2.6 ± 0.8 cm^2) or Duran ring (2.8 ± 0.8 cm^2) when compared with patients who received no ring (3.2 ± 0.7 cm^2). No significant differences were observed for peak transmitral diastolic velocity, peak transmitral diastolic gradient, or the grade of mitral regurgitation by color flow Doppler mapping between patients with and without rings. The etiology of mitral disease and concomitant surgical procedures accompanying mitral valve repair did not significantly influence mitral valve area, peak velocity or peak gradient. These data suggest that Carpentier and Duran rings decrease the hemodynamic mitral valve area; however, the decrease in valve area is small and not associated with a clinically important increase in transvalvular gradient.

To study the natural history of the hemodynamic performance of bioprosthetic heart valves, Reimold and associates[49] from Boston, Massachusetts, and Atlanta, Georgia, recorded Doppler echocardiograms in a group of clinically stable patients at 2 and 5 years after replacement of native aortic valves with porcine bioprostheses. Eighteen patients completed a 2-year and 26 patients a 5-year follow-up examination. The effective orifice areas of identical models of bioprosthetic valves (Hancock II) were determined in vitro in a left-sided heart pulse duplicator system. In vivo Doppler-derived effective orifice areas were compared with the in vitro measurements for the same valve size. At both the 2- and 5-year followup examinations, the Doppler-derived effective orifice area was significantly less than the in vitro area. Ten of 16 valves evaluated serially decreased >0.20 cm^2 in the Doppler-derived effective orifice area between studies. The mean decrease in effective orifice area in valves evaluated serially was 0.25 ± 0.29 cm^2. The peak transaortic gradient increased from 21 ± 6 to 27 ± 8 mm Hg. The mean transaortic gradient increased from 12 ± 4 to 15 + 7 mm Hg. It is concluded that serial Doppler echocardiographic studies demonstrate a deterioration in the hemodynamic performance of bioprosthetic valves over time in patients with no symptoms or signs of valvular dysfunction and that Doppler echocardiography may be useful for identifying subclinical bioprosthetic valvular dysfunction.

Transesophageal and transthoracic echocardiography and color flow Doppler were performed in patients with 42 normal and 20 dysfunctioning bioprosthetic mitral and aortic valves in a study carried out by Alam and associates[50] from Detroit, Michigan. Transesophageal echocardiography was superior to the transthoracic approach in delineating bioprosthetic valve cusps and the presence of valve thickening due to valve degeneration. In 27 clinically normal bioprosthetic mitral valves, MR was demonstrated in 3 patients by the transthoracic approach and in 7 by transesophageal study. Both transesophageal and transthoracic color flow Doppler demonstrated MR in 17 clinically regurgitant valves. The severity of MR was accurately assessed by the transesophageal study in all 13 patients who underwent angiography, whereas the transthoracic imaging underestimated MR in 7 of the 13 cases (54%). Bioprosthetic aortic valves were normal on clinical examination in 15 patients and were regurgitant in 3 others. Both transthoracic and transesophageal color flow Doppler were of equal value in observing and quantifying AR. In 5 clinically normal and regurgitant mitral and aortic valves, transesophageal color flow Doppler revealed eccentric regurgitant jets suggestive of paravalvular leak. This feature was not evident by the transthoracic approach. In conclusion, transesophageal echocardiography and color flow Doppler are superior to transthoracic imaging in estimating bioprosthetic MR, but not AR, in differentiating valvular from paravalvular regurgitation, and in demonstrating thickened valves due to cusp degeneration.

To determine the diagnostic accuracy of transesophageal echocardiography in prosthetic valve dysfunction, the pathologic and/or angiographic data from 37 valves were compared with that obtained by transesophageal and transthoracic echocardiography in an investigation performed by Chaudhry and associates[51] from Chicago, Illinois, and San Antonio, Texas. Of the 21 prostheses with severe regurgitation, transesophageal echocardiography identified all 14 mitral, the 5 aortic, and 1 of the 2 tricuspid valves; on the other hand, transthoracic echocardiography identified 2 of the 14 mitral, the 5 aortic, and 1 of the 2 tricuspid valves. Of the 10 prostheses with flail cusp(s), 9 (90%) were correctly identified by transesophageal echocardiography and 4 (40%) were correctly identified by transthoracic echocardiography. All 5 prostheses with paravalvular regurgitation were detected through the esophageal window and 1 detected through the precordial window. Transesophageal echocardiography was unable to document the 2 prosthetic aortic stenoses, whereas the transthoracic examination correctly quantified the gradient in 1 but underestimated it in the other case. Seven patients underwent valve replacement on the basis of the clinical and transesophageal echocardiographic information alone. In assessing cause, origin, and severity of prosthetic MR, transesophageal echocardiography was the method of choice. In selected cases, transesophageal echocardiography can avoid angiography and facilitate optimal timing of reoperation. In suspected aortic and tricuspid dysfunction, transesophageal echocardiography may provide additional morphologic, but limited hemodynamic information.

Low-dose warfarin

Wilson and associates[52] from Kansas City, Kansas, reviewed the charts of 101 patients who received low intensity (a prothrombin time ratio of 1.3 to 1.5 times control) anticoagulation for mechanical prosthetic valves implanted over a 17 year period. The mean duration of follow-up was 4.6 years and the total duration of follow-up was 466 patient years. There were 3 thromboembolic events or 2.9/100 patient years of follow-up at a prothrombin time ratio of less than 1.3, 4 thromboembolic events or 2.5/100 patient-year of follow-up at 1.3 to 1.5 times control, 4 thromboembolic events or 2.2/100 patient-year of follow-up at 1.6 to 2.0 times control, and no thromboembolic events at prothrombin time ratios greater than 2.0 times control. Hemorrhagic events occurred in 3 patients at a prothrombin time ratio of less than 1.3 times control or 2.8/100 patient-year of follow-up, in 6 patients at 1.3 to 1.5 times control or 3.8/100 patient-year of follow-up, in 10 patients at 1.6 to 2.0 times control or 5.5/100 patient-year of follow-up, and in 2 patients at 2.1 to 2.5 times control or 12.2/100 patient-year of follow-up. The rate of hemorrhagic events at 2.5 times control was 470/100 patient-years of follow-up. While not providing definitive proof, the authors believe that our retrospective study provides supportive evidence for the use of low-intensity anticoagulation in patients with mechanical cardiac prostheses.

Pregnancy and delivery with biologic valve

Badduke and associates[53] from Vancouver, Canada, evaluated long-term performance of biological prostheses and course of pregnancy, labor, and delivery in women less than 35 years of age. Between 1975 and 1987, 87 female patients received a porcine (n = 86) or pericardial valve (n = 1); the mean patient age was 27 years, with a range of 8 to 35 years. A total of 17 of these patients experienced 37 pregnancies. A total of 25 babies were delivered, of which 19 were babies of normal birth weight born at term and 6 were born prematurely (2 of these were stillborn). There were 6 spontaneous abortions and 5 therapeutic abortions. The mean time from primary operation to first delivery was 29 months. Of the 17 pregnant patients, 14 were in normal sinus rhythm and 3 were in AF. One of those in fibrillation had a therapeutic abortion while receiving warfarin therapy, and another was successfully delivered of her neonate after 7 months of warfarin therapy. The remaining 15 patients were treated through 35 pregnancies without anticoagulants or antiplatelet agents. Of the total population of 87 patients, 32 (37%) were treated for valve-related complications. Structural valve deterioration occurred in 8 patients (47.1%) of the pregnancy group and 10 patients (14.3%) of the nonpregnancy group. The freedom from structural valve deterioration at 10 years was 23% ± 14% for the pregnancy group and 74% ± 8% for the nonpregnancy group. There were 8 valve-related deaths (1.5%/patient-year). Reoperation was performed in 59% of the pregnancy group and 19% of the nonpregnancy group, primarily for structural valve deterioration manifested as valvular obstruction from aggressive calcification. The freedom from reoperation at 10 years paralleled freedom from structural valve deterioration (20% ± 12% and 64 ± 9% for the pregnancy and nonpregnancy groups. The overall reoperative mortality was 9% (2 patients).

Combined mitral and aortic valve replacement

Bortolotti and associates[54] from Padova, Italy, analyzed the influence of type of prosthesis on the late outcome of patients with combined MVR + AVR by comparing, at a 14-year follow-up, patients receiving 2 biologic prostheses (group 1; n = 135), 2 mechanical prostheses (group 2; n = 221) or a mechanical prosthesis in the aortic position and a bioprosthesis in the mitral position (group 3; n = 97). No difference was found among the 3 groups in terms of actuarial survival and incidence of and freedom from valve-related deaths, thromboemboli, and hemorrhages. Patients with biological prostheses had a significantly greater incidence of structural valve deterioration, reoperations, and overall complications when compared with patients with only mechanical prostheses. The results of an extended follow-up of patients with combined MVR + AVR indicate that mechanical prostheses perform better in the long-term owing to their superior durability when compared with biological valves. The use of bioprostheses should be confined to old patients with limited life expectancy because of their cardiac disease, provided that anticoagulants are not used. Combination of mechanical and biological prostheses in the same patient should be avoided because the advantages of each type of prosthesis are lost.

Left ventricular outflow after mitral replacement

LV outflow obstruction may result from retaining the anterior mitral leaflet when a mitral prosthesis is inserted in the mitral anulus. Waggoner and associates[55] from St. Louis, Missouri, retrospectively reviewed the echocardiograms (2-dimensional Doppler and Doppler color flow imaging, or transesophageal with color flow imaging) obtained in 7 patients with preoperative MR who had a prosthesis implanted with the native mitral leaflets left intact. Systolic anterior motion of the native anterior mitral leaflet, as seen in dynamic LV outflow tract obstruction, was observed in 6 of 7 patients. LV fractional shortening preoperatively was $\leq$0.25 in all (mean 0.20 ± 0.04) and did not significantly increase postoperatively (mean 0.27 ± 0.12). Color flow imaging revealed disturbed systolic flow in the LV outflow tract in 5 patients, and all had systolic anterior motion of the native anterior mitral leaflet. Continuous wave Doppler detected significant systolic LV outflow tract jets in 5 patients averaging 4.1 ± 0.9 m/sec. Mitral prosthetic function was normal (pressure half-time of 81 ± 25 msec and mean gradient of 7 ± 3 mm Hg) in 5 patients. Clinical follow-up revealed that all had died, 6 of them within 2 months of their operation. Thus systolic anterior motion of the native anterior mitral leaflet occurs commonly after prosthetic mitral valve insertion with the native leaflets left intact. Continuous wave Doppler often demonstrates increased systolic LV outflow tract velocities consistent with dynamic LV outflow obstruction. Therefore, the presence of LV outflow obstruction in patients after prosthetic mitral valve insertion with retained native leaflets may result in adverse postoperative course and requires close follow-up.

The Marfan syndrome

Gott and associates[56] from Baltimore, Maryland, reported outcome in 100 consecutive patients with the Marfan syndrome who underwent composite graft repair of the ascending aortic aneurysm between September

1976 and June 1989. Twenty-two patients had ascending aortic dissection at the time of composite graft repair; 18 patients also had a mitral valve procedure. There were no hospital deaths among 92 patients undergoing elective repair. One of 8 patients undergoing emergency repair of a ruptured aneurysm died in the operating room. The overall hospital mortality rate was 1%. There have been 10 late deaths among the 99 hospital survivors (10%). Five deaths occurred among the first 11 patients in this series and 5 occurred among the last 88 patients (6%). Three late deaths resulted from composite graft endocarditis; 3 other patients with endocarditis are alive after aortic root replacement with cryopreserved homografts. Late coronary dehiscence caused death in 1 patient and was successfully repaired in a second. Actuarial survival for the 100 patients was 93% at 5 years and 76% at 10 years (Figure 6-8). Currently, composite graft repair of Marfan type aneurysms of the ascending aorta can be performed with low hospital and late mortality. Marfan aneurysms with a diameter of 6 cm or greater should be repaired with the Bentall composite graft procedure, even if the patient is asymptomatic.

Aortic-"root" replacement

Kouchoukos and associates[57] from St. Louis, Missouri, described results during a 16-year interval ending October, 1990, of aortic root replacement in 168 patients who had 172 aortic root replacements. Thirty patients (18%) had the Marfan syndrome. Annuloaortic ectasia (81 patients) and aortic dissection (63 patients) were the principal indications for operation. Twenty-seven patients (16%) had previous operations on the ascending aorta or aortic valve. The hospital mortality rate was 5% and the duration of cardiopulmonary bypass was the only significant independent predictor of early death. Major modifications in technique were made in 1981, when the inclusion/wrap technique employing a composite graft (used in the first 105 procedures), and in 1988, when aortic allografts and pulmonary autografts were introduced for selected conditions (reoperations, dissection, endocarditis, isolated aortic valve disease) in 16 patients. The mean duration of follow-up was 81 months. Forty-six patients were followed for >10 years. The actuarial survival rate was 61% at 7 years and 48% at 12 years (Figure 6-9). No significant difference in survival rate was observed between the patients with annu-

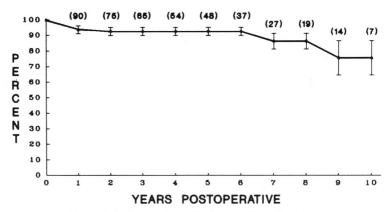

Fig. 6-8. Actuarial survival of 99 patients discharged from the hospital after composite graft repair. Number of patients at risk is shown in parentheses; error bars enclose 70% confidence level. Reprinted with permission from Gott, et al.[56]

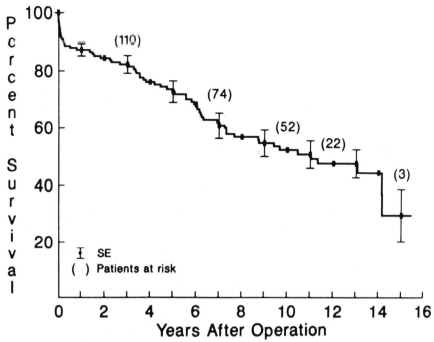

Fig. 6-9. Actuarial survival rates of the 168 patients. The vertical bars enclose the standard error (SE). The numbers in parentheses indicate the number of patients traced at that time. Reprinted with permission from Kouchoukas, et al.[57]

loaortic ectasia and aortic dissection, or between the inclusion/wrap and open techniques. The frequency of pseudoaneurysm formation at suture lines and the frequency of reoperations on the ascending aorta and aortic valve were less with the open technique. The actuarial freedom from thromboembolism for the 153 patients with prosthetic valves was 82% at 12 years. One early and one late death occurred among the 16 patients with allograft or autograft root replacement. Anticoagulant therapy was not used in these patients and no thromboembolic episodes occurred in the follow-up period (mean, 7 months). The satisfactory results observed with extended follow-up support the continued use of the composite graft technique as the preferred method of treatment for patients with annuloaortic ectasia, persistent aneurysms of the sinuses of Valsalva following previous operations, and for patients with ascending aortic dissection who require aortic valve replacement. The availability of aortic root allografts and the perfection of techniques for safe implantation of the autologous pulmonary root into the aortic position have broadened the indications for aortic root replacement.

References

1. Slater J, Gindea AJ, Freedberg RS, Chinitz LA, Tunick PA, Rosenzweig BP, Winer HE, Goldfarb A, Perez JL, Glassman E, Kronzon I: Comparison of cardiac catheterization

and Doppler echocardiography in the decision to operate in aortic and mitral valve disease. J Am Coll Cardiol 1991 (April);17:1026–36.

2. Conway MA, Allis J, Ouwerkerk R, Nhoka T, Rajagopalan B, Radda GK: Lancet 1991 (Oct 1991)338:973–976.

3. Uchida Y, Oshima T, Fujimori Y, Hirose J, Mukai H, Kawashima M: Percutaneous fiber-optic angioscopy of the cardiac valves. Am Heart J 1991 (June);121:1791–1798.

4. Guilherme L, Weidebach W, Kiss MH, Snitcowsky R, and Kalil J: Association of Human Leukocyte Class II Antigens with Rheumatic Fever or Rheumatic Heart Disease in a Brazilian Population. Circulation 1991; (June)83:1995–1998.

5. Fontana ME, Sparks EA, Boudoulas H: Mitral valve prolapse and the mitral valve prolapse syndrome. Current Problems in Cardiology 1991 (May);16:315–375.

6. Wooley CF, Baker PB, Kolibash AJ, Kilman JW, Sparks EA, Boudoulas H: The floppy, myxomatous mitral valve, mitral valve prolapse, and mitral regurgitation. Progress in Cardiovascular Disease (1991); May/June;33:397–433.

7. Sochowski RA, Chan KL, Ascah KJ, Bedard P: Comparison of accuracy of transesophageal versus transthoracic echocardiography for the detection of mitral valve prolapse with ruptured chordae tendineae (flail mitral leaflet). Am J Cardiol 1991 (June 1);67:1251–1255.

8. Jabi H, Burger AJ, Orawiec B, Touchon RC: Late potentials in mitral valve prolapse. Am Heart J 1991 (November);122:1340–1345.

9. Wisenbaugh T, Essop R and Sareli P: Short-term Vasodilator Effect of Captopril in Patients With Severe Mitral Regurgitation Is Parasympathetically Mediated. Circulation 1991 (November);84:2049–2053.

10. Reed D, Abott RD, Smucker ML, and Kaul S: Prediction of Outcome After Mitral Valve Replacement in Patients With Symptomatic Chronic Mitral Regurgitation—The Importance of Left Atrial Size. Circulation 1991 (July);84:23–34.

11. Roberts WC, Eways EA: Clinical and anatomic observations in patients having mitral valve replacement for pure mitral regurgitation and simultaneous tricuspid valve replacement. Am J Cardiol 1991 (Oct 15);68:1107–1111.

12. Meisner JS, Keren G, Pajaro DE, Mani A, Strom JA, Frater RWM, Laniado S, and Yellin EL: Atrial Contribution to Ventricular Filling in Mitral Stenosis. Circulation 1991 (October);84:1469–1480.

13. Kawahara T, Yamagishi M, Seo H, Mitani M, Nakatani S, Beppu S, Nagata S, Miyatake K: Application of Doppler color flow imaging to determine valve area in mitral stenosis. J Am Coll Cardiol 1991;18:85–92.

14. Casale PN, Stewart WJ, Whitlow PL: Percutaneous balloon valvotomy for patients with mitral stenosis: Initial and follow-up results. Am Heart J 1991 (February);121:476–479.

15. Lefèvre T, Bonan R, Serra A, Crépeau J, Dydra I, Petitclerc R, Leclerc Y, Vanderperren O, Waters D. Percutaneous mitral valvuloplasty in surgical high risk patients. J Am Coll Cardiol 1991 (February);17:348–54.

16. Turi ZG, Reyes VP, Raju BS, Raju AR, Kumar DN, Rajagopal P, Sathyanarayana PV, Rao P, Srinath K, Peters P, Connors B, Fromm B, Farkas P, Wynne J: Percutaneous Balloon Versus Surgical Closed Commissurotomy for Mitral Stenosis—A Prospective, Randomized Trial. Circulation 1991; (April)83:1179–1185.

17. Hung JS, Chern MS, Wu JJ, Fu M, Yeh KH, Wu YC, Cherng WJ, Chua S, Lee CB: Short- and long-term results of catheter balloon percutaneous transvenous mitral commissurotomy. Am J Cardiol 1991 (Apr 15);67:854–862.

18. Shrivastava S, Dev V, Ramachandran DM, Vasan S, Das GS, Rajani M: Percutaneous balloon mitral valvuloplasty in juvenile rheumatic mitral stenosis. Am J Cardiol 1991 (Apr 15);67:892–894.

19. Eways EA, Roberts WC: Clinical and anatomic observations in patients having mitral valve replacement for mitral stenosis and simultaneous tricuspid valve replacement. Am J Cardiol 1991 (Nov 15);68:1367–1371.

20. Kennedy KD, Nishimura RA, Holmes Jr. DR, Bailey KR: Natural history of moderate aortic stenosis. J Am Coll Cardiol 1991 (February);17:313–9.

21. Davies SW, Gershlick AH, Balcon R: Progression of valvular aortic stenosis: A long-term retrospective study. Br Heart J 1991 (Jan);12:10–14.

22. Pachulski RT, Weinberg AL, Chan KL: Aortic aneurysm in patients with functionally normal or minimally stenotic bicuspid aortic valve. Am J Cardiol 1991 (Apr 1);67:781–782.

23. Clyne CA, Arrighi JA, Maron BJ, Dilsizian V, Bonow RO, Cannon RO III: Systemic and left ventricular responses to exercise stress in asymptomatic patients with valvular aortic stenosis. Am J Cardiol 1991 (Dec 1);68:1469–1476.

24. Galan A, Zoghbi WA, Quinones MA: Determination of severity of valvular aortic stenosis by Doppler echocardiography and relation of findings to clinical outcome and agreement with hemodynamic measurements determined at cardiac catheterization. Am J Cardiol 1991 (May 1);67:1007–1012.

25. Otto CM, Nishimura RA, Davis KB, Kisslo KB, Bashore TM, Balloon Valvuloplasty Registry Echocardiographers: Doppler echocardiographic findings in adults with severe symptomatic valvular aortic stenosis. Am J Cardiol 1991 (Dec 1);68:1477–1484.

26. Stoddard MF, Arce J, Liddell NE, Peters G, Dillon DS, Kupersmith J: Two-dimensional transesophageal echocardiographic determination of aortic valve area in adults with aortic stenosis. Am Heart J 1991 (November);122:1415–1422.

27. Davidson CJ, Harrison JK, Pieper KS, Harding M, Hermiller JB, Kisslo K, Pierce C, Bashore TM: Determinants of one-year outcome from balloon aortic valvuloplasty. Am J Cardiol 1991 (July 1);68:75–80.

28. Kuntz RE, Tosteson ANA, Berman AD, Goldman L, Gordon PC, Leonard BM, McKay RG, Diver DJ, Safian RD: Predictors of event-free survival after balloon aortic valvuloplasty. N Engl J Med 1991 (July 4);325:17–23.

29. Letac B, Cribier A, Eltchaninoff H, Koning R, Derumeaux G: Evaluation of restenosis after balloon dilatation in adult aortic stenosis by repeat catheterization. Am Heart J 1991 (July);122:55–60.

30. NHLBI Balloon Valvuloplasty Registry Participants: Percutaneous Balloon Aortic Valvuloplasty Acute and 30-Day Follow-up Results in 674 Patients From the NHLBI Balloon Valvuloplasty Registry. Circulation 1991 (December);84:2383–2397.

31. Culliford AT, Galloway AC, Colvin SB, Grossi EA, Baumann FG, Esposito R, Ribakove GH, Spencer FC: Aortic valve replacement for aortic stenosis in persons aged 80 years and over. Am J Cardiol 1991 (June 1);67:1256–1260.

32. Bonow PO, Lakatos E, Maron BJ, Epstein SE: Serial Long-term Assessment of the Natural History of Asymptomatic Patients With Chronic Aortic Regurgitation and Normal Left Ventricular Systolic Function. Circulation 1991 (October);84:1625–1635.

33. Rahko PS: Doppler and Echocardiographic Characteristics of Patients Having an Austin Flint Murmur. Circulation 1991; (June)83:1940–1950.

34. Starling MR, Kirsh MM, Montgomery DG, Gross MD: Mechanisms for left ventricular systolic dysfunction in aortic regurgitation: importance for predicting the functional response to aortic valve replacement. J Am Coll Cardiol 1991 (March);17:887–97.

35. Wilson R, Perlmutter N, Jacobson N, Siemienczuk D, Szlachcic J, Bristow JD, Cheitlin M, Massie B, Greenberg B: Effects of long-term vasodilator therapy on electrocardiographic abnormalities in chronic aortic regurgitation. Am J Cardiol 1991 (Oct 1);68:935–939.

36. Sanfilippo AJ, Picard MH, Newell JB, Rosas E, Davidoff R, Thomas JD, Weyman AE: Echocardiographic assessment of patients with infectious endocarditis: Prediction of risk for complications. J Am Coll Cardiol 1991 (November);18:1191–9.

37. Daniel WG, Mugge A, Martin RP, Lindert O, Hausmann D, Nonnast-Daniel B, Laas J, Lichtlen PR: Improvement in the diagnosis of abscesses associated with endocarditis by transesophageal echocardiography. N Engl J Med 1991 (Mar 21);324:795–800.

38. Pearlman AS: Transesophageal echocardiography—sound diagnostic technique or two-edged sword? N Engl J Med 1991 (Mar 21)324:841–843.

39. Shively BK, Gurule FT, Roldan CA, Leggett JH, Schiller NB: Diagnostic value of transesophageal compared with transthoracic echocardiography in infective endocarditis. J Am Coll Cardiol 1991 (August):18;391–7.

40. Steckelberg JM, Murphy JG, Ballard D, Bailey K, Tajik AJ, Taliercio CP, Giuliani ER, Wilson WR: Emboli in infective endocarditis: The prognostic value of echocardiography. An Intern Med 1991 (Apr 15);114:635–640.

41. Ting W, Silverman N, Levitsky S: Valve replacement in patients with endocarditis and cerebral septic emboli. Ann Thorac Surg 1991 (Jan);51:18–22.

42. Middlemost S, Wisenbaugh T, Meyerowitz C, Teeger S, Essop R, Skoularigis J, Cronje S, Sareli P: A case for early surgery in native left-sided endocarditis complicated by heart failure: Results in 203 patients. J Am Coll Cardiol 1991 (September);18:663–7.

43. Arbulu A, Holmes RJ, Asfaw I: Tricuspid valvulectomy without replacement. J Thorac Cardiovasc Surg 1991 (Dec);102:917–922.

44. Marwick TH, Stewart WJ, Currie PJ, Cosgrove DM: Mechanisms of failure of mitral valve repair: An echocardiographic study. Am Heart J 1991 (July);122:149–156.

45. Taylor KM: Heart valve surgery in the United Kingdom: Present practice and future trends. Br Heart J 1991 (Nov);66:335–336.

46. Akins CW: Mechanical cardiac valvular prostheses. An Thorac Surg 1991 (July);52:161–172.

47. Solymar L, Rao PS, Mardini MK, Fawzy, ME, Guinn G: Prosthetic valves in children and adolescents. Am Heart J 1991 (February);121:557–568.

48. Unger-Graeber B, Lee RT, Sutton MSJ, Plappert M, Collins JJ, Cohn LE: Doppler echocardiographic comparison of the carpentier and duran anuloplasty rings versus no ring after mitral valve repair for mitral regurgitation. Am J Cardiol 1991 (Mar 1);67:517–519.

49. Reimold SC, Yoganathan AP, Sung HW, Cohn LH, Sutton MGS, Lee RT: Doppler echocardiographic study of porcine bioprosthetic heart valves in the aortic valve position in patients without evidence of cardiac dysfunction. Am J Cardiol 1991 (Mar 15);67:611–615.

50. Alam M, Serwin JB, Rosman HS, Polando GA, Sun I, Silverman NA: Transesophageal echocardiographic features of normal and dysfunctioning bioprosthetic valves. Am Heart J 1991 (April);121:1149–1155.

51. Chaudhry FA, Herrera C, DeFrino PF, Mehlman DJ, Zabalgoitia M: Pathologic and angiographic correlations of transesophageal echocardiography in prosthetic heart valve dysfunction. Am Heart J 1991 (October);122:1057–1064.

52. Wilson DB, Dunn MI, Hassanein K: Low-intensity anticoagulation in mechanical cardiac prosthetic valves. Chest 1991 (Dec);100:1553–1557.

53. Badduke BR, Jamieson WRE, Miyagishima RT, Munro AI, Gerein AN, MacNab J, Tyers GFO: Pregnancy and childbearing in a population with biologic valvular prostheses. J Thorac Cardiovasc Surg 1991 (Aug);102:179–186.

54. Bortolotti U, Milano A, Testolin L, Tursi V, Mazzucco A, Gallucci V: Influence of type of prosthesis on late results after combined mitral-aortic valve replacement. An Thorac Surg 1991 (July);52:84–91.

55. Waggoner AD, Perez JE, Barzilai B, Rosenbloom M, Eaton MH, Cox JL: Left ventricular outflow obstruction resulting from insertion of mitral prostheses leaving the native leaflets intact: Adverse clinical outcome in seven patients. Am Heart J 1991 (August);122:483–488.

56. Gott VL, Pyeritz RE, Cameron DE, Greene PS, McKusick VA: Composite graft repair of Marfan aneurysm of the ascending aorta: Results in 100 patients. An Thorac Surg 1991 (July);52:38–45.

57. Kouchoukos NT, Wareing TH, Murphy SF, Perillo JB: Sixteen-year experience with aortic root replacement: Results of 172 operations. An Surg 1991 (Sept);214:308–320.

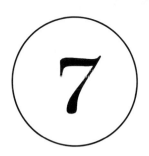

Myocardial Heart Disease

In infants and children

To assess the natural history and potential risk factors in childhood dilated cardiomyopathy, Akagi and associates[1] from Toronto, Canada, investigated 25 patients (ages 9.6 ± 4.4 years) who presented after they were 2 years old. All patients had symptoms of CHF and reduced contractility with a dilated left ventricle at presentation. Two factors at presentation were significantly different between patients who died <1 year after presentation (n = 14) and those who survived >1 years (n = 9); cardiothoracic ratio (65% ± 6.8% vs 57% ± 6.1%) and LVEF (31% ± 7.0% vs 40% ± 6.2%). Irrespective of intensive medical therapy, dilated cardiomyopathy in children had a poor prognosis; the actuarial survival rate was 41% at 1 year and 20% at 3 years. Other forms of therapy should be considered in the early stages of dilated cardiomyopathy in this high-risk group.

Freidman and associates[2] from Houston, Texas, performed a retrospective analysis of 63 children with idiopathic dilated cardiomyopathy to determine prognostic significance of arrhythmias. The mean age at diagnosis was 5 years and overall mortality rate was 16% over a 10 year follow-up period. Persistent CHF and ST-T wave changes correlated with increased mortality but no other variables affected outcome. Arrhythmia were found in 46% of the patients; of the arrhythmias, 48% were atrial arrhythmias. VT was present in 6 patients. Death occurred in 4 of 29 patients with known arrhythmia; 1 of the 5 died suddenly. The remaining 6 deaths occurred in the 34 patients without a documented arrhythmia. The authors conclude that arrhythmias are frequently seen in children with dilated cardiomyopathy but are not predictive of outcome. Sudden death in children is rare and persistent CHF portends a poor prognosis. The question of treatment of rhythm disturbances that are not symptomatic in this patient group remains a difficult one. Many times the treatment options have significant side effects that may be potentially detrimental, including proarrhythmic effects. This continues to be an unanswered problem in this patient group.

Lewis and Chabot[3] from Los Angeles, California, analyzed 81 infants and children with dilated, poorly contracting left ventricles without associated structural abnormalities to identify risk factors for poor outcome, which could be used in selecting candidates for cardiac transplantation. Significant atrial or ventricular dysrhythmias, or both, were detected on presentation or during follow-up in 24 patients. Arrhythmias were present in only 8 of 51 survivors (16%) but were detected in 16 of 30 patients (53%) who died. Patients dying suddenly were even more likely to have had documented dysrhythmias (8 of 11). LV shortening fraction was similar in survivors and non survivors (15 ± 1% vs 15 ± 2%). LV end-diastolic pressure in 44 patients who had cardiac catheterization averaged 21 ± 2 mm Hg. LV end-diastolic pressure was significantly higher in patients who died than in those who survived (29 ± 2 vs 15 ± 2 mm Hg). Analysis of actuarial survival revealed that mortality was highest during the first 6 months after presentation (19% mortality). Survival declined more gradually thereafter and was 70% at 2 years, 64% at 5 years and 52% after 11.5 years. Age at initial presentation did not have any significant impact on survival. However, LV end-diastolic pressure >25 torr was associated with a significantly increased mortality rate. Early cardiac transplantation should be considered in patients with markedly elevated LV end-diastolic pressure or complex atrial or ventricular arrhythmias.

Wiles and associates[4] from Charleston, South Carolina, studied presenting features and long-term outcome of 39 children, age 1 day to 16 years, presenting with idiopathic dilated cardiomyopathy. Four outcome groups were identified: those who died, improved, had resolution, or received transplants. Presenting clinical features of age, sex, race, CHF, cardiomegaly, and degree of systolic ventricular dysfunction did not predict final outcome. LV hypertrophy on the electrocardiogram was present more often in children who improved than in those who died or in whom signs and symptoms resolved. A rhythm disturbance was also seen more often in those who died than in those who survived. Of patients treated medically, 33% died, 42% improved, and 25% resolved. These authors show a lack of dependence on age at presentation on survival. This finding is in agreement with 2 prior studies but in marked contrast to 2 other studies. It remains unclear as to which children presenting with dilated cardiomyopathy have such a low survival rate at 1 year that heart transplantation needs to become an immediate option. There is suggestive evidence in the accompanying article that lack of improvement in clinical and noninvasive assessment at follow-up in 3 to 6 months after initial diagnosis may provide prognostic information in this regard.

Effects of subsequent pregnancy

Pregnancy has been discouraged in patients with peripartum cardiomyopathy to avoid the risk of precipitating recurrent or progressive LV dysfunction. St. John Sutton and associates[5] from Boston, Massachusetts, assessed LV size and contractile function using echocardiography in 4 peripartum cardiomyopathy patients prior to pregnancy, during the third trimester, and a mean of 6 weeks postpartum. LV mean diameters at end-diastole and at end-systole prior to pregnancy (5.2 ± 0.3 and 3.0

± 0.2 cm, respectively) did not change during pregnancy (5.2 ± 0.3 and 3.1 + 0.2 cm). Similarly, LV fractional shortening did not alter significantly during pregnancy or postpartum. Furthermore, no patient developed any symptoms or signs of LV failure. All patients had normal babies, including one who had twins. It was concluded that peripartum cardiomyopathy patients whose LV function returns to normal may undertake further pregnancy with a normal fetal outcome and a low risk of recurrent LV dysfunction.

Electrocardiographic correlates

Pelliccia and associates[6] from Rome, Italy, performed a study to verify whether the electrocardiographic pattern of patients with idiopathic dilated cardiomyopathy might be useful in predicting measurements of LV morphology. A total of 12 electrocardiographic criteria for LV enlargement were evaluated in 67 patients with IDC, aged 14 to 68 years (mean 48), and were correlated to LV wall thickness, volume and mass, as assessed at angiography (all patients) and echocardiography (50 patients). Linear regression analysis showed weak correlations between multiple electrocardiographic criteria and LV wall thickness, volume and mass. Multiple logistic regression analysis showed that total 12-lead QRS amplitude, voltage criteria of Sokolow and Lyon, overshoot and U-wave inversion were the variables significantly related to LV wall thickness, as assessed by angiography and echocardiography. The sum of T/R-wave ratios, the RV_6/RV_5 ratio and the Romhilt-Estes score were predictors of LV end-diastolic volume, as determined by angiography and echocardiography. Total 12-lead QRS amplitude and the sum of T/R-wave ratios were the only independent predictors of LV mass, either angiographically or echocardiographically measured (Figure 7-1). The authors concluded that a single electrocardiographic criterion for prediction of LV morphology in patients with IDC is barely effective. Multiple electrocardiographic criteria should be utilized to better predict LV mass and distinguish reliably between LV wall thickening and dilatation.

Value of programmed ventricular stimulation

To assess the response to programmed ventricular stimulation and the clinical outcome, Brembilla-Perrot and colleagues[7] from Nancy, France, performed a prospective study in 103 patients with idiopathic dilated cardiomyopathy. The protocol used ≤3 extrastimuli delivered at 2 RV sites during sinus rhythm and ventricular pacing at 100 and 150 beats/min and was repeated during infusion of 1 to 4 µg/min of isoproterenol. Sustained monomorphic VT was induced in 8 of 11 patients with spontaneous sustained VT, in none of 35 patients without significant ventricular arrhythmias during Holter monitoring, and in 9 of 56 patients with salvos of VPCs. Isoproterenol infusion facilitated the induction of 2 episodes of sustained VT in patients with spontaneous sustained VT; however, in all but 1 of the remaining patients, induction of ventricular tachyarrhythmias was not impaired. During the follow-up period there were 8 sudden deaths among patients who initially had syncope, inducible sustained VT, or both and 3 episodes of sustained VT in patients who initially had nonsustained VT but inducible sustained VT. Isoproterenol infusion can be used to safely facilitate induction of ventricular tachyarrhythmias in patients with dilated cardiomyopathy. The induction of sustained VT was associated with a poor prognosis.

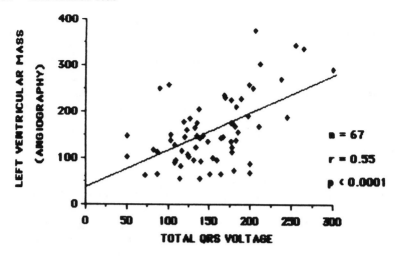

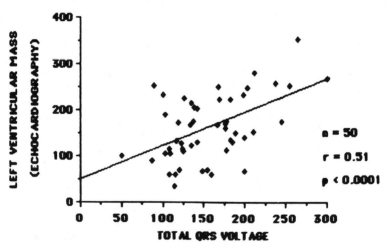

Fig. 7-1. The relation between total 12-lead QRS amplitude and left ventricular mass at assessed wither at angiography (upper level) or at echocardiography (lower panel) in patients with idiopathic dilated cardiomyopathy. Reprinted with permission from Pelliccia, et al.[6]

MYOCARDITIS

Classification

Lieberman and associates[8] in Baltimore, Maryland, analyzed histologic findings and clinical course in the 35 of 348 patients who had endomyocardial biopsies during a 5-year period whose biopsies demonstrated histologic evidence of myocarditis. Analysis of the histologic findings and clinical course of these patients resulted in a new clinical pathologic classification of myocarditis in which 4 distinct subgroups were identified. Patients with fulminant myocarditis become acutely ill after a distinct viral prodrome. They had severe cardiovascular compromise, multiple foci of active myocarditis by histologic study and ventricular dysfunction that either resolved spontaneously or led to their deaths. Patients with acute, chronic active and chronic persistent myocarditis had a less distinct onset of illness. Patients with acute myocarditis presented with established ventricular dysfunction and either responded to immunosuppressive therapy or their condition progressed to dilated cardiomyopathy. Those with chronic active myocarditis initially responded to immunosuppressive therapy, but they had clinical and histologic relapses and developed ventricular dysfunction associated with chronic inflammatory changes, including giant cells on histologic study. Chronic persistent myocarditis was characterized by a persistent histologic infiltrate, often with foci of myocyte necrosis, but without ventricular dysfunction despite other cardiovascular symptoms, including chest pain and palpitations.

Hypersensitivity type

Burke and associates[9] from Washington, D.C., and Mobile, Alabama, studied autopsy tissue specimens of 69 cases of hypersensitivity myocarditis to determine drug association, spectrum of histologic findings, distribution of infiltrates, and correlation between degree of infiltrates and cardiac symptoms. Hypersensitivity myocarditis was defined by the presence of eosinophils, a mixed lympho-histiocytic infiltrate along natural planes of separation, and an absence of fibrosis or granulation tissue in areas of infiltrate. Commonly implicated drugs were methyldopa, hydrochlorothiazide, ampicillin, furosemide, digoxin, tetracycline, aminophylline, phenytoin, benzodiazepines, and tricyclic antidepressants. Histiocytes composed the predominant cell type (in addition to eosinophils and lymphocytes). Lymphocytes were predominantly T cells in 12 cases studied immunohistochemically. Small foci of myocyte necrosis were present in 37 cases, and they correlated with the degree of infiltrate. A nonnecrotizing vasculitis was present in 28 cases. The right ventricle was involved in all but 3 cases. Cardiac arrhythmias or unexplained death occurred in 29 patients and did not correlate with the degree of myocardial infiltrate or presence of necrosis. Eosinophils were present in the livers of 30 of 58 patients, and their presence correlated with the degree of cardiac infiltration. A causative association between histologic findings and drugs is difficult to prove because of the common usage of many of the drugs implicated, multiple drug use, and the absence of clinical criteria of hypersensitivity. Symptoms do not appear related to the degree of infiltrate. In more than half the cases, infiltrates may be missed by endomyocardial biopsy due to focality of lesions.

Immunosuppressive therapy

Chan and associates[10] from Toronto, Canada, used steroid therapy in 13 consecutive infants and children with biopsy-proven myocarditis. The mean age was 5.7 years with a range of 1 to 15 years. CHF was present in all as were ST-T wave changes, cardiomegaly and pulmonary edema on chest roentgenogram. Echocardiography demonstrated pericardial effusion in 5 patients and MR in 8. Mean LVEF was 34%. Prednisone was administered to all patients and one patient also received azathioprine. There was 1 death. All survivors showed clinical improvement with normalization of ECG, heart size and systolic function. No side effects occurred. Repeat biopsy in 8 patients demonstrated improvement in all 8 and elimination of inflammatory infiltrate in 6. In 2 patients signs and symptoms of myocarditis returned after gradual discontinuation of therapy and 1 patient showed persistent inflammation. Reinstitution of therapy improved symptoms; the treatment was continued for another 3 months and discontinued after normal biopsy. These authors show good result in treatment of acute myocarditis in children. Unfortunately there is no control series. A large number of patients in this clinical setting will show spontaneous improvement without therapy. There is a real need for a placebo controlled trial of immunosuppression therapy in children.

HYPERTROPHIC CARDIOMYOPATHY

Genetic analysis

Familial HC, an inherited primary cardiac abnormality characterized by ventricular hypertrophy, is the leading cause of sudden death in the young. Recent application of restriction fragment length polymorphism makers has proved provocative results, with localization to chromosome 18 (Japanese studies), 16 (Italian studies), 14 (US and French-Canadian studies), and two (National Institutes of Health studies) indicating genetic heterogeneity. Interpretation remains speculative until at least one of these loci is confirmed in unrelated pedigrees by independent investigators. Hejtmancik and co-investigators[11] in Houston, Texas, studied eight unrelated families of varied ethnic origins across the United States. DNA from each individual was digested with restriction enzymes TAq1 or BamHI and analyzed by Southern blots followed by hybridization with probes T cell receptor alpha, myosin heavy chain beta, D14S25, and D14S26. Multipoint linkage analysis showed a maximum lod score of 4.3, placing the locus 10 cM from D14S26 between D14S26 and T cell receptor alpha, with an odds ratio of 20,000:1 and 90% confidence limits of 12 cM proximal to D14S25 to 4 cM distal to T cell receptor alpha. The probability of linkage to 14q1 was more than 99%. These results indicate that the loci for familial HC in these families were primarily 14q1 but did not exclude other loci in a small proportion of the families. Thus, 14q1 appears to be the locus for familial HC in a significant proportion of the US population.

The clinical diagnosis of familial HC is usually made on the basis of the physical examination, electrocardiogram, and echocardiogram. Making an accurate diagnosis can be particularly difficult in children, who may not have cardiac hypertrophy until adulthood. Recently, it was demonstrated that mutations in the cardiac myosin heavy-chain genes cause familial HC in some families. In the present report Rosenzweig and associates[12] from Boston, Massachusetts, London, UK, Taichung, Taiwan, and Baltimore, Maryland, reported a diagnostic test for familial HC that relies on the detection of mutations in the B myosin heavy-chain gene in circulating lymphocytes, and they used this test to evaluate 3 generations of a family, including the children. Using the polymerase chain reaction, the authors found that normal and mutant B cardiac myosin heavy-chain genes are transcribed in circulating lymphocytes. This allowed them to examine B cardiac myosin heavy-chain messenger RNA from blood lymphocytes, even though ordinary expression of the gene is virtually restricted to the heart. Base sequences amplified from this messenger RNA were analyzed with a ribonuclease protection assay to identify small deletions, abnormal splicing, or missense mutations. Using this technique the authors identified a novel missense mutation in a patient with familial HC. They evaluated 15 of the patient's adult relatives and found perfect agreement with the clinical diagnosis (8 affected and 7 not affected). Clinical analysis of 14 of the children (age, 1 to 20 years) of these affected family members revealed 1 child with echocardiographic findings diagnostic of familial HC. However, genetic analyses showed that 6 other children had also inherited the missense mutation and might later manifest the disease. Transcripts of B cardiac myosin heavy-chain gene can be detected in blood lymphocytes and used to screen for mutations that cause familial HC. This approach makes practical the identification of mutations responsible for this disorder and may be applicable to other diseases in which direct analysis is difficult because the mutated gene is expressed only in certain tissues. Preclinical or prenatal screening in an affected family will make it possible to study the disease longitudinally and to develop preventive interventions.

With marked hypertrophy of the left ventricular posterior wall

Lewis and Maron[13] in Bethesda, Maryland, and Washington, D.C., studied a subgroup of 17 patients with HC and an unusual and distinctive pattern of LV hypertrophy characterized on echocardiography by marked thickening of the posterior LV free wall and virtually normal or only modestly increased ventricular septal thickness. This distribution of hypertrophy often created a distinctive pattern of "inverted" asymmetry of the posterior wall relative to the septum. The thickness of the posterior wall was 20 to 42 mm (mean 25), whereas that of the basal ventricular septum was only 12 to 24 mm (mean 17). The LV outflow tract was narrowed because of anterior displacement of the mitral valve within the small LV cavity. Systolic anterior motion of the mitral valve was present in 16 of the 17 patients. These patients ranged in age from 13 to 54 years at the time of their evaluation. Most were symptomatic and had experienced important symptoms early in life. The condition of only 4 of these 11 patients improved with medical therapy over an average follow-up period of 9 years. However, 6 of the 7 patients who had unsuccessful medical treatment had MVR (5 patients) or ventricular septal myotomy-myectomy (1 patient) and experienced symptomatic benefit. Thus, a subgroup of patients described in this report identifies the morphologic and clinical diversity that exists within the overall disease spectrum of HC. Characteristically, these patients were young, severely symptomatic, and demonstrated evidence of outflow obstruction and an "inverted" asymmetric pattern of posterior free wall LV hypertrophy.

Mitral valve prolapse with systolic anterior motion

Panza and Maron[14] from Bethesda, Maryland, described the simultaneous occurrence of MVP and systolic anterior motion (SAM) in HC. In 25 patients (aged 7 to 62 years, mean 29), 15 (60%) of whom were male, distal portions of the anterior or posterior mitral leaflets approached or made midsystolic contact with the ventricular septum, whereas the proximal portion of the mitral leaflets showed marked cephalad excursion into the left atrium, 5 to 15 mm beyond the mitral anular plane. Three mitral valves that were available for gross visual inspection were not morphologically typical of patients with primary MVP. Clinical features and natural history (1 to 14 years [mean 6] of follow-up), cardiac dimensions, and distribution of LV hypertrophy defined in the study patients did not appear to differ distinctly from those in the overall referral population of patients with HC evaluated at our institution. Hence, patients with HC may show a striking pattern of mitral valvular motion involving SAM into the LV outflow tract, as well as MVP; this prolapse motion is probably due to anatomic disproportion between the mitral valve and the small LV cavity rather than to the coexistence of 2 separate disease entities.

Adrenergic hypersensitivity after Beta-blocker withdrawal

Withdrawal of B-blocker therapy has been associated with the development of adrenergic hypersensitivity and adverse clinical effects in patients with CAD and systemic hypertension. Gilligan and associates[15] from London, UK, examined the occurrence and clinical significance of adrenergic hypersensitivity after abrupt withdrawal of long-term B blockade in HC. Beta-adrenergic sensitivity was measured using the isoprenaline chronotropic dose$_{25}$. Symptom assessment chronotropic dose$_{25}$ calculation, bicycle exercise, echocardiography and Holter monitoring were performed while the patient received B-blocker therapy and repeated on days 2, 4, 6, 8 (acute withdrawal period) and on day 21 after abrupt withdrawal. The study was terminated after 7 patients had been studied because all patients experienced a marked deterioration in symptoms and several clinical events had occurred. The chronotropic dose$_{25}$ demonstrated B$_1$-adrenergic hypersensitivity with a minimal value of 1.6 $\pm$ 0.8 µg during the acute withdrawal period compared with 3.8 $\pm$ 1.7 µg on day 21. Heart rates during rest and exercise showed an overshoot increase during the acute withdrawal period. The maximal 24-hour ventricular ectopic count was higher during the acute withdrawal period than during the day 21. Of 3 patients with inducible outflow tract gradients, 2 developed resting gradients >30 mm Hg during the acute withdrawal period. There was an increase in peak late filling velocity of mitral inflow after B-blocker withdrawal. In conclusion, transient B-adrenergic hypersensitivity occurs after B-blocker withdrawal in HC and is associated with significant physiologic changes and adverse clinical consequences.

Evaluation after cardiac arrest

Fananapazir and Epstein[16] from Bethesda, Maryland, performed hemodynamic and electrophysiologic studies in 30 survivors of sudden cardiac arrest with HC to determine responsible factors. Electrophysiologic abnormalities alone were present in 27 patients (90%): sinus node dysfunction in 14 (47%), delayed AV nodal conduction in 1 (3%), abnormal His-Purkinje conduction in 7 (23%), an inducible AT in 7 (23%), and inducible sustained ventricular arrhythmia in 21 (70%). Sustained ventricular arrhythmia was polymorphic VT in 18 patients (86%), monomorphic VT in 2 patients (7%) and VF in 1 patient (3%). In 1 patient the arrhythmia recorded during an episode of cardiac arrest and induced at electrophysiologic study was polymorphic VT. VT was induced with 2 extra-stimuli in only 1 patient (3%) but with 3 extra-stimuli in 20 patients (97%). Potential causes of sudden cardiac arrest were found in all patients and were multiple in 13 patients (43%). These were (1) ventricular electrical instability in 21 patients (70%), (2) severe LV outflow tract obstruction in 8 patients (27%), (3) bradycardia in 5 patients (17%), (4) myocardial ischemia associated with hypotension in 5 patients (17%), and (5) atrial tachycardia resulting in hypotension in 4 patients (13%). Of the 21 patients with inducible sustained ventricular arrhythmia, 17 received an implantable defibrillator device and 4 were treated with antiarrhythmic drugs. Seven patients underwent LV septal myectomy. Three patients with atrial tachycardia received antiarrhythmic medication. One patient had catheter ablation of a concealed posteroseptal accessory pathway. Three patients with myocardial ischemia as the only abnormality were treated with verapamil and propranolol (2 also received implantable defibrillators). During a mean follow-up period of 18 ± 19 months (maximum 75), 4 patients died suddenly and 4 patients received a total of 13 defibrillator shocks (1-year survival rate of 93% and a 1-year event-free rate of 80%). Thus, electrophysiologic studies identify potential mechanisms for cardiac arrest in most patients with HC.

Amiodarone therapy

Amiodarone is reported to improve symptoms and to prevent sudden death in patients with HC. Fananapazir and associates[17] from Bethesda, Maryland, administered amiodarone (loading dose 30 g given over 6 weeks; maintenance dose 400 mg/day) to 50 patients with HC in whom the drug was initiated because of symptoms refractory to conventional drug therapy (calcium antagonists and B blockers). Twenty-one (42%) of the patients had VT during Holter monitoring. Amiodarone significantly and often markedly improved the patients' New York Heart Association functional class status (from 3.3 to 2.7 at 2 months and treadmill exercise duration. Eight patients, however, died (7 suddenly) during a mean follow-up period of 2.2 ± 1.8 years. Of the 7 sudden deaths, 6 occurred within 5 months of initiation of treatment. The 6-month and 1- and 2-year survival rates were 87, 85 and 80%, respectively. The survival rate of patients with VT was significantly worse than that of patients without VT (61 vs 97% at 2 years) (Figure 7-2). Sudden death occurred despite abolition of VT on Holter monitoring. Amiodarone increased LV peak filling rate by radionuclide angiography in 20 of 33 patients (61%). Decrease in peak LV filling rate within 10 days of amiodarone therapy (8 of 33 patients) was associated with subsequent sudden death. It is concluded that although amiodarone results in significant functional improvement in most symptomatic patients with HC and reduces VT on ambulatory monitoring, empiric therapy with this potent antiarrhythmic drug may result in a high early incidence of sudden death. Amiodarone may provoke malignant arrhythmias or conduction abnormalities in this subgroup of patients, particularly in patients in whom LV diastolic filling is reduced by the drug.

Fananapazir and Epstein[18] from Bethesda, Maryland, studied the relation of electrophysiologic effects of amiodarone to long-term outcome in 35 patients with HC. Indications for electrophysiologic studies were: cardiac arrest (n = 3), syncope/presyncope (n = 27) and asymptomatic VT (n = 5). Twenty-eight patients (80%) had VT, 3 (9%) AT and 3 (9%) paroxysmal AF during 24-hour Holter monitoring. The studies were repeated after a total amiodarone dose of 58 ± 122 g and during a maintenance median daily dose of 400 mg. Amiodarone abolished paroxysmal atrial arrhythmias in all 6 patients. However, it caused marked atrio-

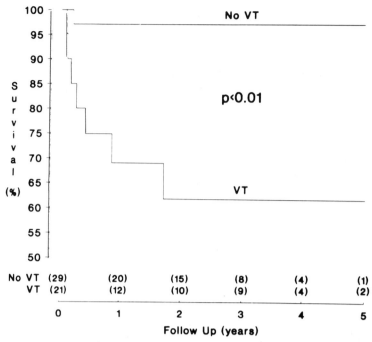

Fig. 7-2. Comparison of product-limit survival rates in patients with hypertrophic cardiomyopathy with and without ventricular tachycardia (VT) during ambulatory Holter monitoring who were treated with amiodarone. Numbers in parentheses are the number of patients remaining at each time interval. Reprinted with permission from Fananapazir, et al.[17]

ventricular nodal conduction abnormality in 3 patients and heart block or marked HV interval prolongation (to ≥100 ms) in 4 patients. Sustained VT was induced in 26 patients (74%) at baseline study and in 23 patients (66%) taking amiodarone therapy. With amiodarone, VT was no longer inducible or was more difficult to induce in 11 patients (31%), and the drug abolished VT during Holter monitoring in all patients (Figure 7-3). However, VT was easier to induce with amiodarone or was induced only with amiodarone in 18 (51%) patients. Amiodarone significantly slowed the rate of induced VT (from 248 ± 29 to 214 ± 37 beats/min). This was associated with a change in its morphology from polymorphic to monomorphic VT in 7 patients. During a follow up of 18 ± 14 months (range 2 to 56), amiodarone was discontinued because of adverse effects in 8 patients (23%). Additionally, 4 of 18 patients in whom amiodarone facilitated induction of VT either died (n = 2) or received appropriate electric shocks from an implanted defibrillator device compared with none of the remaining 17 patients taking amiodarone in whom VT induction was not possible, unchanged or more difficult (1-year event-free rates: 71 vs 100%). All 4 patients had presented with syncope or cardiac arrest. Thus, although amiodarone effectively suppresses atrial arrhythmias and reduces or prevents VT induction in about one-third of patients with HC, it causes important conduction abnormalities in about 20% of patients and facilitates induction of VT in about half of patients. This latter group of patients may be prone to malignant VT and amiodarone, and cannot be identified by Holter recordings. Electrophysiologic studies are there-

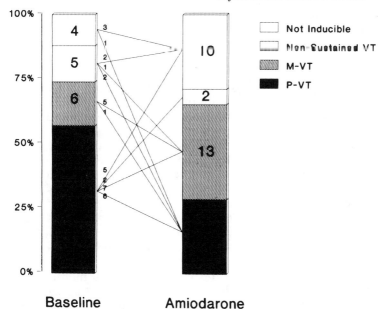

Fig. 7-3. Inducibility of nonstained ventricular tachycardia (VT) and various morphologic types of sustained VT at baseline electrophysiologic study and during amiodarone therapy. M-VT = monomorphic ventricular tachycardia; P-VT = polymorphic ventricular tachycardia. Reprinted with permission from Fananapazir, et al.[18]

fore necessary when initiating amiodarone, because the results identify patients with HC who should receive a pacemaker with the drug, as well as those in whom amiodarone should be discontinued because of serious proarrhythmic effects.

Persistent outflow obstruction after myotomy-myectomy

Roberts and associates[19] from Bethesda, Maryland, compared results of a second LV myotomy and myectomy (M+M) with those of MVR as reoperative procedures for persistent LV outflow obstruction after M+M in HC. Comparison of the second M+M group (n = 12) with the MVR group (n = 11) disclosed significant differences in mean age at the initial operation (29 ± 11 years versus 40 ± 8 years), interval between operations (46 ± 57 months versus 18 ± 13 months), and age at reoperation (33 ± 10 years versus 42 ± 8 years); and insignificant differences in mean preoperative functional class, cardiac index, LV outflow gradients at rest or with provocation, and hospital mortality at reoperation (2/12 versus 1/11). At 6 months after reoperation, comparison of results of a second M+M with MVR showed that mean functional class, cardiac index, and LV outflow gradient at rest were similarly improved, but the outflow gradient with provocation was significantly higher in the second M+M group (57 ± 44 mm Hg versus 14 ± 9 mm Hg). Total follow-up was 108 patient-years (100% complete) with an average of 5.9 years per patient in the second M+M group and 3.4 years per patient in the MVR group. Actuarial survival, including hospital mortality, at 3 and 5 years was 83% and 76%, respectively, after the second M+M, which was similar to 92% and 77% after MVR. Thus, either a second M+M or MVR is effective in relieving the hemodynamic obstruction and decreasing symptoms, but a second M + M is preferable because complications of anticoagulation and substitute valves are avoided.

Aortic regurgitation after myotomy-myectomy

Brown and associates[20] from Bethesda, Maryland, analyzed 525 patients with HC who underwent LV myotomy and myectomy from 1960 to 1990 to determine the frequency of AR post-operatively. Four hundred ninety-six had nonregurgitant tricuspid aortic valves before LV myotomy and myectomy. In 19 (4%) of these patients, AR developed after LV myotomy and myectomy. Age of the 19 patients ranged from 10 to 58 years (mean age, 35 ± 3 years). Seven were male and 12, female. Five patients underwent LV myotomy and myectomy followed immediately by AVR or valvuloplasty. AR developed in 14 patients at a later date. The average New York Heart Association functional class improved from 3.2 ± 0.1 to 1.3 ± 0.1 after operation. The average peak systolic LV outflow tract gradient at rest and with provocation decreased from 65 ± 8 to 14 ± 5 mm Hg and 108 ± 9 to 45 ± 7 mm Hg, respectively, 6 to 8 months after operation. AR occurred in 7 of the 14 patients at ≤6 months after operation, and 3 required operative repair. In the other 7 patients, AR developed 3 years or more after LV myotomy and myectomy, and 3 of them also required operative repair. All 12 patients in whom AR developed at operation or within 6 months post-operatively had either a very small aortic "annulus" (≤21 mm, 5 patients), a low mitral-septal contact lesion (≥35 mm below the aortic "annulus," 3 patients), or both (4 patients). None of the patients in whom AR occurred ≥3 years postoperatively had an aortic "annulus" of ≤21 mm, and only 1 had a low mitral-septal contact point. A small aortic "annulus" or a low mitral-septal contact lesion greatly increased the difficulty of the operation and resulted in increased retraction of the aortic valve and "annulus" (with increased possibility of damage to the valve) to gain exposure to the ventricular septum. The authors recommend in patients with a small aortic annulus, a low mitral-septal contact lesion, or both, that caution be exercised when operating through the aortic valve and that the valve be routinely evaluated post-operatively. If myotomy and myectomy cannot be performed easily in these patients, consideration should be given to using another means of access to the ventricular septum or performing MVR.

ASSOCIATION WITH A CONDITION AFFECTING PRIMARILY A NON-CARDIAC STRUCTURE(S)

Acquired immunodeficiency syndrome

Blanchard and associates[21] in San Diego, California, studied 70 adults who tested positive for human immunodeficiency virus with serial echocardiography to define the prevalence and progression of cardiac disease. Fifty outpatients (Group A) including 44 with acquired immunodeficiency syndrome (AIDS) and 6 with AIDS-related complex and 20 additional patients (Group B) with asymptomatic HIV infection had baseline echocardiographic studies at a time when no patient had symptomatic evidence of heart disease. Follow-up studies were performed at 9 ± 3 months in 52 patients (74%) and again at 15 ± 3 months after baseline studies in 29 patients (41%). During the study, 22 patients (44%) in Group A and 1 patient (5%) in Group B died. Cardiac abnormalities were noted in 26 patients (52%) in Group A and 8 patients (10%) in Group B on initial or follow-up study. An abnormal LVEF (<45%) or fractional shortening (<28%) was seen in seven patients in Group A. Among these, three had normal LV function on a later echocardiogram. One patient in Group B had persistent LV dysfunction. All patients in Group A with LV dysfunction on two serial studies died within 1 year after the initial echocardiogram. LVEF did not change between baseline and two follow-up studies in either group. Right-sided cardiac enlargement resolved in 18 patients, including 5 of 10 in Group A and 3 of 18 in Group B. Pericardial effusions resolved without specific intervention in 5 (42%) of 12 patients in Group A and 2 (50%) of 4 in Group B. Analysis of CD4 counts revealed no relation with the presence of LV dysfunction or RV enlargement. In patients with AIDS with pericardial effusions, CD4 counts were significantly lower (68 ± 74/mm³) than in those without effusion (290 ± 248/mm³). Therefore, echocardiographic abnormalities are common in asymptomatic patients with HIV infection and persistent LV dysfunction identifies an especially poor prognosis in patients with AIDS. In these patients, cardiac abnormalities may be transient in nature and are not consistently associated with clinically apparent intercurrent illness.

Diabetes mellitus

Although several reports have described early changes of cardiac structure and function in diabetic patients, controversy persists regarding the existence of a clinically distinct diabetic cardiomyopathy. To this end, Galderisi and associates[22] of the Framingham Heart Study used sex-specific linear regression analyses to examine the contribution of diabetes mellitus and glucose intolerance to age-adjusted echocardiographic parameters in 1,986 men (mean age 48 years) and in 2,529 women (mean age 50 years) from the original Framingham Study cohort and the Framingham Offspring Study. Subjects with evidence of cardiovascular disease at the time of echocardiogram were excluded. Diabetics had higher heart rates than nondiabetics (68 vs 64 beats/min in men, and 73 vs 68 beats/min in women). Diabetic women had increased LV wall thickness (19 vs 17 mm), relative wall thickness (0.403 vs 0.377), LV end-diastolic dimension (47 vs 46 mm) and LV mass corrected for height (100 vs 82 g/m). Women with glucose intolerance showed similar, less significant trends. In diabetic men, fractional shortening was slightly reduced (0.35 vs 0.36). In a multivariate model that included potentially confounding factors, diabetes remained an independent contributor to LV mass and wall thickness in women. In a separate linear regression model, which assessed the association of age with LV mass, the age-coefficient for diabetic women was much higher than that for nondiabetics (13.6 vs 6.6 g/m per 10-year increment in age). In conclusion, many echocardiographic differences in diabetics are explained by the contributions of other concomitant factors such as obesity, hypertension and smoking, but an independent association of diabetes with LV mass and LV wall thickness is evident in women.

Chagas' disease

Chagas' heart disease is believed to be rare in the USA, although many persons from countries where the disease is endemic reside here. Hagar and Rahimtoola[23] from Los Angeles, California, performed a retrospective case review and prospective follow-up of 25 patients with Chagas' heart disease and no obstructive CAD on angiography. The patients mainly presented with symptomatic AV block, CHF, anginal chest pain, sudden death averted by resuscitation, or sustained VT. Of the 25 patients, 18 had been treated for CAD or idiopathic dilated cardiomyopathy for up to 108 months before the diagnosis of Chagas' disease was considered. The electrocardiograms frequently suggested CAD. Six of the 7 patients who had exercise thallium-perfusion scans had abnormalities suggesting ischemia or infarction. A LV aneurysm was found in 14 of the 25 patients, segmental akinesia or hypokinesia in 5, and diffuse hypokinesia in 3. Programmed ventricular stimulation performed in 13 patients induced sustained VT in 9 and nonsustained VT in 2. Actuarial survival (mean ± SE) after 4 years for the entire group was 56 ± 12%; it was 32 ± 16% among those with global LV dysfunction, and 78 ± 14% among those without such dysfunction (Figure 7-4). Only patients with LV dysfunction or an aneurysm died (4-year survival, 45 ± 14%, as compared with 100% for the remaining patients. Heart failure and LV aneurysm or dysfunction were the only independent predictors of death. Nine patients required permanent pacemakers. In the United States, Chagas' heart disease commonly mimics CAD or idiopathic dilated cardiomyopathy. The prognosis is poor for patients with CHF or LV aneurysm or dysfunction. The disease may be underdiagnosed in the United States.

To date, there is no effective pharmacologic treatment for Chagas' cardioneuropathy, 1 of the most common causes of CHF and sudden death in the world. In an investigation carried out by Iosa and colleagues[24] from Còrdoba, Argentina, Abano Terme, Italy, and Washington, D.C., 58 adults with positive serology for Chagas' disease and abnormal autonomic nervous system tests participated in this placebo-controlled clinical trial with Cronassial (mixed gangliosides), 40 mg daily intramuscular injection

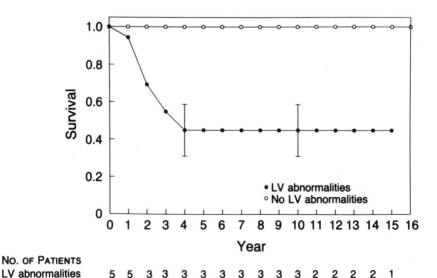

NO. OF PATIENTS

LV abnormalities	5	5	3	3	3	3	3	3	3	3	3	2	2	2	2	1
No LV abnormalities	20	15	11	6	4	2	2	2	2	2	2	2	2	2	2	1	1

Fig. 7-4. Survival of patients in the angiography group who had left ventricular (LV) dysfunction or aneurysm and those who did not. Bars indicate standard error. P = 0.0002 for the comparison between groups after four years. Reprinted with permission from Hagar, et al.[23]

for 4 or 8 weeks. The investigators measured postural response (heart rate, systolic and diastolic arterial BP changes in response to standing); heart rate changes induced by cough and hyperventilation reflex tests; dizziness on standing; number of stress-induced arrhythmias; and periodic acid-Schiff-positive T-lymphocyte percentage in blood samples. Cronassial was safe and significantly improved systolic BP and double product responses to postural stress, hyperventilation heart rate response, frequency of dizziness episodes, number of arrhythmias, and percentage of periodic acid-Schiff-positive T-lymphocyte counts compared with placebo.

Sickle cell anemia

Lewis and colleagues[25] in Washington, D.C., evaluated whether LV diastolic abnormalities are an early feature of cardiac dysfunction in patients with sickle cell anemia. Indices of diastolic filling were obtained with pulsed Doppler echocardiography in 30 consecutive patients with sickle cell anemia who had a mean age of 29 years who had not experienced symptoms of CHF and had normal LVEFs. Data were compared with those from 30 normal control subjects of similar ages. Seventeen of the 30 patients with sickle cell anemia had evidence of abnormal LV diastolic filling. Six of these patients had a Doppler pattern consistent with "restrictive" filling, characterized by reduced early diastolic deceleration time or an increased rate of decline of early flow velocity, or both. Another 11 patients demonstrated a Doppler waveform consistent with impaired LV relaxation. Thus, Doppler echocardiographic analysis demonstrates that LV diastolic filling patterns are altered in patients with sickle cell anemia and these diastolic abnormalities may be present in the absence of symptoms of CHF.

Sarcoidosis

Winters and associates[26] in New York, New York, studied the presentation, cardiac anatomy and utility of programmed ventricular stimulation in 7 patients with sustained VT associated with sarcoidosis. The mean patient age was 38 ± 8 years. Pulmonary involvement was apparent in three patients and no systemic manifestation of sarcoidosis was present in 1 patient. All patients had electrocardiogram abnormalities at rest and 6 had an LVEF <45%. All 7 patients had LV wall motion abnormalities and 5 had mitral valve dysfunction. Sustained VT was easily induced in all patients. Spontaneous sustained VT was not prevented with corticosteroid administration. Despite antiarrhythmic drug therapy, 2 patients had sudden cardiac death and an additional 4 had recurrence of VT. Four patients had an automatic cardioverter-defibrillator implanted and received drug therapy and all 4 received appropriate shocks. Thus, sustained VT may occur in patients with sarcoidosis. Antiarrhythmic drug therapy of VT in patients with this entity is associated with a high rate of arrhythmia recurrence, sudden death, or both. Thus, implantation of an automatic antitachycardia device should be considered as primary therapy in such patients.

Acromegaly

Heart disease frequency occurs in advanced acromegaly. To investigate cardiac mass and function in acromegaly in the absence of obvious cardiac disease, Morvan and associates[27] from Paris, France, performed Doppler echocardiography in 15 asymptomatic acromegalic patients (6 of whom had systemic hypertension). The data were compared with those of a group of 10 age-matched controls. LV mass index was increased in acromegaly (110 ± 32 vs 32 ± 12 g m^{-2}), but shortening fraction and systolic time intervals did not differ. Mitral EF slope was decreased (80 ± 21 vs 101 ± 30 mms^{-1}), while the duration of the isovolumic relaxation period was increased (92 ± 13 vs 69 ± 16 ms). Hypertensive acromegalic patients (n = 6) had a higher LV mass index than normotensive acromegalic patients (n = 9) (133 ± 27 vs 94 ± m^{-2}) and this was confirmed by a meta-analysis of data in previous publications. The prevalence of hypertrophy was 76% in the presence of hypertension vs 50% in its absence. Isovolumic relaxation period was prolonged in normotensive acromegalic patients vs normal controls (90 ± 11 vs 69 ± 16 ms). In conclusion, subclinical cardiac abnormalities occur frequently in acromegaly in the absence of obvious heart disease, and hypertrophy is observed in asymptomatic hypertensive acromegaly.

Muscular dystrophy (Duchenne)

This study by Yotsukura and associates[28] from Tokyo, Japan, describes the late potentials obtained by signal-averaged electrocardiography in 66 patients with Duchenne's progressive muscular dystrophy. It also assesses the possible relations between late potentials and the severity of Duchenne's muscular dystrophy, and the findings of 2-dimensional echocardiography, as well as ventricular arrhythmias examined with the Holter system. The total wall motion index was significantly more abnormal in the patients with late potentials than in those without late potentials. The incidence of late potentials was found to be higher in the dilated cardiomyopathy type (8 of 12) than in the normal type (9 of 41; 22%). The incidence of VPCs was significantly higher in patients with late potentials (13 of 21; 62%) than in those without late potentials (13 of 45; 29%). No sustained VT was observed, although nonsustained VT was noted in 3 patients with late potentials. The late potentials in patients with Duchenne's muscular dystrophy were thus associated with LV dysfunction, and the presence of late potentials might be correlated with the extent of myocardial derangement in Duchenne's muscular dystrophy.

Myotonic dystrophy

To determine the prevalence of ventricular late potentials, as determined by signal-averaged electrocardiography, in patients with myotonic dystrophy, Milner and associates[29] from Washington, D.C., performed a cross-sectional, with blinded analysis of all electrocardiographic data, in 24 patients with myotonic dystrophy. Patients were excluded from the study if they had either a history suggestive of significant ventricular arrhythmias or electrocardiographic evidence of a BBB. Two comparison groups were also formed; 1 group included 44 healthy employees at the tertiary hospital and the other, 30 cardiac patients with inducible VT. A time-domain analysis of the signal-averaged electrocardiograms showed that 75% of patients with myotonic dystrophy met 1 criterion for the presence of late potentials, 67% met 2 criteria, and 29% met all 3 criteria. Spectrotemporal mapping in these patients showed markedly abnormal spectral peaks with a mean factor of normality that was significantly lower than that of the normal volunteers; the frequency of electrocardiographic abnormalities approached that seen in patients with known VT. The presence of late potentials correlated directly with the length of the PR interval and inversely with LV fractional shortening. In the study, the prevalence of late potentials on signal-averaged electrocardiography in patients with myotonic dystrophy approached that seen in cardiac patients with inducible VT. It is possible that ventricular arrhythmias play a role in the occurrence of sudden death in some patients with myotonic dystrophy.

MISCELLANEOUS TOPICS

Cardiac "toxicity" late after anthracycline or doxorubicin therapy

To assess the cardiac status of long-term survivors of pediatric malignancies who received chemotherapy, including anthracyclines, Steinherz and associates[30] from New York, New York, evaluated 201 patients who had received a total anthracycline dose of 200–1275 mg/m² (median = 450 mg/m²) and 51 patients having mediastinal radiotherapy by echocardiogram from 4–20 years (median 7) after completion of anthracycline therapy. The overall incidence and severity of abnormal systolic cardiac function were determined for the entire cohort. Twenty-three percent (47 of 201 patients) of the cohort had abnormal cardiac function on noninvasive testing at long-term follow-up. Correlation between total cumulative dose, length of follow-up, and mediastinal irradiation with incidence of abnormalities was significant. Fifty-six patients were followed up for 10 years or more (median, 12 years), with a median anthracycline dose of 495 mg/m². Thirty-eight percent (21/56) of these patients, compared with 18% (26/145) of patients evaluated after less than 10 years, had abnormal findings. Sixty-three percent of patients followed up for 10 years or more after receiving 500 mg/m² or more of anthracyclines had abnormal findings. Nine of 201 patients had late symptoms, including cardiac failure and dysrhythmia, and 3 patients died suddenly. Microscopic examination of the myocardium on biopsy and autopsy revealed fibrosis. The 23% incidence of late cardiac abnormalities warrants continued evaluation of patients after anthracyclines to guide patient care and the design of future chemotherapeutic protocols.

Lipshultz and associates[31] from Boston, Massachusetts, assessed the cardiac status of 115 children who had been treated for acute lymphoblastic leukemia with doxorubicin 1 to 15 years earlier in whom the disease was in continuous remission. Eighteen patients received 1 dose of doxorubicin (45 mg/m²/BSA), and 97 received multiple doses totaling 228 to 550 mg/m² (median, 360). The median interval between the end of treatment and the cardiac evaluation was 6.4 years. Our evaluation consisted of a history, 24-hour ambulatory electrocardiographic recording, exercise testing, and echocardiography. Fifty-seven percent of the patients had abnormalities of LV afterload (measured as end-systolic wall stress) or contractility (measured as the stress-velocity index). The cumulative dose of doxorubicin was the most significant predictor of abnormal cardiac function. Seventeen percent of patients who received one dose of doxorubicin had slightly elevated age-adjusted afterload, and none had decreased contractility. In contrast, 65% of patients who received at least 228 mg of doxorubicin per square meter had increased afterload (59% of patients), decreased contractility (23%), or both. Increased afterload was due to reduced ventricular wall thickness, not to hypertension or ventricular dilatation. In multivariate analyses restricted to patients who received at least 228 mg of doxorubicin/m², the only significant predictive factors were a highly cumulative dose, which predicted decreased contractility, and an age of less than 4 years at treatment, which predicted increased afterload. Afterload increased progressively in 24 of 34 patients evaluated serially (71%). Reported symptoms correlated poorly with indexes of exercise tolerance or ventricular function. Eleven patients had CAD within 1 year of treatment with doxorubicin; 5 of them had recurrent CHF 3.7 to 10.3 years after completing doxorubicin treatment, and 2 required heart transplantation. No patient had late CHF as a new event. Doxorubicin therapy in childhood impairs myocardial growth in a dose-related fashion and results in a progressive increase in LV afterload, sometimes accompanied by reduced contractility. The authors hypothesized that the loss of myocytes during doxorubicin therapy in childhood might result in inadequate LV mass and clinically important heart disease in later years.

References

1. Akagi T, Benson LN, Lightfoot NE, Chin K, Wilson G, Freedom RM: Natural history of dilated cardiomyopathy in children. Am Heart J 1991 (May);121:1502–1506.
2. Friedman RA, Moak JP, Garson A Jr: Clinical Course of Idiopathic Dilated Cardiomyopathy in Children. J Am Coll Cardiol (July) 1991;18:152–157.
3. Lewis AB, Chabot M: Outcome of infants and children with dilated cardiomyopathy. Am J Cardiol 1991 (Aug 1);68:365–369.
4. Wiles HB, McArthur PD, Taylor AB, Gillette PC, Fyfe DA, Matthews JP, Shelton LW: Prognostic Features of Children with Idiopathic Dilated Cardiomyopathy. Am J Cardiol (November 15) 1991;68:1372–1376.
5. St. John Sutton M, Cole P, Plappert M, Saltzman D, Goldhaber S: Effects of subsequent pregnancy on left ventricular function in peripartum cardiomyopathy. Am Heart J 1991 (June);121:1776–1778.
6. Pelliccia F, Critelli G, Cianfrocca C, Nigri A, Reale A: Electrocardiographic correlates with left ventricular morphology in idiopathic dilated cardiomyopathy. Am J Cardiol 1991 (Sept 1);68:642–647.
7. Brembilla-Perrot B, Donetti J, Terrier de la Chaise A, Sadoul N, Aliot E, Juilliere Y: Diagnostic value of ventricular stimulation in patients with idiopathic dilated cardiomyopathy. Am Heart J 1991 (April);121:1124–1131.
8. Lieberman EB, Hutchins GM, Herskowitz A, Rose NR, Baughman KL: Clinicopathologic description of myocarditis. J Am Coll Cardiol 1991 (December);18:1617–26.
9. Burke AP, Saenger J, Mullick F, Virmani R: Hypersensitivity myocarditis. Arch Pathol Lab Med 1991 (Aug);115:764–769.
10. Chan KY, Iwahara M, Benson LN, Wilson GJ, Freedom RM: Immunosuppressive Therapy in the Management of Acute Myocarditis in Children: A Clinical Trial. J Am Coll Cardiol (February) 1991;17:458–460.
11. Hejtmancik JF, Brink PA, Towbin J, Hill R, Brink L, Tapscott T, Trakhtenbroit A, Roberts R: Localization of Gene for Familial Hypertrophic Cardiomyopathy to Chromosome 14q1 in A Diverse US Population. Circulation 1991; (May) 83:1592–1597.
12. Rosenzweig A, Watkins H, Hwang DS, Miri M, McKenna W, Traill TA, Seidman JG, Seidman CE: Preclinical diagnosis of familial hypertrophic cardiomyopathy by genetic analysis of blood lymphocytes. N Engl J Med 1991 (Dec 19);325:1753–1760.

13. Lewis JF, Maron BJ: Hypertrophic cardiomyopathy characterized by marked hypertrophy of the posterior left ventricular free wall: Significance and clinical implications. J Am Coll Cardiol 1991 (August);18:421–8

14. Panza JA, Maron BJ: Simultaneous occurrence of mitral valve prolapse and systolic anterior motion in hypertrophic cardiomyopathy. Am J Cardiol 1991 (Feb 15);67:404–410.

15. Gilligan DM, Chan WL, Stewart R, Oakley CM, Krikler S, Joshi J: Adrenergic hypersensitivity after beta-blocker withdrawal in hypertrophic cardiomyopathy. Am J Cardiol 1991 (Sept 15);68:766–772.

16. Fananapazir L, Epstein S: Hemodynamic and electrophysiologic evaluation of patients with hypertrophic cardiomyopathy surviving cardiac arrest. Am J Cardiol 1991 (Feb 1);67:280–287.

17. Fananapazir L, Leon MB, Bonow RO, Tracy CM, Cannon RO III, Epstein SE: Sudden death during empiric amiodarone therapy in symptomatic hypertrophic cardiomyopathy. Am J Cardiol 1991 (Jan 15);67:169–174.

18. Fananapazir L, Epstein SE: Value of electrophysiologic studies in hypertrophic cardiomyopathy treated with amiodarone. Am J Cardiol 1991 (Jan 15);67:175–182.

19. Roberts CS, McIntosh CL, Brown PS Jr, Cannon RO III, Gertz SD, Clark RE: Reoperation for persistent outflow obstruction in hypertrophic cardiomyopathy. Ann Thorac Surg 1991 (Mar);51:455–460.

20. Brown PS Jr, Roberts CS, McIntosh CL, Clark RE: Aortic regurgitation after left ventricular myotomy and myectomy. Ann Thorac Surg 1991 (Apr);51:585–592.

21. Blanchard DG, Hagenhoff C, Chow LC, McCann HA, Dittrich HC: Reversibility of cardiac abnormalities in human immunodeficiency virus (HIV)-infected individuals: A serial echocardiographic study. J Am Coll Cardiol 1991 (May);17:1270–6.

22. Galderisi M, Anderson KM, Wilson PWF, Levy D: Echocardiographic evidence for the existence of a distinct diabetic cardiomyopathy (The Framingham Heart Study). Am J Cardiol 1991 (July 1);68:85–89.

23. Hagar JM, Rahimtoola SH: Chagas' heart disease in the United States. N Engl J Med 1991 (Sept 12);325:763–768.

24. Iosa D, Massari DC, Dorsey FC. Chagas' cardioneuropathy: Effect of ganglioside treatment in chronic dysautonomic patients—A randomized, double-blind, parallel, placebo-controlled study. Am Heart J 1991 (September);122:775–785.

25. Lewis JF, Maron BJ, Castro O, Moosa YA: Left ventricular diastolic filling abnormalities identified by Doppler echocardiography in asymptomatic patients with sickle cell anemia. J Am Coll Cardiol 1991;17:1473–8.

26. Winters SL, Cohen M, Greenberg S, Stein B, Curwin J, Pe E, Gomes JA: Sustained ventricular tachycardia associated with sarcoidosis: Assessment of the underlying cardiac anatomy and the prospective utility of programmed ventricular stimulation, drug therapy and an implantable antitachycardia device. J Am Coll Cardiol 1991 (October);18:937–43.

27. Morvan D, Komajda M, Grimaldi A, Turpin G, Grosgogeat Y: Cardiac hypertrophy and function in asymptomatic acromegaly. European Heart Journal 1991 (June);12:666–672.

28. Yotsukura M, Ishizuka T, Shimada T, Ishikawa K: Late potentials in progressive muscular dystrophy of the Duchenne type. Am Heart J 1991 (April);121:1137–1142.

29. Milner MR, Hawley RJ, Jachim M, Lindsay J Jr, Fletcher RD: Ventricular late potentials in myotonic dystrophy. An Intern Med 1991 (Oct 15);115:607–613.

30. Steinherz LJ, Steinherz PG, Tan CTC, Heller G, Murphy L: Cardiac toxicity 4 to 20 years after completing anthracycline therapy. JAMA 1991 (Sept 25);266:1672–1677.

31. Lipshultz SE, Colan SD, Gelber RD, Perez-Atayde AR, Sallan SE, Sanders SP: Late cardiac effect of doxorubicin therapy for acute lymphoblastic leukemia in childhood. N Engl J Med 1991 (Mar 21);324:808–815.

8

Congenital
Heart Disease

ATRIAL SEPTAL DEFECT

Cardiorespiratory exercise capacity

To study the influence of age at the time of the operation on long-term functional performance in children undergoing surgery for ASD of the secundum type, exercise tolerance was assessed in 24 patients and values were compared with those of normal individuals in an investigation performed by Reybrouck and associates[1] from Leuven, Belgium. Patients were divided into 2 groups: 11 patients had surgery <age of 5 years (group 1) and 13 patients had surgery at a later age (group 2). There were no significant differences between groups 1 and 2 with regard to the pulmonary-to-systemic flow ratio, PA pressure, and the interval between surgery and exercise testing. Performance capacity was assessed by determination of the ventilatory threshold during submaximal exercise. The mean value for the ventilatory threshold in group 1 was normal (99 ± 15% of the age-predicted normal value). In the children who were >5 years of age at the time of the operation, the ventilatory threshold was below normal (85 ± 11% of the age-predicted normal value). Furthermore, in group 2 more patients (77%) had values that were below normal compared with group 1 (27%). It was concluded that functional performance capacity is better when surgical closure of ASD is performed in early childhood and <age of 5 years rather than at a later age.

ATRIOVENTRICULAR CANAL

Prenatal diagnosis

Fourteen fetuses with A-V canal malformations were examined by 2-dimensional echocardiography, pulsed-wave Doppler echocardiography, and color Doppler flow mapping, in a study performed by Gembruch and associates[2] from Bonn, Germany. Eleven fetuses had complete and 3 fetuses had partial A-V canal malformations. Nonimmune hydrops fetalis was associated with 6 cases, and fetal arrhythmia was seen in 3 cases. With 2-dimensional echocardiography, the A-V canal malformations could be diagnosed accurately. The inclusion of color Doppler flow mapping, however, provided additional hemodynamic information that was important from the prognostic point of view. Incompetence of A-V valves could be demonstrated in 10 of 14 cases by Doppler echocardiography. In 9 cases, detailed Doppler echocardiographic evaluation of the regurgitation jet was possible. The proportion of systolic time during which A-V valve insufficiency was demonstrated was related to the occurrence of nonimmune hydrops fetalis. When insufficiency of A-V valves was associated with hydrops (4 cases), a pansystolic insufficiency was always present. In cases without hydrops (5), regurgitation was confined to early systole. Thus a reliable method for semiquantitative evaluation of the degree of insufficiency seems to have been found. Moreoever, an association appeared to exist between the occurrence of hydrops fetalis and the proportion of atrial area that was taken up by regurgitant jet area, as determined by planimetry in the 4-chamber view. Prenatal diagnosis was confirmed by autopsy or neonatal cardiac evaluation. Only 1 neonate survived. Two were stillborn, 4 died during the neonatal period, 2 died during infancy, and pregnancy was electively terminated prematurely in 5 cases. Eight fetuses were found to have a karyotypic abnormality.

VENTRICULAR SEPTAL DEFECT

Relation of symptoms to defect size

Kimball and associates[3] from Cincinnati, Ohio, studied 42 infants with VSD to determine if symptoms of CHF were due to depressed contractility or defect size or both. Echocardiographic indexes of defect size, LV performance, preload, afterload, and contractility were measured in 21 symptomatic and 21 asymptomatic patients and compared with 17 control infants. Although there was no significant difference in age, the symptomatic group had lower weight and a higher respiratory rate compared with control subjects. The mean pulmonary to systemic flow ratio in the symptomatic group was 2.9. Preload indexed for body surface area was significantly higher in the group with VSD compared with control subjects but shortening fraction, afterload and contractility were not significantly different among all groups. Defect size $>.5$ cm or >1.8 cm/m^2 was predictive of the presence of symptoms. These authors conclude that contractility is normal in infants with a VSD and symptoms probably related to pulmonary overcirculation.

Effect of digoxin in infancy

Kimball and associates[4] from Cincinnati, Ohio, studied the effect of digoxin on 19 infants with CHF and large VSD. Infants were studied before medication, while on chronic diuretics, while on both diuretics and digoxin, and while on diuretics alone, to determine if digoxin increases contractility and improves symptoms. Symptoms, heart rate, respiratory rate, weight gain, shortening fraction, LV end-diastolic dimension, LV end-systolic wall stress and contractility were measured at each period. The difference between measured and predicted velocities of circumferential fiber shortening for measured wall stress served as an index of contractility. Eighteen patients also underwent catheterization and mean pulmonary-to-systemic blood flow ratio was 3:1. When digoxin was added to diuretics, contractility index was significantly > in controls. Symptoms and signs were not significantly improved by either diuretics or digoxin. This study showed that infants with large VSD prior to therapy had contractility indices that were normal to slightly above normal. Although the contractility index in VSD patients with diuretics and digoxin was > controls, it was not > VSD patients on no medication. These authors thus question the value of digoxin in infants with symptoms due to large VSD and suggest that afterload reducing agents may deserve further consideration for medical treatment in this patient group.

Surgery of the supracristal defect

Backer and associates[5] from Chicago, Illinois, reviewed data on 36 children with conal VSD who underwent intracardiac repair. Preoperative evaluation showed that 72% of patients had aortic valve prolapse and 44% had AR. Pulmonary to systemic flow ratios ranged from 1.1 to 3.5. Only 10 patients were believed to have clinical CHF. Age at the time of operation ranged from 2 weeks to 18 years. Operative exposure was through the pulmonary artery in 26, aorta in 4, right ventricle in 3, or right atrium in 3. Simultaneous aortic valve suspensions for AR was performed in 4 patients. There were no deaths and follow-up from .5 to 9 years was available in all patients. There were no residual VSDs and 64% had no evidence of AR. Thirty-three percent had trivial or mild AR. One patient with initial severe AR underwent repeat aortic valvuloplasty 3 years later. No patients required aortic valve replacement. The authors believe that the operative approach should be through the pulmonary artery and that conal VSDs should undergo early closure regardless of shunt volumes to prevent progressive aortic valve prolapse and AR. It is unclear that all patients with small conal VSDs need this approach since a number of them may continue to have small shunts without AR. Further data regarding patients with small conal VSDs with long-term follow-up will be necessary to determine the optimal management for such patients.

PULMONIC VALVE STENOSIS

Balloon valvuloplasty

McCrindle and Kan[6] from Baltimore, Maryland, reported follow-up data of 46 patients with a mean age of 5 years who had balloon pulmonary valvuloplasty at one institution and had a followup for an average of 5 years. Mean systolic gradient from right ventricle to PA before procedure was 70 ± 36 mmHg, immediately after procedure 23 ± 14 mmHg, at intermediate follow-up at <2 years after procedure 23 ± 16 mmHg and at long-term followup by Doppler at more than 2 years after valvuloplasty 20 ± 13 mmHg. Valvuloplasty acutely reduced the gradient to <36 mmHg for 89% of patients. A patient age of <2 years at the initial procedure, as well as a higher initial gradient were risk factors for gradients over 36 mmHg at followup. Six patients had significant gradients at intermediate followup and 3 of 6 had successful repeat valvuloplasty. These authors also presented effective use of this procedure in 4 of 5 patients with Noonan's syndrome and varying degrees of pulmonary valve dysplasia.

TETRALOGY OF FALLOT

Repair in neonates

Di Donato and associates[7] from Boston, Massachusetts, reported results for 27 neonates with symptomatic TF or TF with valvar pulmonary atresia who underwent repair. Mean age at repair was 8 ± 8 days and mean weight was 3 ± .7 kg. Unsatisfactory shunts had been placed elsewhere in 4 patients. There were 25 transannular patches and 2 conduits used. There were 5 hospital deaths and all deaths occurred with the pulmonary artery (Nakata) index <150 mm^2/m^2. Actuarial survival at 5 years was 74%. There was a single rapidly declining hazard phase for death with the hazard approaching 0 at 1½ years after repair. Actuarial freedom from reoperation was 76% at 5 years. Postoperative catheterization of 15 survivors showed RV pressure <70% systemic in 13 patients. All patients are symptomatically well and in sinus rhythm 1 to 15 years (mean 5 years) after repair. These authors show good results for repair of the neonate with severe tetralogy. At present they do not support neonatal repair of asymptomatic patients. Most infants with tetralogy do not become symptomatic before 3 months of age and repair is probably best performed in the 3 to 18 month age range.

PULMONIC VALVE ATRESIA

Survival

Hofbeck and associates[8] from Toronto, Canada, studied the clinical course of 104 consecutive patients with pulmonary valve atresia and VSD who were diagnosed in the first year of life and followed for a mean period of 5 years with a range of 2 days to 14 years. Confluent pulmonary arteries supplied by a single PDA were present in 69%, whereas 31% had a pulmonary blood supply that was partially or exclusively dependent on systemic collateral arteries. An estimate of the probability of survival at 10 years was 69% of the entire cohort with no differences between groups. Definitive repair was performed in 46% of patients with PDA and confluent pulmonary arteries, compared with 16% in patients with pulmonary flow dependent on collateral arteries. Arborization and distribution abnormalities of the pulmonary arteries, as well as intrapulmonary stenoses that were exclusively present in patients with systemic collateral arteries accounted for the significantly lower probability of undergoing reparative operation in the latter patient group. These authors show much improved survival for this group than has previously been reported in the era prior to the use of prostaglandins. Of interest is the identical survival, at least during the first 5 years, for patients in these disparate groups. One would predict that with late follow-up the group with multiple systemic collateral arteries who could not have reparative operation will not do as well. These data are valuable in presenting some prognostic information for parents and patients. The outlook is obviously better than for patients with pulmonary atresia and intact ventricular septum who have been shown to have a 34% probability of survival at 10 years, as well as patients with tricuspid atresia who show a 55% survival at 8 years as reported by this same group.

Balloon "valvuloplasty"

Qureshi and associates[9] from London, UK, performed laser-assisted pulmonary valve dilation in 5 infants with pulmonary atresia who ranged in age from 5 days to 2 years and in weight from 2 to 9 kilograms. Two patients had ventricular septal defect and 3 had intact ventricular septum. All had confluent central pulmonary arteries and 3 had had previously placed Blalock-Taussig shunts. All patients had a RV catheter positioned close to the valve and a retrograde catheter through a patent ductus or shunt positioned just distal to the valve. One catheter was used to pass the laser guide while the other was used as a landmark. The route was through the right ventricle for the laser wire in 3 patients and from pulmonary artery to right ventricle in 2 patients. Once the laser wire was across the valve a predilating catheter was passed over it and this was followed by serial dilation of the valve using appropriate sized balloons. in 1 patient the laser wire did not cross the valve but entered the pericardial cavity. Cardiac tamponade resulted which responded to needle aspiration and the patient then underwent a systemic to pulmonary artery shunt. During a 2 to 6 month follow-up of the 4 successful procedures, estimated pressure gradient across the RV outflow tract ranged between 50 and 70 mmHg and there was evidence of PR in all patients. Transcutaneous oxygen saturation ranged from 70 to 87%. This short report may well represent a landmark paper in the treatment of some of these very difficult patients. Obviously patients with infundibular atresia will not be candidates for this procedure but others may well benefit. How far this technique can be extended for this difficult group of patients will be of great interest to the Pediatric Cardiology community.

Staged surgical repair

Iyer and Mee[10] from Parkville, Australia, reported a staged surgical approach for 58 consecutive patients with pulmonary atresia, VSD, hypoplastic pulmonary arteries with arborization defects, and major aortopulmonary collaterals. Prerepair procedures were designed to encourage native pulmonary artery growth by increasing blood flow and unifocalize pulmonary blood supply by transplanting or ligating major collaterals. A total of 121 staging procedures were performed with an overall mortality of 10%. Ligation or transplantation of 134 major collaterals was performed and 30 patients eventually underwent repair with an early mortality of 3% and late mortality of 10%. Survivors remain well after a mean follow-up of 3.6 years. There was failure to achieve minimum requirements for repair after staging in 12 patients and these patients await further palliation or heart-lung transplantation. The current technique is usually mid-line sternotomy and central aorta to pulmonary artery shunt. This is followed by bilateral thoracotomy and transplantation or ligation of major aortopulmonary collaterals. Repeat sternotomy with closure of VSD and insertion of a valve conduit between the RV outflow tract and the reconstruction of pulmonary arteries is the reparative operation when adequate growth of the pulmonary arteries is achieved. These authors show excellent early result for this very difficult group of patients. They argue against early connection of right ventricle to pulmonary arteries with severely hypoplastic pulmonary arteries. They found aneurysmal dilatation and bifurcation stenosis as frequent complications of this procedure with the additional disadvantage of requiring cardiopulmonary bypass for the connection of the outflow tract to the pulmonary artery. Careful follow-up of the procedure advocated here versus early outflow tract connection will be important to asses the relative merits of these two methods of treatment.

Thromboexclusion of the right ventricle

Williams and associates[11] from Toronto, Canada, performed closure of the tricuspid valve as a part of a new surgical procedure in 12 children with pulmonary atresia and intact ventricular septum. In 2 cases a concomitant Fontan operation was performed. In each patient the right ventricle was small and RV pressure higher than systemic pressure. Ventricle-coronary connections provided flow of desaturated blood from the right ventricle into the coronary arteries in 11 of 12 patients. There were 5 deaths in 12 children and postmortem exam revealed severe acute and chronic myocardial ischemic damage and high-grade obstruction or interruption of the proximal left anterior descending coronary artery. Preoperative angiography demonstrated occlusive changes in the coronary arteries, resulting in RV dependent circulation in all 5 children who died and in 1 child who survived operation. Survivors are well 4 months to 3.5 years later and 2 have undergone successful Fontan operation and 2 others are suitable candidates. Tricuspid valve closure and thromboexclusion with coils or other material is recommended for a carefully selected group of infants with pulmonary atresia and an intact ventricular septum provided a RV-dependent coronary circulation can be excluded on the basis of preoperative coronary angiography. These patients continue to be extremely difficult to treat. Preoperative catheterization should include not only some estimate of RV size but most importantly the demonstration of ventricular-coronary connections. In addition, it is necessary to determine whether or not there are stenotic or obstructive lesions in the coronaries and whether a RV-dependent circulation is present before RV decompression or exclusion is attempted.

COMPLETE TRANSPOSITION OF THE GREAT ARTERIES

Atrial repair results

Merlo and associates[12] from Bergamo, Italy, presented the late results for the first 104 consecutive patients surviving atrial repair for TGA between 1971 and 1978. Mean follow-up time was 12 years and ranged from .1 to 18 years. The actuarial survival rate at 18 years was 84% for simple TGA and 94% for complex TGA. Nine of the 11 deaths were sudden. Symptomatic ventricular dysfunction occurred in 3% of the 78 late survivals with simple TGA and 27% of the 15 late survivors with complex TGA. Ambulatory electrocardiographic monitoring was performed in 33 patients and showed stable sinus rhythm in only 49%. Pathological rhythm disturbances were present in 30%. Radionuclide angiography revealed an abnormal RV response in 11 of 13 and an abnormal left ventricular response in 2 of 13. These authors show a low prevalence for symptomatic RV dysfunction in simple TGA, but a much higher prevalence in complex TGA. Rhythm disturbances were common in both groups. Despite these problems, the survival rate at 18 years was 84%. It will be increasingly important to determine the prevalence of further ventricular dysfunction abnormalities and rhythm disturbances in the next 20 years.

DOUBLE INLET VENTRICLE

Echocardiographic anatomy

Bevilacqua and associates[13] from Boston, Massachusetts, studied the echocardiographic anatomy of double-inlet left ventricle in 57 patients ages 1 day to 27 years. The visceroatrial situs was solitus and the heart was on the left side of the chest in all patients. A d-loop ventricle was present in 21 patients and an l-loop ventricle in 26 patients. The great arteries were normally related in 8 and transposed in 49. In all hearts, the right AV valve was anterior to the left AV valve. In 53 patients the tricuspid valve was closer to and had attachments on the septum. The tricuspid valve straddled the outflow chamber in 8 patients. No significant difference was noted in the mean AV valve diameter when comparing mitral and tricuspid valves within the same group or between the groups with a d- or l-loop ventricle. The right AV valve diameter had a significant direct correlation with the aortic valve diameter and the size of the VSD regardless of ventricular loop. Both AV valves were functionally normal in 34 patients. Among patients with AV valve dysfunction, the tricuspid valve tended to be stenotic in patients with an l-loop ventricle and regurgitant in patients with a d-loop ventricle. Mitral valve dysfunction was uncommon. The VSD was separated from the semilunar valves in 24 patients and adjacent to the anterior semilunar valve as a result of hypoplasia or malalignment, or both, of the infundibular septum in 19 patients with a subaortic defect. Multiple defects were present in 3 patients. The defect was unrestrictive in 26 patients, restrictive in 23 and could not be evaluated in 8. Pulmonary artery banding had been performed in 8 of 26 patients with an unrestrictive defect and in 10 of 23 patients with a restrictive defect. Only 4 of 19 subaortic defects, compared with 16 of 24 muscular defects, were restrictive. Among patients with transposition, only 2 of 13 with pulmonary stenosis had a restrictive VSD compared with 15 of 30 without pulmonary stenosis. In patients with transposition, the defect size was significantly smaller if coarctation was present. These complex patients are potential candidates for Fontan operation and in all instances must be evaluated meticulously before being sent for this procedure. Echocardiographic data frequently is as helpful or more helpful than angiographic data for this purpose and always is complementary to catheterization evaluation.

Operative results

Franklin and associates[14] from London and Cambridge, United Kingdom, studied the survival before definitive operation in 191 infants with double inlet ventricle presenting before 1 year of age with a median followup of 8.5 years. The morphologic spectrum was broad with a great prevalence of associated lesions. The actuarial survival rate before definitive repair was 57% at 1 year, 49% at 5 years, and 42% at 10 years. Univariate risk factors established that RA isomerism, common AV orifice, pulmonary atresia, obstruction of the systemic outflow tract, and extracardiac anomalous pulmonary venous connection were strongly associated with poorer survival. Pulmonary stenosis, balanced pulmonary blood flow, and presentation at an older age were beneficial. These findings are in agreement with the poor prognosis reported from smaller series that have focused on patients with the adverse features of atrial isomerism and common AV orifice. The survival rate was worse than in prior reports because of the younger age of entry into the series. This type of analysis is useful in terms of attempting to find better long-term strategy for dealing with this complex condition.

Franklin and associates[15] from London and Cambridge, UK, studied the influence of palliation on survival of 191 consecutive infants presenting under 1 year of age with double inlet ventricle. Palliative operations were performed on 54 occasions in 121 patients. Survival after a systemic-pulmonary artery shunt (n = 57) and banding of the pulmonary trunk (n = 35) was comparable at 84 and 77% respectively at 1 year and 62% at 5 years. Those who underwent repair of aortic arch obstruction fared worse (n = 18 with survival 44% and 22% at 1 and 5 years). The remainder did not undergo an operation because of balanced physiology, complex anatomy or irreversible low output. Palliative surgery overall had a deleterious effect on immediate survival but in the survivors, medium-term outcome was improved. This effect was most marked for those undergoing a systemic-PA shunt; by contrast, after banding of the pulmonary trunk, without or without additional repair of the aortic arch, medium-term risk was not altered. These data indicate that palliative operations enable patients to reach an age when definitive repair procedures are currently undertaken but are not of themselves a means for ensuring long-term survival. It was notable that patients who underwent banding of the pulmonary trunk with and without repair of an aortic arch lesion did not appear to show a benefit from palliation even in the medium-term. This was due to the subsequent early and usually fatal development of subaortic stenosis in many of these patients, particularly in those who required surgery to the aortic arch.

Franklin and associates[16] from London and Cambridge, UK, studied the fate of 191 infants with double inlet ventricle to determine the influence of morphologlical characteristics at presentation and subsequent management on the potential for and timing of definitive repair by the Fontan operation or ventricular septation. At presentation, 136 (71%) were potential candidates for Fontan procedure. Actuarial survival was better than for those deemed unsuitable for either definitive option but still only 78 patients were known to be alive and unsuitable candidates at 2 years of age. This was largely due to death after presentation with low cardiac output in 19 and death at palliative operation in 20 of 98 surgically treated patients. The adverse events of late sudden death occurred in 14 and development of new features precluding a Fontan operation occurred in 18 mostly before 4 years of age. Patients requiring no operation and those who underwent a systemic-pulmonary arterial shunt fared better than those who underwent isolated banding of the pulmonary trunk. Development of subaortic stenosis was common in patients with aortic arch repair associated with banding. These authors suggest that management in infancy should be aimed at maintaining potential for a future Fontan operation which should not be delayed for most patients beyond 3 years of age because of the prevalence of adverse events with increasing age.

AORTIC-VALVE STENOSIS

Critical stenosis in infancy

Leung and associates[17] from Liverpool, UK, examined 20 heart specimens from infants under 3 months of age and reviewed the clinical course and echocardiograms of 20 patients in the same age group. All 20 patients underwent open valvotomy and in 5 cases both echocardiographic and postmortem measurements were available for the same heart. Anatomic specimens showed a spectrum of valvular, ventricular, and vascular abnormalities that could be accurately identified by echocardiography. A small LV cavity was usually associated with a narrow ventriculoarterial junction, small ascending aorta, and narrow subaortic region. In these hearts, the mitral valve had a single or grossly hypoplastic papillary muscle with short or "arcuate" tendinous cords. The 5 nonsurvivors and the 15 survivors of open valvotomy showed significant differences in echocardiographic dimension of the left ventricle, the subaortic region, the ventriculoaortic junction, the ascending aorta, and the mitral valve annulus. The papillary muscle of the mitral valve was invariably single or hypoplastic in the early nonsurvivors. Infants with unfavorable cardiac anatomy tended to present earlier and to have a lower systemic blood pressure. This study suggests that patients with a LV inflow dimension of <25 mm, a narrow ventriculoaortic junction of <5 mm, and a mitral valve orifice of <9 mm may have hypoplastic left ventricles more suited for cardiac transplantation or Norwood palliation. These authors have made a further attempt for a noninvasive estimation of the hypoplastic left ventricle. These data would have been more useful if they had included patient weight and body surface area to go with their echocardiographic estimations. The inflow mentioned which is measured from the mitral valve annulus to the apex has not previously been used extensively in terms of determining the small left ventricle and may be of use in prospective studies. Unfortunately there still remains significant overlap with survivors and nonsurvivors for most of these dimensions and further prospective analysis will be needed to more accurately quantify the truly hypoplastic left ventricle.

Left ventricular size in infants

Parsons and associates[18] from Nashville, Tennessee, studied the echocardiograms and catheterization data of 25 infants <3 months of age undergoing aortic valvotomy of isolated AS over a 10 year period in an attempt to develop echocardiographic criteria for adequacy of left ventricular size. Significant differences between survivors and nonsurvivors were noted for age at operation, mitral valve diameter, LV end diastolic dimension, left atrial dimension, LV cross-sectional area and angiographically determined LV volume. There was no difference with respect to patient weight, body surface area, aortic root dimension or LV ejection fraction. LV cross-sectional area <2 cm², as measured on the parasternal long axis echocardiogram was found in 5 of 7 nonsurvivors and 0 of 12 survivors. LV end diastolic dimension <13mm was found in 5 of 6 non-survivors and 2 of 17 survivors. There was a good correlation between angiographic LV volume and LV cross sectional area. With the advent of therapy for patients with hypoplastic left ventricle other than valvulotomy (transplant or Norwood operation), the need for rapid noninvasive determination of criteria for hypoplastic left ventricle becomes critical. These data serve as a useful adjunct in this diagnosis.

Balloon valvuloplasty

Beekman and associates[19] from Ann Arbor, Michigan, attempted balloon valvuloplasty in 8 newborns <28 days of age with critical AS. This procedure was unsuccessful in 3 infants presenting before 1989, when improved catheter technology became available. Subsequently 5 patients have had successful balloon valvuloplasty as evidenced by a decrease in valve gradient and improvement in LV function and cardiac output. Peak gradient was reduced from 69 ± 8 to 25 ± 3 mmHg and LV systolic pressure decreased from 128 ± 9 to 95 ± 9 mmHg. LV end-diastolic pressure decreased from 20 ± 2 to 11 ± 1 mmHg. Moderate AR was documented in 2 of 5 infants after valvuloplasty. These authors have utilized new catheter technology to allow a transumbilical approach to the majority of the infants. This approach may prove useful in this very difficult clinical problem.

Use of pulmonary homograft

Gerosa and associates[20] from London, UK, reported 34 patients ages 3 to 18 years who underwent replacement of the aortic valve or root with their own pulmonic valve. The indication for operation was LV outflow obstruction in 16 patients, AR in 14, mixed aortic valve disease in 3 and failure of a previously implanted aortic homograft in 1. There were 4 early deaths, all before 1971, giving a hospital mortality of 12%. Surviving patients have been followed a cumulative total of 214 patient years with the longest observation being 16.5 years. Late mortality was 13% and 4 other patients required removal of the autograft for endocarditis. Actuarial rates at 16 years were 74% freedom from reoperation on the LV outflow tract, 80% freedom from reoperation on the RV outflow tract and 77% for late survival. There was no instance of primary structural degeneration in the pulmonary autograft and all patients were without symptoms. This procedure represents an interesting option for treatment of severe aortic outflow problems. Although most of these patients had AR apparently it was not severe. The long-term followup of this group will be extremely important in terms of finding another applicable operation for these difficult patients.

SUBAORTIC STENOSIS

Balloon dilatation

Suarez de Lezo and associates[21] from Cordoba and las Palmas de Gran Canaria, Spain, presented findings of 33 patients with discrete subaortic stenosis who were treated by percutaneous balloon dilation and followed up for 2 months to 6 years with mean follow-up of 34 months. The mean age was 13 years and associated malformations were observed in 9 patients. Mean valve to membrane distance was 4.5 mm/m². After balloon dilation the pressure gradient from left ventricle to aorta decreased from 68 to 20; there was no significant change in the degree of AR. A fluttering and widely mobile remaining membrane was clearly visualized after dilation. Better immediate results were obtained in patients with a smaller baseline gradient, a larger aortic anulus, and a longer valve to membrane distance. Serial echocardiographic studies were available in 30 patients and 18 hemodynamic evaluations were performed in 13 patients. Restenosis occurred in 7 patients who underwent redilation at a mean of 29 months. Redilation in 6 of 7 patients obtained benefits similar to those obtained at the first dilation. Only 1 patient had unsuccessful redilation and required surgery. The mean value of the last residual gradient on hemodynamic or Doppler study in the remaining 32 patients was 21 ± 10 mmHg. These authors show excellent results from balloon dilatation of discrete subaortic stenosis of the non-tunnel type. The data suggest that the discrete fibrous ridge or membrane is torn by the balloon dilatation. This results in significant improvement of orifice size. Because of the progressive nature of the disease, this problem needs considerable long-term followup in other groups attempting to obtain similar results. Several previous studies have suggested only short term benefits from this procedure.

Associated obstructive lesions and operative therapy

Rychik and associates[22] from Philadelphia, Pennsylvania, reported 50 infants with a variety of congenital cardiac lesions other than hypoplastic left heart syndrome who underwent surgical relief of aortic outflow obstruction by creation of a PA to aorta anastomosis. Nineteen patients had normally aligned great arteries; 25 had TGA, all with a univentricular heart of LV morphology; and 6 had a double-outlet right ventricle. All patients had either aortic stenosis or atresia, subaortic stenosis or a restrictive VSD. Sixteen had normal arch anatomy; 34 had arch anomalies consisting of arch hypoplasia in 17, coarctation in 11, interruption of the arch in 4, and complex anomalies in 2. Surgery was performed at a median age of 10 days with 33 of 50 surviving. No significant difference in early survival was noted among the groups of varying ventriculoarterial alignment. Overall actuarial survival was 63% at 18 months. Of the 33 survivors, 26 have proceeded to the next surgical stage, including the Fontan procedure in 8, superior cavopulmonary anastomosis in 13 and biventricular repair in 5. This type of radical surgery obviously can be useful for patients with severe anomalies of obstruction as presented. The decision as to when to use this type of surgery is a difficult one and the exact criteria for its use needs to be developed.

In single ventricle "equivalents"

Ilbawi and associates[23] from Oak Lawn, Illinois, reviewed data on 13 patients with single ventricle equivalents and subaortic stenosis who underwent relief of the stenosis and subsequent Fontan operation. Nine patients constituting group 1 had the obstruction relieved at 4 ± 2 years of age whenever the pressure gradient became apparent. Four patients constituting group 2 had the stenosis operated on at an average age of 11 days before hemodynamic evidence of obstruction. Preoperative pressure gradient was 44 ± 5 in group 1 versus 5 ± 5 in group 2. Ventricular muscle mass was 186% of normal in group 1 versus 114% of normal in group 2 and mass/volume ratio was 1.12 in group 1 versus 0.62 in group 2. Relief of subaortic stenosis was achieved by proximal PA to ascending aorta or aortic arch anastomosis and systemic to PA shunt. There were no hospital mortality or complications related to this procedure. At evaluation before Fontan operation, 4 years later in group 1 and 3 years later in group 2, the pressure gradient across the outflow tract was 4 mmHg in group 1 and 3 mmHg in group 2. Ventricular muscle mass was 184% of normal in group 1 and 114% of normal in group 2 and mass/volume ratio was 1.2 in group 1 versus 0.62 in group 2. After Fontan operation there were two perioperative deaths and two takedowns of Fontan in group 1 and none in group 2. Postoperative mean RA pressure was 18 in group 1 versus 11 in group 2. Serious postoperative effusions were present in 4 of 5 patients in group 1 versus 0 of 4 patients in group 2. These preliminary data suggest that early relief of subaortic stenosis in single ventricle equivalent decreases ventricular muscle mass which may have a favorable effect on ventricular compliance as well as a favorable effect on eventual Fontan operation.

AORTIC ISTHMIC COARCTATION

Neural crest as pathogenetic factor

Kappetein and associates[24] from Leiden, The Netherlands, analyzed 109 patients operated on for coarctation of the aorta for occurrence of associated cardiac and noncardiac anomalies. Attention was also paid to the prevalence of cardiac anomalies in the relatives of these patients. Of the patients with coarctation of the aorta, 57 (52%) had a bicuspid aortic valve. Forty-three (39%) of the 109 patients had one or more noncardiac anomalies. In 29 (27%) patients the noncardiac anomaly involved the head/neck structures. Noncardiac anomalies were much more prevalent in patients with coarctation and bicuspid aortic valve, especially anomalies involving the head/neck structures: 44% compared to 8% of patients with a normal aortic valve. Congenital cardiac malformations were present in relatives in the first or second degree of 18% of the patients. Bicuspid aortic valve was more prevalent in patients with an affected relative (75%) than in patients with unaffected relatives (47%). Recent studies showed that the neural crest plays an important role in the development of cardiac and a variety of noncardiac structures. The cardiac structures derived from the neural crest involve the outflow tract of the heart and the aortic arch system. Maldevelopment of neural crest cells could therefore be responsible for the combined occurrence of outflow tract (e.g., bicuspid aortic valve), aortic arch (e.g., coarctation), and noncardiac anomalies. This study supports the concept that some anomalies of the aortic arch system, including aortic coarctation, are cardiovascular manifestations of a spectrum of anomalies involving the head and neck region that may be due to a genetic-environmental disorder of the neural crest.

Patterns of ductal tissue

Russell and associates[25] from Bristol, United Kingdom, studied ductal tissue in aortic segments removed from 23 patients <3 months of age who underwent resection of coarctation of the aorta. The surgical policy was to perform extensive excision of the coarctation, including a wide margin of descending aorta beyond the ductus arteriosus. Histologic examination showed a circumferential sling of ductal tissue extending from the ductus arteriosus and surrounding the aorta at the level of the coarctation shelf in 22 specimens. In 15 of 22, 1 or 2 tongue-like prolongations of ductal tissue extended distally and onto the aortic wall. Incomplete excision of ductal tissue was found in 11 specimens. These authors show a marked difference from normal in the extension of ductal tissue onto the aorta in patients with coarctation. This pathologic review is consistent with wide distribution of ductal tissue onto the aorta in the young infant and provides the basis for a pathophysiologic mechanism both for primary coarctation and recoarctation.

Balloon angioplasty

Hijazi and associates[26] from New Haven, Connecticut, reviewed balloon angioplasty for recurrent coarctation of the aorta which they performed 29 times in 26 patients with a median age of 4 years and 9 months and a range from 4 months to 29 years. Initial surgical techniques were end-to-end anastomosis in 11, subclavian angioplasty in 11 and patch aortoplasty in 4. Angioplasty was performed at a median interval of 2 years and 7 months with a range of 4 months to 23 years after surgery. Mean peak systolic pressure across the coarctation decreased from 40 ± 17 to 10 ± 10 mmHg after the initial angioplasty and the mean diameter of the coarctation site increased from 6 ± 4 to 9 ± 4 mm. There was no mortality and only 1 patient developed an aneurysm. Three patients underwent repeat angioplasty for a pressure difference of more than 20 mmHg. Long-term follow-up on 24 of 26 patients with a mean follow-up of 42 months revealed mean systolic difference across the area of coarctation decreased from 40 ± 17 to 9 ± 8 mmHg after final angioplasty and 8 ± 8 mmHg at follow-up. Mean peak systolic pressure in the upper extremities decreased from 133 ± 15 before angioplasty to 111 ± 14 mmHg at long-term follow-up. These authors show convincing data for effective treatment of recurrent coarctation by balloon dilatation. This modality should be considered as an alternative to surgery in this group of patients.

Late operative results

To study early and late mortality after surgical correction of aortic isthmic coarctation, Bobby and associates[27] from London, UK, collected data on 223 patients operated on at a single hospital in London, UK, between 1946 and 1981. The data was collected and updated by questionnaire. All 223 patients were recorded as undergoing operation for aortic coarctation up to the end of 1981. Fifteen of 197 survivors were lost to follow up; most of them were patients from overseas. The early mortality (within 1 month of operation) was 12% overall, 2.6% for elective surgery, and 0% for the 77 patients undergoing surgery since 1968. Survivors were followed up for a total of 3,288 patient years; in 27 follow-up lasted more than 30 years. In a few it reached 40 years. Twenty-two patients died during this period, 18 from causes that could be attributed to coarctation or its repair. Mortality was highest more than 20 years after the operation. Repair increased life expectancy in patients with aortic coarctation. Late problems caused by persistent hypertension or recoarctation became apparent in long term survivors. The increased risk of late mortality associated with the duration of preoperative hypertension was not statistically significant. There were no deaths from cerebrovascular accidents. (In an earlier necropsy series cerebrovascular accidents accounted for 12% of deaths.) The incidence of deaths from aneurysms resembled that in the earlier necropsy series.

Results of patch angioplasty

Malan and associates[28] from Johannesburg, South Africa, report the long-term complications of patch angioplasty repair for coarctation of the aorta in 119 patients operated from 4 days to 13 years. There were 7 late deaths and 17 patients were lost to follow-up. Follow-up for a minimum of 3 years was obtained in 95 patients with a mean of 6 years. Hypertension occurred in 17% and 26 had a resting systolic arm-leg gradient >20 mmHg. Recoarctation occurred more frequently with surgery before 1 month of age. Calcification of the patch occurred in 4 patients, 1 of whom subsequently had aneurysm formation. In a second child aneurysm was detected at repeat operation. Exercise tests in 15 patients showed significantly higher systolic arm pressure in patients (165 mmHg) when compared to controls (139 mmHg) and a significant increase in arm-leg systolic gradient, 36 versus 6mmHg. These authors conclude that the most important long-term complication following aortic patch angioplasty is re-stenosis. Aneurysm was detected only twice. Although aneurysm has been reported after patch angioplasty for coarctation, there are no prior series with significant numbers of patients to document the true prevalence. These authors feel that repair at a younger age may be associated with a lower prevalence of this problem. It should be noted that 53% of their patients were repaired under 1 year of age. The re-stenosis rate of 26% and the reoperation rate of 15% would favor the consideration of either subclavian flap angioplasty for a young infant or resection and end-to-end anastomosis for young infants.

Sciolaro and associates[29] from Tucson, Arizona, retrospectively reviewed 56 children under 4 years of age with coarctation repair between 1977 and 1986. Subclavian flap angioplasty was used in 34 and 22 had resection with oblique end-to-end anastomosis. The group was further subdivided to study 23 infants <3 months of age: 8 with resection and 15 with subclavian angioplasty. The remaining 33 patients older than 3 months of age were divided into 14 patients with resection and 19 patients with subclavian angioplasty. Mortality was not different between the 2 techniques. Postoperative hypertension was more prevalent with resection than with angioplasty and 7 patients had recurrent coarctation. The 6 year actuarial freedom from recoarctation was 93 ± 6% in the infant subclavian flap group compared with 53 ± 20% in the infant resection group. There was no difference in recoarctation in children operated <3 months of age in regard to the type of repair. There continues to be controversy regarding which is the best operation in terms of preventing recoarctation. There are a number of strong advocates for subclavian angioplasty in the young infant, and only 1 report to suggest significant problems with arm ischemia following this technique. These recommendations for subclavian flap in patients <3 months of age seem reasonable although some infants in this age have favorable anatomy that would be well-suited for end-to-end anastomosis.

AORTIC VALVE ATRESIA

Fetal echocardiography

Allan and associates[30] from London, UK, diagnosed hypoplastic left heart syndrome prenatally and confirmed it in 105 fetuses since 1983 at a regional referral center. An increased detection rate since 1988 is probably related to increased experience in the use of a 4-chamber view of the fetal heart during routine obstetric ultrasound scanning. When the diagnosis was made sufficiently early, most parents chose to terminate the pregnancy after the prognosis and surgical options were explained. By contrast, after an increase in the mid 1980s, since 1988 there has been a striking fall in the number of newborn babies with hypoplastic left heart syndrome treated at a supraregional referral center. More widespread use of 4-chamber cardiac screening during routine fetal ultrasonography may reduce the number of newborn babies with hypoplastic left heart syndrome—a factor which should be taken into account when the likely requirements for neonatal cardiac transplantation facilities are calculated.

Assessment after initial reconstructive operation

Chang and associates[31] from Philadelphia, Pennsylvania, reported catheterization data from 59 patients who underwent initial reconstructive surgery for hypoplastic left heart syndrome. Ages ranged from 3 to 27 months, with a mean of 14 months and all patients were evaluated for an anticipated modified Fontan procedure. Five hemodynamic and anatomic features which are considered components of successful initial surgery were addressed. These included interatrial communication with only 2 patients with a measured pressure difference >4 mmHg across the atrial septum, tricuspid valve function with only 5 patients showing significant TR, aortic arch with only 2 patients showing a gradient from right ventricle to descending aorta >25 mmHg, pulmonary vasculature with 10 patients having calculated pulmonary vascular resistance >4 $U \cdot m^2$ and 86% of the 59 patients having no evidence of distortion of either the left or right PA, RV function with only 5 patients having end-diastolic pressure >12 mmHg and 2 patients having qualitative assessment of decreased RV function. Comparison of catheterization data between survivors and nonsurvivors of the subsequent modified Fontan procedure showed that only significant TR was a possible predictor of poor outcome. These authors show reasonably good outcome of the first stage Norwood procedure. Unfortunately, the qualitative evaluation of systolic function may be misleading in terms of overall myocardial performance. The overall survival rate for the modified Fontan procedure was 58%. This mortality is one of the reasons for the new strategy for reducing the volume load on the ventricle with a superior cavo-pulmonary anastomosis in the first 6 to 18 months of life. It is still unclear as to whether overall survival and morbidity will be improved with this strategy but early results are promising.

Cardiac transplantation

Neonatal cardiac transplantation offers the prospect of survival for babies with aortic valve atresia but only if suitable donors are available.

In a retrospective survey in the Northern health region of England and Wales, Stuart and associates[32] from Newcastle upon Tyne, UK, found that the likely need for neonatal cardiac transplantation far outweighed the potential availability of donors. Over 8 years (1983–1990) hypoplastic left heart syndrome was identified in 38 newborn babies and in 9 fetuses in utero. Of 41 live births (including 3 diagnosed prenatally) 31 would have been candidates for a cardiac transplant but only 4 suitable donors could be identified (3 with anencephaly born alive during the same period and 1 who died between 1979 and 1986 after a head injury). Analysis of all infant deaths in 1987–1989 revealed only 3 potential donors from 426 deaths in the 3 years. Although more widespread antenatal diagnosis may lead to fewer liveborn babies with hypoplastic left heart syndrome, these findings indicate that an alternative source of donors needs to be identified before neonatal cardiac transplantation can be widely used in the treatment of this disorder.

TRICUSPID VALVE ATRESIA

Ventricular function during exercise

Akagi and associates[33] from Toronto, Canada, studied 14 patients with tricuspid atresia and normally related great arteries using rest and supine bicycle exercise equilibrium radionuclide studies. EF, heart rate, blood pressure and oxygen saturation were measured. Mean age was 15 years and ranged from 6 to 21 years. Eight patients had systemic to pulmonary shunts placed as palliation 8 years before study and 6 patients had caval to pulmonary shunts placed 12 years previously. EF was abnormal at rest and with exercise averaging 54% of rest and 55% at peak exercise. EF was slightly higher at rest in patients with systemic shunts but this difference was not present at peak exercise. There was a significant negative correlation between EF at peak exercise and interval since palliative surgery. These data further indicate that ventricular function is compromised during exercise and abnormal performance is influenced by longstanding volume overload. In this particular group, the choice of palliative shunting procedure appeared to have little effect on normalizing pump performance. These data did not show a potential benefit of the Glenn shunt in preventing long-term volume overload and decreasing the prevalence of ventricular dysfunction with time. This study does support early repair to reduce the influence of volume overload and hypoxemia both of which may contribute to abnormal ventricular function.

TRUNCUS ARTERIOSUS

Repair in infancy

Pearl and associates[34] from Los Angeles, California, reported results of primary repair of truncus arteriosus in 32 patients under the age of 12 months. The average age was 3.5 months and range was <1 to 12 months. Three patients had interrupted aortic arch. Early mortality was 5 of 32 (16%). For those older than 1 month early mortality was 2 of 28

(7%). In the past 4 years, early mortality has decreased to 2 of 24 or 8% and both of these patients had interrupted aortic arch. Excluding patients with interrupted aortic arch, there were no early deaths in the last 22 patients. Late mortality overall was 2 of 27 or 7%. In a mean follow-up of 73 months, 71% of survivors with porcine-valved conduits required conduit replacement secondary to obstruction. In a mean follow-up of 36 months only 14% of patients with homographs required replacement secondary to obstruction. These authors show outstanding results in repair of truncus arteriosus. The early results suggest improvement in progressive outflow obstruction with homografts although it is obvious that these grafts will be obstructed with increasing growth in all patients and will need eventual replacement.

EBSTEIN'S ANOMALY

Surgery

Starnes and associates[35] from Stanford and Sacramento, California, report a new surgical procedure for 5 newborn infants with severe Ebstein's anomaly. At initial examination patients weighed 3.6 ± 1.8 kg and had a mean oxygen tension of 30 ± 2 mmHg. Chest films demonstrated a mean cardiothoracic ratio of .81. Echocardiography demonstrated massive RA enlargement, severe TR, and pulmonary valves which were not opening. All infants were dependent on prostaglandin E_1 and attempts to wean them were unsuccessful. Palliative treatment consisted of tricuspid closure with autologous pericardium and an aortopulmonary shunt of 4 mm polytetrafluoroethylene tubing. There were no operative or late deaths. One infant has had a successful Glenn anastomosis and 2 infants have had successful Fontan repairs. This new management strategy for infants with severe Ebstein's anomaly who are refractory to medical management deserves further trial. Since most neonates with Ebstein's anomaly spontaneously improve in the first month of life with the fall in pulmonary vascular resistance, the decision about when to operate remains difficult.

Quaegebeur and associates[36] from Rotterdam, The Netherlands, reported 10 consecutive patients ages 4 to 44 years who underwent surgical repair of Ebstein's anomaly by vertical plication of the right ventricle and reimplantation of the tricuspid valve leaflets. No patient died during the operation. Intraoperative postbypass echocardiography documented a good result in 9 patients but severe TR in 1 patient who then underwent prosthetic valve replacement. All patients were evaluated clinically and by echocardiography 2 to 23 months later. All patients showed clinical improvement, 7 by 1 functional class and 3 by 2 classes. All were in sinus rhythm. The mean cardiothoracic ratio decreased by 6%. TR diminished in 8 patients by 3 grades in 2 patients, by 2 grades in 5 and by 1 grade in 1 patient. These authors show excellent early results for this type of repair which is a modification of that suggested by Carpentier (J Thorac Cardiovasc Surg, 1988;96:92–108). It requires a reasonable sized distal RV chamber which is present in most patients who have reached the age of 4 to 5 years without severe symptomatology. It will be important to compare the long-term results of this operation versus the results achieved by Danielson, et al (Ann Surg 1982;196:499–503).

Intrauterine echocardiographic diagnosis

Sharland and associates[37] from London, UK, reported echocardiographic prenatal studies in 38 fetuses with either a dysplastic or a displaced tricuspid valve. The valve was dysplastic in 22 fetuses, all of which had evidence of TR resulting in right atrial dilatation and increased cardiothoracic ratio. An associated abnormality of the pulmonary valve occurred in 16 fetuses. The remaining 16 fetuses had Ebstein's malformation, 14 with evidence of TR at presentation and 10 with an associated abnormality of the pulmonary valve. Pregnancy was interrupted in 17 of 38, intrauterine fetal death occurred in 8 of 38, 11 of 38 died postnatally and 2 of 38 are still alive. Additional abnormalities were found in 8 patients, including chromosomal anomalies in 2, VSD in 2, corrected transposition in 2, Chiari malformation in 2, SVT in 1 and coarctation in 1. These authors also show a high rate of natural loss both intrauterine and immediately after birth in patients with severe tricuspid valve abnormalities resulting in enlargement of the right heart and probable decrease in right lung size. They stress the importance of sequential studies during pregnancy to be important in terms of predicting prognosis because cardiac malformations may show progressive deterioration during fetal life.

With tricuspid regurgitation in the fetus

Hornberger and associates[38] from San Diego, California, New Haven, Connecticut, and Tucson, Arizona, studied the clinical course of 26 fetuses with tricuspid valve disease and significant TR. Ebstein's anomaly was present in 17, tricuspid valve dysplasia in 7, and unguarded tricuspid orifice in 2. All fetuses had massive right atrial dilation and most had progressive right-sided cardiomegaly. Hydrops fetalis was found in 6 patients and atrial flutter in 5. Associated cardiac lesions included PS in 5 and pulmonary atresia in 6. Normal forward pulmonary flow was found in 4 fetuses at initial study who subsequently had retrograde pulmonary artery and ductal flow associated with the development of severe PS or pulmonary atresia. The clinical course of 23 fetuses (excluding 3 with elective abortion) revealed that 48% died in utero and 35% who were liveborn died despite vigorous medical or surgical management. There were 4 survivors with 3 having a benign neonatal course with mild to moderate Ebstein's anomaly. An additional finding at autopsy was significant lung hypoplasia in 19 of 19 patients. The prognosis for the fetus diagnosed in utero with severe tricuspid valve disease and progressive right heart dilation is extremely poor, with cardiac failure and lung hypoplasia in many and development of PS or atresia later in a few.

CORONARY ANOMALY

Left main from the pulmonary trunk

Previous studies have indicated that the definitive diagnosis of anomalous origin of the left coronary artery from the pulmonary trunk should be made by cardiac catheterization and angiography. Jureidini and associates[39] from St. Louis, Missouri, evaluated echocardiography (2-dimensional, pulsed Doppler, and color flow mapping) as a method to establish the diagnosis of anomalous left coronary artery origin. To diagnose this condition, a modified parasternal short-axis view was used to demonstrate continuity of the anomalous origin of the left coronary artery with the pulmonary trunk and to detect the retrograde flow through the anomalous origin of the left coronary artery into the pulmonary trunk. Absence of these imaging characteristics ruled out anomalous origin of the left coronary artery. From June 1985 to January 1990, 16 patients who presented with or had previously had a dilated poorly contracting left ventricle were prospectively assessed by echocardiography to rule out anomalous origin of the left coronary artery. Four patients had anomalous left coronary origin (ages 2 to 120 months, mean 32 ± 59) and 12 patients (ages 1 to 192 months, mean 57 ± 80) had myocardiopathy. Two other patients with known anomalous left coronary origin were evaluated by an observer unaware of the diagnosis. All coronary anatomy was confirmed by angiography, surgery, or autopsy. The correct diagnosis of coronary anatomy was obtained by echocardiography in all instances without false positive or false negative diagnosis of anomalous origin of the left coronary artery. Three infants underwent surgical repair of anomalous left coronary origin based only on the echocardiographic diagnosis. Echocardiography can be used to establish the diagnosis of anomalous origin of the left coronary artery from the pulmonary trunk. Therefore, surgical repair can be undertaken in some critically sick infants based on the echocardiographic diagnosis alone.

Origin of both the left anterior descending and left circumflex coronary arteries directly from the left aortic sinus

Among 20,332 adult patients who underwent consecutive cardiac catheterization and coronary arteriography, 83 (0.4%) were angiographically identified as having an absent LM in a report by Topaz and colleagues[40] from Richmond, Virginia. The angiographic characteristics of this coronary anomaly include: 1) the presence of 2 well-separated coronary ostia at the left aortic sinus resulting in separate origin of the LAD and LC; 2) an increased incidence of left coronary dominance; 3) a higher (6%) than usual (0.5% to 1.5%) incidence of myocardial bridging; 4) lack of a high incidence of congenital heart anomalies; and 5) an incidence of atherosclerotic CAD similar to that of patients whose LM is intact. In 39% of the patients, difficulties in selectively cannulating the separate ostium of the LC and adequately opacifying this vessel resulted in a need to change the diagnostic catheter size. Recognition of this coronary anomaly is needed to insure accurate angiographic interpretation and is important for patients undergoing cardiac surgery to selectively perfuse these separate vessels during cardiopulmonary bypass.

PATENT DUCTUS ARTERIOSUS

Transcatheter closure

Bridges and associates[41] from Boston, Massachusetts, attempted closure of a large PDA (>4 mm diameter) with a clamshell septal umbrella. Patient ages ranged from .7 to 30 years. An isolated PDA was present in

11 patients and 3 patients had additional congenital heart lesions. Moderate or severe pulmonary hypertension was present in 4 patients. The diameter of the PDA ranged from 4.5 to 14 mm, as determined by contrast injection through an 11F sheath or by balloon sizing; it appeared larger by this method than by standard angiography. All 14 lesions were successfully closed. Prior embolization of a Rashkind umbrella was the reason for using a Clamshell device in 3 patients; 1 additional embolization of a Clamshell device occurred. All errant devices were retrieved at cardiac catheterization, without hemodynamic instability. Among the 14 patients, 11 had complete ductal closure by Doppler color mapping at last follow-up and 3 had trivial residual flow. All 4 patients having associated complex lesions or pulmonary hypertension had symptomatic improvement although 1 child with Shone's anomaly died 3 months later. This device provides stable and effective closure of a large PDA and allows transcatheter closure to be offered to some patients who were felt unsuitable for this technique.

THE FONTAN OPERATION

Ventricular function

Parikh and associates[42] from Indianapolis, Indiana, studied 47 patients with single ventricle before and after the Fontan procedure using radionuclide angiography. Before Fontan surgery EF averaged 57% and was significantly different from a normal value of 68%. Age, ventricular morphology and the presence of pulmonary atresia and or systemic to PA shunt had no statistical relation to EF. Serial evaluation in 15 patients preoperatively over 4 years revealed no significant change in EF. Modified Fontan procedure was performed in 24 of 47 patients with 7 deaths, 1 transplant and 1 patient facing transplant. No difference was noted in preoperative EF between survivors and nonsurvivors. Ventricular morphology, age at surgery and operative factors, including bypass and cross-clamp time, were not related to functional outcome. Preoperative EF in the subgroup with postoperative study averaged 52% and decreased to 39% when evaluated 1.2 years after surgery. These authors do show a decrease in EF following Fontan repair. Other studies have shown stability of EF or even an improvement. Obviously, further data will be needed on this important assessment in continuing to evaluate this form of palliative surgery.

Right-sided hemodynamics

Nakazawa and associates[43] from Tokyo, Japan, compared right sided heart hemodynamics in 7 patients after direct AV anastamosis for Fontan procedure with 8 patients after direct atriopulmonary anastomosis. The average age at operation (9 years) was not different between groups. In the RV group cardiac index was 2.7 ± 0.6; mean right atrial and pulmonary artery pressures were both 13 ± 3 mmHg. Mean PA wedge pressure was 7 ± 5 mmHg; LV end diastolic volume 129 ± 40% of normal and ejection fraction 0.5 ± .09. In the RA group, data were similar except for slightly higher right heart pressure. These authors utilized a direct atrial to ventricular communication without the use of a valved conduit in these Fontan operations. There was no clear evidence that the lower right sided heart pressures in the AV connection group were advantageous, at least short-term, which was only 3 to 4 weeks after operation. Backward flow into the inferior vena cava with RV contraction limits the effectiveness of this approach. The authors conclude that good postoperative hemodynamics result from normal or larger than normal PA size and low PA resistance and not necessarily from inclusion of the right ventricle in the Fontan repair. There are probably occasional patients with large right ventricles and somewhat small PAs or slight elevated pulmonary vascular resistance in whom inclusion of the right ventricle with the use of a valved conduit might improve their survival and postoperative hemodynamics. Unfortunately, these patients may be at a disadvantage because of the probable need for late reoperation to replace an obstructed homograft or conduit.

Doppler assessment

Frommelt and associates[44] from Ann Arbor, Michigan, studied ventricular systolic and diastolic function and PA flow patterns after the Fontan operation in 15 postoperative patients. Indexes of diastolic function were measured from the systemic atrioventricular valve inflow and compared with 15 age matched control subjects. The patients who had undergone the Fontan procedure had decreased peak E velocity, decreased E/A velocity ratio, and decreased normalized peak filling rate. These diastolic filling abnormalities are consistent with impaired ventricular relaxation and decreased early diastolic transvalvular pressure gradients. Pattern I, observed in 9 patients, showed biphasic forward flow with peak velocities in mid to late systole and mid-diastole. Pattern II, shown in the remaining 6 patients, showed decreased systolic forward flow, a late systolic to early diastolic flow reversal, and delayed onset of diastolic forward flow. Pattern II patients had a significantly lower ejection fraction than Pattern I patients and 3 of these 6 patients have had a poor outcome after the Fontan procedures. Many patients undergoing the Fontan procedure have impaired ventricular relaxation, but in the presence of a normal ejection fraction, biphasic forward PA flow is maintained. With the development of decreased ejection fraction, atrial systolic filling pressures are likely increased, the ventricular suction effect is decreased, and PA flow is diminished or absent in systole or early diastole. These patterns can be of interest to physicians caring for patients with the Fontan operation.

Transesophageal echocardiographic assessment

Stumper and associates[45] from Rotterdam, The Netherlands, used transesophageal echocardiography in 18 patients ages 2 to 34 years to assess the immediate or intermediate results after a Fontan-type procedure. The results were correlated with precordial echocardiography in all patients and cardiac catheterization in 11 patients. Atrial shunting was documented by transesophageal studies in 3 patients versus 1 by precordial study. Confirmation was obtained by cardiac catheterization in 2 and reoperation in 1. Pulmonary artery obstruction was documented in 3 patients by transesophageal study versus 1 patient by precordial. Evaluation of anterior Fontan connection was successful in 5 of 8 patients by transesophageal study and in 6 of 8 patients by precordial study. Posterior connections were evaluated in 10 of 10 patients by esophageal study and in 5 of 10 patients by precordial study. A Glenn shunt was evaluated in 8 of 9 patients by transesophageal study versus 3 of 9 by precordial study. Thrombus formation was detected by transesophageal study in 3 patients versus only 1 by precordial study. AV regurgitation was better evaluated by transesophageal study in 11 of 18 patients versus of 5 of 18 by precordial study. These authors show the usefulness of transesophageal study for evaluating the intracardiac hemodynamics and shunting, as well as thrombus formation. These studies are particularly helpful in the older patient with complex heart disease.

In an investigation of Fyfe and associates[46] from Charleston, South Carolina, transesophageal echocardiography with Doppler examination was performed intraoperatively in 19 children undergoing modified Fontan operations and in 10 patients postoperatively. Comparisons were made with results of intraoperative epicardial imaging (9 patients) and with postoperative transthoracic imaging (10 patients). Transesophageal echocardiography optimally visualized atriopulmonary and cavopulmonary anastomoses. Epicardial echocardiography was successful in only 3 of 9 patients. Intraoperative transesophageal echocardiography showed residua in 8 of 19 studies and led directly to surgical revision or medical therapy. These residua included stenosis of the cavopulmonary anastomosis (1 patient), unsatisfactory atrial fenestration (2 patients), PDA (1 patient), residual cavoatrial shunting (1 patient), atrial thrombi (1 patient), and poor ventricular function (2 patients). Results of examination in the postoperative intensive care unit showed significant abnormalities in 4 of 10 patients. This investigation demonstrates that transesophageal echocardiography provides unique anatomic and physiologic information during and after modified Fontan operations in small children and therefore may have significant impact on patient management.

Electrophysiologic findings

Kürer and associates[47] from Philadelphia, Pennsylvania, studied the electrophysiological effects of the Fontan procedure in 30 patients who underwent catheterization a mean of 1.9 years after operation. Abnormalities of sinus node or ectopic pacemaker automaticity were detected in 59% with a prolonged sinus node or pacemaker recovery time. Total sinoatrial conduction was prolonged in 50% of patients with normal sinus rhythm. The predominant atrial rhythm was sinus in 70% and ectopic atrial or junctional in 30%. Abnormalities of atrial effective and functional refractory periods were noted in 43% and were most pronounced at faster paced cycle lengths. Intraatrial conduction delay between adjacent sites was found in 76% of patients tested and in 8 of 9 patients with inducible intraatrial reentry. Programmed atrial stimulation induced nonsustained SVT in 10% of the 30 patients and sustained arrhythmias in 27%. Intraatrial reentry was the most common inducible arrhythmia and was present in 7 or 8 patients with sustained and 2 of the 3 patients with nonsustained atrial arrhythmia. Atrioventricular conduction abnormalities were noted in 10%. No patient had inducible ventricular arrhythmias with programmed stimulation. These authors show similar electrophysiological findings in patients following Fontan repair as those previously reported after atrial repair of transposition. Sick sinus syndrome associated with intraatrial reentry tachycardia, particularly in patients with poor cardiac function, is a potentially lethal combination.

MISCELLANEOUS TOPICS

Twenty-five year mortality after surgical repair in childhood

To determine long-term survival and the cause of death after repair of 1 of 8 congenital heart defects in childhood (TF, VSD, ASD, coarctation of the aorta, AS, PS, TGA, and PDA) Morris and Menashe[48] from Portland, Oregon, followed up 2701 individuals having repair of 1 of the 8 defects when the patient was aged 18 years or younger (Table 8-1). Age at surgery and operative mortality have decreased significantly over the last 30 years. Late cardiac mortality at 25 years after surgery was 5% for TF and isolated VSD, 10% for coarctation of the aorta, 17% for AS, 5% for PS, and less than 1% for PDA; there were no late cardiac deaths after ASD repair. For TGA, late cardiac mortality was 15% at 15 years after the Mustard operation and was 2% at 10 years after the Senning operation. Surgical repair of most congenital heart defects is associated with lingering cardiac mortality, particularly for AS, coarctation, and TGA.

Aortico-left ventricular tunnel

Sreeram and associates[49] from Liverpool, United Kingdom, studied 4 children with aortico-LV tunnel over a 14 year period. All presented in infancy from 5 days to 9 months of age with a systolic and diastolic murmur. The first 2 patients had inconclusive echocardiographic data and the diagnosis was confirmed at cardiac catheterization at 10 and 23 months of age. The latter 2 patients were diagnosed by echocardiography and all 4 patients underwent surgery by patch closure of the aortic end of the tunnel in 3 patients and direct suture closure in 1 patient. There

TABLE 8-1. *Overall survival and cardiac death-free survival by cardiac defect. Reproduced with permission from Morris, et al.[50]*

Cardiac Defect	30 d	1 y	5 y	10 y	15 y	20 y	25 y
Tetralogy of Fallot (n = 425)							
Overall survival	0.88 ± 0.02	0.87 ± 0.02	0.86 ± 0.02	0.86 ± 0.02	0.86 ± 0.02	0.84 ± 0.02	0.82 ± 0.02
Cardiac death-free survival	0.89 ± 0.02	0.88 ± 0.02	0.87 ± 0.02	0.87 ± 0.02	0.87 ± 0.02	0.85 ± 0.02	0.84 ± 0.02
No. at risk	371	362	308	240	190	118	62
Ventricular septal defect (n = 378)							
Overall survival	0.93 ± 0.01	0.92 ± 0.01	0.91 ± 0.02	0.90 ± 0.02	0.90 ± 0.02	0.87 ± 0.02	0.86 ± 0.03
Cardiac death-free survival	0.93 ± 0.01	0.92 ± 0.01	0.92 ± 0.01	0.91 ± 0.02	0.91 ± 0.02	0.90 ± 0.02	0.88 ± 0.02
No. at risk	343	328	267	200	134	81	44
Atrial septal defect (n = 472)							
Overall survival	0.99 ± 0.004	0.99 ± 0.004	0.99 ± 0.01	0.98 ± 0.01	0.98 ± 0.01	0.96 ± 0.02	0.92 ± 0.03
Cardiac death-free survival	0.99 ± 0.004	0.99 ± 0.004	0.99 ± 0.004	0.99 ± 0.004	0.99 ± 0.004	0.99 ± 0.004	0.99 ± 0.004
No. at risk	462	447	352	267	176	100	43
Coarctation of the aorta (n = 447)							
Overall survival	0.94 ± 0.01	0.91 ± 0.01	0.90 ± 0.01	0.90 ± 0.02	0.89 ± 0.02	0.88 ± 0.02	0.79 ± 0.04
Cardiac death-free survival	0.94 ± 0.01	0.92 ± 0.01	0.91 ± 0.01	0.90 ± 0.02	0.90 ± 0.02	0.90 ± 0.02	0.84 ± 0.04
No. at risk	415	391	325	218	122	68	36
Aortic stenosis (n = 133)							
Overall survival	0.93 ± 0.02	0.91 ± 0.02	0.88 ± 0.03	0.85 ± 0.03	0.83 ± 0.04	0.76 ± 0.06	0.76 ± 0.06
Cardiac death-free survival	0.93 ± 0.02	0.91 ± 0.02	0.88 ± 0.03	0.86 ± 0.03	0.84 ± 0.04	0.76 ± 0.06	0.76 ± 0.06
No. at risk	121	116	80	58	32	12	8
Pulmonic stenosis (n = 192)							
Overall survival	0.95 ± 0.02	0.95 ± 0.02	0.94 ± 0.02	0.94 ± 0.02	0.93 ± 0.02	0.93 ± 0.02	0.90 ± 0.04
Cardiac death-free survival	0.95 ± 0.02	0.95 ± 0.02	0.95 ± 0.02	0.95 ± 0.02	0.94 ± 0.02	0.94 ± 0.02	0.90 ± 0.04
No. at risk	181	172	147	116	98	56	23
Transposition of the great arteries (n = 152)							
Overall survival	0.78 ± 0.03	0.74 ± 0.04	0.69 ± 0.04	0.64 ± 0.04	0.61 ± 0.05	...	...
Cardiac death-free survival	0.78 ± 0.03	0.76 ± 0.04	0.71 ± 0.04	0.67 ± 0.04	0.64 ± 0.05	...	...
No. at risk	118	103	69	36	18	...	...
Patent ductus arteriosus (n = 501)							
Overall survival	1.0	0.99 ± 0.004	0.99 ± 0.005	0.98 ± 0.01	0.98 ± 0.01	0.96 ± 0.01	0.96 ± 0.01
Cardiac death-free survival	1.0	1.0	0.997 ± 0.003	0.995 ± 0.004	0.99 ± 0.004	0.99 ± 0.01	0.99 ± 0.01
No. at risk	473	452	378	281	209	129	79

were no deaths. The mean age at operation was 11 months and during a mean follow-up of 71 months 3 patients have trivial AR which was noted in the immediate postoperative period in 1 and at early follow up in the other 2. All are symptom-free, are taking no medications, and are growing and developing normally. These authors show excellent results for this rare abnormality. Currently diagnosis by echocardiography with color flow mapping is much easier than in the past and these patients should not be misdiagnosed.

Balloon dilatation of restrictive atrial septal defect

Webber and associates[50] from Vancouver, Canada, presented data for balloon dilatation of restrictive atrial defects in 3 patients with complex conditions consisting of pulmonary atresia with intact septum, mitral atresia with intact ventricular septum, and double outlet right ventricle. For various reasons of small left atrium, thickened atrial septum, or inability to manipulate a blade septostomy catheter, these patients were not candidates for standard septostomy procedures. Balloon dilatation of the atrial defect was successfully performed using valvuloplasty catheters ranging from 8 to 18 mm in diameter and 3 cm in length. This procedure is useful for patients in whom standard septostomy techniques are not possible. This includes patients with hypoplastic left heart syndrome and small left atria to whom this technique can be applied.

Balloon dilatation of blalock-taussig "shunts"

Marks and associates[51] from Philadelphia, Pennsylvania and Kingsport, Tennessee, attempted balloon dilation of stenotic standard Blalock-Taussig shunts in 5 patients ages 11 to 67 months with cyanotic heart disease who were becoming progressively cyanotic because of discrete shunt stenosis at the site of the pulmonary anastomosis. Balloon diameters selected were equal to or within 1 mm of the unobstructed proximal shunt diameter. The diameter at the site of stenosis was 3 mm prior to procedure and 6 mm after procedure. The diameter increased in all patients; the mean increase was 3 mm with percentage increase ranging from 80 to 182%. Oxygen saturation increased from 73 to 84% with a satisfactory increase of >5% seen in all patients; the mean increase was 11%. At 6 months follow-up, oxygen saturation by pulse oximetry was 86%. These authors show the potential from prolonging shunt life in patients with stenotic Blalock-Taussig shunts. These authors used large balloon diameters ranging from 250 to 470% of the diameter of the stenosis. They achieved good results without complications. They do not feel that this procedure could be used in modified Blalock-Taussig shunts because of the severe angulation of the shunt. Clearly this can be useful in certain patients and further study of this procedure is indicated in a large number of patients.

Endovascular stents

O'Laughlin and associates[52] from Houston, Texas and Boston, Massachusetts, reported the use of 45 endovascular stents in 30 patients ages .2–30 years of age with congenital heart disease. Stents were mounted over balloons and placed by standard catheterization techniques. PA stenosis was present in 23 patients and 36 stents were placed successfully with reduction of pressure gradients from 51 ± 24 to 16 ± 13 mmHg.

Stents were placed after atrial surgery in 5 patients: 3 in obstructed Fontan repairs, 1 at the superior vena cava-RA junction after sinus venous defect repair, and 1 at the site of a Glenn shunt. Atrial stents reduced pressure gradients from 10 ± 8 to 2 ± 3 mmHg. One patient had a stent placed in the descending aorta after coarctation dilation and the pressure gradient was reduced from 50 to 25 mmHg. One patient had successful dilation of stenotic pulmonary veins but later developed parenchymal pulmonary vein stenosis. Two stents migrated at the time of placement; 1 required surgical removal and 1 was anchored in place by balloon dilation. One patient died within 24 hours because of thrombus obstruction of the Fontan repair. Nine patients had recatheterization and all stented vessels have remained at the same caliber as the original placement. These authors show outstanding results in the early use of endovascular stents in conditions that are difficult to treat by any other methodology. Hopefully this will continue to prove a useful modality for treatment of these very difficult patient problems.

Total cavopulmonary connection in single ventricle

Stein and associates[53] from Los Angeles, California, reported total cavopulmonary connection as a modification of the Fontan procedure and reviewed 38 patients, aged 17 months to 30 years, who underwent this procedure. There were 32 patients with univentricular heart, 2 with pulmonary atresia and intact ventricular septum, 3 with tricuspid atresia, and 1 with hypoplastic left heart syndrome. One or more previous palliative procedures were performed in 34 patients, including 19 shunts, 16 pulmonary artery bandings, 7 atrial septectomies/septostomies, 7 Glenn shunts, and 1 PDA ligation. Preoperative hemodynamics showed a pulmonary artery pressure of 12 with a range of 6 to 22, pulmonary-systemic flow ratios ranging from .4 to 3.0, LV end diastolic pressure from 3 to 15 mmHg and systemic arterial oxygen saturation ranging from 67 to 94%. Concomitant with cavopulmonary connection, 13 patients underwent additional procedures, including 9 atrioventricular valve annuloplasties, 4 Damus-Stansel-Kaye procedures, and 2 resections of subaortic membranes. Modifying the Fontan procedure in this fashion was particularly useful in the management of 2 patients with pulmonary atresia who had right ventricular-dependent coronary blood flow. Cavopulmonary anastomosis and atrial septectomy were performed in both patients, with resultant inflow of oxygenated blood to the right ventricle and coronary arteries. Excellent postoperative results were noted in each. Postextubation hemodynamics for the entire group included a mean right atrial pressure ranging from 11 to 17 mmHg, a left atrial pressure from 3 to 12 mmHg, and a room air oxygen saturation of from 92 to 98%. Seven patients had pleural effusions, 3 required pacemaker placement, and 2 required reoperation for tamponade. One early death occurred in a patient who had intractable ventricular fibrillation 2 days after operation. There was 1 late cardiac death caused by ventricular failure and 1 late noncardiac death. These authors present excellent results for this modification of the Fontan procedure. Adjustable atrial defects were used in 2 patients with elevated PA pressure and appeared to be useful.

Changing patterns of infective endocarditis

Awadallah and associates[54] from Syracuse, New York, reported 48 cases of infective endocarditis occurring in 42 patients with congenital heart disease from 1970 through 1990. These data were compared with a 20 year review of 108 cases diagnosed between 1953 and 1972. The natural history of endocarditis in children has changed over the last 2 decades, with half of the cases occurring now after surgery for congenital heart disease. In the postoperative group, 46% of patients had undergone valve replacement and 7 of these had a RV to PA valve conduit as the site for endocarditis. Among patients with nonsurgically treated heart disease, MVP has emerged as an important underlying heart lesion occurring in 29% of patients. The bacterial spectrum has shifted, with a significant increase in the uncommon causative organisms. The mortality has continued to decline with survivorship of 90% in this series. These authors have 7 patients with MVP who developed endocarditis in childhood. Three of these did not have the diagnosis known prior to the development of endocarditis and 1 additional patient has known MVP without MR. This gives further credence to the use of endocarditis prophylaxis for MVP whether or not MR is present.

Conversion of atrial flutter

Cunningham and associates[55] from London, UK, used intracardiac atrial stimulation protocols in 16 patients presenting on 21 occasions with atrial flutter in association in complex congenital heart disease. Successful conversion to sinus rhythm occurred in 19 of 21 and in the remaining 2 atrial fibrillation was induced with spontaneous conversion to sinus rhythm within 12 hours in 1 patient and immediate DC cardioversion to sinus rhythm in the other. This represents an important modality for this problem which unfortunately remains common in patients following palliation of complex congenital heart disease. Many patients break through medical therapy and require frequent DC cardioversion. This seems a much more kinder and gentler method for treatment of this problem.

References

1. Reybrouck T, Bisschop A, Dumoulin M, van der Hauwaert LG: Cardiorespiratory exercise capacity after surgical closure of atrial septal defect is influenced by the age at surgery. Am Heart J 1991 (October);122:1073–1078.

2. Gembruch U, Knöpfle G, Chatterjee M, Bald R, Redel DA, Födisch H-J, Hansmann M: Prenatal diagnosis of atrioventricular canal malformations with up-to-date echocardiographic technology: report of 14 cases. Am Heart J 1991 (May);121:1489–1497.

3. Kimball TR, Daniels SR, Meyer RA, Hannon DW, Khoury P, Schwartz DC: Relation of symptoms to contractility and defect size in infants with ventricular septal defect. Am J Cardiol (May 15) 1991;67:1097–1102.

4. Kimball TR, Daniels SR, Meyer RA, Hannon DW, Tian J, Skukla R, Schwartz DC: Effect of Digoxin on Contractility and Symptoms in Infants with a Large Ventricular Septal Defect. Am J Cardiol (November 15) 1991;68:1377–1382.

5. Backer CL, Idriss FS, Zales VR, Ilbawi MN, DeLeon SY, Muster AJ, Mavroudis C: Surgical Management of the Conal (Supracristal) Ventricular Septal Defect. J Thorac Cardiovasc Surg (August) 1991;102:288–296.

6. McCrindle BW and Kan JS: Long-term results after balloon pulmonary valvuloplasty. Circulation (June) 1991;83:1915–1922.

7. Di Donato RM, Jonas RA, Lang P, Rome JJ, Mayer JE, Castaneda AR: Neonatal Repair of Tetralogy of Fallot with and without Pulmonary Atresia. J Thorac Cardiovasc Surg (January) 1991;101:126–137.

8. Hofbeck M, Sunnegård JT, Burrows PE, Moes CAF, Lightfoot N, Williams WG, Trusler GA, Freedom RM: Analysis of Survival in Patients with Pulmonic Valve Atresia and Ventricular Septal Defect. Am J Cardiol (April 1) 1991;67:737–743.

9. Qureshi SA, Rosenthal E, Tynan M, Anjos R, Baker EJ: Transcatheter Laser-Assisted Balloon Pulmonary Valve Dilation in Pulmonic Valve Atresia. Am J Cardiol (February) 1991;67:428–431.

10. Iyer KS and Mee RBB: Staged Repair of Pulmonary Atresia with Ventricular Septal Defect and Major Systemic to Pulmonary Artery Collaterals. Ann Thorac Surg (January) 1991;51:65–72.

11. Williams WG, Burrows P, Freedom RM, Trusler GA, Coles JG, Moes CAF, Smallhorn J: Thromboexclusion of the Right Ventricle in Children with Pulmonary Atresia and Intact Ventricular Septum. J Thorac Cardiovasc Surg (February) 1991;101:222–229.

12. Merlo M, De Tommasi SM, Brunelli F, Abbruzzese PA, Crupi G, Ghidoni I, Casari A, Piti A, Mamprin F, Parenzan L: Long-Term Results after Atrial Correction of Complete Transposition of the Great Arteries. Ann Thorac Surg (February) 1991;51:227–231.

13. Bevilacqua M, Sanders SP, Van Praagh S, Colan SD, Parness I: Double-Inlet Single Left Ventricle: Echocardiographic Anatomy with Emphasis on the Morphology of the Atrioventricular Valves and Ventricular Septal Defect. J Am Coll Cardiol (August) 1991;18:559–568.

14. Franklin RCG, Spiegelhalter DJ, Anderson RH, Macartney FJ, Filho RIR, Douglas JM, Rigby ML, Deanfield JE: Double-inlet ventricle presenting in infancy. I. Survival without definitive repair. J Thorac Cardiovasc Surg (May) 1991;101:767–776.

15. Franklin RCG, Spiegelhalter DJ, Anderson RH, Macartney FJ, Filho RIR, Douglas JM, Rigby ML, Deanfield JE: Double-inlet ventricle presenting in infancy. II. Results of palliative operations. J Thorac Cardiovasc Surg (May) 1991;101:917–923.

16. Franklin RCG, Spiegelhalter DJ, Anderson RH, Macartney FJ, Filho RIR, Douglas JM, Rigby ML, Deanfield JE: Double-inlet ventricle presenting in infancy. III. Outcome and potential for definitive repair. J Thorac Cardiovasc Surg (May) 1991;101:924–934.

17. Leung MP, McKay R, Smith A, Anderson RH, Arnold R: Critical Aortic Stenosis in Early Infancy. J Thorac Cardiovasc Surgery (March) 1991;101:526–535.

18. Parsons MK, Moreau GA, Graham TP, Johns JA, Boucek RJ Jr: Echocardiographic Estimation of Critical Left Ventricular Size in Infants with Isolated Aortic Valve Stenosis. J Am Coll Cardiol (October) 1991;18:1049–1055.

19. Beekman RJ, Rocchini AP, Andes A: Balloon Valvuloplasty for Critical Aortic Stenosis in the Newborn: Influence of New Catheter Technology. J Am Coll Cardiol (April) 1991;17:1172–1176.

20. Gerosa G, McKay R, Ross DN: Replacement of the Aortic Valve or Root with a Pulmonary Autograft in Children. Ann Thorac Surg (March) 1991;51:424–429.

21. Suarez de Lezo J, Pan M, Medina A, Romero M, Melian F, Seguar J, Hernandez E, Pavlovic D, Morales J, Vivancos R, Ortego JR: Immediate and Follow-Up of Transluminal Balloon Dilation for Discrete Subaortic Stenosis. J Am Coll Cardiol (November 1) 1991;18:1309–1315.

22. Rychik J, Murdison KA, Chin AJ, Norwood WI: Surgical Management of Severe Aortic Outflow Obstruction in Lesions Other than the Hypoplastic Left Heart Syndrome: Use of a Pulmonary Artery to Aorta Anastomosis. J Am Coll Cardiol (September) 1991;18:809–816.

23. Ilbawi MN, DeLeon SY, Wilson WR, Quinones JA, Roberson DA, Husayni TS, Thilenius OG, Arcilla RA: Advantages of Early Relief of Subaortic Stenosis in Single Ventricle Equivalents. Ann Thorac Surg (October) 1991;52:842–849.

24. Kappetein AP, Gittenberger-De Groot AC, Zwinderman AH, Rohmer J, Poelmann RE, Huysmans HA: The neural crest as a possible pathogenetic factor in coarctation of the aorta and bicuspid aortic valve. J Thorac Cardiovasc Surg 1991 (Dec); 102:830–836.

25. Russell GA, Berry PJ, Watterson K, Dhasmana JP, Wisheart JD: Patterns of Ductal Tissue in Coarctation of the Aorta in the First Three Months of Life. J Thorac Cardiovasc Surg (October) 1991;102:596–601.

26. Hijazi ZM, Fahey JT, Kleinman CS, Hellenbrand WE: Balloon Angioplasty for Recurrent Coarctation of Aorta. Circulation (September) 1991;84:1150–1156.

27. Bobby JJ, Emami JM, Farmer RDT, Newman CGH: Operative survival and 40 year follow-up of surgical repair of aortic coarctation. Br Heart J 1991 (May) 65:271–276.

28. Malan JE, Benatar A, Levin SE: Long-Term Followup of Coarctation of the Aorta Repaired by Patch Angioplasty. Int J Cardiol (January) 1991;30:23–32.

29. Sciolaro C, Copeland J, Cork R, Barkenbush M, Donnerstein R, Goldberg S: Long-term Follow-up Comparing Subclavian Flap Angioplasty to Resection with Modified Oblique End-to-End Anastomosis. J Thorac Cardiovasc Surg (January) 1991;101:1–13.

30. Allan LD, Cook A, Sullivan I, Sharland GK: Hypoplastic left heart syndrome: Effects of fetal echocardiography on birth prevalence. Lancet 1991 (Apr 20);337:959–960.

31. Chang AC, Farrell PE, Murdison KA, Baffa JM, Barber G, Norwood WI, Murphy JD: Hypoplastic Left Heart Syndrome: Hemodynamic and Angiographic Assessment after Initial Reconstructive Surgery and Relevance to Modified Fontan Procedure. J Am Coll Cardiol (April) 1991;17:1143–1149.

32. Stuart AG, Wren C, Sharples PM, Hunter S, Hey EN: Hypoplastic left heart syndrome: more potential transplant recipients than suitable donors. Lancet 1991 (Apr 20);337:957–959.

33. Akagi T, Benson LN, Green M, DeSouza M, Harder JR, Gilday DL, Freedom RM: Ventricular function during supine bicycle exercise in univentricular connection with absent right atrioventricular connection. Am J Cardiol (June 1) 1991;67:1273–1278.

34. Pearl JM, Laks H, Drinkwater, Jr. DC, Milgalter E, Orrini-Ailloni-Charas, Fiacobetti F, George B, Williams R: Repair of Truncus Arteriosus in Infancy. Ann Thorac Surg (October) 1991;52:780–786.

35. Starnes VA, Pitlick PT, Bernstein D, Griffin ML, Choy M, Shumway NE: Ebstein's anomaly appearing in the neonate. J Thorac Cardiovasc Surg (June) 1991;101:1082–1087.

36. Quaegebeur JM, Sreeram N, Fraser AG, Bogers JJC, Stümper OFW, Jess J, Bos E, Sutherland GR: Surgery for Ebstein's Anomaly: The Clinical and Echocardiographic Evaluation of a New Technique. J Am Coll Cardiol (March) 1991;17:722–728.

37. Sharland GK, Chita SK, Allan LD: Tricuspid Valve Dysplasia or Displacement in Intrauterine Life. J Am College Cardiol (March 15) 1991;17:944–949.

38. Hornberger LK, Sahn DJ, Kleinman CS, Copel JA, Reed KL: Tricuspid Valve Disease with Significant Tricuspid Insufficiency in the Fetus: Diagnosis and Outcome. J Am Coll Cardiol (January) 1991;17:167–173.

39. Jureidini SB, Nouri S, Crawford CJ, Chen S, Pennington DG, Fiore A: Reliability of echocardiography in the diagnosis of anomalous origin of the left coronary artery from the pulmonary trunk. Am Heart J 1991 (July);122:61–68.

40. Topaz O, DiSciascio G, Cowley MJ, Soffer A, Lanter P, Goudreau E, Nath AM, Warner M, Vetrovec GW. Absent left main coronary artery: Angiographic findings in 83 patients with separate ostia of the left anterior descending and circumflex arteries at the left aortic sinus. Am Heart J 1991 (August); 122:447–452.

41. Bridges ND, Perry SB, Parness I, Keane JF, Lock JE: Transcatheter Closure of a Large Patent Ductus Arteriosus with the Clamshell Septal Umbrella. J Am Coll Cardiol (November 1) 1991;18:1297–302.

42. Parikh SR, Hurwitz RA, Caldwell RL, Girod DA: Ventricular function in the single ventricle before and after Fontan surgery. Am J Cardiol (June 15) 1991;67:1390–1395.

43. Nakazawa M, Katayama H, Imai Y, Nojima K, Nakanishi T, Kurosawa H, Takao A, Okuda H: A Quantitative Analysis of Hemodynamic Effects of Right Ventricle Included in the Circulation of the Fontan Procedure. Circulation (March) 1991;83:822–826.

44. Frommelt PC, Snider AR, Meliones JN, Vermillon RP: Doppler Assessment of Pulmonary Artery Flow Patterns and Ventricular Function after the Fontan Operation. Am J Cardiol (November 1) 1991;68:1211–1215.

45. Stumper O, Sutherland GR, Geuskens R, Roelandt JRTC, Bos E, Hess J: Transesophageal Echocardiography in Evaluation and Management after a Fontan Procedure. J Am Coll Cardiol (April) 1991;17:1152–1160.

46. Fyfe DA, Kline CH, Sade RM, Greene CA, Gillette PC: The utility of transesophageal echocardiography during and after Fontan operations in small children. Am Heart J 1991 (November); 122:1403–1415.

47. Kürer CC, Tanner CS, Vetter VL: Electrophysiologic Findings after Fontan Repair of Functional Single Ventricle. J Am Coll Cardiol (January) 1991;17:174–181.

48. Morris CD, Menashe VD: 25-year mortality after surgical repair of congenital heart defect in childhood: A population-based cohort study. JAMA 1991 (Dec 25);266:3447–3452.

49. Sreeram N, Franks R, Arnold R, Walsh K: Aortico-Left Ventricular Tunnel: Long-Term Outcome after Surgical Repair. J Am Coll Cardiol (March 15) 1991;17:950–955.

50. Webber SA, Culham JAG, Sandro GGS, Patterson MWH: Balloon dilatation of restrictive interatrial communications in congenital heart disease. Br Heart J (June) 1991;65:346–348.

51. Marks LA, Mehta AV, Marangi D: Percutaneous Transluminal Balloon Angioplasty of Stenotic Standard Blalock-Taussig Shunts: Effects on Choice of Initial Palliation in Cyanotic Congenital Heart Disease. J Am Coll Cardiol (August) 1991;18:546–551.

52. O'Laughlin MP, Perry SB, Lock JE, Mullins CE: Use of endovascular stents in congenital heart disease. Circulation (June) 1991;83:1923–1939.

53. Stein DG, Laks H, Drinkwater DC, Permut LC, Louis HW, Pearl JM, Geroge BL, Williams RG: Results of Total Cavopulmonary Connection in the Treatment of Patients with a Functional Single Ventricle. J Thorac Cardiovasc Surg (August) 1991;102:280–287.

54. Awadallah SM, Kavey R-EW, Byrum CJ, Smith FC, Kveselis DA, Blackman MS: The Changing Pattern of Infective Endocarditis in Childhood. Am J Cardiol (July 1) 1991;68:90–94.

55. Cunningham D, Somerville J, Kennedy JA, Rowland E, Rickards AF: Successful intracardiac electrical conversion of atrial flutter in patients with complex congenital heart disease. Br Heart J (June) 1991;65:349–354.

9

Congestive Heart Failure

History

Braunwald[1] from Boston, Massachusetts, compared key sections of Harrison's classic article in 1935 to current views on CHF expressed in 2 chapters on the subject in the current (12th) edition of *Harrison's Principles of Internal Medicine*, which were prepared by Dr. Braunwald. The 12th edition appeared in 1991. This is an interesting article.

Erythrocyte sedimentation rate

Physicians have long believed that the erythrocyte sedimentation rate is low in patients with CHF, but this concept is based on a misinterpretation of the results in a single report published in 1936. To reevaluate this concept, Haber and associates[2] from New York, New York, measured the sedimentation rate in 242 patients who were referred for treatment of chronic CHF (Figure 9-1). The cause of the CHF was CAD in 142 patients, ideopathic dilated cardiomyopathy in 82 patients and severe MR or AR or both in 18 patients. All 242 patients had a LVEF of <35% as assessed by either echocardiography or radionuclide ventriculography within the previous 12 months. The sedimentation rate was low (<5 mm/hour) in only 24 patients (10%) but was increased (>25 mm/hour) in 50%. Patients with low or normal sedimentation rates (<25 mm per hour) had more severe hemodynamic abnormalities than patients with elevated rates: lower cardiac index (mean ± SEM, 1.7 ± 0.1 vs 2.0 ± 0.1 L/min/m² BSA and higher mean RA pressure (mean ± SEM, 12 ± 1 vs 9 ± 1 mm Hg). New York Heart Association functional class IV symptoms were present in 66% of the patients with a low or normal sedimentation rate, as compared with 42% of those with elevated rates. After 1 to 3 months of therapy, patients whose sedimentation rates decreased showed little hemodynamic or clinical response to treatment, whereas both cardiac perfor-

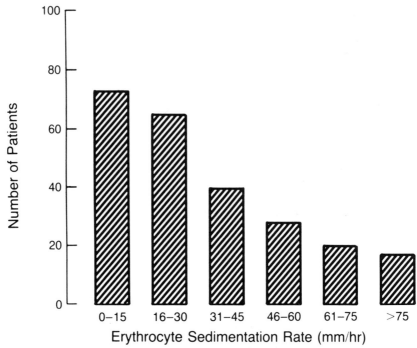

Fig. 9-1. Distribution of values for the Erythrocyte sedimentation rate in all 242 patients with chronic heart failure. The values ranged from 0 to 122 mm per hour (mean, 32; median, 25). Reprinted with permission from Haber, et al.[2]

mance and functional status improved in patients whose rates increased. The sedimentation rate was correlated with the plasma fibrinogen level, and changes in the sedimentation rate during treatment were correlated inversely with changes in mean RA pressure. During long-term follow-up, patients with low or normal sedimentation rates had a worse 1-year survival than patients with elevated rates. These data indicate that the erythrocyte sedimentation rate is correlated with the severity of illness in patients with CHF. Because of its lack of discriminatory power, however, the test is of limited value in the clinical management of this disorder.

Atrial fibrillation

AF is common in advanced CHF, but its prognostic significance is controversial. Middlekauff and colleagues[3] in Los Angeles, California, evaluated the relation of atrial rhythm to overall survival and sudden death in 390 consecutive advanced CHF patients. Etiology of CHF was CAD in 177 patients and nonischemic cardiomyopathy or valvular heart disease in 213 patients. Mean LVEF was 0.19. Seventy-five patients had paroxysmal (26 patients) or chronic (49 patients) AF. Compared with patients with sinus rhythm, patients with AF did not differ in etiology of CHF, mean PA wedge pressure on therapy, or embolic events but were more likely to be receiving warfarin and antiarrhythmic drugs and had a slightly higher LVEF. After a mean follow-up of 236 days, 98 patients died: 56 died suddenly, and 36 died of progressive CHF. Actuarial 1-year overall survival was 68%, and sudden death-free survival was 79%. Actuarial survival was significantly worse for AF than for sinus rhythm patients (52% versus 71%) (Figure 9-2). Similarly, sudden death-free survival was significantly worse for AF than for sinus rhythm patients (69% vs 82%). By Cox pro-

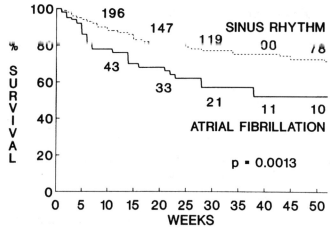

Fig. 9-2. Plots of actuarial 1-year total survival patients with sinus rhythm (n = 315, broken line) compared with those with atrial fibrillation (n = 75, solid line). Numbers along each curve present number of patients at risk. By the Breslow test, survival in atrial fibrillation patients was significantly worse than in sinus rhythm patients (52% vs 71%, p = 0.0013). SEM for sinus rhythm and atrial fibrillation patients' survival, respectively, at 25 weeks ±3% and ±8% and at 50 weeks is ±5% and ±9%. Reprinted with permission from Middlekauff, et al.[3]

portional hazards model, PA wedge pressure on therapy, LVEF, CAD and AF were independent risk factors for total mortality and sudden death. For patients who had PA wedge pressure <16 mm Hg on therapy, AF was associated with poorer 1-year survival (44% vs 83%); however, in the high PA wedge pressure group, AF did not confer an increased risk. (58% vs 57%). AF is a marker for increased risk of death, especially in CHF patients who have lower filling pressures on vasodilator and diuretic therapy. Whether aggressive attempts to maintain sinus rhythm will reduce this risk is unknown.

Ventricular arrhythmias

Spontaneous variability of ventricular arrhythmia in patients with chronic CHF is not well described. Anastasiou-Nana and associates[4] from Salt Lake City, Utah, measured this variability in 23 consecutive patients with chronic CHF who were prospectively enrolled in the placebo limb of a trial concerned with treatment of CHF. Patients underwent from 1 to 3 periods of ambulatory monitoring separated by 1 to 3 months while they were not receiving antiarrhythmic drug treatment. The variability in frequency of VPCs was determined at interrecording intervals of 1, 2, and 3 months. The percentage reduction in total VPCs required to exceed the 95% confidence limits of spontaneous variability at these intervals were 91%, 90%, and 97%, respectively. Corresponding values for repetitive beats (beats in couplets and beats in VT events) were 98%, 80%, and 97%, and for VT events 98%, 83%, and 98%, respectively. The percentage increases in total VPCs, repetitive beats, and VT events required to identify aggravation of arrhythmia in this study population were 1301%, 4050%, and 6147%, respectively, at 1-month intervals and 2950%, 2868%, and 5938%, respectively, at 3-month intervals. The percentage reductions required to show a true drug effect at 2- and 3-month intervals were 63% and 84% for patients with an EF <0.22 and 89% and 98% for those with an EF ≥0.22. Ventricular arrhythmia would have been missed in 6 (26%) of the

23 patients if only 1 screening ambulatory recording was available. Thus marked variability in VPCs occurs in patients with chronic CHF. Suppression must exceed 90% of total VPCs, 80% of repetitive beats, and 83% of VT events at 1 to 3 months after a baseline recording to be confidently considered a true drug effect.

Exercise capability

Cowley and associates[5] studied exercise capability in 39 patients with severe chronic CHF (secondary to CAD in 26 patients, to dilated cardiomyopathy in 5 patients, and to MR and/or AR in 8 patients) in several ways and compared the exercise capability with measurements of cardiac output. The relation between cardiac index and exercise tolerance measured on a treadmill was poor. Exercise tolerance, however, measured with a series of self-paced corridor walk tests showed moderate correlations with cardiac index and customary activity assessed by step counting correlated better with cardiac index. The authors concluded that cardiac output seems to be a factor determining patients' exercise capability when they choose their own walking speed but not when they undergo formal treadmill tests in the laboratory.

Plasma beta-endorphin

Kawashima and associates[6] in Nishinomiya, Japan, measured plasma beta-endorphin levels in 37 patients with CHF and compared them to those 21 age- and gender-matched normal subjects. The relation of plasma beta-endorphin levels and cardiac function at rest and exercise capability was assessed in 17 of the patients with dilated cardiomyopathy. Exercise capacity was determined by symptom-limited maximal treadmill exercise with expired gas analysis. Plasma beta-endorphin levels were elevated and correlated with the patient's New York Heart Association functional cardiac status (Figure 9-3). There was no relationship demonstrated between plasma beta-endorphin levels and LV systolic performance as assessed by M-mode and Doppler echocardiography. There is a good correlation between plasma beta-endorphin levels at rest and exercise capacity. These data show that plasma beta-endorphin levels are elevated in patients with CHF and appear to correlate with the severity of CHF.

Coronary sinus oxygen content

White and colleagues[7] in Montreal and Ottawa, Canada, and San Francisco, California, determined that patients with CHF have abnormal coronary hemodynamics, characterized by decreased coronary sinus oxygen content, increased coronary sinus blood flow, and increased myocardial oxygen consumption. To evaluate their prognostic importance, the clinical characteristics and systemic coronary hemodynamics were related to survival in 91 patients with severe CHF and decreased LVEFs (26 ± 10%). In 69 patients, CHF was due to CAD (group 1) and in 22 it was associated with idiopathic dilated cardiomyopathy (group 2). Five patients were in New York Heart functional class II, 48 in class III and 38 in class IV. The median survival time was 21 months. Coronary sinus oxygen content was most strongly associated with a poor prognosis (Figure 9-4). The low coronary sinus oxygen content was associated with a 2.3-fold increased risk of dying. A low systolic BP and high diastolic PA pressure were also associated with increased mortality. Patients in the subgroup with a low coronary sinus

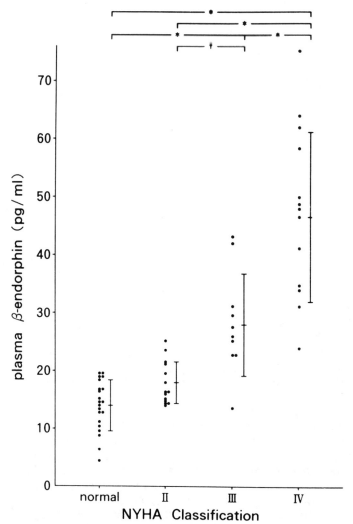

Fig. 9-3. Functional cardiac status (New York Heart Association [NYHA] classification) versus plasma beta-endorphin levels in 21 control subjects and 37 patients with congestive heart failure. The mean ± SD is indicated by the solid bar for each functional class. *p < 0.01; tp < 0.05. Reprinted with permission from Kawashima, et al.[6]

oxygen content had values for functional class, LVEFs and systemic hemo-dynamics similar to those of patients in the subgroup with high coronary sinus oxygen content. Thus, a low coronary sinus oxygen content is indic-ative of noncompensated metabolic demand and suggests a poor prognosis in patients with severe CHF.

TREATMENT

Furosemide

To test the hypothesis that long-term furosemide therapy in patients with CHF is associated with clinically significant thiamine deficiency via urinary loss, Seligmann and associates[8] from Tel Hashomer, Haifa, and

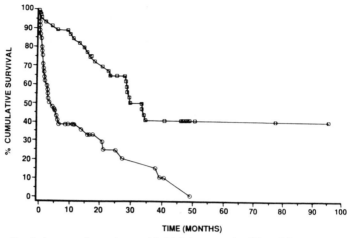

Fig. 9-4. Survival curves for patients with high (>4.44 vol%; ■) and low (≤4.44 vol%; ○) coronary sinus oxygen content (generalized Wilcoxon statistic, p ≤ 0.001). Reprinted with permission from White, et al.[7]

Jerusalem, Israel, studied 23 patients with chronic CHF receiving furo-semide and 16 age-matched control patients without CHF and not taking diuretics. Daily furosemide doses were 80 to 240 mg and duration of furosemide therapy was 3 to 14 months. Patients with identifiable causes of inadequate thiamine intake, absorption, or utilization or increased metabolic requirements were excluded. A 7-day course of intravenous thiamine, 100 mg twice daily, in 6 consenting patients with CHF. A high thiamine pyrophosphate effect (TPPE), indicating thiamine deficiency, was found in 21 of 23 furosemide-treated patients and in 2 of 16 controls. The mean (± SE) TPPE (normal: 0% to 15%) in furosemide-treated and control patients was 28 ± 2% and 7 ± 2%, respectively. Despite the high TPPE, the mean (± SE) urinary thiamine excretion in the furosemide-treated patients (n = 18) was inappropriately high (defined as greater than 130 μg/g creatinine), 410 ± 95 μg/g creatinine, even in comparison with that in the controls (n = 14): 236 ± 69 μg/g creatinine. In 6 patients treated with intravenous thiamine, the elevated TPPE decreased to normal, from a mean (± SE) of 27.0 ± 3.8% to 4.5 ± 1.3%, indicating normal thiamine utilization capacity. LVEF increased in 4 of 5 of these patients studied by echocardiography. These preliminary findings suggest that long-term furosemide therapy may be associated with clinically significant thiamine deficiency due to urinary loss and contribute to impaired cardiac performance in patients with CHF. This deficit may be prevented or corrected by appropriate thiamine supplements.

Digitalis

Digitalis, of course, has been used for treatment of chronic CHF for 215 years. Kulick and Rahimtoola[9] from Los Angeles, California, evaluated numerous clinical studies and trials on the efficacy of digitalis in the treatment of patients with CHF. The data indicate that digitalis is a valu-able therapeutic agent for relieving symptoms and improving exercise performance and LV function in patients with CHF. Comparison of the various advantages and disadvantages of digitalis with alternative ther-apies in patients with CHF shows an important continuing role for dig-italis therapy.

Digoxin is commonly used to treat congestive heart failure. Digoxin augments ventricular systolic performance, but it does not benefit patients whose CHF is caused by poor diastolic function. Forman and associates[10] from Boston, Massachusetts, studied 47 patients aged 65 years or older in 2 urban nursing homes who were receiving long-term digoxin therapy. The LVEF was measured using both a standard and a highly portable echocardiographic machine. Thirty-five of 47 patients had a normal EF (>50%). In this subgroup, 23 patients were in normal sinus rhythm. Digoxin was discontinued in 14 patients with good systolic function and normal sinus rhythm, but in 9 cases physicians refused to stop the digoxin. Follow-up evaluations showed no deterioration off digoxin. Excellent correlations existed between estimated LVEF from the 2 echocardiography machines. Many nursing home patients taking digoxin do not need it. Physician reluctance to discontinue digoxin may change with the availability of highly portable echocardiography.

Hickey and colleagues[11] in the Research Triangle Park, Durham, Winston-Salem, North Carolina, Denver, Colorado, and Boston, Massachusetts, performed an observational surveillance study to monitor the safety and effectiveness of treatment with Digoxin Immune Fab (Ovine) (Digibind) in patients with digitalis intoxication. Before April 1986, a relatively limited number of patients received treatment with digoxin-specific Fab fragments through a multi-center clinical trial. Beginning with its commercial availability in July, 1986, this study evaluated additional, voluntarily reported clinical data pertinent to treatment through a 3 week follow-up. The study included 717 adults who received Digoxin Immune Fab (Ovine). Most patients were ≥70 years of age and developed toxicity during maintenance dosing with digoxin. Fifty percent of patients were reported to have a complete response to treatment, 24% a partial response and 12% no response. The response for 14% of patients was not reported or was reported as uncertain. Six patients (0.8%) had an allergic reaction to digoxin-specific antibody fragments. Three of the six had a history of allergy to antibiotics. Twenty patients (2.8%) developed recrudescent toxicity. The risk of recrudescent toxicity increased by sixfold when <50% of the estimated dose of the antibody had been given. In 215 patients, there were posttreatment adverse events. The events for 76% of these patients were judged to result from manifestations of underlying disease and therefore were considered unrelated to Fab treatment. Thus, digoxin-specific antibody fragments were generally well tolerated and clinically effective in patients judged by treating physicians to have potentially life-threatening digitalis intoxication.

Enalapril

Patients with CHF have a high mortality rate and are also hospitalized frequently. The SOLVD Investigators[12] studied the effect of the angiotensin-converting-enzyme inhibitor, enalapril, on mortality and hospitalization in patients with chronic CHF and EF ≤0.35. Patients receiving conventional treatment for CHF were randomly assigned to receive either placebo (n = 1284) or enalapril (n = 1285) at doses of 2.5 to 20 mg per day in a double-blind trial. Approximately 90% of the patients were in New York Heart Association functional classes II and III. The follow-up averaged 41.4 months. There were 510 deaths in the placebo group (40%), as compared with 452 in the enalapril group (35%) (reduction in risk, 16%) (Figure 9-5). Although reductions in mortality were observed in several categories of cardiac deaths, the largest reduction occurred among

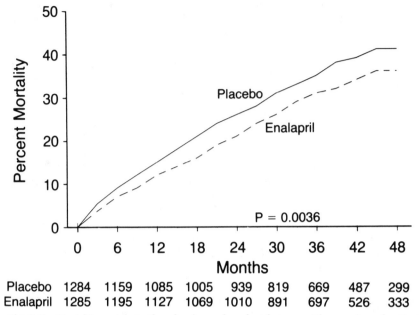

Fig. 9-5. Mortality curves in the placebo and enalapril groups. The number of patients alive in each group at the end of each period are shown at the bottom of the figure. P = 0.0036 for the comparison between groups by the log-rank test. Reprinted with permission from New England Journal of Medicine.[12]

the deaths attributed to progressive CHF (251 in the placebo group vs 209 in the enalapril group; reduction in risk, 22%) (Figure 9-6). There was little apparent effect of treatment on deaths classified as due to arrhythmia without pump failure. Fewer patients died or were hospitalized for worsening heart failure (736 in the placebo group and 613 in the enalapril group; risk reduction, 26%). The addition of enalapril to conventional therapy significantly reduced mortality and hospitalizations for CHF in patients with chronic CHF and low EF.

Studies of Left Ventricular Dysfunction (SOLVD) is a randomized trial of enalapril versus placebo in reducing mortality in patients with LVEF ≤35%.[13] Before administration, patients at risk for hypotension were hospitalized for a test dose of 2.5 mg of enalapril administered orally at baseline and again 12 hours later. As of February 1989, 89 of 7,539 (1.2%) patients had been studied during hospitalization. Baseline systolic and diastolic BP were 115 ± 18 and 73 ± 10 mm Hg, respectively. After enalapril, systolic BP decreased slightly but significantly 8 to 20 hours after the initial dose (mean reduction 8 to 11 mm Hg). It is emphasized that most patients with cardiac dysfunction readily tolerate enalapril. However, the agent should be administered with caution to patients with advanced CHF and diminished baseline BP, owing to a significant incidence of symptomatic hypotension.

Enalapril vs digoxin

Davies and associates[14] in Ottawa, Canada, conducted a randomized control trial comparing enalapril (n = 72) and digoxin (n = 73) in patients with New York Heart Association functional classification II or III CHF who had been stabilized on furosemide therapy. End points were clinical outcome, exercise capacity, and echocardiographic LV dimension. Im-

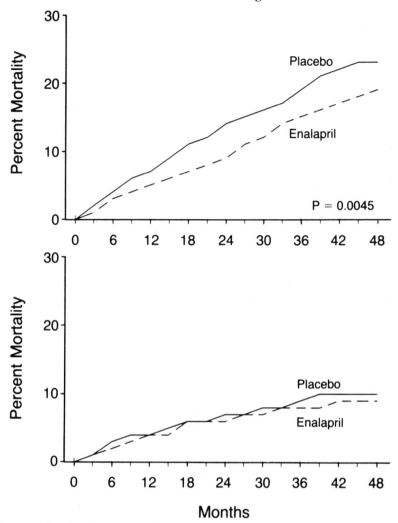

Fig. 9-6. Mortality due to progressive heart failure (upper panel) (P = 0.0045) and presumed to be due to an arrhythmia but not preceded by worsening congestive heart failure (lower panel) (P not significant). Reprinted with permission from New England Journal of Medicine.[12]

provement in clinical outcome was defined as a reduction of at least one functional class, and deterioration as an increase of at least one functional class or withdrawal because of an adverse clinical event. After 4 weeks, 13 patients treated with enalapril showed improvement; 55 had no change and 9 had deteriorated as compared with 7, 49 and 17, respectively in the digoxin treated group. After 14 weeks, 13 patients receiving enalapril showed improvement, 50 had not changed and 9 had deteriorated compared with 14, 37 and 22, respectively in the digoxin treated group. Most patients in the digoxin group were withdrawn because of an adverse clinical event. Exercise time and percent fractional shortening improved in both groups with no significant difference between groups. Both rate-pressure product and subjectively evaluated exertion during submaximal exercise were reduced only in the enalapril group. Most patients receiving enalapril experienced fewer adverse clinical events and had less fatigue during submaximal exercise. Thus, this study suggests that afterload reduction with enalapril is a very good alternative treatment to digoxin in patients with class II or III CHF. In some patients, it may be superior.

Enalapril vs hydralazine isosorbide dinitrate

To define better the efficacy of vasodilator therapy in the treatment of chronic CHF, Cohn and associates[15] of the Vasodilator-Heart Failure Veterans Affairs Cooperative Study Group compared the effects of hydralazine and isosorbide dinitrate with those of enalapril in 804 men receiving digoxin and diuretic therapy for CHF. The patients were randomly assigned in a double-blind manner to receive 20 mg of enalapril daily or 300 mg of hydralazine plus 160 mg of isosorbide dinitrate daily. The latter regimen was identical to that used with a similar patient population in the effective-treatment arm of the previous Vasodilator—Heart Failure Trial. Mortality after 2 years was significantly lower in the enalapril arm (18%) than in the hydralazine-isosorbide dinitrate arm (25%), and overall mortality tended to be lower (Figure 9-7). The lower mortality in the enalapril arm was attributable to a reduction in the incidence of sudden death, and this beneficial effect was more prominent in patients with less severe symptoms (New York Heart Association class I or II). In contrast, body oxygen consumption at peak exercise was increased only by hydralazine-isosorbide dinitrate treatment, and LVEF, which increased

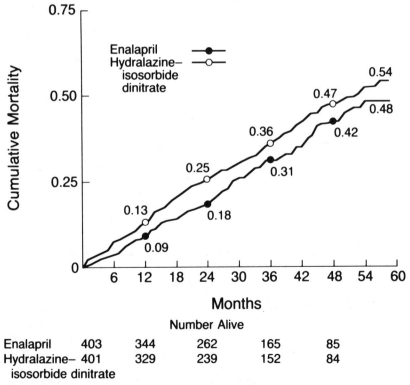

Fig. 9-7. Cumulative mortality in the enalapril and hydralazine-isosorbide dinitrate treatment arms over the entire follow-up period. Cumulative mortality rates are shown after each 12-month period. For comparison of the treatment arms after two years and overall, P = 0.016 and P = 0.08, respectively (log-rank test). The number of patients alive after each year is shown below the graph. Reprinted with permission from Cohn, et al.[15]

with both regimens during the 2 years after randomization, increased more during the first 13 weeks in the hydralazine-isosorbide dinitrate group (Figure 9-8). The similar 2-year mortality in the hydralazine isosorbide dinitrate arms in our previous Vasodilator-Heart Failure Trial (26%) and in the present trial (25%), as compared with that in the placebo arm in the previous trial (34%), and the further survival benefit with enalapril in the present trial (18%) strengthen the conclusion that vasodilator therapy should be included in the standard treatment for CHF. The different effects of the 2 regimens (enalapril and hydralazine-isosorbide dinitrate) on mortality and physiologic end points suggest that the profile of effects might be enhanced if the regimens were used in combination.

This article was followed by an editorial entitled "Ace Inhibitors—A Cornerstone of the Treatment of Heart Failure" by Eugene Braunwald[16] from Boston, Massachusetts. Braunwald emphasized that these 2 new trials (SOLVD and V-HeFT II) have now shown benefit from therapy with 1 or more vasodilators. On the basis of the consistent results in these independent, well conducted trials, vasodilators can now be considered 1 of the 3 cornerstones of the pharmacologic treatment of CHF, the others being cardiac glycosides and diuretic agents. Indeed, this relatively new form of treatment rests on much firmer ground than do the other 2, much older cornerstones, whose value in prolonging survival in CHF has still not been clearly established. A randomized, placebo-controlled trial that is just beginning should clarify the effects on mortality of adding digoxin to a regimen of diuretic agents and ACE inhibitors. Braunwald further states, "Since ACE inhibitors are beneficial both hemodynamically and clinically in severe CHF and since they prolong survival in mild, moderate, and severe chronic CHF, the question naturally arises whether they are also indicated in patients with heart disease and LV dysfunction who do not have overt CHF. Although this possibility is intriguing, it

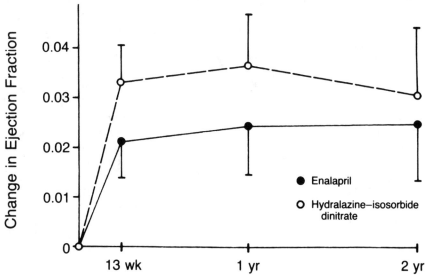

Fig. 9-8. Mean change from base line in left ventricular ejection fraction over the first two years of the study in each treatment arm. Vertical bars represent 95 percent confidence intervals. The crease after the first 13 weeks in the hydralazine-isosorbide dinitrate arm was greater than in the enalapril arm (P < 0.05). Reprinted with permission from Cohn, et al.[15]

would be inappropriate at this time to extend the results of trials conducted in patients with CHF to those without this condition. It will be another 7 years before the role of ACE inhibitors in the prevention and treatment of ventricular dysfunction, with or without accompanying CHF, will have been clearly delineated."

Cilazapril

In an investigation by Kiowski and associates[17] from Basel, Switzerland, the effects of angiotensin converting enzyme inhibition on systemic and coronary hemodynamics and on myocardial lactate metabolism were investigated before and 2 and 6 hours after *cilazapril* at rest and during supine submaximal exercise in 10 patients with New York Heart Association class II or III chronic CHF. Angiotensin converting enzyme inhibition, indicated by a significant increase in plasma renin activity, resulted in significant reductions in BP and systemic vascular resistance. Myocardial oxygen demand decreased (resting double product), but coronary sinus blood flow remained unchanged and calculated coronary resistance decreased suggesting coronary vasodilatation. Changes in coronary vascular resistance were directly related to changes in systemic vascular resistance. Myocardial lactate extraction increased at rest and during exercise both in patients with CAD (n = 5) and idiopathic dilated cardiomyopathy (n = 5). Resting lactate production was converted to lactate extraction in 2 patients with CAD. Neither plasma catecholamine nor atrial natriuretic peptide concentrations changed significantly. These results suggest coronary vasodilation and improved aerobic myocardial metabolism by angiotensin converting enzyme inhibition in patients with CHF.

Bucindolol

Woodley and co-workers[18] in Salt Lake City, Utah, investigated the effects of bucindolol, a nonselective, non ISA B-blocker with mild vasodilatory properties, in patients with CAD from ischemic dilated cardiomyopathy and compared the results with those in subjects with CHF from idiopathic dilated cardiomyopathy. Patients were randomized in a double-blind fashion to receive 12 weeks treatment with either bucindolol or placebo, with randomization stratified for idiopathic or ischemic cardiomyopathy. Invasive (right heart catheterization) and noninvasive (echo, MUGA < central venous norepinephrine, exercise treadmill studies, and symptom scores) tests of CHF severity were determined at baseline and end of the study. For all subjects relative to placebo treatment, bucindolol-related patients had significant improvement in EF, LV size and filling pressure, stroke work index, symptom score, and central venous norepinephrine. However, most of these differences could be attributed to improvement in the idiopathic cardiomyopathy subgroup, as the only parameter with a statistically significant degree of improvement in the bucindolol-treated ischemic cardiomyopathy subgroup was LV size. The investigators concluded that B-blockade may produce quantitatively different degrees of response in different kinds of heart muscle disease.

Isosorbide dinitrate

Early development of nitrate tolerance has been shown in patients with CHF receiving continuous nitroglycerin therapy. The influence of dosing interval of oral isosorbide dinitrate, the nitrate preparation most widely used for the treatment of CHF, has not been investigated. Elkayam and coworkers[19] in Los Angeles, California, performed a prospective, randomized study to evaluate the effect of various regimens of oral Isosorbide dinitrate on the development of early tolerance to its effect on LV filling pressure in patients with moderate to severe CHF. Forty-four responders were divided into 4 groups of 11 patients each, and randomized to receive their effective isosorbide dinitrate dose (40–120 mg) every 4 hours, every 6 hours, every 8 hours, or 3 times daily. All groups demonstrated a significant and comparable reduction in LV filling pressure following administration of the first isosorbide dinitrate dose. Early attenuation of hemodynamic response was demonstrated with frequent dosing (every 4 hours and every 6 hours) of isosorbide dinitrate. Tolerance was prevented with a Q 8-hour regimen as demonstrated by preserved hemodynamic response to each dose. The effect of each dose, however, was short-term, with return of pulmonary artery wedge pressure to baseline level at 2 to 4 hours, resulting in an intermittent effect totaling no longer than 12 hours of the 30-hour study period. The use of a three times daily regimen resulted in marked attenuation of response after the third dose with complete restoration of nitrate effect following a 12-hour washout period between the third and fourth doses. These data demonstrate the development of tolerance and early attenuation of effect on LV filling pressure with frequent oral dosing (every 4 and every 6 hours) with Isosorbide dinitrate in patients with chronic CHF, which may be related to persistently elevated trough blood levels of isosorbide dinitrate. The development of tolerance can be reversed after a washout period of 12 hours and can be prevented with a Q 8-hour administration. These regimens, however, are limited by an inconsistent effect. Although long-term implications of these findings need further clarification, the present study demonstrates the difficulty of maintaining a persistent isosorbide dinitrate-mediated reduction in LV filling pressure in patients with chronic, moderate to severe CHF. These results suggest the need to use intermittent isosorbide dinitrate therapy during a daily nitrate washout interval and the rationale for combined vasodilator therapy in patients with CHF.

Dobutamine

Parker and colleagues[20] in Boston, Massachusetts, tested the hypothesis that B-adrenergic receptor-stimulated acceleration of LV isovolumic relaxation is attenuated in patients with severe CHF compared with patients without LV dysfunction or CHF. The B-adrenergic agonist dobutamine was infused by the intracoronary route in 14 subjects (normal group 6; CHF patients, 8) and by the intravenous route in a second group of 14 subjects (normal group, 4; CHF patients, 10). The positive inotropic response to intracoronary or intravenous dobutamine was substantially and significantly reduced in the patients with CHF. LV isovolumic relaxation assessed by all three methods was significantly prolonged in CHF patients compared with normal subjects. Intracoronary and intravenous infusions of dobutamine caused significant acceleration of LV isovolumic relaxation in both normal subjects and patients with CHF. The magnitude of the dobutamine-stimulated acceleration of isovolumic relaxation in patients with CHF was comparable with that in normal subjects. These data demonstrate that B-adrenergic receptor stimulation causes significant acceleration of LV isovolumic relaxation in both normal subjects and patients with severe CHF. Contrary to the investigators hypothesis, the lusitropic response to B-adrenergic stimulation is well preserved in patients with severe CHF despite substantial attenuation of the B-adrenergic positive inotropic response. These findings have potentially important implications regarding the physiology and pharmacology of adrenergically mediated LV relaxation in humans.

Dopexamine

Gollub and colleagues[21] in Kansas City, Kansas, Los Angeles, California, Houston, Texas, and Saint Louis, Missouri, studied the effects of dopexamine hydrochloride a new synthetic catecholamine that provides a unique profile of adrenergic and dopaminergic activity. This multicenter, parallel design, placebo-controlled study, included 45 patients with functional class III or IV chronic CHF randomized to receive a placebo or one of three different doses of dopexamine. After a 2 hour dose titration sequence, patients received a 6 hour constant dose infusion. During this 6 hour period, dopexamine was infused at rates of 1, 2, and 4 µg/kg body weight/minute. In patients receiving the higher infusion rate, dopexamine produced a 78% increase in cardiac index and a 43% decrease in SVR and 24% in heart rate. There was a trend toward a moderate increase in cardiac index at low and intermediate doses. In patients randomized to receive dopexamine, RA, systemic arterial, PA, and PA wedge pressures showed minimal changes from baseline. Few patients developed adverse reactions related to dopexamine, although five patients randomized to receive high dose and 3 patients randomized to receive intermediate dose dopexamine required dose reduction because hemodynamic variables exceeded arbitrary safe limits or the patients developed symptoms. Thus, dopexamine in higher doses effectively increases cardiac index and reduces systemic vascular resistance and may be useful in the short-term treatment of patients with severe CHF.

Enoximone

In a parallel study design, 164 patients with New York Heart Association Functional class II or III CHF were randomized to receive either enoximone given as 50 mg 3 times a day, or 100 mg 3 times a day, or a matching placebo, in an investigation carried out by Narahara[22] from Torrance, California, and the Western Enoximone Study Group. All patients were receiving digitalis and/or diuretics and had LVEF ≤45. Exercise tests were performed after 1, 4, 8, and 12 weeks of treatment. Enoximone produced significantly greater increases in exercise time than placebo treatment at weeks 4 and 8 but not after 12 weeks. LVEF increased significantly after the first dose of enoximone but not after 12 weeks of long-term therapy. Heart failure symptoms and the physicians' evaluations of cardiac status were significantly improved in both enoximone therapy groups during the first 4 weeks of evaluation when compared with evaluations of cardiac status in the placebo group. Diuretic doses were increased more frequently for patients who were receiving a placebo. Adverse events were reported with similar frequency in the placebo and 50 mg enoximone treatment groups; 100 mg enoximone resulted in a significantly greater incidence of adverse events. Mean heart rate and ventricular ectopic activity were not different among the 3 treatment regimens. Enoximone appears to improve exercise tolerance, ventricular function, and symptoms of CHF for 4 to 8 weeks. Heart rate, ventricular ectopic activity, and mortality rate were not increased. Enoximone, in a dosage of 50 mg 3 times a day was well tolerated and may be a useful short-term therapy for patients with chronic CHF.

Pimobendan

In an investigation reported by Hagemeijer[23] from Rotterdam, The Netherlands, in 25 patients whose chronic CHF had recently worsened to New York Heart Association class IV, pimobendan (5 to 20 mg/day), a new phosphodiesterase inhibitor, was added to maximum conventional therapy consisting of digoxin, diuretics, angiotensin-converting enzyme inhibitors, coumadin derivatives to prevent thromboembolic complications, and amiodarone to suppress serious ventricular rhythm disturbances. CHF was fatal in <1 month in 5 patients (2 had shown some initial improvement). The other 20 had sustained improvement by ≥1 functional class, interrupted by episodes of CHF that usually responded to intravenous therapy. Median survival was 12 months (range 10 days to >3 years); 5 patients died suddenly, 12 died of intractable CHF, and 2 died of other causes. Six patients were alive 3 years after the onset of treatment with pimobendan. Add-on therapy with pimobendan produced a sustained improvement in many patients with severe CHF that was no longer responding to a combination of digoxin, diuretics, and angiotensin-converting enzyme inhibitors.

Mexiletine vs quinidine

Mexiletine and quinidine are often administered to patients with severe CHF, but their hemodynamic effects have not been adequately studied in these individuals. In a randomized, crossover study carried out by Gottlieb and Weinberg[24] from Baltimore, Maryland, the hemodynamic responses to single oral doses of quinidine (600 mg) and mexiletine (400 mg) were compared in 20 patients with marked LV dysfunction. Quinidine predominantly caused vasodilation, with mean arterial, LV filling, and RA pressures all decreasing (-7 ± 2, -2.3 ± 1.0, and -1.1 ± 0.5 mm Hg, respectively) and the systemic vascular resistance also declining (-308 ± 84 dynes·sec·cm^5). In contrast, the systemic vascular resistance increased (314 ± 84 dynes·sec·cm^{-5}) and the mean arterial, LV filling, and RA pressures also increased ($+2 \pm 2$, $+6.1 \pm 1.8$, and $+1.8 \pm 0.6$ mm Hg, respectively) after mexiletine. Cardiac performance declined with mexiletine (cardiac and stroke work indexes decreasing -0.3 ± 0.1 L/min/m^2 and -5 ± 1 gm·m/m^2, respectively), but there was no significant change in cardiac or stroke work indexes with quinidine. The response to the 2 agents significantly differed for all parameters measured. These hemodynamic changes were accompanied by clinical effects. Mexiletine induced increased dyspnea in 5 patients and quinidine led to symptomatic hypotension in 2 patients. Plasma concentrations of mexiletine and serum concentrations of quinidine were within or below the therapeutic range in all patients. In conclusion, mexiletine and quinidine exert different hemodynamic effects when given to patients with severe CHF. Mexiletine is more likely than quinidine to cause exacerbation of heart failure, and quinidine is more likely to provoke hypotension.

Amiodarone

Sudden cardiac death is a common cause of mortality in patients with CHF. To determine if low-dose amiodarone could reduce sudden death among these patients, a prospective, placebo-controlled, double-blind pilot trial was conducted by Nicklas and associates from Ann Arbor, Michigan, and London, UK.[25] One hundred and one patients with ejection fractions <30%, New York Heart Association class III or IV symptoms, and frequent but asymptomatic spontaneous ventricular ectopy (Lown class II to V) were randomly assigned to treatment with low-dose amiodarone (400 mg/day for 4 weeks and then 200 mg/day) or placebo. Mean follow-up was 357 days (range 4 to 1009 days). Side effects were infrequent and there was no difference in the incidence of side effects between the treatment groups. The frequency of spontaneous ventricular ectopy in the group receiving amiodarone fell from 4992 ± 1240 beats/24 hours at baseline to 1135 ± 494 beats/24 hours after 1 month of treatment and remained low after 6 months, while there was no change in ventricular ectopy among the patients receiving placebo. Despite the reduction in ectopy, there was no improvement in mortality or decrease in the incidence of sudden death. One-year mortality by Kaplan-Meier analysis was 28% in the group receiving amiodarone and not significantly different at 19% in the group receiving placebo. One-year mortality in patients with >75% reduction in ventricular ectopy after 1 month of treatment was not significantly different at 31% versus 17% in patients with ≤75% ectopic suppression. Although the size of the trial and its statistical power do not eliminate the possibility of a significant reduction in mortality with low-dose amiodarone, any effect is likely to be modest. Therefore, low-dose amiodarone can be safely administered to patients with severely impaired myocardial function and will significantly suppress spontaneous ventricular ectopy. However, despite arrhythmia suppression, low-dose amiodarone may not reduce or may have only a modest effect on the incidence of sudden death in patients with CHF and asymptomatic ventricular ectopy.

References

1. Braunwald E: "The pathogenesis of congestive heart failure": Then and now. Medicine 1991;70:68–81.
2. Haber HL, Leavy JA, Kessler PD, Kukin ML, Gottlieb SS, Packer M: The erythrocyte sedimentation rate in congestive heart failure. N Engl J Med 1991 (Feb 7);324:353–358.
3. Middlekauff HR, Stevenson WG, and Stevenson LW: Prognostic Significance of Atrial Fibrillation in Advanced Heart Failure—A Study of 390 Patients. Circulation 1991 (July);84:40–48.
4. Anastasiou-Nana MI, Menlove RL, Nanas JN, Mason JW: Spontaneous variability of ventricular arrhythmias in patients with chronic heart failure. Am Heart J 1991 (October);122:1007–1015.
5. Cowley AJ, Fullwood LJ, Muller AF, Stainer K, Skene AM, Hampton JR: Exercise capability in heart failure: Is cardiac output important after all? Lancet 1991 (Mar 30);337:771–773.
6. Kawashima S, Fukutake N, Nishian K, Asakuma S, Iwasaki T: Elevated plasma beta-endorphin levels in patients with congestive heart failure. J Am Coll Cardiol 1991 (January);17:53–8.
7. White M, Rouleau JL, Ruddy TD, de Marco T, Moher D, Chatterjee K: Decreased coronary sinus oxygen content: a predictor of adverse prognosis in patients with severe congestive heart failure. J Am Coll Cardiol 1991 (December);18:1631–7.
8. Seligmann H, Halkin H, Rauchfleisch Shmuel, Kaufmann N, Tal R, Motro M, Vered Z, Ezra D: Thiamine deficiency in patients with congestive heart failure receiving long-term furosemide therapy: A pilot study. Am J Med 1991 (Aug);91:151–155.
9. Kulick DL, Rahimtoola SH: Current role of digitalis therapy in patients with congestive heart failure. JAMA 1991 (June 12);265:2995–2997.

10. Forman DE, Coletta D, Kenny D, Kosowsky BD, Stoukides J, Rohrer M, Pastore JO: Clinical issues related to discontinuing digoxin therapy in elderly nursing home patients. Arch Intern Med 1991 (Nov);151:2194–2198.

11. Hickey AR, Wenger TL, Carpenter VP, Tilson HH, Hlatky MA, Furberg CD, Kirkpatrick CH, Strauss HC, Smith TW: Digoxin immune fab therapy in the management of digitalis intoxication: safety and efficacy results of an observational surveillance study. J Am Coll Cardiol 1991 (March);17:590–8.

12. SOLVD Investigators: Effect of enalapril on survival in patients with reduced left ventricular ejection fractions and congestive heart failure. N Engl J Med 1991 (Aug 1);325:293–302.

13. Hood WB Jr, Youngblood M, Ghali JK, Reid M, Rogers WJ, Howe D, Teo KK, Lejemtel TH: Initial blood pressure response to enalapril in hospitalized patients (Studies of Left Ventricular Dysfunction [SOLVD]). Am J Cardiol 1991 (Dec 1);68:1465–1468.

14. Davies RF, Beanlands DS, Nadeau C, Phaneuf D, Morris A, Arnold JM, Parker JO, Baigrie R, Latour P, Klinke P, Bernstein V, Leblanc M, Mizgala H, Stevens A, Boisvert G, for the Canadian Enalapril Versus Digoxin Study Group: Enalapril versus digoxin in patients with congestive heart failure: a multi-center study. J Am Coll Cardiol 1991 (December);18:1602–9.

15. Cohn JN, Johnson G, Ziesche S, Cobb F, Francis G, Tristani F, Smith R, Dunkman WB, Loeb H, Wong M, Bhat G, Goldman S, Fletcher RD, Doherty J, Hughes CV, Carson P, Cintron G, Shabetai R, Haakenson C: A comparison of enalapril with hydralazine-isosorbide dinitrate in the treatment of chronic congestive heart failure. N Engl J Med 1991 (Aug 1);325:303–310.

16. Braunwald E: ACE inhibitors—a cornerstone of the treatment of heart failure. N Engl J Med 1991 (Aug 1);325:351–353.

17. Kiowski W, Zuber M, Elsasser S, Erne P, Pfisterer M, Burkart F: Coronary vasodilation and improved myocardial lactate metabolism after angiotensin converting enzyme inhibition with cilazapril in patients with congestive heart failure. Am Heart J 1991 (November);122:1382–1388.

18. Woodley SL, Gilbert EM, Anderson JL, O'Connell JB, Deitchman D, Yanowitz FG, Mealey PC, Volkman K, Renlund DG, Menlove R, Bristow M: B-Blockade With Bucindolol in Heart Failure Caused by Ischemic Versus Idiopathic Dilated Cardiomyopathy. Circulation 1991 (December);84:2426–2441.

19. Elkayam U, Roth A, Mehra A, Ostrzega E, Shotan A, Kulick D, Jamison M, Johnson JV and Rahimtoola SH: Randomized Study to Evaluate the Relation Between Oral Isosorbide Dinitrate Dosing Interval and the Development of Early Tolerance to Its Effect on Left Ventricular Filling Pressure in Patients With Chronic Heart Failure. Circulation 1991 (November)84;2040–2048.

20. Parker JD, Landzberg JS, Bittl JA, Mirsky I, and Colucci WS: Effects of B-Adrenergic Stimulation With Dobutamine on Isovolumic Relaxation in the Normal and Failing Human Left Ventricle. Circulation 1991 (September);84:1040–1048.

21. Gollub SB, Elkayam U, Young JB, Miller LW, Haffey KA, for the Dopexamine Investigators and Their Associates: Efficacy and safety of a short-term (6-h) intravenous infusion of dopexamine in patients with severe congestive heart failure: A randomized, double-blind, parallel, placebo-controlled multicenter study. J Am Coll Cardiol 1991 (August);18:383–90.

22. Narahara KA, and the Western Enoximone Study Group: Oral enoximone therapy in chronic heart failure: A placebo-controlled randomized trial. Am Heart J 1991 (May);121:1471–1479.

23. Hagemeijer F: Intractable heart failure despite angiotensin-converting enzyme inhibitors, digoxin, and diuretics: Long-term effectiveness of add-on therapy with pimobendan. Am Heart J 1991 (August);122:517–522.

24. Gottlieb SS, Weinberg M: Comparative hemodynamic effects of mexiletine and quinidine in patients with severe left ventricular dysfunction. Am Heart J 1991 (November);122:1368–1374.

25. Nicklas JM, McKenna WJ, Stewart RA, Mickelson JK, Das SK, Schork MA, Krikler SJ, Quain LA, Morady F, Pitt B: Prospective, double-blind, placebo-controlled trial of low-dose amiodarone in patients with severe heart failure and asymptomatic frequent ventricular ectopy. Am Heart J 1991 (October);122:1016–1021.

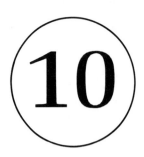

Miscellaneous Topics

Effusion

During the past 20 years only a few studies have been published concerning large pericardial effusions. Ilan and associates[1] from Jerusalem, Israel, reviewed 34 patients who presented with large pericardial effusions not associated with trauma. Their analysis revealed that 52% had pericardial effusion of unknown origin. Four patients had postmyocardial infarction pericardial effusion, 3 had associated malignant neoplasms, 3 suffered from collagen diseases, and 2 had infectious agents. Uremia and irradiation accounted for a single case each. Twenty-seven (79%) of the patients underwent pericardiocentesis and 2 (6%) had a pericardial window operation. The overall prognosis of the patients was excellent.

Tamponade

Levine and associates[2] in Boston, Massachusetts, used two-dimensional echocardiography to study 50 consecutive medical patients who were identified by echocardiography to have probable tamponade as evidenced by the presence of right heart chamber collapse in the presence of pericardial effusion and who underwent combined right heart cardiac catheterization and percutaneous pericardiocentesis. All patients had elevated pericardial pressures. However, many had minimal evidence of hemodynamic compromise, including 94% with systolic pressures ≥100 mm Hg and 58% with a cardiac index ≥2.3 liters/min per m². Pericardiocentesis resulted in hemodynamic improvement, but frequently did not alleviate dyspnea or correct tachycardia. Patients with malignancy as the cause of tamponade had a high mortality rate (Figure 10-1). Thus, echocardiography assisted diagnosis of pericardial tamponade in medical patients results in the identification of a substantial subset of patients with only subtle evidence of hemodynamic compromise. This subset of patients differs sharply from medical patients described in previous reports with classic tamponade. The natural history and the optimal management strategy for this group are not resolved.

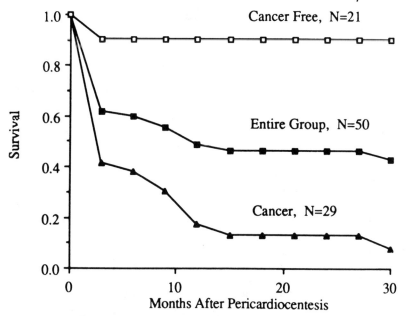

Fig. 10-1. Cumulative probability of survival after pericardiocentris in 50 cases of cardiac tamponade. Reprinted with permission from Levine, et al.[2]

Cardiac tamponade after cardiac surgical procedures is often associated with hemodynamically significant localized pericardial effusions. The localized collection of pericardial effusion in the postoperative period and the atypical presentation of cardiac tamponade limit the use of conventional clinical and echocardiographic signs usually seen with a circumferential pericardial effusion. Observation of LV diastolic collapse in the echocardiogram of a patient with postoperative regional cardiac tamponade prompted Chuttani and colleagues[3] in Boston, Massachusetts, to explore the frequency of this sign in regional cardiac tamponade. The investigators retrospectively analyzed the echocardiograms of 18 patients with postoperative cardiac tamponade for the following echocardiographic findings: RA collapse, RV diastolic collapse, LA collapse, and LV diastolic collapse. Three of the 18 patients had circumferential pericardial effusion, and 15 had loculated pericardial effusion; in 10, the effusion was predominantly posterior, and in the other 5, it was extended laterally or inferiorly. The conventional echocardiographic signs of cardiac tamponade such as RA collapse, RV diastolic collapse, and LA collapse were present in only 3, 1, and 3 of these 15 patients, respectively, but all had LV diastolic collapse. Increasing pressure within the compartment of a loculated pericardial effusion reaching the limit of pericardial distensibility and consequent transient reversal of transmural LV pressure during diastole are most likely the basis for diastolic collapse of the thick-wall ventricle in a setting of regional cardiac tamponade. The investigators concluded that LV diastolic collapse is a frequent sign of regional cardiac tamponade and could be a useful marker of tamponade in postoperative patients.

Constriction

The pathogenesis of sodium and water accumulation in chronic constrictive pericarditis is not well understood and may differ from that in patients with CHF due to myocardial disease. Using standard techniques Anand and co-investigators[4] in Chandigarh, India, measured the hemodynamics, water and electrolyte spaces, renal function, and plasma concentrations of hormones in 16 patients with untreated constrictive pericarditis and repeated these measurements in 8 patients after pericardiectomy. The average hemodynamic measurements were as follows: cardiac output, 2.0 l/min/m_2; RA pressure, 23 mm Hg; PA wedge pressure, 24 mm Hg; and mean PA pressure 30 mm Hg. The systemic and pulmonary vascular resistances were increased. Significant increases occurred in body water, extracellular volume, plasma volume, and exchangeable sodium. The renal plasma flow was only moderately decreased and the glomerular filtration rate was normal. Significant increases also occurred in plasma concentrations of norepinephrine, renin activity, aldosterone, cortisol, growth hormone, and atrial natriuretic peptide. The ratio of LA to aortic diameter measured by echocardiography was only minimally increased, indicating that in constrictive pericarditis the atria are prevented from expanding. The studies repeated after pericardiectomy in the 8 patients showed that all measurements returned toward normal. The investigators concluded that the restricted distensibility of the atria, in constrictive pericarditis, limits the secretion of atrial natriuretic factor and, thus, reduces its natriuretic and diuretic effects. This results in retention of water and sodium greater than that occurring in patients with edema from myocardial disease. The arterial pressure is maintained more by the expansion of the blood volume than by an increase in the peripheral vascular resistance.

Pericardiectomy

De Valeria and associates[5] from Baltimore, Maryland, retrospectively analyzed records of 60 patients who underwent pericardiectomy over a 10-year period (1980–1990) at The Johns Hopkins Hospital (Figure 10-2). Indications for operation were effusive disease in 24 patients and constriction in 36 patients (Table 10-1). Six patients (10%) with pericardial effusion had pain as the primary symptom necessitating intervention. The operative approach for pericardiectomy was median sternotomy in 52 patients (4 patients required cardiopulmonary bypass) and left anterior thoracotomy in 8 patients. Nine patients (5 with constriction and 4 with effusion) with a poor limited pericardial procedure required formal pericardiectomy. The operative mortality rate for pericardial effusion and constriction was 4.2% and 5.6%, respectively. Follow-up (median follow-up, 56.9 ± 38.2 months) was obtained on 56 patients (93.3%). Actuarial survival at 1 year, 5 years, and 10 years for all patients was 82% ± 5%, 72% ±7%, and 60% ± 12%, respectively (Figure 10-3). A Cox proportional hazards regression analysis was performed using 20 clinical variables. A history of malignancy, previous pericardial procedure, and preoperative New York Heart Association class IV were found to be predictors of poor survival. All patients who underwent operation primarily for effusion with associated pain are alive and have improved functional capacity without steroid use. The authors concluded that pericardiectomy can be performed with low mortality and can result in good long-term survival and improved functional capacity. Patients who are seen primarily with pain refractory to steroid therapy can be relieved of symptoms with operation.

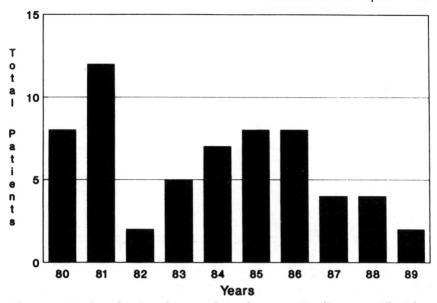

Fig. 10-2. Number of patients by year who underwent pericardiectomy at The Johns Hopkins Hospital between January 1, 1980, and December 31, 1989. Reprinted with permission from Devaleria, et al.[5]

TABLE 10-1. *Etiology of pericarditis. Reproduced with permission from Devaleria, et al.[5]*

Cause	Effusion	Constriction	Total
Idiopathic or viral	10	17	27
Infection	3	0	3
Radiation-induced	1	4	5
Previous cardiac operation	2	8	10
Neoplasm	1	1	2
Uremia	2	1	3
Connective-tissue disease	3	0	3
Previous Dressler's syndrome	1	3	4
Tuberculosis	1	2	3
Total	24	36	60

CARDIAC AND/OR PULMONARY TRANSPLANTATION

Review

An excellent review on Cardiac Transplantation by Stevenson and Miller[6] from Los Angeles, California, and St. Louis, Missouri, appeared in April, 1991, *Current Problems in Cardiology.*

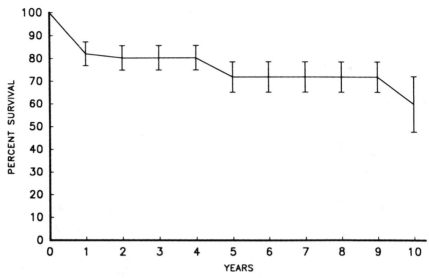

Fig. 10-3. Actuarial survival for all patients who underwent pericardiectomy (including operative deaths). Reprinted with permission from Devaleria, et al.[5]

Predictors of pulmonary vascular resistance

Elevated pulmonary vascular resistance is a known risk factor for early death after acute RV failure after orthotopic cardiac transplantation. Patients in whom the elevated pulmonary vascular resistance is due primarily to increased LA pressure ("reactive") frequently have normalization of resistance after transplantation, but few studies have detailed the time course and magnitude of these changes. To analyze the response of pulmonary vascular resistance to cardiac transplantation, Bourge and associates[7] from Birmingham, Alabama, analyzed data from 4,353 right-sided cardiac catheterizations on all 182 patients undergoing cardiac transplantation between 1981 and January 1, 1990. Before transplantation 18% of patients had a pulmonary vascular resistance greater than 4 WU, 16% had a pulmonary artery systolic pressure greater than 60 mm Hg, and 16% had a transpulmonary gradient greater than 14 mm Hg. In the overall group of patients, pulmonary vascular resistance (mean value 2.63 WU), transpulmonary gradient (mean value 10 mm Hg), and PA systolic pressure (mean value 48 mm Hg) were normalized within 1 week of cardiac transplantation. In patients with a high preoperative pulmonary vascular resistance (≥4 WU), the resistance fell promptly within 1 week of transplantation but continued to be slightly elevated throughout the period of follow-up. By multiple regression analysis, pulmonary vascular resistance at 1 week and 1 year after transplantation was significantly correlated with the pretransplantation resistance. Pulmonary vascular resistance anytime after transplantation was related to preoperative resistance, body surface area, and PA diastolic pressure. Inferences: (1) As a group, cardiac transplant recipients have a normal pulmonary vascular resistance, transpulmonary gradient, and PA systolic pressure within 1 week after transplantation with little change thereafter for at least several years. (2) Patients with reversible elevation of pulmonary vascular resistance before cardiac transplantation typically have a reactive and a fixed component. Cardiac transplantation relieves the reactive but not the fixed component. As a result, pulmonary vascular resistance early (within 1 week) and late after transplantation will have fallen but not completely normalized.

Coronary endothelial function

Kushwaha and colleagues[8] in Harefield, Middlesex, and London, UK, evaluated the endothelium-dependent vasodilator substance P in 12 cardiac transplant recipients to determine whether intracoronary infusions of substance P allowed one to identify normal and diseased coronary vessels in humans in vivo. All patients were well with no evidence of rejection and with angiographically normal coronary arteries. Substance P was infused at 2 ml/min for 2 minutes into the coronary artery, starting at a dose of 1.4 pmol/min and increasing by doubling increments, and followed by isosorbide dinitrate as 1 mg/min infused over 2 min. Coronary artery diameters were measured in 23 vessel segments from 12 transplant recipients. The following doses were infused: saline solution, substance P, and isosorbide dinitrate. The mean percent increase in diameter in response to increasing doses of substance P was as follows: 0, 6.5 ± 2.9%, 10.9 ± 2.9%, 12.1 ± 2.9%, 16.5 ± 2.6%, 19.2 ± 3.1%, and 25.8 ± 2.2%, respectively. Half maximal dilation was produced with 1.4 to 2.8 pmol/min of substance P. The maximal response in mean percent diameter change was 22 ± 2.5%. This was not significantly different from that achieved with isosorbide dinitrate. Thus, coronary endothelial function as assessed by response to substance P is preserved in cardiac transplant recipients with angiographically normal coronary arteries. Substance P may be a suitable agent for testing endothelial function in these patients.

Effects of anti-hypertensive therapy

Angermann and colleagues[9] in Munich, Germany, designed a prospective study to examine whether LV hypertrophy of the denervated transplanted heart may be reversed by medical therapy and, if so, to investigate the time course of this process and its effect on exercise capacity, myocardial function, and cardiac hemodynamics. Ten hypertensive heart transplant recipients with LV hypertrophy were evaluated before therapy with enalapril plus furosemide alone or combined with verapamil, at initial BP control and after 3, 6, 9, and 12 months, using 24-hour noninvasive ambulatory BP monitoring, m-mode and two-dimensional endocardiography, and supine bicycle ergometry. Average 24-hour systolic and diastolic BP declined from 158 and 102 mm Hg to 129 and 84 mm Hg at initial BP control and total peripheral resistance from 1,687 to 1,376 dyne sec cm^{-5}, remaining normal thereafter. Exercise capacity remained unchanged during the study period. LV mass, mass-to-volume ratio, and end-diastolic septal plus posterior wall thickness decreased progressively from 211 g, 2.5 g/ml, and 26 mm to 184 g, 2.2 g/ml and 23 mm after 3 months and 174 g, 2.1 g/ml, and 22 mm after 6 months, remaining unaltered at 9 and 12 months. A correlation was found between the decrease in average 24-hour mean BP and LV mass after 3 months of antihypertensive therapy. Systolic meridional wall stress, LV end-diastolic and stroke volume, EF, and cardiac output remained unchanged throughout the observation period. The results indicate that regression of LV hypertrophy is induced by effective antihypertensive therapy in the denervated transplanted heart. The extent of decrease in average 24-hour

BP appears to be the main determinant for the extent of reduction in LV mass. LV afterload as characterized by systolic meridional wall stress, LV size and pump function, and physical exercise capacity of the transplant patients are not influenced by the therapeutic regimen chosen in this study.

Ventricular function with rejection

Attempts to identify noninvasive markers of ventricular dysfunction accompanying acute rejection have been hampered by a lack of detailed simultaneous hemodynamic data. Therefore, Showronski and co-workers[10] in San Diego, California prospectively performed serial monitoring of detailed LV and RV hemodynamic parameters in cardiac transplant recipients at the time of routine endomyocardial biopsy to better define the physiology of the allograft heart during and after acute rejection. To better assess the pathophysiology of the rejection process, 18 cardiac transplant patients were prospectively studied by serial right heart micromanometer catheterization and digital image processing at the time of routine endomyocardial biopsy. Eleven patients had 18 episodes of rejection. Studies of baseline (negative biopsy preceding rejection), rejection (acute moderate rejection), and resolved (first negative biopsy after rejection) states were compared. Seven patients who did not experience an episode of rejection served as the control group. RV minimum and end-diastolic pressures increased from baseline values of 0.1 and 7 mm Hg, respectively, to 3 and 10 mm Hg, respectively, with rejection and remained elevated despite histological resolution of rejection. Concurrently, RV end-diastolic volumes and LV end-diastolic volumes significantly decreased during rejection and remained decreased after resolution of rejection. RV chamber stiffness increased with rejection and remained elevated after resolution of rejection. RV peak filling rate also increased from a baseline value of 2.5 to 2.8 ml end-diastolic volumes per second with rejection. Elevation of RV filling pressures, peak filling rate, and chamber stiffness with a concomitant decrease in end-diastolic volume is consistent with a restrictive/constrictive physiology. Mean arterial BP and systemic vascular resistance were elevated after the resolution of rejection associated with a higher mean daily dose of prednisone. The control group experienced a time-dependent increase in mean and diastolic systemic arterial pressures without detectable diastolic dysfunction. Persistence of biventricular diastolic dysfunction may be due to an irreversible effect of rejection, although mutlifactorial changes in LV afterload occur that may complicate serial assessment of ventricular function.

Cytomegalovirus pneumonitis

To evaluate the incidence and clinical features of cytomegalovirus (CMV) pneumonitis after cardiac transplantation, Schulman and associates[11] from New York, New York, identified 27 (16%) of 171 consecutive patients in whom CMV pneumonitis was confirmed by straight diagnostic criteria. Cytomegalovirus pneumonitis occurred in 6 (30%) of 20 patients treated with azathioprine and prednisone, and 8 (25%) of 32 patients treated with azathioprine, cyclosporine, and prednisone, but only 13 (11%) of 119 patients treated with cyclosporine and prednisone. The incidence of CMV pneumonitis was not related to recipient preoperative CMV titers or to postoperative cardiac rejection, but there was a trend toward increased CMV pneumonitis in patients who received organs from CMV-positive donors. Mean onset of CMV pneumonitis was 2.9 ± 1.6 months after transplantation. In the azathioprine-prednisone group, CMV was always associated with at least 1 other respiratory pathogen (Aspergillus, n = 5; Pneumocystis carinii, n = 2). In the 2 cyclosporine groups, CMV was either the sole respiratory pathogen (n = 9), or associated with P carnii (n = 11). Roentgenographically, diffuse bilateral hazy pulmonary opacities were present in 19 (70%) of 27 patients, but focal subsegmental opacity (26%), small pleural effusion (26%), and lobar consolidation (7%) were also observed. When bronchoscopy was performed, bronchoalveolar lavage was the most sensitive technique for detecting CMV (72%), whereas transbronchial biopsy (39%) and combined washings and brushings (33%) were relatively insensitive techniques. Respiratory failure and death occurred in 52% and 44%, respectively, of patients with CMV pneumonitis. In this population of immunocompromised hosts: (1) CMV pneumonitis, alone or with other respiratory pathogens, was a major cause of morbidity and mortality; (2) localized roentgenographic opacity did not exclude CMV pneumonitis; (3) bronchoalveolar lavage was the most sensitive bronchoscopic technique for detecting CMV pneumonitis.

Single-lung transplantation

Shorter waiting times, relative technical simplicity, and satisfactory application to a broad spectrum of patients has made single-lung transplantation an attractive option in the treatment of patients with end-stage pulmonary hypertension. Pasque and co-workers[12] in St. Louis, Missouri examined the acute and 3 month follow-up hemodynamics in 7 patients with pulmonary hypertension who underwent single-lung transplantation. Simultaneous closure of associated ASDS was accomplished in 2 patients. Despite severely compromised pretransplant RV function in all patients, there was no early or late mortality. RV functional recovery as characterized by hemodynamic assessment before and at a mean of 13 weeks posttransplant was nearly uniform and characterized by a drop in 1) PA systolic pressure from 97 to 29 mm Hg, 2) central venous pressure from 10 to 1 mm Hg and 3) pulmonary vascular resistance index from 1,924 to 232 dyne-sec-cm^{-9}. Radionuclide ventriculography before and at a mean of 17 weeks posttransplant documented a significant increase in RV EF from 22 to 51%. Quantitative pulmonary perfusion scintigraphy at a mean of 17 weeks posttransplant demonstrated a significant increase in perfusion to the transplanted lung from 56 to 97%. There was a concomitant, slight but significant decrease in ventilation to the transplanted side from 56 to 49%. After transplantation, all patients returned to New York Heart Association functional class I or II from their preoperative levels of class III or IV. These early follow-up data cautiously support the option of single-lung transplantation in patients with pulmonary hypertension, although long-term durability of these hemodynamic changes deserve documentation before widespread application.

Heart and lung

Heart-lung transplantation and lung transplantation (LT) are effective in patients with advanced pulmonary parenchymal or vascular disease. Lung transplantation offers potential advantages over heart-lung transplantation, including reduced pretransplant waiting time and improved efficiency of organ utilization, and is currently being offered to patients formerly treated by heart-lung transplantation. To explore the relative merits of these procedures, Bolman and associates[13] from Minneapolis, Minnesota, examined the results of 44 procedures (23 heart-lung transplantations and 21 lung transplantations) in 42 patients transplanted at their institution. Heart-lung transplant recipients included 20 adults and 3 children (ages 5, 5 and 3). Most heart-lung transplantation patients had primary pulmonary hypertension (n = 9) or Eisenmenger's syndrome (n = 8). Twenty-two of 23 patients have been long-term survivors (mean follow-up = 18 months, Kaplan-Meier survival at 12 months = 85%) (Figure 10-4). Obliterative bronchiolitis has occurred in 5 patients (22%), and all have died. Of 21 lung transplantations in 19 patients, 9 had obstructive and 8 had restrictive lung diseases. Three single-lung transplantation patients had primary pulmonary hypertension, and 1 had Eisenmenger's syndrome secondary to a VSD. Mean PA pressures fell from 55 ± 6 mm Hg before single-lung transplantation to 21 ± 3 mm Hg after single-lung transplantation. Three pediatric patients (ages 4, 10, 17, and 17 [re-transplant] have undergone 4 single transplantations. With mean follow-up of 6.4 months, lung transplantation patients have survival at 12 months of 80% (Kaplan-Meier). Lung transplant patients wait a far shorter time for their transplant than do heart-lung transplantation patients (166 vs 384 days). Three patients (19%) have evidence of OB after single-lung transplantation with 1 death. By virtue of equal intermediate-term outcomes, shorter waiting times, and better use of donor organs in comparison with heart-lung transplantation, lung transplantation should be offered whenever possible to patients with end-stage pulmonary parenchymal or vascular disease. The authors' pediatric lung transplantation and heart-lung transplantation experience (7 treatments in 6 patients) is the largest reported to date and demonstrates the utility of these procedures in this group. Chronic rejection remains the greatest impediment to long-term survival in both lung transplantation and heart-lung transplantation patients.

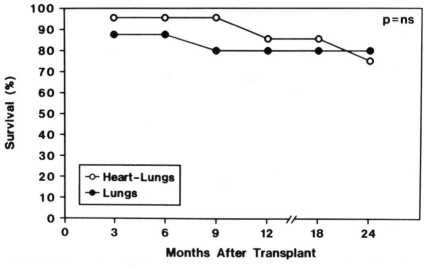

Fig. 10-4. Comparison of Kaplan-Meier survival of patients after lung-only and heart-lung transplant. Reprinted with permission from Bolman, et al.[13]

AORTIC DISSECTION

Transesophageal echocardiography

In a study reported by Chan[14] from Ontario, Canada, between September 1987 and April 1989, 40 patients suspected of having aortic dissection were evaluated by transesophageal echocardiography. Aortic dissection was identified in 18 patients. This study evaluated the ability of transesophageal echocardiography in the assessment of the 22 patients in whom aortic dissection was not found. A range of pathologic conditions was diagnosed in these patients. Five patients had ischemic heart disease when they were initially seen. Among the remaining 17, only 1 patient had a normal aorta. Aortic disease was present in the other 16 patients with aortic dilatation in 10. Atheromas were detected in 7 patients with concomitant aortic dilatation in 5 of them. An extrinsic aortic mass was present in 2 patients. Transesophageal echocardiography correctly identified an anastomotic leak at the site of left coronary artery implantation in a patient with a recent Bentall procedure, and a large mobile clot within the proximal descending aorta in a patient with blunt chest trauma. These findings obviated the need for other tests in 15 patients and led to surgery in 4 with no ancillary tests performed in 3 of them. Thus transesophageal echocardiography has an important role in assessing patients with suspected dissection. Aortic disease is common even in patients in whom aortic dissection is excluded, and some of the conditions can be just as life-threatening as dissection. Transesophageal echocardiography not only reliably identifies dissection, but can also detect luminal and extraluminal diseases not adequately visualized by other modalities.

Ballal and colleagues[15] in Birmingham, Alabama, studied the value of transesophageal echocardiography in the assessment of patients with aortic dissection. Group 1 (34 patients) represented all patients studied at their institution with this technique in whom aortic dissection was proven by aortography, surgery, or autopsy. Group 2 (27 patients) represented all patients studied with this technique at their institution in whom aortic dissection was excluded by aortography. Transesophageal echocardiography made a correct diagnosis of aortic dissection in 33 of 34 patients (sensitivity, 97%; specificity, 100%). It also correctly demonstrated the type of dissection in all 29 patients with aortographic or surgical proof. On the other hand, computed tomography scanning, performed in 24 of 34 patients in group 1, made a correct diagnosis in only 67% of patients and misclassified the type of dissection in 33%. Transesophageal echocardiography correctly identified involvement of the coronary arteries by aortic dissection in six of seven patients as well as absence of both left and right coronary artery involvement in 10 patients with aortic dissection. This technique was also useful in detecting communications between the true and false lumens, presence of thrombi in the false lumen, and, in two patients, localized dissection rupture with formation of a false aneurysm. In both groups 1 and 2, transesophageal echocardiography correctly identified patients with moderate to severe AR. Transesophageal echocardiography is very useful in the assessment of aortic dissection.

Operative therapy

Glower and associates[16] from Durham, North Carolina, reviewed 163 patients admitted to Duke University Medical Center between 1975 and 1988 with aortic dissection. Type I and Type II patients received grafting of the ascending aorta, with an intraoperative mortality rate of 11%. For Type III dissection, management was medical in 53 patients, while 19 required surgery for aortic rupture or expansion, with an intraoperative mortality rate of 11%. The 9- or 10-year survival rates were 29%, 46%, and 29% for types I, II, and III respectively (Figure 10-5). Of 135 patients with primary aortic dissection, 17 (13%) required subsequent aortic surgery. Cause of late death was other cardiovascular disease in 38%, rupture of another aortic segment in 18%, sudden death in 24%, and other medical conditions in 21% (Figure 10-6). Although operative therapy for types I and II dissections and reserving operation for selected type III dissections provides acceptable long-term survival, careful follow-up is necessary due to concurrent cardiovascular disease and residual aortic disease (Figure 10-7).

Fann and associates[17] from Stanford, California, and Durham, North Carolina, described findings in 252 patients who underwent operation for type A aortic dissection at Stanford University Medical Center from 1963 to 1987 and at Duke University Medical Center from 1975 to 1988. Sixty-seven percent had an acute type A dissection and 33% had a chronic type A dissection. In addition to repair or replacement of the ascending aorta, 121 patients (48%) required an aortic valve procedure. Valve resuspension was performed in 46 (39 acute type A and 7 chronic type A), with an operative mortality rate of 13% ± 5%, and AVR in 75 (36 acute type A and 39 chronic type A), with an operative mortality rate of 20% ± 5%. The operative mortality rate for patients requiring only repair or replacement of the ascending aorta was 32% ± 4%. Indications for AVR included coexistent (nonacute) aortic valve disease, the Marfan syndrome, annuloaortic ectasia, and cases in which successful resuspension could not be accomplished. The overall actuarial survival rate for all patients

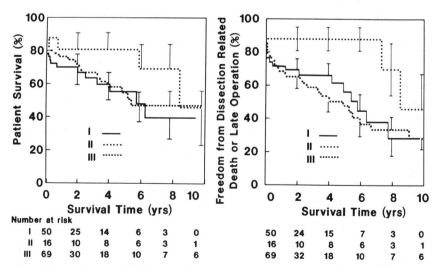

Fig. 10-5. Patient survival (left panel) and freedom from dissection-related death or late operation (right panel) for type I, type II, and type III aortic dissections. Reprinted with permission from Glower, et al.[16]

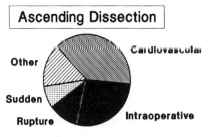

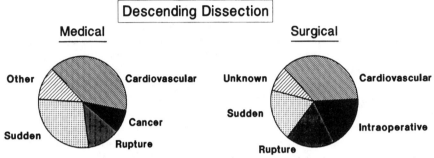

Fig. 10-6. Cause of death for patients with ascending dissection (top panel) or descending dissection with medical or surgical therapy (bottom panel). Reprinted with permission from Glower, et al.[16]

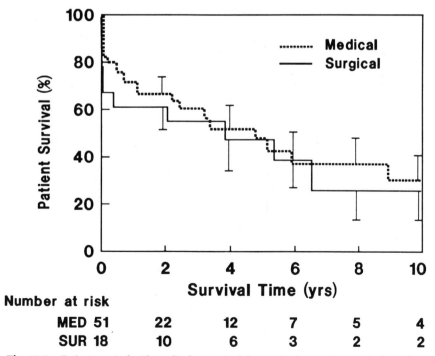

Fig. 10-7. Patient survival with medical or surgical therapy in descending aortic dissection. Reprinted with permission from Glower, et al.[16]

was 59% ± 3%, 40% ± 4%, and 25% ± 5% at 5, 10, and 15 years, respectively. Survival rates at these same times for patients with valve resuspension were 67% ± 8%, 52% ± 10%, and 26% ± 19%, respectively; for patients who required AVR, these survival rates were 70% ± 5%, 39% ± 8%, and 21% ± 11%; finally, patients who received only an ascending aortic procedure had survival probabilities of 51% ± 5%, 37% ± 6%, and 23% ± 6% (Figure 10-8). Multivariate analysis showed advanced age, previous cardiac or aortic operation, more preoperative dissection complications, and earlier operative date to be the only significant, independent factors that increased the likelihood of early or late death. The type of aortic valve procedure (resuspension versus AVR versus none) was not a significant predictor of mortality. Two of 46 patients with valve resuspension required late AVR (freedom from AVR: 100% and 80% ± 13% at 5 and 10 years, respectively), as did 4 of 75 patients with initial AVR (freedom from repeat AVR: 98% ± 2% and 73% ± 13%, respectively). Five of the 131 patients who underwent isolated ascending aortic repair or replacement required AVR (freedom from AVR was 94% ± 3% and 91% ± 4%) at these same times. This demonstrated satisfactory durability of aortic valve resuspension, coupled with the absence of potential prosthetic valve-related complications and need for indefinite anticoagulation, argue for preserving the native valve whenever possible in most patients. Exceptions include individuals with the Marfan syndrome or gross annuloaortic ectasia.

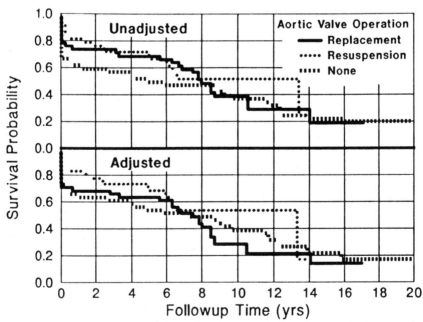

Fig. 10-8. Unadjusted actuarial survival curves according to type on initial aortic valve procedure and actuarial survival adjusted by the four significant determinants of mortality. As indicated by the similarities between the unadjusted and adjusted curves, the type of initial aortic valve procedure (aortic valve replacement versus resuspension versus none) had no significant influence on overall survival. Reprinted with permission from Fann, et al.[17]

CAROTID ARTERY DISEASE

Endarterectomy

Without strong evidence of benefit, the use of carotid endarterectomy for prophylaxis against stroke rose dramatically until the mid-1980s, then declined. The North American Symptomatic Carotid Endarterectomy Trial Collaborators[18] from 50 centers in the USA and Canada sought to determine whether carotid endarterectomy reduces the risk of stroke among patients with a recent adverse cerebrovascular event and ipsilateral carotid stenosis. The authors conducted a randomized trial at 50 clinical centers throughout the USA and Canada, in patients in 2 predetermined strata based on the severity of carotid stenosis—30 to 69% and 70 to 99%. The authors reported the results in the 659 patients in the latter stratum, who had had a hemispheric or retinal transient ischemic attack or a nondisabling stroke within the 120 days before entry and had stenosis of 70 to 99% in the symptomatic carotid artery. All patients received optimal medical care, including antiplatelet therapy. Those assigned to surgical treatment underwent carotid endarterectomy performed by neurosurgeons or vascular surgeons. All patients were examined by neurologists 1, 3, 6, 9, and 12 months after entry and then every 4 months. End points were assessed by blinded, independent case review. No patient was lost to follow-up. Life-table estimates of the cumulative risk of any ipsilateral stroke at 2 years were 26% in the 331 medical patients and 9% in the 328 surgical patients—an absolute risk reduction ($\pm$ SE) of 17 $\pm$ 3.5%. For a major or fatal ipsilateral stroke, the corresponding estimates were 13.1% and 2.5%—an absolute risk reduction of 10.6 $\pm$ 2.6%. Carotid endarterectomy was still found to be beneficial when all strokes and deaths were included in the analysis. Carotid endarterectomy is highly beneficial to patients with recent hemispheric and retinal transient ischemic attacks or nondisabling strokes and ipsilateral high-grade stenosis (70 to 99%) of the internal carotid artery.

This article was followed by an editorial entitled "Carotid Endarterectomy—Specific Therapy Based on Pathophysiology" by Kistler and associates[19] from Boston, Massachusetts. These authors provided the following recommendation: " . . . a randomized trial comparing medical and surgical therapy that specifically targets hemodynamically important but asymptomatic carotid stenosis is needed: 2 are going on now. Until it is possible to assess accurately the efficacy of endarterectomy under these circumstances, physicians may consider surgery, but only after an asymptomatic stenosis has become hemodynamically important. Progression of the stenosis can be monitored noninvasively; such evaluation should be combined with the transcranial Doppler assessment of blood flow through the ophthalmic artery and the circle of Willis. Even when the lesion is hemodynamically important, however, surgery is not an attractive option in asymptomatic patients unless the surgical and medical teams' previous experience is characterized by the same low rates of perioperative morbidity and mortality achieved by those participating in the NASCET study. When this is not the case, it may be better simply to prescribe 325 mg or less of aspirin a day."

To determine whether carotid endarterectomy provides protection against subsequent cerebral ischemia in men with ischemic symptoms in the distribution of >50% diameter narrowing of the ipsilateral internal carotid artery, Mayberg and associates[20] for the Veterans Affairs Cooperative Studies Program 309 Trialist Group involving 16 university affiliated Veterans Affairs medical centers randomized 189 men with angiographic internal carotid artery stenosis >50% ipsilateral to the presenting symptoms. Cerebral infarction or crescendo transient ischemic attacks in the vascular distribution of the original symptoms or death within 30 days of randomization were the outcome measures. Carotid endarterectomy plus the best medical care was performed in 91 patients versus the best medical care alone in 98 patients. At a mean follow-up of 11.9 months, there was a significant reduction in stroke or crescendo transient ischemic attacks in patients who received carotid endarterectomy (8%) compared with nonsurgical patients (19%) or an absolute reduction of 12% (Figure 10-9). The benefit of surgery was more profound in patients with internal carotid stenosis >70% (absolute risk reduction = 18%). The benefit of surgery was apparent within 2 months after randomization,

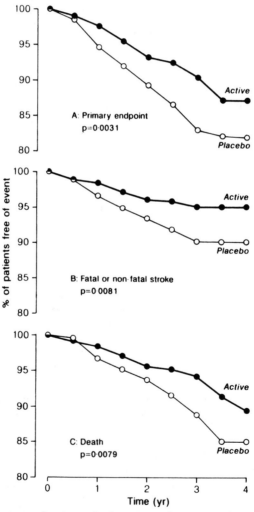

Fig. 10-9. Percentages of patients who have escaped a primary endpoint (A), fatal or non-fatal stroke (B), or death (C) during four years of treatment. Survival functions estimated by maximum likelihood methods assuming constant hazard functions within 6-month periods. P values apply to total study period. Reprinted with permission from Mayberg, et al.[20]

and only 1 stroke occurred in the surgical group beyond the 30 day perioperative period.

PERIPHERAL VASCULAR DISEASE

Muscle carnitine deficiency

Brevetti and co-investigators[21] in Padua, Italy, evaluated the effect of severe peripheral arterial insufficiency on carnitine concentrations and carnitine acetyltransferase and palmitoyltransferase activities in the ischemic skeletal muscles of patients with severe peripheral vascular disease. Nine muscle biopsy specimens of ischemic muscles were obtained from five patients undergoing reconstructive vascular surgery. Biopsies from 35 normal subjects served as controls. Ischemic muscles showed a significant reduction in total carnitine from the control value of 21 to 12 nmol/mg noncollagen protein. A significantly lower free carnitine and acylcarnitines content contributed to this reduction. Similarly, carnitine acetyltransferase activity was reduced in the ischemic muscles from the control value of 102 to 53 mnmol/min/mg noncollagen protein. On the contrary, carnitine palmitoyltransferase activity did show any change. Carnitine, acylcarnitines, and enzyme activities were also measured in the ischemic muscles in four additional patients 2 days after intravenous administration of L-propionylcarnitine (1.5 as a single bolus followed by an infusion of 1 mg/kg/min for 30 minutes). Treatment restored normal levels of carnitine and its esters in the ischemic muscles but did not affect enzyme activities. Demonstration of carnitine deficiency in severe peripheral vascular disease substantiates previous findings showing the efficacy of carnitine supplementation to ischemic muscles. Furthermore, the feasibility of restoring carnitine homeostasis with L-propionylcarnitine provides the basis for clinical trials aimed at assessing the efficacy of this carnitine ester in the treatment of peripheral vascular disease.

Beta-Adrenergic blocker therapy

B-Adrenergic blockers have been considered relatively contraindicated in peripheral arterial disease because of the perceived risk that these drugs could worsen intermittent claudication. Radack and Deck[22] from Cincinnati, Ohio, conducted a meta-analysis of available randomized controlled trials from the English-language to determine whether or not B-blockers exacerbate intermittent claudication. The primary focus of this analysis was the effect of B-blockers on exercise duration, measured as walking capacity or endurance time. Outcomes were pooled where appropriate. Of 11 eligible reports, 6 included 11 individual controlled treatment comparisons that provided data for an analysis of pain-free exercise capacity; no effect size was statistically significant. The pooled effect size for pain-free walking distance was -0.24, indicating no significant impairment of walking capacity compared with placebo. Only one study reported that certain B-blockers were associated with worsening of intermittent claudication. These results strongly suggest that B-blockers do not adversely affect walking capacity or symptoms of intermittent claudication in patients with mild to moderate peripheral arterial disease. In the absence of other contraindications, B-blockers can probably be used safely in such patients.

Angioplasty, bypass, and amputation

Percutaneous transluminal angioplasty has been adopted widely as a treatment for patients with peripheral vascular disease. The effect of these procedures on the overall management, however, and on the outcomes of patients with peripheral vascular disease has not been clearly delineated. To assess the extent to which angioplasty is used and the associated changes in the surgical management of peripheral vascular disease of the lower extremities, Tunis and associates[23] from Baltimore, Maryland, used data on hospital discharges in Maryland to identify all angioplasty procedures, peripheral bypass operations, and lower extremity amputations performed for peripheral vascular disease in Maryland hospitals between 1979 and 1989. The authors estimated that from 1979 to 1989 the annual rate of percutaneous transluminal angioplasty for peripheral vascular disease of the lower extremities, adjusted for age and sex, rose from 1 to 24 per 100,000 Maryland residents. Despite this increase in the use of angioplasty, the adjusted annual rate of peripheral bypass surgery also rose substantially, from 32 to 65 per 100,000, whereas the adjusted annual rate of lower-extremity amputation remained stable at about 30 per 100,000 (Figure 10-10). Total charges for hospitalizations during which a peripheral revascularization procedure was performed increased from $14.7 million in 1979 (in 1989 dollars) to $30.5 million in 1989. In Maryland, the adoption of percutaneous transluminal angioplasty for peripheral vascular disease of the lower extremities has been associated with an increase in the use of peripheral bypass surgery and with no decline in lower-extremity amputations. These results could be due to increased diagnosis of peripheral vascular disease, expanded indications for procedural interventions, or an increased number of repeat procedures performed in patients with peripheral vascular disease of the lower extremities.

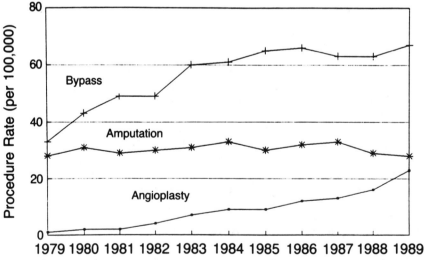

Fig. 10-10. Adjusted annual rates of angioplasty, bypass surgery, and amputation for peripheral vascular disease of the lower extremities in Maryland, 1979 through 1989. Rates have been adjusted for age and sex and are expressed as number of procedures per 100,000 Maryland residents. P<0.0001 for the increase in the rate of angioplasty between 1979 and 1989. P<0.001 for the increase in the rate of bypass between 1979 and 1989. Reprinted with permission from Tunis, et al.[23]

This article was followed by an editorial entitled, "Intermittent Claudication—Be Conservative" by J. D. Coffman[24] from Boston, Massachusetts. His conclusion was the following: "The treatment of patients with intermittent claudication alone should be conservative, because the prognosis for the limb is favorable, because surgical mortality from cardiovascular events is high among such patients, and because the use of interventions has not decreased the rate of amputation in many hospitals. Invasive procedures are indicated only for the severely ischemic limb and should be performed in an institution and by a team with a good track record."

Ultrasonic angioplasty

Ultrasonic PTCA was recently shown to ablate thrombi and atherosclerotic plaques in vitro and to recanalize occluded arteries in experimental animal models. The goal of this study was to examine the clinical feasibility of ultrasonic PTCA. Rosenschein and co-workers[25] in Ann Arbor, Michigan, performed intraoperative ultrasonic angioplasty PTCA in vivo on totally occluded peripheral arteries. The ultrasonic PTCA device consists of a 1.6 mm diameter flexible wire attached to a piezoelectric crystal generating ultrasound at 20 kHz. The controls, totally occluded human atherosclerotic femoral arterial segments, were crossed mechanically with the ultrasound wire ex vivo but without application of ultrasonic energy. Ultrasonic PTCA achieved successful recanalization without perforation in all vessels. Angiograms of the treated arteries showed an average lumen patency of 83%. Histological examination of the recanalized arteries revealed that the recanalization had taken place through intima diffusely involved with complicated plaque. The treated arteries, compared with the controls, had greater area of recanalized lumen and more flow. The damage in treated and control arteries was similar. Size-distribution analysis of the plaque debris from the treated arteries showed that 41% of the debris was less than 8 micro meters, 48% was 8–30 micro meters and the remainder was 30–100 micro meters. In the mechanically crossed arteries, there was a shift in the distribution to larger size debris with 47% >100 micro meter. Ultrasonic PTCA may be a useful clinical method for recanalization of total occlusions in patients with peripheral vascular disease. Ultrasonic energy appears to cause controlled injury to the atherosclerotic intima by selectively disrupting the ultrasound-sensitive occlusion.

PULMONARY DISEASE

Acute pulmonary embolism

Stein and associates[26] from 6 different USA medical centers evaluated the history, physical examination, chest radiograph, electrocardiogram, and blood gases with suspected acute pulmonary embolism and no history or evidence of pre-existing cardiac or pulmonary disease. The investigation focused upon patients with no previous cardiac or pulmonary disease in order to evaluate the clinical characteristics that were due only to pulmonary embolism. Acute pulmonary embolism was present in 117 patients and pulmonary embolism was excluded in 248 patients. Among the patients with pulmonary embolism, dyspnea or tachypnea

(≥20/min) was present in 105 of 117 (90%). Dyspnea, hemoptysis, or pleuritic pain was present in 107 of 117 (91%). The partial pressure of oxygen in arterial blood on room air was <80 mm Hg in 65 of 88 (74%). The alveolar-arterial oxygen gradient was >20 mm Hg in 76 of 88 (86%). Atelectasis and/or pulmonary parenchymal abnormalities were most common, 79 of 117 (68%). Nonspecific ST segment or T wave change was the most common electrocardiographic abnormality, in 44 of 89 (49%). Dyspnea, tachypnea, or signs of deep venous thrombosis was present in 107 of 117 (91%). Dyspnea or tachypnea or pleuritic pain was present in 113 of 117 (97%). Dyspnea or tachypnea or pleuritic pain or atelectasis or a parenchymal abnormality on the chest radiograph was present in 115 of 117 (98%). In conclusion, among the patients with pulmonary embolism that were identified, only a small percentage did not have these important manifestations or combinations of manifestations. Clinical evaluation, though nonspecific, is of considerable value in the selection of patients in whom there is a need for further diagnostic studies.

Stein and colleagues[27] in Detroit, Michigan, New Haven, Connecticut, Durham, North Carolina, and Baltimore, Maryland, studied the diagnostic features of acute pulmonary embolism among 72 patients ≥70 years of age and compared them to similar characteristics among 144 patients, 40 to 69 years of age and 44 patients <44 years old. Syndromes characterized by either 1) pleuritic pain or hemoptysis, 2) isolated dyspnea, or 3) circulatory collapse were observed with comparable frequency among patients ≥70 years old and younger patients. One of the presenting syndromes occurred in 64 (89%) of the 72 patients ≥70 years old. Those who did not show these clinical symptoms were identified on the basis of unexpected radiographic abnormalities, which may have been accompanied by tachypnea or a history of thrombophlebitis. Among the 72 patients ≥70 years with pulmonary embolism, dyspnea or tachypnea (respiratory rate ≥20/min) developed in 66 patients (92%), dyspnea or tachypnea or pleuritic pain in 68 (94%) and dyspnea or tachypnea or radiographic evidence of atelectasis or a parenchymal abnormality in 72 (100%). Complications of angiography were evaluated among patients with and without pulmonary embolism. Major complications of pulmonary angiography among patients ≥70 years of age (2 of 200) were no more frequent than among younger patients (6 of 562). Renal failure, major or minor, was more frequent in patients that were aged occurring in 6 of 200 patients versus 4 of 562 patients who are younger. Nonspecific manifestations of pulmonary embolism were often present in elderly patients. Thus, whenever necessary, pulmonary angiography may be performed with no greater overall frequency of complication in elderly patients, although renal failure after angiography is a problem in this patient group.

Hsu and associates[28] from New York, New York, monitored 62 consecutive patients awaiting heart transplantation for evidence of acute pulmonary embolism. Acute pulmonary infarction was documented by ventilation-perfusion scan, pulmonary angiography or pathologic examination in 6 patients. This complication occurred in 5 of 36 patients with dilated cardiomyopathy and 1 of 20 patients with congenital heart disease. Neither age at the time of transplantation evaluation, duration of CHF, presence of arrhythmia nor degree of cardiac dysfunction were seen as risk factors for pulmonary embolism. Echocardiography failed to detect intracardiac thrombus in 4 of 6 patients. Successful heart transplantation was performed in 2 patients following pulmonary infarction and 4 died within 6 weeks of initiation of anticoagulant therapy before transplantation could safely be performed. These authors strongly suggest the use of anticoagulant therapy in patients who are candidates for cardiac transplantation with careful monitoring to maintain the therapeutic prothrombin between 1.3 to 1.5 × control values to minimize the risk of bleeding.

Rapid restoration of pulmonary blood flow is important in preventing death due to a massive pulmonary embolus. Devices developed specifically for percutaneous transvenous removal of pulmonary emboli are bulky and their insertion through a cut down or by the use of a large venous sheath can lead to bleeding at the entry site. Brady and associates[29] from London, UK, in 3 patients with acute massive pulmonary embolism, used conventional cardiac catheters to break up the embolis and disperse the fragments distally. Cardiac output was rapidly restored in all 3 patients. There were no serious complications. This technique requires no more specialist equipment or skill than those needed for temporary cardiac pacing and could be important for the emergency management of patients with acute severe pulmonary embolism.

High-altitude pulmonary edema

Exaggerated PA pressure due to hypoxic vasoconstriction is considered an important pathogenetic factor in high-altitude pulmonary edema. Bartsch and associates[30] from Zurich and Bern, Switzerland, previously found that nifedipine lowered PA pressure and improved exercise performance, gas exchange, and the radiographic manifestations of disease in patients with high-altitude pulmonary edema. They further hypothesized in the present report that the prophylactic administration of nifedipine would prevent its recurrence. Accordingly, 21 mountaineers (1 woman and 20 men) with a history of radiographically documented high-altitude pulmonary edema were randomly assigned to receive either 20 mg of a slow-release preparation of nifedipine (n = 10) or placebo (n = 11) every 8 hours while ascending rapidly (within 22 hours) from a low altitude to 4,559 m and during the following 3 days at this altitude. Both the subjects and the investigators were blinded to the assigned treatment. The diagnosis of pulmonary edema was based on chest radiography. PA pressure was measured by Doppler echocardiography and the difference between alveolar and arterial oxygen pressure was measured in simultaneously sampled arterial blood and end-expiratory air. Seven of the 11 subjects who received placebo but only 1 of the 10 subjects who received nifedipine had pulmonary edema at 4,559 m. As compared with the subjects who received placebo, those who received nifedipine had a significantly lower mean (± SD) systolic PA pressure (41 ± 8 vs 53 ± 16 mm Hg), alveolar-arterial pressure gradient (7 ± 4 vs 12 ± 4 mm Hg), and symptom score of acute mountain sickness (2.0 ± 0.7 vs 3.9 ± 1.9) at 4,559 m. The prophylactic administration of nifedipine is effective in lowering PA pressure and preventing high-altitude pulmonary edema in susceptible subjects. These findings support the concept that high PA pressure has an important role in the development of high-altitude pulmonary edema.

MISCELLANEOUS TOPICS

Frequency of cardiologic procedures

The Cardiology Working Group[31] co-chaired by Thomas J. Ryan and Charles D. Baker from Boston, Massachusetts, and the Cardiology Working Group of the American Medical Association prepared an article entitled, "Cardiology and the Quality of Medical Practice." The Working Group presented the background and current status of 3 important and expensive technologies; namely, cardiac pacemaker implantation, coronary angioplasty following thrombolytic therapy, and CABG (Table 10-2). The Working Group attempted to define the quality of practice of these 3 technologies in the USA and to make appropriate changes, if necessary, in the practice utilizing these 3 technologies.

Computer electrocardiographic interpretation

Computer programs for the interpretation of electrocardiograms are now widely used. A systematic assessment of various computer programs for the interpretation of electrocardiograms has not been performed. Willems and associates[32] from several European centers undertook a large international study to compare the performance of 9 electrocardiographic computer programs with that of 8 cardiologists interpreting electrocardiograms in 1,220 clinically validated cases of various cardiac disorders. Electrocardiograms from the following groups were included in the sample: control patients (n = 382); patients with LV hypertrophy (n = 183), RV hypertrophy (n = 55), or biventricular hypertrophy (n = 53); patients

TABLE 10-2. *Regional utilization rates for cardiovascular procedures (rate per 100,000 population)—National Center for Health Statistics, 1987.* Reproduced with permission from Cardiology Working Group.*[31]

	Cardiologists per 100 000 Population†	PTCA‡	CABG	MI	CHF
Northeast	8.2	35.8	79.1	34.9	27.8
Midwest	4.6	78.0	163.0	31.1	25.1
South	4.8	59.7	125.3	30.1	23.9
West	5.4	42.6	94.8	29.2	20.3
National rate	5.6	55.8	137.3	31.7	24.3

*Data are from the National Center for Health Statistics, 1987.
†These data are from reference 17.
‡PTCA indicates percutaneous transluminal coronary angioplasty; CABG, coronary artery bypass graft; MI, myocardial infarction; and CHF, congestive heart failure.

Utilization of cardiovascular procedures in the United States*

	1981	1982	1983	1984	1985	1986	1987	1988
CABG[17]	159	170	188	202	200 247†	210 284†	230 324†	235
PTCA[17]	6	12	32	63	106	133	188	235
Pace makers‡	108 (122.0)§	102 (121.0)	99 (117.0)	91 (117.0)	88 (119.0)	85 (109.4)	88 (109.3)	90 (111.3)

*Numbers given are in thousands. CABG indicates coronary artery bypass graft; and PTCA, percutaneous transluminal coronary angioplasty.
†Figures frequently reported for these years when internal mammary artery grafts were counted as separate procedures.
‡Commission on Professional and Hospital Activities (Healthcare Knowledge Systems, Inc).
§Figures in parentheses are based on Medtronic actual sales and IMS data, a secondary market research source (J. Warren Harthorne, MD, personal communication).

with anterior AMI (n = 170), inferior AMI (n = 273), or combined AMI (n = 72); and patients with combined infarction and hypertrophy (n = 31). The interpretations of the computer programs and the cardiologists were compared with the clinical diagnoses made independently of the electrocardiograms, and the computer interpretations were compared with those of the cardiologists. The percentage of electrocardiograms correctly classified by the computer programs (median, 91.3%) was lower than that for the cardiologists (median, 96.0%). The median sensitivity of the computer programs was also significantly lower than that of the cardiologists in diagnosing LV hypertrophy (57% vs 64%), RV hypertrophy (32% vs 47%), anterior AMI (77% vs 85%), and inferior AMI (59% vs 72%). The median total accuracy level (the percentage of correct classifications) was 7% lower for the computer programs (70%) than for the cardiologists (76%). However, the performance of the best programs nearly matched that of the most accurate cardiologists. The study shows that some but not all computer programs for the interpretation of electrocardiograms perform almost as well as cardiologists in identifying seven major cardiac disorders.

Transesophageal echocardiography for detecting cardiac masses, sources of cerebral emboli, aortic atheroma, atrial septal aneurysm and causing bacteremia

Although transthoracic 2-dimensional echocardiography has been a procedure of choice for diagnosing cardiac masses, the advent of transesophageal echocardiography (TEE) provided better visualization of cardiac structures, especially those at a considerable depth from the chest wall, and lesions that involve the LA appendage. Reeder and associates[33] from Rochester, Minnesota, examined their experience at the Mayo Clinic with TEE imaging of cardiac masses (excluding valvular vegetations) from April 1988 to July 1990. TEE studies detected 83 lesions (in 80 patients), which the authors characterized by type and site: 46 left atrial, 16 right atrial, 7 LV, 2 RV, and 12 extracardiac mass lesions. Of the 46 left atrial lesions, 9 were tumors and 37 were thrombi that involved the LA body, the LA appendage, or both. Associated mitral valve disease, chronic AF, or spontaneous microcavitations were common. Of the 16 RA mass lesions, 4 were tumors and 12 were thrombi, including "string" thrombi characteristic of venous thromboembolism. Of the 7 LV mass lesions, 6 were thrombi and 1 was a papilloma. Of the 12 extracardiac mass lesions, 2 were pericardial cysts and the rest were solid lesions. TEE added new or important clinical information beyond that derived from transthoracic echocardiography in LA thrombi, RA masses, and extracardiac lesions and was assessed to have influenced the management of patients most in these areas also. TEE is a useful addition to transthoracic echocardiography for diagnosis and clarification of cardiac mass lesions in selected patients.

Pearson and associates[34] in St. Louis, Missouri, used transesophageal and transthoracic echocardiography for identifying a cardiac source of embolism in 79 patients presenting with unexplained stroke or transient ischemic attacks. There were 35 men and 44 women with a mean age of 59 years. Fifty-two percent had clinical cardiac disease. Both transthoracic and transesophageal echocardiograms were performed using Doppler color flow and contrast imaging. TEE identified a potential cardiac source of embolism in 57% of the overall study group compared with only 15% of transthoracic echocardiography. Compared with transthoracic echocardiography, TEE more frequently identified atrial septal aneurysm, LA thrombus or tumor, and LA spontaneous contrast. All cases of LA thrombus or spontaneous contrast were identified in patients with clinically identified cardiac disease. In the 38 patients with no cardiac disease, TEE identified isolated atrial septal aneurysm and atrial septal aneurysm with a patent foramen ovale more frequently than transthoracic echocardiography (8 versus 2 of 38 patients). The 2 techniques had a similar rate of identifying apical thrombus and MVP. TEE identified abnormalities in 39% of patients with no cardiac disease versus 19% for transthoracic echocardiography. Therefore, TEE identifies potential cardiac sources of embolism in the many patients with unexplained stroke.

Karalis and associates[35] in Philadelphia, Pennsylvania, studied 556 patients with TEE to identify the prevalence, clinical significance and embolic potential of intraaortic atherosclerotic debris. An embolic event occurred among 11 (31%) of the 36 study patients with intraaortic atherosclerotic debris. The incidence of the embolic event was higher when the debris was pedunculated and highly mobile (8 of 11 patients) than when it was layered and immobile (3 of 25 patients). Among 15 patients having an invasive procedure of the aorta, the incidence of embolism was 27%. Thus, in a patient with an embolic event, the thoracic aorta should be considered as a potential source. TEE may reliably detect intraaortic atherosclerotic debris, and when it is identified, an invasive aortic procedure should be avoided if possible.

To determine whether protruding atheromas in the thoracic aorta diagnosed by TEE are risk factors for systemic emboli, Tunick and associates[36] from New York, New York, performed TEE in 122 patients with a history of stroke, transient ischemic attack, or peripheral emboli and an equal number of age- and sex-matched control subjects. Matched logistic regression showed that the presence of protruding atheromas was strongly related to the occurrence of systemic emboli. Furthermore, atheromas with mobile components were present only in case patients. When known risk factors for stroke (hypertension and diabetes) were added to the model, the presence of protruding atheromas remained an independent risk factor for embolic symptoms. Hypertension was also independently associated with embolic symptoms, but diabetes was not. Protruding atheromas in the thoracic aorta can be detected by TEE and should be considered as a cause of strokes, transient ischemic attacks, and peripheral emboli.

Pearson and associates[37] in Columbus, Ohio, and St. Louis, Missouri, studied the prevalence and morphologic characteristics of atrial septal aneurysm identified by TEE in 410 consecutive patients. Two groups of patients were compared: Group I consisted of 133 patients referred for evaluation of the potential source of an embolus and Group II consisted of 277 patients referred for other reasons. An atrial septal aneurysm was diagnosed by TEE in 32 (8%) of the 410 patients. Surface echocardiogram identified only 12 of these aneurysms. Atrial septal aneurysm was significantly more common in patients with strokes (20, 15% of 133 vs 12, 4% of 277 patients); right-to-left shunting at the atrial level was demonstrated in 70% of patients in Group I and 75% of patients in Group II. Four patients in Group I had an ASD with additional left-to-right flow. There were no differences between the 2 groups in aneurysm base width, total excursion, or LA or RA excursion. Group I patients had a thinner atrial septal aneurysm than did Group II patients. Thus, atrial septal aneurysms occur commonly in patients with unexplained strokes, they are more frequently detected by TEE than by surface echo, and they are usually associated with right-to-left shunt. The benefits of specific types of therapy in patients with atrial septal aneurysms needs to be determined.

Melendez and associates[55] in London and Ottawa, Canada, studied the incidence of bacteremia related to TEE in 140 consecutive patients. Thirty-four patients had one or more prosthetic heart valves. Blood cultures were obtained from each patient through separate venipuncture sites immediately before and after TEE. An additional late blood culture was obtained in 114 patients 1 hour later. The skin was cleaned with povidone-iodine and venipunctures were performed with separate butterfly needles with the use of sterile gloves and drapes. Blood samples were drawn into separate syringes, transferred to aerobic and anaerobic culture bottles and processed with the use of a semiautomated system. The overall incidence of blood cultures positive for bacteremia was 2% and all positive cultures grew in a single blood culture bottle. Positive cultures occurred in 4 (1.4%) of 280 bottles before the procedure, in 2 (0.7%) of 280 bottles immediately after the procedure and in 2 (0.9%) of 228 late blood culture bottles. Bacterial isolates were coagulase-negative staphylococci (n = 5), Propionibacterium (n = 2) and Moraxella (n = 1). All were considered contaminants. Mean endoscopic times in these patients were not significantly different from those in others. Follow-up of patients with positive blood cultures positive for bacteremia revealed no clinical evidence of systemic infection. Thus, these data suggest that the incidence of bacteremia related to TEE is low, and the incidence of blood cultures positive for bacteremia after TEE is indistinguishable from the anticipated contamination rate.

Aspirin for cerebral ischemia

Aspirin is known to improve the outcome of patients who have had a cerebral transient ischemic attack, but the optimal dose of aspirin remains uncertain. The Dutch TIA Trial Study Group[39] assessed the effects of 2 doses of acetylsalicylic acid, or aspirin (30 mg vs 283 mg a day), on the occurrence of death from all vascular causes, nonfatal stroke, or nonfatal AMI in a double-blind, randomized, controlled clinical trial in patients who had had a transient ischemic attack or minor stroke. A total of 3,131 patients participated in the study. The mean follow-up was 2.6 years. In the group assigned to receive 30 mg of aspirin, the frequency of death from vascular causes, nonfatal stroke, or nonfatal AMI was 228 of 1,555 (14.7%), as compared with 240 of 1,576 (15.2%) in the group assigned to receive 283 mg. The age- and sex-adjusted hazard ratio for the group receiving the lower dose was 0.91. There were slightly fewer major bleeding complications in the 30-mg group than in the 283-mg group (40 vs 53), and significantly fewer reports of minor bleeding (49 vs 84). Fewer patients receiving 30 mg of aspirin reported gastrointestinal symptoms (164 vs 179) and other adverse effects (73 vs 90). Our data indicate that 30 mg of aspirin daily is no less effective in the prevention of vascular events than a 283-mg dose in patients with a transient ischemic attack or minor stroke, and has fewer adverse effects (Figure 10-11).

The efficacy of aspirin in daily doses of 300 mg and more as secondary prophylaxis after cerebrovascular events is well established. Since much lower doses of aspirin can inhibit platelet function, and carry a lower risk of adverse effects, the Swedish Aspirin Low-dose Trial (SALT) was set up to study the efficacy of 75 mg aspirin daily in prevention of stroke and death after transient ischemic attack (TIA) or minor stroke.[40] One

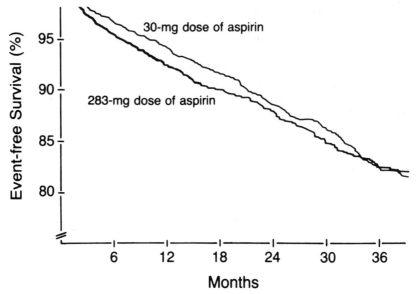

Fig. 10-11. Kaplan-Meier curves for the combined outcome event of death from vascular causes, nonfatal stroke, or nonfatal myocardial infarction, according to assigned treatment. Reprinted with permission from New England Journal of Medicine.[39]

thousand three hundred sixty patients entered the study 1–4 months after the qualifying event: 676 were randomly assigned to aspirin treatment and 684 to placebo treatment. The median duration of follow-up was 32 months. Compared with the placebo group, the aspirin group showed a reduction of 18% in the risk of primary outcome events (stroke or death; relative risk 0.82), and reductions of 16–20% in the risks of secondary outcome events (stroke; stroke or 2 or more TIAs within a week of each other necessitating a change of treatment; or AMI). Adverse drug effects were reported by 147 aspirin-treated and 123 placebo-treated patients. Gastrointestinal side-effects were only slightly more common in the aspirin-treated patients, but that group had a significant excess of bleeding episodes. Thus, the authors found that a low dose (75 mg/day) of aspirin significantly reduces the risk of stroke or death in patients with cerebrovascular ischemic events.

Physiologic cardiac hypertrophy in athletes

In some highly trained athletes, the thickness of the LV wall may increase as a consequence of exercise training and resemble that found in cardiac diseases associated with LV hypertrophy, such as HC. In these athletes, the differential diagnosis between physiologic and pathologic hypertrophy may be difficult. To address this issue, Pelliccia and associates[41] from Rome, Italy, and Bethesda, Maryland, measured LV dimensions by echocardiography in 947 elite, highly trained athletes who participated in a wide variety of sports. The thickest LV wall among the athletes measured 16 mm. Wall thicknesses within a range compatible with the diagnosis of HC (≥13 mm) were identified in only 16 of the 947 athletes (1.7%); 15 were rowers or canoeists, and 1 was a cyclist. Therefore, the wall was ≥13 mm thick in 7% of 219 rowers, canoeists, and cyclists but in none of 728 participants in 22 other sports. All athletes with walls ≥13 mm thick also had enlarged LV end-diastolic cavities (dimensions, 55 to 63 mm). On the basis of these data, a LV wall thickness of >13 mm is very uncommon in highly trained athletes, virtually confined to athletes training in rowing sports, and associated with an enlarged LV cavity. In addition, the upper limit to which the thickness of the LV wall may be increased by athletic training appears to be 16 mm. Therefore, athletes with a wall thickness of >16 mm and a nondilated LV cavity are likely to have primary forms of pathologic hypertrophy, such as HC.

Takayasu's arteritis

Talwar and associates[42] from New Delhi, India, studied 54 patients (18 males and 36 females, ages 2 to 37 years) with nonspecific aortoarteritis. Evaluation revealed hypertension in 35, CHF in 24, mild to moderate MR in 6, and mild AR in 2. Erythrocyte sedimentation rate was raised (>35 mm in the first hour) in 38 patients. PA involvement was present in 4 of the 20 patients in whom it was studied. Selective coronary angiography was done in 11 patients and revealed 90% LM stenosis in 1 patient. Hemodynamic data revealed raised (>7 mm Hg) mean RA pressure in 9, raised mean PA pressure (>20 mm Hg) in 29, and raised LV filling pressure (>12 mm Hg) in 27 patients. Radionuclide ventriculography revealed reduced (<45%) LVEF in 27 patients. The myocardial morphology as evaluated on RV endomyocardial biopsy revealed normal histology in 9, features of inflammatory myocarditis in 24, and nonspecific changes suggestive of dilated cardiomyopathy in 6 patients. Marked RV endocardial thickening was present in 3. All patients with CHF had some histologic abnormality. It was concluded that myocardial involvement including myocarditis is common in nonspecific aortoarteritis and may precipitate CHF in these patients.

Comparison of 4 USA cardiology journals

Roberts[43] from Bethesda, Maryland, summarized results of counting the numbers of editorial pages published and the types of articles published in 1990 in *The American Heart Journal, The American Journal of Cardiology, Circulation,* and *The Journal of the American College of Cardiology.* The results are presented in Table 10-3.

Some good cardiologic books published in 1991

Roberts[44] described some good cardiologic books published in 1991.

MAJOR TEXTBOOKS

1. Braunwald E, editor. *Heart Disease. A Textbook of Cardiovascular Medicine.* Philadelphia: WB Saunders Company, 1992:1918, $110.00 (single volume), $125.00 (double volume).

2. Chatterjee K, Cheitlin MD, Karliner J, Parmley WW, Rapaport E, Scheinman M, editors. *CARDIOLOGY. An Illustrated Text/Reference, Volume 1, Physiology, Pharmacology, Diagnosis* (approximately 1400 pages) and *Volume 2, Cardiovascular Disease* (approximately 1320 pages). Philadelphia: JB Lippincott, and New York: Gower Medical Publishing, 1991: approximately 2720 pages, $225.00 (both volumes).

TABLE 10-3. *Numbers of editorial (non-advertising) pages and articles published in the regular issues (excludes symposia issues) of the four major USA cardiology journals in 1990. Reproduced with permission from Roberts.*[43]

TABLE II Numbers of Editorial (non-advertising) Pages and Articles Published in the Regular Issues (excludes symposia issues) of the Four Major USA Cardiology Journals in 1990

	American Heart Journal	American Journal of Cardiology	Circulation	Journal of the American College of Cardiology	Totals
Numbers of pages	2,911	3,498	4,967	3,753	15,129
For articles	2,715 (93.27%)	3,001 (85.79%)	4,346 (87.50%)	3,426 (91.21%)	13,488 (89.15%)
For "letters"	17	20	33	12	82
For staff, editorial board	12	24	24	42	102
For contents in brief	59 (2.03%)	83 (2.37%)	46 (0.93%)	28 (0.75%)	216 (1.43%)
For contents with abstracts	0	233 (6.66%)	120 (2.42%)	121 (3.22%)	474 (3.13%)
For boxed abstracts	0	0	137 (2.76%)	0	137 (0.91%)
For information for authors	24	24	24	42ᵍ	114 (0.75%)
For meeting abstracts	0	10ᵇ	19ᵈ	0	29 (0.19%)
For erratum	0	0	4		4
For miscellaneous	10ᵃ (0.34%)	0	150ᵉ (3.02%)	18ʰ (0.48%)	178 (1.18%)
For volume indexes	74 (2.54%)	103 (2.94%)	64 (1.29%)	64 (1.70%)	305 (2.02%)
Numbers of articles	489 (41/month)	662 (55/month)	528 (44/month)	540 (45/month)	2,219
Long reports	277	448	388	373	1,486
Concerning humans	248 (50.72%)	448 (67.67%)	256 (48.48%)	323 (59.81%)	1,275 (57.46%)
Concerning non-humans	29 (5.93%)	0	132 (25.00%)	50 (9.26%)	211 (9.51%)
Brief reports	12 (2.45%)	158 (23.87%)	0	0	170 (7.66%)
Case reports	168 (34.36%)	23 (3.47%)	0	6 (1.11%)	197 (8.88%)
Reviews	23 (4.70%)	0	31ᶠ (5.87%)	20 (3.70%)	74 (3.33%)
Editorials	9 (1.84%)	25 (3.78%)	109 (20.64%)	141 (26.11%)	284 (12.80%)
From the editor	0	8 (1.21%)	0	0	8 (0.36%)
Numbers of "letters" (replies)	17 (9)	40 (11)ᶜ	17 (12)	12 (5)	86 (37)
Annual subscription cost in USA	$65.00	$66.00	$84.00	$82.00	$297.00
Individual journals/year	12	24	12	14	62
Weight of journals/year in kg (lbs)ⁱ	7.65 (16.86)	10.20 (22.49)	12.26 (27.03)	13.14 (28.97)	43.25 (95.35)

ᵃ Includes "Bookshelf" and "Acknowledgment to Reviewers."
ᵇ Includes 38 abstracts of the annual meeting of the Section on Cardiology of the American Academy of Pediatrics.
ᶜ Letters to the Editor are called "Readers' Comments" in this journal.
ᵈ Includes abstracts of the 30th Annual Conference on Cardiovascular Disease Epidemiology.
ᵉ Includes "News from the American Heart Association," "Meetings Calendar" (domestic and abroad), and table of contents of 4 other American Heart Association journals (*Arteriosclerosis, Circulation Research, Hypertension* and *Stroke*), and "In Appreciation" to non-board reviewers.
ᶠ Includes American Heart Association Medical/Scientific Statements.
ᵍ Fourteen of the pages (The reference format one . . .) is included among the numbered editorial pages; the other 28, among the "A" (advertising) pages.
ʰ Includes "newly elected members of the College, Board of Governors, Books Received, American College of Cardiology News, Committee appointments, and Participants in Bethesda Conference.
ⁱ Includes journal as received from the printer. Therefore, it includes the advertisements, covers, etc.

3. Giuliani ER, Fuster V, Gersh BJ, McGoon MD, McGoon DC, editors. *Cardiology: Fundamentals and Practice*, Second Edition. St. Louis: Mosby Year Book, 1991:2261 (Volumes 1 and 2), $125.00

All 3 are good. One originates from Boston (Harvard), 1 from San Francisco (University of California), and 1 from Rochester, Minnesota (Mayo Clinic). I prefer the Braunwald book because it contains the most information proportional to size and price. Each page is fully packed. Although it has 69 contributors, Braunwald is the author or coauthor of 23 (37%) of the 62 chapters, and he vigorously edited the other 39 (63%). Although the Braunwald book now has single-colored lines in illustrations, reddish background for tables, and red subheadings, the Chatterjee et al book has taken color much further to produce a beautiful 2-volume text on thick paper. The tradeoff, however, is that the Chatterjee text is twice the cost of the Braunwald book. The Chatterjee text actually represents a hardbound edition of the looseleaf *Cardiology* text edited by Drs. William Parmley and Kanu Chatterjee, published originally in 1987 and updated yearly since. The Giuliani book is a single institution one that is in the price range of the Braunwald book. All 3 texts are heavy, especially the Chatterjee one. If any of these volumes slip off a desk they can break a toe.

4. Fozzard HA, Haber E, Jennings RB, Katz AM, Morgan HE, editors. *The Heart and Cardiovascular System. Scientific Foundations.* Second Edition. Volumes I and II. New York: Raven Press, 1991:2335, $340.00.

These 2 volumes provide comprehensive reviews of principles and methods of cardiovascular research. The first edition was well received and this second edition looks even more comprehensive.

5. Flyer DC, editor. *Nadas' Pediatric Cardiology.* Philadelphia: Hanley & Belfus (also St. Louis: Mosby Year Book), 1992:784, $75.00.

Although it has Dr. Alexander S. Nadas' name in the title, this book represents a near complete new text and is written to honor Dr. Nadas who was chief to most of the contributors to this volume. The book remains easily readable. If one has a single textbook on pediatric cardiology, I would vote for this one, which is reasonably priced.

CARDIAC IMAGING

6. Marcus ML, Skorton DJ, Schelbert HR, Wolf GL, editors; Braunwald E, consulting editor. *Cardiac Imaging. A Companion to Braunwald's Heart Disease.* Philadelphia: WB Saunders Company, 1991:1318, $110.00.

7. Pohost GM, O'Rourke RA, editors. *Principles and Practice of Cardiovascular Imaging.* Boston: Little, Brown and Company, 1991:880, $175.00.

The Marcus book has 118 contributors and is published in the same format as the Braunwald book. Thus, each page is fully packed. The Pohost book, which costs 38% more and has 33% fewer pages, is also well-done. The best value here clearly is the Marcus book.

8. Elliott LP, editor. *Cardiac Imaging in Infants, Children, and Adults.* Philadelphia: JB Lippincott, 1991:927, $150.00.

This book focuses primarily on angiography and would appeal most to radiologists.

9. Gerson MC, editor. *Cardiac Nuclear Medicine.* Second Edition. New York: McGraw-Hill, Inc., 1991:653, $100.00.

A good book by 37 contributors.

10. Gutierrez FR, Brown JJ, editors. *Cardiovascular Magnetic Resonance Imaging.* St. Louis: Mosby Year Book, 1992:233, $99.00.

Magnetic resonance imaging represents 1 of the most significant advances in diagnostic imaging in the last decade. This book from the Mallinckrodt Institute of Radiology summarizes current use and future applications of this technique to the cardiovascular system.

THROMBOSIS AND THROMBOLYSIS

11. Fuster V, Verstraete M, editors. *Thrombosis in Cardiovascular Disorders.* Philadelphia: WB Saunders Company, 1992:565, $95.00.

A superb and much needed book by 47 contributors. The best book so far on this subject.

12. Haber E, Braunwald E, editors. *Thrombolysis. Basic Contributions and Clinical Progress.* St. Louis: Mosby Year Book, 1991:357, $57.00.

Drs. Haber and Braunwald served as chairmen of a symposium on thrombolysis sponsored by the National Heart, Lung, and Blood Institute. The 25 chapters in this book are updates of presentations at that symposium. This book is loaded with information on thrombolysis, as one might expect from the editors and the sponsor.

CORONARY ARTERY DISEASE

13. Roberts R, editor. *Coronary Heart Disease and Risk Factors.* Mount Kisco: New York, 1991:346, $59.00.

A quick update book by 21 authors, 14 from Roberts' Baylor College of Medicine.

14. Redmond GP, editor. *Lipids and Women's Health.* New York: Springer-Verlag, 1991:260, $49.00.

A timely book with 14 contributors.

15. Rifkind BM, editor. *Drug Treatment of Hyperlipidemia*. New York: Marcel Dekkar, Inc., 1991:270, $79.75.

A timely book on lipid-lowering therapy by 11 experts in this field.

16. Goldberger AL. *Myocardial Infarction. Electrocardiographic Differential Diagnosis*. Fourth Edition with 210 illustrations. St. Louis: Mosby Year Book, 1991:386, $49.95.

This book focuses on the electrocardiogram in myocardial infarction and its electrocardiographic simulators. As such, it is comprehensive, authoritative and well-done.

17. Rutherford JD, editor. *Unstable Angina*. New York: Marcel Dekker, Inc., 1992:301, $89.75.

Dr. Eugene Braunwald in the foreword states that 750,000 patients are admitted to hospitals in the U.S. each year with unstable angina pectoris and that almost 100,000 each year develop acute myocardial infarction within 1 month after onset of unstable angina. Thus, a single book on a common problem is useful.

18. Abrams J, Pepine CJ, Thadani U, editors. *Medical Therapy of Ischemic Heart Disease. Nitrates, Beta Blockers, and Calcium Antagonists*. Boston: Little, Brown and Company, 1992:527, $75.00.

These 16 contributors and leaders in cardiovascular therapeutics provide a useful book.

19. Leier CV, editor. *Cardiotonic Drugs. A Clinical Review*. Second Edition. New York: Marcel Dekker, 1991:362, $115.00.

A good book on the positive inotropic agents, those that increase cardiac contractility.

20. Vlay SC, editor. *Medical Care of the Cardiac Surgical Patient*. Boston: Blackwell Scientific Publications, 1992:331, $29.95.

The least expensive book of quality in the present list. Very useful. Can be placed in the doctor's white coat.

21. Wenger NK, Hellerstein HK, editors. *Rehabilitation of the Coronary Patient*. Third Edition. New York: Churchill Livingstone, 1992:625, $74.95.

An excellent book with 44 contributors. Much expanded compared with the second edition.

ECHOCARDIOGRAPHY

22. Clements FM, de Bruijn NP. *Transesophageal Echocardiography*. Boston: Little, Brown and Company, 1991:163, $105.00.

23. Sutherland GR, Roelandt Jos RTC, Fraser AG, Anderson RH. *Transesophageal Echocardiography in Clinical Practice*. London: Gower Medical Publishing, 1991: approximately 120 pages, $167.00.

Clements and de Bruijn perform approximately 150 transesophageal echocardiographic studies yearly in awake patients and approximately 500 yearly in the operating room at Duke University. Their first book on this subject appeared in 1987, and at the time, I believe, their book was the first on the subject. This second one now has much competition, but it is still good. The Sutherland et al book is nicely prepared with lots of color illustrations, but its price is 38% more and it has 26% fewer pages than the Clements-de Bruijn book.

ELECTROCARDIOGRAPHY AND ELECTROPHYSIOLOGY

24. Rowlands DJ. *Clinical Electrocardiography*. London: Gower Medical Publishing, 1991:615, $109.00.

A beautifully prepared book in which nearly all of the many illustrations are in color.

25. Fisch C, Surawicz B, editors. *Cardiac Electrophysiology and Arrhythmias.* New York: Elsevier, 1991: 488, $84.00.

26. Naccarelli GV, editor. *Cardiac Arrhythmias: A Practical Approach.* Mount Kisco, New York: Futura Publishing Company, 1991:583, $70.00.

27. Dangman KH, Miura DS, editors. *Electrophysiology and Pharmacology of the Heart. A Clinical Guide.* New York: Marcel Dekker, Inc., 1991:756, $175.00.

The Fisch book is a comprehensive update of present knowledge in the broad field of investigative and practical electrocardiology by 69 contributors.

Dr. Douglas P. Zipes in the foreword of the Naccarelli book states, "While several texts have been published recently that encompass a wide area of cardiac electrophysiology, none have been devoted solely to a practical approach to arrhythmia management." Such is the edited book by Naccarelli and 43 experts in the field.

The Dangman-Miura book by 55 contributors is divided into 4 parts: Part I discusses the 4 major techniques used to investigate the electrical behavior of the heart; Part II discusses electrophysiology of the 5 major types of excitable tissue in the heart; Part III, the common laboratory models of cardiac arrhythmias; and Part IV, the positive inotropic agents and antiarrhythmic drugs. The price is outrageous.

28. Falk RH, Podrid PJ, editors. *Atrial Fibrillation. Mechanisms and Management.* New York: Raven Press, 1992:428, $95.00.

The authors estimate that 1 or 2 million persons living in the U.S. have atrial fibrillation of nonvalvular etiology. Thus, the subject is a very important one, and this entire book is devoted to various aspects of this arrhythmia. It is well done and will be useful.

29. El-Sherif N, Turitto G. *High-Resolution Electrocardiography.* Mount Kisco, New York: Futura Publishing Company, 1992:690, $98.00.

High-resolution electrocardiography (HRE) is a technique that allows detection and analysis of low-amplitude electrocardiographic signals that may not be detected on the body surface by routine measurements. The term "signal-energized electrocardiogram," which is frequently used synonymously with HRE, refers to 1 signal processing technique that enhances the detection of low-amplitude electrocardiographic signals. HRE began in the 1970s and the goal was to record the His-Purkinje signal noninvasively. In the mid-1970s, El-Sherif and associates observed that low-amplitude "fractionated" diastolic potentials—later called "late potentials"—are a potential marker for the anatomic electrophysiologic substrate of recurrent arrhythmias. This book provides a state-of-the-art review of HRE.

30. Lüderitz B, Saksena S, editors. *Interventional Electrophysiology.* Mount Kisco, New York: Futura, 1991:571, $95.00.

A good book.

INTERVENTIONAL CARDIOLOGY

31. Kulick DL, Rahimtoola SH, editors. *Techniques and Applications in Interventional Cardiology.* St. Louis: Mosby Year Book, 1991:527, $62.00.

32. White CJ, Ramee SR, editors. *Interventional Cardiology. Clinical Application of New Technologies.* New York: Raven Press, 1991:252, $75.00.

The Kulick-Rahimtoola book is a comprehensive, edited book divided into 4 parts: 10 chapters on intracoronary and peripheral vascular interventions; 3, on catheter valvuloplasty and dilatation of congenitally stenotic lesions; 5, on pacemakers, antitachycardia pacing, automatic implantable cardioverting and defibrillating devices, catheter ablation for tachyarrhythmias and transcoronary ablation of arrhythmogenic areas or pathways; and 2 on endomyocardial biopsy and pericardiocentesis. A fine book.

The White-Ramee book has 52% fewer pages and it costs 17% more. No comparison.

33. Clark DA. *Coronary Angioplasty.* Second Edition. New York: Wiley-Liss, 1991:302, $69.00 (with 5-hour videos, $495.00).

A fine book but the printer did not do justice to the many pictures. The price is very reasonable. Dr. Clark wrote 9 of the 13 chapters.

34. Black AJR, Anderson HV, Ellis SG, editors. *Complications of Coronary Angioplasty.* New York: Marcel Dekker, Inc., 1991:261, $99.75.

Of the many books on coronary angioplasty, relatively little attention has been given to its complications. This book is devoted exclusively to them and as such it is useful.

35. Shawl FA, editor. *Supported Complex and High Risk Coronary Angioplasty.* Boston: Kluwer Academic Publishers, 1991:261, $97.50.

Dr. Shawl has been a leader in the clinical application of percutaneous cardiopulmonary bypass support techniques, and this edited book provides to the interventionist the basic principles of cardiopulmonary bypass and other alternate support devices for myocardial protection. Dr. Shawl is joined by 15 other contributors, also leaders in this field.

36. Holmes DR Jr, Garratt KN, editors. *Atherectomy.* Boston: Blackwell Scientific Publications, 1992:230, $59.95.

Twenty-two leaders in this field author this book that probably is the best so far on this subject.

37. Karsh KR, Haase KK, editors. *Coronary Laser Angioplasty. An Update.* New York: Springer-Verlag, 1991:178, $49.00.

This book focuses exclusively on laser techniques in coronary artery stenosis, and for those still interested it would be useful.

VALVULAR HEART DISEASE

38. Emery RW, Arom KV, editors. *The Aortic Valve.* Philadelphia: Hanley & Belfus, Inc. (St. Louis: Mosby Year Book), 1991:336, $65.00.

This book is edited by 2 cardiovascular surgeons. It is well done and I highly recommend it.

39. Bodnar E, Frater R, editors. *Replacement Cardiac Valves.* New York: Pergamon Press, 1991:482, $94.50.

This multiauthored book may be the best of the more recent books on this subject. It is very comprehensive.

40. Bashore TM, Davidson CJ, editors. *Percutaneous Balloon Valvuloplasty and Related Techniques.* Baltimore: Williams & Wilkins, 1991:351, $62.00.

Surely this book is the best one on this subject. Of the 19 chapters by the 29 contributors, 15 focus on the mitral and aortic valves.

ANNUAL CARDIOLOGY REVIEWS

41. Schlant RC (editor in chief), Collins JJ Jr, Engle MA, Frye RL, Kaplan NM, O'Rourke RA (editors). *1991 The Year Book of Cardiology.* St. Louis: Mosby Year Book, 1991:379, $57.95.

42. Roberts WC (editor), Willerson JT, Mason DT, Rackley CE, Graham TP Jr. *Cardiology 1991.* Boston: Butterworth-Heinemann, 1991:494, $80.00.

The Schlant book is the thirty-first in the series. It contains summaries and comments on 305 clinically relevant articles. The Roberts book is the eleventh in the series beginning in 1981. A total of 801 articles are summarized and all articles had appeared in 1990. Additionally, the book contains 120 figures and 61 tables. Each page is fully packed. Although obviously biased I prefer the Roberts book, which summarizes 63% more articles and costs only 28% more than the Schlant book.

MISCELLANEOUS

43. Fowler NO. *Diagnosis of Heart Disease*. New York: Springer-Verlag, 1991:429, $79.00.

It is nice to see a single-authored book. This one by a masterful clinician is a good one, too.

44. Perloff JK, Child JS, editors. *Congenital Heart Disease in Adults*. Philadelphia: WB Saunders, 1991:342, $75.00.

I was fortunate to have edited in 1979 a book entitled *Congenital Heart Disease in Adults* and a new version in 1987 entitled *Adult Congenital Heart Disease*. Thus, I feel comfortable in evaluating the new book by Drs. Perloff and Child with 19 contributors, 14 of whom are at UCLA with the 2 editors. Dr. Perloff is the author or coauthor of 17 of the book's 20 chapters. This book is unique among textbooks on congenital heart disease in that it does not focus on the specific varieties of congenital anomalies, but rather on general concepts and problems in adults. For physicians seeing adults with congenital heart disease, this is the book to have.

45. Opie LH. *The Heart, Physiology and Metabolism*. Second Edition. New York: Raven Press, 1991:513, $72.00.

A single-authored book on the fundamentals of cardiac cellular physiology.

46. Wilcox BR, Anderson RH. *Surgical Anatomy of the Heart*. Second Edition. London: Gower Medical Publishing, 1992: approximately 120 pages, $125.00.

Dr. David C. Sabiston, Jr. states in the foreword: "The second edition embraces all the excellence of its predecessor and in addition contains new data on the previous subjects as well as the addition of detailed anatomy of the tricuspid, pulmonary, mitral and aortic valves and much new material on the surgical anatomy of the coronary circulation." The illustrations in this book are truly magnificent. I believe that Dr. Wilcox gets the best photographs in the operating room of any surgeon.

47. Kapoor AS, Laks H, Schroeder JS, Yacoub MH, editors. *Cardiomyopathies and Heart-Lung Transplantation*. New York: McGraw-Hill, 1991:511, $120.00.

This book provides up-to-date comprehensive coverage of developments in cardiomyopathies, cardiac assist devices and heart-lung transplantation. A fine book by 61 contributors.

48. O'Rourke MF, Kelly RP, Avolio AP. *The Arterial Pulse*. Philadelphia: Lea & Febiger, 1992:239, $49.95.

It's all here on this single topic.

49. Master GT, Pinciroli F, editors. *Databases For Cardiology*. Dordrecht, the Netherlands: Kluwer Academic Publishers, 1991:418, $196.00.

The editors, 1 a cardiologist and 1 an information scientist, have provided "an extensive overview of the medical cardiological database field, with examples of design, construction and data-analysis, while not omitting possible problems and pitfalls."

COMMENTS

Of the 49 books reviewed here, 36 (73%) contained a 1991 publication date and 13 (27%), a 1992 publication date. The numbers of pages in these 49 books ranged from 120 to 2720 (mean 600), and the costs of the books ranged from $29.95 to $340.00 (mean $100.00). There was no relation between the number of pages a book contained and its cost (r = .42, p = 0.1). Thirty-seven books (76%) were multiauthored (>10) and 12 (24%) had ≤6 authors; only 2 books had a single author.

Most books unfortunately continue to be published on acid paper. Of the 49 books, only 11 (22%) (numbers 14, 15, 17, 19, 25, 27, 34, 37, 42, 43 and 49) were stated to have been published on acid-free paper, but only 1 (number 42) of them contained the permanent-paper insignia (infinity symbol within a circle) on the verso of the title page of the book indicating that the paper used was alkaline (i.e., permanent). None of the books published by American publishers were on acid-free paper! In contrast, all books published by Butterworth-Heinemann, Elsevier, Kluwen Academic, Marcel Dekker, and Springer-Verlag were on permanent (acid-free) paper. I encourage all authors to require in their book contracts that the paper used for their books be acid-free!

References

1. Ilan Y, Oren R, Ben-Chetrit E: Etiology, treatment, and prognosis of large pericardial effusions: A study of 34 patients. Chest 1991 (Oct); 100:985–987.

2. Levine MJ, Lorell BH, Diver DJ, Come PC: Implications of echocardiographically assisted diagnosis of pericardial tamponade in contemporary medical patients: detection before hemodynamic embarrassment. J Am Coll Cardiol 1991 (January); 17:59–65.

3. Chuttani K, Pandian NG, Mohanty PK, Rosenfield K, Schwartz SL, Udelson JE, Simonetti J, Kusay BS, Caldeira ME: Left Ventricular Diastolic Collapse—An Echocardiographic Sign of Regional Cardiac Tamponade. Circulation 1991; (June) 83:1999–2006.

4. Anand IS, Ferrari R, Kalra G, Wahi PL, Poole-Wilson PA, Harris PC: Pathogenesis of Edema in Constrictive Pericarditis—Studies of Body Water and Sodium, Renal Function, Hemodynamics, and Plasma Hormones Before and After Pericardiectomy. Circulation 1991; (June) 83:1880–1887.

5. Devaleria PA, Baumgartner WA, Casale AS, Greene PS, Cameron DE, Gardner TJ, Gott VL, Watkins L Jr, Reitz BA: Current indications, risks, and outcome after pericardiectomy. An Thorac Surg 1991 (Aug); 52:219–224.

6. Stevenson LW, Miller LW: Cardiac transplantation as therapy for heart failure. Current Problems in Cardiology 1991 (April); 16:223–30.

7. Bourge RC, Kirklin JK, Naftel DC, White C, Mason DA, Epstein AE: Analysis and predictors of pulmonary vascular resistance after cardiac transplantation. J Thorac Cardiovasc Surg 1991 (Mar); 101:432–445.

8. Kushwaha SS, Crossman DC, Bustami M, Davies GJ, Mitchell AG, Maseri A, Yacoub MH: Substance P for evaluation of coronary endothelial function after cardiac transplantation. J Am Coll Cardiol 1991; 17:1537–44.

9. Angermann CE, Spes CH, Willems S, Dominiak P, Kemkes BM, Theisen K: Regression of Left Ventricular Hypertrophy in Hypertensive Heart Transplant Recipients Treated With Enalapril, Furosemide, and Verapamil. Circulation 1991 (August);84:583–593.

10. Skowronski EW, Epstein M, Ota D, Hoagland PM, Gordon JB, Adamson RM, McDaniel M, Peterson KL, Smith SC, Jaski BE: Right and Left Ventricular Function After Cardiac Transplantation Changes During and After Rejection. Circulation 1991 (December);84:2409–2417.

11. Schulman LL, Reison DS, Austin JHM, Rose EA: Cytomegalovirus pneumonitis after cardiac transplantation. Arch Intern Med 1991 (June);151:1118–1124.

12. Pasque MK, Trulock EP, Kaiser LR, Cooper JD: Single Lung Transplantation for Pulmonary Hypertension Three-Month Hemodynamic Follow-up. Circulation 1991 (December);84:2275–2279.

13. Bolman RM III, Shumway SJ, Estrin JA, Hertz MI: Lung and heart-lung transplantation. An of Surg 1991 (Oct); 214:456–470.

14. Chan K-L: Usefulness of transesophageal echocardiography in the diagnosis of conditions mimicking aortic dissection. Am Heart J 1991 (August); 122:495–504.

15. Balla RS, Nanda NC, Gatewood R, D'Arcy B, Samdarshi TE, Holman WL, Kirklin JE, Pacifico AD: Usefulness of Transesophageal Echocardiography in Assessment of Aortic Dissection. Circulation 1991 (November); 84:1903–1914.

16. Glower DD, Speier RH, White WD, Smith LR, Rankin JS, Wolfe WG: Management and long-term outcome of aortic dissection. An of Surg 1991 (July); 214:31–41.

17. Fann JI, Glower DD, Miller DC, Yun KL, Rankin JS, White WD, Smith LR, Wolfe WG, Shumway NE: Preservation of aortic valve in type A aortic dissection complicated by aortic regurgitation. J Thorac Cardiovas Surg 1991 (July); 102:62–75.

18. North American Symptomatic Carotid Endarterectomy Trial Collaborators: Beneficial effect of carotid endarterectomy in symptomatic patients with high-grade carotid stenosis. N Engl J Med 1991 (Aug 15); 325:445–453.

19. Kistler JP, Buonanno FS, Gress DR: Carotid endarterectomy—specific therapy based on pathophysiology. N Engl J Med 1991 (Aug 15); 325:505–507.

20. Mayberg MR, Wilson E, Yatsu F, Weiss DG, Messina L, Hershey LA, Colling C, Eskridge J, Deykin D, Winn HR: Carotid endarterectomy and prevention of cerebral ischemia in symptomatic carotid stenosis. JAMA 1991 (Dec 18); 266:3289–3294.

21. Brevetti G, Angelini C, Rosa M, Carrozzo R, Perna S, Corsi M, Matarazzo A, Marcialis A: Muscle Carnitine Deficiency in Patients With Severe Peripheral Vascular. Circulation 1991 (October); 84:1490–1495.

22. Radack K, Deck C: B-Adrenergic blocker therapy does not worsen intermittent claudication in subjects with peripheral arterial disease: A meta-analysis of randomized controlled trials. Arch Intern Med 1991 (Sept); 151:1769–1776.

23. Tunis SR, Bass EB, Steinberg EP: The use of angioplasty, bypass surgery, and amputation in the management of peripheral vascular disease. N Engl J Med 1991 (Aug 22); 325:556–562.

24. Coffman JD: Intermittent claudication—be conservative. N Engl J Med 1991 (Aug 22); 325:577–578.

25. Rosenschein U, Rozenszajn LA, Kraus L, Marboe CC, Watkins JF, Rose EA, David D, Cannon PJ, Weinstein JS: Ultrasonic Angioplasty in Totally Occluded Peripheral Arteries—Initial Clinical, Histological, and Angiographic Results. Circulation 1991; (June) 83:1976–1986.

26. Stein PD, Terrin ML, Hales CA, Palevsky HI, Saltzman HA, Thompson T, Weg JG: Clinical, laboratory, roentgenographic, and electrocardiographic findings in patients with acute pulmonary embolism and no pre-existing cardiac or pulmonary disease. Chest 1991 (Sept); 100:598–603.

27. Stein PD, Gottschalk A, Saltzman HA, Terrin ML: Diagnosis of acute pulmonary embolism in the elderly. J Am Coll Cardiol 1991 (November); 18:1452–7.

28. Hsu DT, Addonizio LJ, Hordof AJ, Gersony WM: Acute pulmonary embolism in pediatric patients awaiting heart transplantation. J Am Coll Cardiol (June) 1991;17:1621–1625.

29. Brady AJB, Crake T, Oakley CM: Percutaneous catheter fragmentation and distal dispersion of proximal pulmonary embolus. Lancet 1991 (Nov 9); 338:1186–1188.

30. Bartsch P, Maggiorini M, Ritter M, Noti C, Vock P, Oelz O: Prevention of high-altitude pulmonary edema by nifedipine. N Engl J Med 1991 (Oct 31); 325:1284–1289.

31. Cardiology Working Group: Cardiology and the quality of medical practice. JAMA 1991 (Jan 23/30); 265:482–485.

32. Willems JL, Abreu-Lima C, Arnaud P, Van Bemmel JH, Brohet C, Degani R, Denis B, Gehring J, Graham I, Van Herpen G, Machado H, MacFarlane PW, Michaelis J, Moulopoulos SD, Rubel P, Zywietz C: The diagnostic performance of computer programs for the interpretation of electrocardiograms. N Engl J Med 1991 (Dec 19); 325:1767–1773.

33. Reeder GS, Khandheria BK, Seward JB, Tajik AJ: Transesophageal echocardiography and cardiac masses. Mayo Clin Proc 1991 (Nov); 66:1101–1109.

34. Pearson AC, Labovitz AJ, Tatineni S, Gomez CR: Superiority of transesophageal echocardiography in detecting cardiac source of embolism in patients with cerebral ischemia of uncertain etiology. J Am Coll Cardiol 1991 (January); 17:66–72.

35. Karalis DG, Chandrasekaran K, Victor MF, Ross Jr JJ, Mintz GS: Recognition and embolic potential of intraaortic atherosclerotic debris. J Am Coll Cardiol 1991 (January); 17:73–8.

36. Tunick PA, Perez JL, Kronzon I: Protruding atheromas in the thoracic aorta and systemic embolization. An Intern Med 1991 (Sept 15); 115:423–427.

37. Pearson AC, Nagelhout D, Castello R, Gomez CR, Labovitz AJ: Atrial septal aneurysm and stroke: A transesophageal echocardiographic study. J Am Coll Cardiol 1991 (November); 18:1223–9.

38. Melendez LJ, Chan K, Cheung PK, Sochowski RA, Wong S, Austin TW: Incidence of bacteremia in transesophageal echocardiography: a prospective study of 140 consecutive patients. J Am Coll Cardiol 1991 (December); 18:1650–4.

39. Dutch TIA Trial Study Group: A comparison of two doses of aspirin (30 mg vs. 283 mg a day) in patients after a transient ischemic attack or minor ischemic stroke. N Engl J Med 1991 (Oct 31); 325:1261–1266.

40. SALT Collaborative Group: Swedish aspirin low-dose trial of 75 mg aspirin as secondary prophylaxis after cerebrovascular ischemic events. Lancet 1991 (Nov 30); 338:1345–1349.

41. Pelliccia A, Maron BJ, Spataro A, Proschan MA, Spirito P: The upper limit of physiologic cardiac hypertrophy in highly trained elite athletes. N Engl J Med 1991 (Jan 31); 324:295–301.

42. Talwar KK, Kumar K, Chopra P, Sharma S, Shrivastava S, Wasir HS, Rajani M, Tandon R: Cardiac involvement in nonspecific aortoarteritis (Takayasu's arteritis). Am Heart J 1991 (December); 122:1666–1670.

43. Roberts WC: Comparison of the four major USA cardiology journals in 1990: A look at 51 kilograms (112 pounds) of journals and over 15,000 editorial pages. Am J Cardiol 1991 (Mar 1); 67:551.

44. Roberts WC: Some good cardiologic books published in 1991. Am J Cardiol 1992;69:141–144.

Author Index

459

Subject Index

Numbers in italic indicate figures. Page numbers followed by a t indicate tables.